Essentials of Cardiac Anesthesia

Joel A. Kaplan, MD, CPE, FACC

Dean Emeritus, School of Medicine
Former Chancellor, Health Sciences Center
Professor of Clinical Anesthesiology
University of Louisville School of Medicine
Louisville, Kentucky
Professor, Clinical Anesthesiology
University of California, San Diego, School of Medicine
San Diego, California

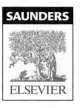

SAUNDERS

ELSEVIER

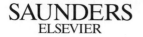

SAUNDERS
ELSEVIER

1600 John F. Kennedy Boulevard
Suite 1800
Philadelphia, PA 19103-2899

Essentials of Cardiac Anesthesia   ISBN: 978-1-4160-3786-6

Notice

Knowledge and best practice in this field are constantly changing. As new research and
experience broaden our knowledge, changes in practice, treatment, and drug therapy
may become necessary or appropriate. Readers are advised to check the most current
information provided (i) on procedures featured or (ii) by the manufacturer of each
product to be administered, to verify the recommended dose or formula, the method
and duration of administration, and contraindications. It is the responsibility of the
practitioner, relying on his or her own experience and knowledge of the patient, to make
diagnoses, to determine dosages and the best treatment for each individual patient,
and to take all appropriate safety precautions. To the fullest extent of the law, neither
the publisher nor the authors assume any liability for any injury and/or damage to
persons or property arising out of or related to any use of the material contained in
this book.

The Publisher

Library of Congress Cataloging-in-Publication Data
Essentials of cardiac anesthesia / [edited by] Joel A. Kaplan. – 1st ed.
  p. ; cm.
Includes bibliographical references.
ISBN 978-1-4160-3786-6
1. Anesthesia in cardiology. 2. Heart–Surgery. I. Kaplan, Joel A.
[DNLM: 1. Anesthesia. 2. Cardiac Surgical Procedures.
3. Heart–drug effects. WO 245 E78 2008]

RD87.3.H43E87 2008
617.9'6741–dc22   2007038046

Acquisitions Editor: Natasha Andjelkovic
Developmental Editor: Isabel Trudeau
Publishing Services Manager: Joan Sinclair
Project Manager: Lawrence Shanmugaraj
Text Designer: Karen O'Keefe Owens

Working together to grow
libraries in developing countries

www.elsevier.com | www.bookaid.org | www.sabre.org

ELSEVIER   BOOK AID International   Sabre Foundation

Printed in China
Last digit is the print number: 9 8 7 6 5 4 3 2 1

Dedication

TO ALL OF THE RESIDENTS AND FELLOWS IN CARDIAC

ANESTHESIA WITH WHOM I HAVE BEEN FORTUNATE TO WORK

OVER THE PAST 30 YEARS.

JAK

Contributors

Maher Adi, MD

Staff Anesthesiologist
Department of Cardiothoracic
Anesthesiology
The Cleveland Clinic Foundation
Cleveland, Ohio
3: Cardiac Physiology

Lishan Aklog, MD

Chair, The Cardiovascular Center
Chief of Cardiovascular Surgery
The Heart and Lung Institute
St. Joseph's Hospital and
Medical Center
Phoenix, Arizona
15: Minimally Invasive Cardiac Surgery

James M. Bailey, MD, PhD

Clinical Associate Professor
Department of Anesthesiology
Emory University School of Medicine
Atlanta, Georgia
*27: Postoperative Cardiovascular
Management*

Daniel Bainbridge, MD, FRCPC

Assistant Professor
Department of Anesthesia and
Perioperative Medicine
The University of Western Ontario
Active Staff Anesthesiologist
Department of Anesthesia and
Perioperative Medicine
London Health Sciences
Centre–University Hospital
London, Ontario, Canada
*26: Postoperative Cardiac Recovery
and Outcomes*

Victor C. Baum, MD

Professor of Anesthesiology
and Pediatrics
Director of Cardiac Anesthesia
Executive Vice-Chair
Department of Anesthesiology
University of Virginia School of
Medicine
Charlottesville , Virginia
16: Congenital Heart Disease in Adults

Elliott Bennett-Guerrero, MD

Associate Professor
Department of Anesthesiology
Duke University Medical Center
Director of Perioperative Clinical
Research
Duke Clinical Research Institute
Durham, North Carolina
6: Systemic Inflammation

Dan E. Berkowitz, MD

Associate Professor, Department
of Anesthesiology and Critical Care
Medicine
Associate Professor, Department
of Biomedical Engineering
The Johns Hopkins University School
of Medicine
Baltimore, Maryland
7: Pharmacology of Anesthetic Drugs

John F. Butterworth IV, MD

Robert K. Stoelting Professor
and Chair
Department of Anesthesia
Indiana University School of Medicine
Anesthesiologist
Clarian University Hospital
Indianapolis, Indiana
8: Cardiovascular Pharmacology

Alfonso Casta, MD
Lecturer
Department of Anesthesia
Harvard Medical School
Senior Associate in Cardiac Anesthesia
Department of Anesthesiology,
Perioperative and Pain Medicine
Children's Hospital Boston
Boston, Massachusetts
*20: Anesthesia for Heart, Lung,
and Heart-Lung Transplantation*

Charles E. Chambers, MD
Professor of Medicine and Radiology
Pennsylvania State University School
of Medicine
Director, Cardiac Catheterization
Laboratories
Milton S. Hershey Medical Center
Hershey, Pennsylvania
*2: The Cardiac Catheterization
Laboratory*

Mark A. Chaney, MD
Associate Professor
Director of Cardiac Anesthesia
Department of Anesthesia
and Critical Care
University of Chicago Hospitals
Chicago, Illinois
*31: Pain Management for the
Postoperative Cardiac Patient*

**Davy C. H. Cheng, MD, MSc,
FRCPC**
Professor and Chairman
Department of Anesthesia
and Perioperative Medicine
The University of Western Ontario
Chief
Department of Anesthesia
and Perioperative Medicine
London Health Sciences Centre
St. Joseph's Health Care London
London, Ontario, Canada
*26: Postoperative Cardiac Recovery
and Outcomes*

Albert T. Cheung, MD
Professor
Department of Anesthesiology
and Critical Care Medicine
University of Pennsylvania School
of Medicine
Philadelphia, Pennsylvania
17: Thoracic Aortic Disease

John L. Chow, MD, MS
Assistant Professor
Divisions of Cardiovascular Anesthesia
and Critical Care Medicine
Department of Anesthesia
Stanford University School of Medicine
Stanford, California
*22: Cardiopulmonary Bypass and the
Anesthesiologist*

David J. Cook, MD
Professor
Department of Anesthesiology
Mayo Clinic College of Medicine
Rochester, Minnesota
*14: Valvular Heart Disease:
Replacement and Repair*

Marianne Coutu, MD, FRCSC
Assistant Professor
Cardiac Surgery Department
University of Sherbrooke Medical Center
Fleurimont, Quebec, Canada
15: Minimally Invasive Cardiac Surgery

Marcel E. Durieux, MD, PhD
Professor of Anesthesiology
Clinical Professor, Department
of Neurological Surgery
University of Virginia Health System
Charlottesville, Virginia
5: Molecular Cardiovascular Medicine

Harvey L. Edmonds, Jr., PhD
Director of Cardiovascular Services
Surgical Monitoring Associates, Inc.
Bala Cynwyd, Pennsylvania
*11: Central Nervous System
Monitoring*

Gregory W. Fischer, MD
Instructor in Anesthesiology
Department of Anesthesiology
Mount Sinai School of Medicine
New York, New York
*21: New Approaches to the Surgical
Treatment of End-Stage Heart
Failure*

Lee A. Fleisher, MD, FACC
Robert D. Dripps Professor and Chair
Department of Anesthesiology
and Critical Care
University of Pennsylvania School
of Medicine
Philadelphia, Pennsylvania
1: Assessment of Cardiac Risk

Dean T. Giacobbe, MD
Staff Anesthesiologist
Chesapeake Regional Medical Center
Chesapeake, Virginia
*30: Long-Term Complications and
Management*

Leanne Groban, MD
Associate Professor
Department of Anesthesiology
Wake Forest University School
of Medicine
Winston-Salem, North Carolina
8: Cardiovascular Pharmacology

Hilary P. Grocott, MD, FRCPC
Professsor
Department of Anesthesiology
and Surgery
University of Manitoba
Winnipeg, Manitoba, Canada
Adjunct Professor of Anesthesiology
Duke University
Durham, North Carolina
*23: Organ Protection During
Cardiopulmonary Bypass*

Kelly L. Grogan, MD
Assistant Professor
Department of Anesthesiology and
Critical Care Medicine
The Johns Hopkins University School
of Medicine
Anesthesiologist
The Johns Hopkins Hospital
Baltimore, Maryland
7: Pharmacology of Anesthetic Drugs

**Thomas L. Higgins, MD, MBA,
FCCM**
Professor of Medicine and Surgery
Associate Professor of
Anesthesiology
Tufts University School of Medicine
Boston, Massachusetts
Chief, Critical Care Division
Departments of Medicine, Surgery
and Anesthesiology
Baystate Medical Center
Springfield, Massachusetts
28: Postoperative Respiratory Care

Zak Hillel, MD, PhD
Professor of Clinical Anesthesiology
Columbia University College of
Physicians and Surgeons
Director of Cardiac Anesthesia
St. Luke's–Roosevelt Hospital Center
New York, New york
3: Cardiac Physiology

Roberta L. Hines, MD
Professor and Chair
Department of Anesthesiology
Yale University School of Medicine
Chief of Anesthesia
Yale University School of Medicine
New Haven, Connecticut
3: Cardiac Physiology
*25: Discontinuing Cardiopulmonary
Bypass*

Jiri Horak, MD

Assistant Professor
Department of Anesthesiology
and Critical Care
University of Pennsylvania School
of Medicine
Philadelphia, Pennsylvania
1: Assessment of Cardiac Risk

Jay Horrow, MD

Professor and Chairman
Department of Anesthesiology
Drexel University School of Medicine
Professor of Epidemiology and
Biostatistics
Drexel University School of Public Health
Hahnemann University Hospital
Philadelphia, Pennsylvania
*24: Transfusion Medicine and
Coagulation Disorders*

Philippe R. Housmans, MD, PhD

Professor
Department of Anesthesiology
Mayo Clinic College of Medicine
Rochester, Minnesota
*14: Valvular Heart Disease:
Replacement and Repair*

Ivan Iglesias, MD

Assistant Professor
Department of Anesthesia and
Perioperative Medicine
University of Western Ontario
London Health Sciences Centre–
University Hospital
London, Ontario, Canada
*29: Central Nervous System Dysfunction
After Cardiopulmonary Bypass*

Brian Johnson, MD

Associate Staff Anesthesiologist
Department of General
Anesthesiology
The Cleveland Clinic
Cleveland, Ohio
3: Cardiac Physiology

Ronald A. Kahn, MD

Associate Professor
Department of Anesthesiology
and Surgery
Mount Sinai School of Medicine
New York, New York
10: Intraoperative Echocardiography

Max Kanevsky, MD, PhD

Assistant Professor of Anesthesia
Division of Cardiovascular Anesthesia
Department of Anesthesia
Stanford University School of
Medicine
Stanford, California
*22: Cardiopulmonary Bypass and the
Anesthesiologist*

Joel A. Kaplan, MD, CPE, FACC

Dean Emeritus, School of Medicine
Former Chancellor, Health Sciences
Center
Professor of Clinical Anesthesiology
University of Louisville School of
Medicine
Louisville, Kentucky
Professor, Clinical Anesthesiology
University of California, San Diego,
School of Medicine
San Diego, California
3: Cardiac Physiology
*9: Monitoring of the Heart and
Vascular System*
*13: Anesthesia for Myocardial
Revascularization*
*24: Transfusion Medicine and
Coagulation Disorders*
*25: Discontinuing Cardiopulmonary
Bypass*

Steven N. Konstadt, MD, MBA, FACC

Professor and Chairman
Department of Anesthesiology
Maimonides Medical Center
Brooklyn, New York
10: Intraoperative Echocardiography

Mark Kozak, MD
Associate Professor of Medicine
Department of Medicine
Pennsylvania State University School
of Medicine
Staff Cardiologist
Department of Medicine/Cardiology
Milton S. Hershey Medical Center
Hershey, Pennsylvania
*2: The Cardiac Catheterization
Laboratory*

Jerrold H. Levy, MD
Professor of Anesthesiology
Emory University School of Medicine
Deputy Chair, Research
Department of Anesthesiology, Emory
Healthcare
Atlanta, Georgia
*27: Postoperative Cardiovascular
Management*

Michael G. Licina, MD
Staff Anesthesiologist
Department of Cardiothoracic
Anesthesiology
The Cleveland Clinic
Cleveland, Ohio
3: Cardiac Physiology

Martin J. London, MD
Professor of Clinical Anesthesia
Department of Anesthesia and
Perioperative Care
University of California, San Francisco
Attending Anesthesiologist
San Francisco Veterans Affairs Medical
Center
San Francisco, California
*9: Monitoring of the Heart and
Vascular System*
*13: Anesthesia for Myocardial
Revascularization*

Alexander J. Mittnacht, MD
Assistant Professor
Department of Anesthesiology
Mount Sinai School of Medicine
Assistant Attending
Department of Cardiothoracic
Anesthesiology
Mount Sinai Hospital
New York, New York
*9: Monitoring of the Heart and
Vascular System*
*13: Anesthesia for Myocardial
Revascularization*

Christina Mora-Mangano, MD
Professor of Anesthesia
Stanford University Medical Center
Stanford, California
*22: Cardiopulmonary Bypass and the
Anesthesiologist*

J. Paul Mounsey, BM, BCh, PhD
Associate Professor of Medicine
Department of Internal Medicine
Cardiovascular Division
University of Virginia
Charlottesville, Virginia
5: Molecular Cardiovascular Medicine

John M. Murkin, MD, FRCPC
Professor of Anesthesiology
Director of Cardiac Anesthesiology
Department of Anesthesia and
Perioperative Medicine
The University of Western Ontario
London Health Sciences
Centre – University Hospital
London, Ontario, Canada
*29: Central Nervous System
Dysfunction After Cardiopulmonary
Bypass*

Andrew W. Murray, MD
Assistant Professor
Department of Anesthesiology
University of Pittsburgh
Presbyterian University Hospital
Pittsburgh, Pennsylvania
*20: Anesthesia for Heart, Lung,
and Heart-Lung Transplantation*

Michael J. Murray, MD, PhD, FCCP, FCCM
Professor
Department of Anesthesiology
Mayo Clinic College of Medicine
Consultant, Department of Anesthesiology
Mayo Clinic Arizona
Scottsdale, Arizona
30: Long-Term Complications and Management

Howard J. Nathan, MD
Professor and Vice-Chair (Research)
Department of Anesthesiology
University of Ottawa Heart Institute
Ottawa, Ontario, Canada
4: Coronary Physiology and Atherosclerosis

Gregory A. Nuttall, MD
Associate Professor
Department of Anesthesiology
Mayo Clinic College of Medicine
Rochester, Minnesota
18: Uncommon Cardiac Diseases

Daniel Nyhan, MD
Professor and Chief of Cardiac Anesthesia
Department of Anesthesiology
and Critical Care Medicine
Associate Professor, Department of Surgery
The Johns Hopkins University School of Medicine
Baltimore, Maryland
7: Pharmacology of Anesthetic Drugs

Edward R. M. O'Brien, MD, FRCPC, FACC
Associate Professor of Medicine (Cardiology) and Biochemistry
University of Ottawa
CIHR-Medtronic Research Chair
University of Ottawa Heart Institute
Ottawa, Ontario, Canada
4: Coronary Physiology and Atherosclerosis

William C. Oliver, Jr., MD
Associate Professor
Department of Anesthesiology
Mayo Clinic College of Medicine
Rochester, Minnesota
18: Uncommon Cardiac Diseases

Enrique J. Pantin, MD
Assistant Professor of Anesthesiology
Department of Anesthesia
University of Medicine and Dentistry of New Jersey
Chief, Section of Intraoperative Echocardiography
Chief, Section of Pediatrics Anesthesia
Robert Wood Johnson University Hospital
New Brunswick, New Jersey
17: Thoracic Aortic Disease

Joseph J. Quinlan, MD
Professor
Department of Anesthesiology
University of Pittsburgh
Chief Anesthesiologist
University of Pittsburgh Medical Center
Presbyterian University Hospital
Pittsburgh, Pennsylvania
20: Anesthesia for Heart, Lung, and Heart-Lung Transplantation

James G. Ramsay, MD
Professor
Director, Anesthesiology Critical Care
Department of Anesthesiology
Emory University School of Medicine
Anesthesiology Service Chief
Emory University Hospital
Atlanta, Georgia
27: Postoperative Cardiovascular Management

Kent H. Rehfeldt, MD
Assistant Professor
Department of Anesthesiology
Mayo Clinic College of Medicine
Rochester, Minnesota
14: Valvular Heart Disease: Replacement and Repair

David L. Reich, MD

Horace W. Goldsmith Professor
and Chair
Department of Anesthesiology
Mount Sinai School of Medicine
New York, New York
*9: Monitoring of the Heart and
Vascular System*

Bryan J. Robertson, MD

Staff Cardiologist
Allegheny General Hospital
Pittsburgh Cardiology Associates
Pittsburgh, Pennsylvania
*2: The Cardiac Catheterization
Laboratory*

Roger L. Royster, MD

Professor and Executive Vice Chair
Department of Anesthesiology
Wake Forest University School of Medicine
Cardiac Anesthesiologist
Wake Forest University Baptist
Medical Center
Winston-Salem, North Carolina
8: Cardiovascular Pharmacology

Marc A. Rozner, MD, PhD

Professor
Departments of Anesthesiology
and Cardiology
Department of Anesthesiology
and Pain Medicine
The University of Texas
M. D. Anderson Cancer Center
Adjunct Assistant Professor of
Integrative Biology and Pharmacology
University of Texas Houston Health
Science Center
Houston, Texas
19: Cardiac Pacing and Defibrillation

Joseph S. Savino, MD

Associate Professor
Department of Anesthesiology
and Critical Care
Hospital of the University of
Pennsylvania School of Medicine
Philadelphia, Pennsylvania
10: Intraoperative Echocardiography

Jack S. Shanewise, MD

Associate Professor of Clinical
Anesthesiology
Director, Division of Cardiothoracic
Anesthesiology
Columbia University College of
Physicians and Surgeons
Chief of Cardiac Anesthesia
Columbia-Presbyterian Hospital
New York, New York
*25: Discontinuing Cardiopulmonary
Bypass*

Stanton K. Shernan, MD

Assistant Professor of Anesthesia
Department of Anesthesiology
Perioperative and Pain Medicine
Harvard Medical School
Director of Cardiac Anesthesia
Brigham and Women's Hospital
Boston, Massachusetts
10: Intraoperative Echocardiography

Linda Shore-Lesserson MD

Associate Professor
Department of Anesthesiology
Albert Einstein College of Medicine
Chief, Cardiothoracic
Anesthesiology and Fellowship
Director
Montefiore Medical Center
Bronx, New York
12: Coagulation Monitoring

Thomas F. Slaughter, MD

Professor
Department of Anesthesiology
Section of Cardiothoracic
Anesthesiology
Wake Forest University School
of Medicine
Winston-Salem, North Carolina
8: Cardiovascular Pharmacology

Bruce D. Spiess, MD, FAHA

Director of VCURES
Professor of Anesthesiology
and Emergency Medicine
Department of Anesthesia
Director of Research
Department of Anesthesiology
VCU – Medical College of Virginia
Richmond, Virginia
24: Transfusion Medicine and
Coagulation Disorders

Mark Stafford-Smith, MD, CM, FRCPC

Associate Professor
Department of Anesthesiology
Duke University Medical Center
Durham, North Carolina
23: Organ Protection During
Cardiopulmonary Bypass

Marc E. Stone, MD

Assistant Professor
Department of Anesthesiology
Mount Sinai School of Medicine,
Program Director, Fellowship in
Cardiothoracic Anesthesiology
Co-Director, Division of Cardiothoracic
Anesthesiology
Mount Sinai Medical Center
New York, New york
21: New Approaches to the Surgical
Treatment of End-Stage Heart
Failure

Kenichi Tanaka, MD

Assistant Professor of Anesthesiology
Department of Anesthesiology
Emory University School of Medicine
Atlanta, Georgia
Attending Physician
Department of Anesthesiology
Veterans Affairs Medical Center
Decatur, Georgia
27: Postoperative Cardiovascular
Management

Daniel M. Thys, MD

Professor of Clinical Anesthesiology
Columbia University College
of Physicians and Surgeons
Chairman, Department of
Anesthesiology
St. Luke's–Roosevelt Hospital Center
New York, New york
3: Cardiac Physiology

Mark F. Trankina, MD

Associate Professor
University of Alabama School
of Medicine
Staff Anesthesiologist
St. Vincent's Hospital
Birmingham, Alabama
19: Cardiac Pacing and Defibrillation

Stuart Joel Weiss, MD, PHD

Associate Professor
Department of Anesthesiology
and Critical Care
University of Pennsylvania School
of Medicine
Philadelphia, Pennsylvania
10: Intraoperative Echocardiography

Jean-Pierre Yared, MD

Medical Director, Cardiovascular
Intensive Care Unit
Department of Cardiac
Anesthesiology and Critical Care
The Cleveland Clinic Foundation
Cleveland, Ohio
28: Postoperative Respiratory Care

David A. Zvara, M.D

Jay J. Jacoby Professor and Chair
Department of Anesthesiology
The Ohio State University
Columbus, Ohio
8: Cardiovascular Pharmacology

Preface

Essentials of Cardiac Anesthesia has been written to further improve the anesthetic management of the patient with cardiac disease undergoing cardiac or noncardiac surgery. *Essentials* incorporates much of the clinically relevant material from the standard reference textbook in the field, *Kaplan's Cardiac Anesthesia,* 5th edition, published in 2006. It is intended primarily for the use of residents, clinical fellows, certified registered nurse anesthetists, and attending anesthesiologists participating in cardiac anesthesia on a limited basis, versus the larger text that is designed for the practitioner, teacher, and researcher in cardiac anesthesia.

The chapters have been written by the acknowledged experts in each specific area, and the material has been coordinated to maximize its clinical value. Recent information has been integrated from the fields of anesthesiology, cardiology, cardiac surgery, critical care medicine, and clinical pharmacology to present a complete clinical picture. This "essential" information will enable the clinician to understand the basic principles of each subject and facilitate their application in practice. Because of the large volume of material presented, several teaching aids have been included with the essentials to help highlight the most important clinical information. Teaching boxes have been used, which include many of the "take home messages." In addition, the summary at the end of each chapter highlights the key points in the chapter. Finally, the reference list for each chapter has been limited to a small number of key articles where more in-depth information can be obtained. A more complete list of references for each chapter can be obtained from the larger textbook, *Kaplan's Cardiac Anesthesia,* along with the basic experimental data and translational medicine underlying the clinical approaches covered in this essentials text.

Essentials of Cardiac Anesthesia is organized into six sections: I, Preoperative Evaluation, including diagnostic procedures and therapeutic interventions in the catheterization laboratory; II, Cardiovascular Physiology, Pharmacology, and Molecular Biology, including the latest material on new cardiovascular drugs; III, Monitoring, with an emphasis on 2D transesophageal echocardiography (TEE); IV, Anesthesia for Cardiac Surgical Procedures, which covers the care of most cardiac surgical patients; V, Extracorporeal Circulation, with an emphasis on organ protection; and VI, Postoperative Care and Pain Management in the cardiac patient.

Essentials of Cardiac Anesthesia should also further the care of the large number of cardiac patients undergoing noncardiac surgery. Much of the information learned in the cardiac surgical patient is applicable to similar patients undergoing major or even minor noncardiac surgical procedures. Some of the same monitoring and anesthetic techniques can be used in other high-risk surgical procedures. New modalities that start in cardiac surgery, such as TEE, will eventually have wider application during noncardiac surgery. Therefore, the authors believe that the *Essentials* should be read and used by all practitioners of perioperative care.

I would like to gratefully acknowledge the contributions made by the authors of each of the chapters. They are the clinical experts who have brought the field of cardiac anesthesia to its highly respected place at the present time. In addition, they are the teachers of our residents and students who will carry the subspecialty forward and further improve the care for our progressively older and sicker patients.

Joel A. Kaplan, MD

Contents

Section IV
ANESTHESIA TECHNIQUES FOR CARDIAC SURGICAL PROCEDURES, 291

Section I
Preoperative Assessment

Chapter 1

Assessment of Cardiac Risk

Jiri Horak, MD • Lee A. Fleisher, MD, FACC

The impetus for the development of a risk-adjusted scoring system was the need to compare adult cardiac surgery results in different institutions and to benchmark the observed complication rates.[1] The first risk-scoring scheme for cardiac surgery was introduced by Paiement and colleagues at the Montreal Heart Institute in 1983.[2] Since then, multiple preoperative cardiac surgery risk indices have been developed. The patient characteristics that affected the probability of specific adverse outcomes were identified and weighted, and the resultant risk indices have been used to adjust for case-mix differences among surgeons and centers where performance profiles have been compiled. In addition to comparisons among centers, the preoperative cardiac risk indices have been used to counsel patients and their families in resource planning, in high-risk group identification for special care or research, to determine cost-effectiveness, to determine effectiveness of interventions to improve provider practice, and to assess costs related to severity of disease.[3]

Anesthesiologists are interested in risk indices as a means of identifying patients who are at high risk for intraoperative cardiac injury and, along with the surgeon, to estimate perioperative risk for cardiac surgery, in order to provide objective information to patients and their families during the preoperative discussion.

CARDIAC RISK ASSESSMENT AND CARDIAC RISK STRATIFICATION MODELS

In defining important risk factors and developing risk indices, each of the studies has used different primary outcomes. Postoperative mortality remains the most definitive outcome that is reflective of patient injury in the perioperative period. Death can

---

BOX 1-1 *Common Variables Associated with Increased Risk of Cardiac Surgery*

- Age
- Female gender
- Left ventricular function
- Body habitus
- Reoperation
- Type of surgery
- Urgency of surgery

---

be cardiac or noncardiac and, if cardiac, may be ischemic or nonischemic. Postoperative mortality is reported as either in-hospital or 30-day. The latter represents a more standardized definition, although it is more difficult to capture because of the push to discharge patients early after surgery.

Postoperative morbidity includes acute myocardial infarction and reversible events such as congestive heart failure and need for inotropic support. Because resource utilization has become such an important financial consideration for hospitals, length of stay in an intensive care unit (ICU) increasingly has been used in the development of risk indices.

Consistency among Risk Indices

Many different variables have been found to be associated with the increased risk during cardiac surgery, but only a few variables have consistently been found to be major risk factors across multiple and very diverse study settings. Age, female gender, left ventricular function, body habitus, reoperation, type of surgery, and urgency of surgery were some variables consistently present in most of the models (Box 1-1).

Predictors of Postoperative Morbidity and Mortality

A risk-scoring scheme for cardiac surgery (coronary artery bypass graft [CABG] and valve) was introduced by Paiement and colleagues at the Montreal Heart Institute in 1983.[2] Eight risk factors were identified: (1) poor LV function, (2) congestive heart failure, (3) unstable angina or recent (within 6 weeks) myocardial infarction, (4) age older than 65 years, (5) severe obesity (body mass index > 30 kg/m^2), (6) reoperation, (7) emergency surgery, and (8) other significant or uncontrolled systemic disturbances. Three classifications were identified: patients with none of these factors (normal), those presenting with one risk factor (increased risk), and those with more than one factor (high risk). In a study of 500 consecutive cardiac surgical patients, it was found that operative mortality increased with increasing risk (confirming their scoring system).

One of the most commonly used scoring systems for CABG was developed by Parsonnet and colleagues[4] (Table 1-1). Fourteen risk factors were identified for in-hospital or 30-day mortality after univariate regression analysis of 3500 consecutive operations. An additive model was constructed and prospectively evaluated in 1332 cardiac procedures. Five categories of risk were identified with increasing mortality rates, complication rates, and length of stay. The Parsonnet Index frequently is used as a benchmark for comparison between institutions.

Higgins and associates[5] developed a Clinical Severity Score for CABG at the Cleveland Clinic. Independent predictors of in-hospital and 30-day mortality were

Table 1-1   Components of the Additive Model

Risk Factor	Assigned Weight
Female gender	1
Morbid obesity (≥1.5 × ideal weight)	3
Diabetes (unspecified type)	3
Hypertension (systolic BP > 140 mmHg)	3
Ejection fraction (%): _____(actual value when available)	
Good (≥50)	0
Fair (30-49)	2
Poor (<30)	4
Age (yr): _____	
70-74	7
75-79	12
≥80	20
Reoperation	
First	5
Second	10
Preoperative IABP	2
Left ventricular aneurysm	5
Emergency surgery after PTCA or catheterization complications	10
Dialysis dependency (peritoneal dialysis or hemodialysis)	10
Catastrophic states (eg, acute structural defect, cardiogenic shock, acute renal failure)*	10-50[†]
Other rare circumstances (eg, paraplegia, pacemaker dependency, congenital heart disease in adult, severe asthma)*	2-10[†]
Valve surgery	
Mitral	5
PA pressure≥60 mmHg	8
Aortic	5
Pressure gradient > 120 mmHg	7
CABG at the time of valve surgery	2

BP = blood pressure; IABP = intra-aortic balloon pump; PTCA = percutaneous transluminal coronary angioplasty; PA = pulmonary artery; CABG = coronary artery bypass graft.

From Parsonnet V, Dean D, Bernstein A: A method of uniform stratification of risk for evaluating the results of surgery in acquired adult heart disease. Circulation 79:I3, 1989.

*On the actual worksheet, these risk factors require justification.

†Values were predictive of increased risk of operative mortality in univariate analysis.

emergency procedure, preoperative serum creatinine level of greater than 168 μmol/L, severe left ventricular dysfunction, preoperative hematocrit of less than 34%, increasing age, chronic pulmonary disease, prior vascular surgery, reoperation, and mitral valve insufficiency. Predictors of morbidity (acute myocardial infarction and use of intra-aortic balloon pump [IABP], mechanical ventilation for 3 or more days, neurologic deficit, oliguric or anuric renal failure, or serious infection) included diabetes mellitus, body weight of 65 kg or less, aortic stenosis, and cerebrovascular disease. Each independent predictor was assigned a weight or score, with increasing mortality and morbidity associated with an increasing total score.

The New York State model of Hannan and coworkers[6] collected data from 1989 through 1992, with 57,187 patients in a study with 14 variables. It was validated in 30 institutions. The mortality definition was "in hospital." Observed mortality was 3.7%, and the expected mortality rate was 2.8%. These researchers included only isolated CABG operations.

The Society of Thoracic Surgeons national database represents the most robust source of data for calculating risk-adjusted scoring systems.[7] Established in 1989, the database had grown to include 638 participating hospitals by 2004. This provider-supported database allows participants to benchmark their risk-adjusted results against regional and national standards. New patient data are brought into the Society of Thoracic Surgeons database on an annual and, now, semiannual basis. Since 1990, when more complete data collection was achieved, risk stratification models were developed for both CABG and valve replacement surgery.

European System for Cardiac Operative Risk Evaluation (EuroSCORE) for cardiac operative risk evaluation was constructed from an analysis of 19,030 patients undergoing a diverse group of cardiac surgical procedures from 128 centers across Europe[8] (Tables 1-2 and 1-3). The following risk factors were associated with increased mortality: age, female gender, serum creatinine, extracardiac arteriopathy, chronic airway disease, severe neurologic dysfunction, previous cardiac surgery, recent myocardial infarction, left ventricular ejection fraction, chronic congestive heart failure, pulmonary hypertension, active endocarditis, unstable angina, procedure urgency, critical preoperative condition, ventricular septal rupture, noncoronary surgery, and thoracic aortic surgery.

During the first years of this decade, this additive EuroSCORE has been widely used and validated across different centers in Europe and across the world, making it a primary tool for risk stratification in cardiac surgery.[9] Although its accuracy has been well established for CABG and isolated valve procedures, its predictive ability in combined CABG and valve procedures has been less well studied.

Dupuis and colleagues[10] attempted to simplify the approach to risk of cardiac surgical procedures in a manner similar to the original American Society of Anesthesiologists (ASA) physical status classification. They developed a score that uses a simple continuous categorization, using five classes plus an emergency status (Table 1-4). The Cardiac Anesthesia Evaluation Score (CARE) model collected data from 1996 to 1999 and included 3548 patients to predict both in-hospital mortality and a diverse group of major morbidities. It combined clinical judgment and the recognition of three risk factors previously identified by multifactorial risk indices: comorbid conditions categorized as controlled or uncontrolled, the surgical complexity, and the urgency of the procedure. The CARE score demonstrated similar or superior predictive characteristics compared with the more complex indices.

Hannan and colleagues[11] evaluated predictors of mortality after valve surgery. A total of 18 independent risk factors were identified in the six models of differing combinations of valve and CABG. Shock and dialysis-dependent renal failure were among the most significant risk factors in all models. The risk factors and odds ratios are shown for aortic valve surgery in Table 1-5. Eleven risk factors were found to be independently associated with higher readmission rates: older age, female sex, African American race, greater body surface area, previous acute myocardial infarction within 1 week, and six comorbidities.

CARDIOVASCULAR TESTING

Patients who present for cardiac surgery have extensive cardiovascular imaging before surgery to guide the procedure. Coronary angiography provides a static view of the coronary circulation, whereas exercise and pharmacologic testing provide a more dynamic view. Because both tests may be available, it is useful to review some basics of cardiovascular imaging (Box 1-2).

In patients with a normal baseline ECG without a prior history of coronary artery disease, the exercise ECG response is abnormal in up to 25% and increases

I

Table 1-2 EuroSCORE: Risk Factors, Definitions, and Weights (Score)

Patient-Related Factors	Definition	Score
Age	Per 5 years or part thereof over 60 years	1
Sex	Female	1
Chronic pulmonary disease	Long-term use of bronchodilators or corticosteroids for lung disease	1
Extracardiac arteriopathy	Any one or more of the following: claudication, carotid occlusion or >50% stenosis, previous or planned intervention on the abdominal aorta, limb arteries, or carotid arteries	2
Neurologic dysfunction	Disease severely affecting ambulation or day-to-day functioning	2
Previous cardiac surgery	Requiring opening of the pericardium	3
Serum creatinine level	>200 μmol/L preoperatively	2
Active endocarditis	Patient still under antibiotic treatment for endocarditis at the time of surgery	3
Critical preoperative state	Any one or more of the following: ventricular tachycardia or fibrillation or aborted sudden death, preoperative cardiac massage, preoperative ventilation before arrival in the anesthetic room, preoperative inotropic support, intra-aortic balloon counterpulsation or preoperative acute renal failure (anuria or oliguria <10 mL/hr)	3
Cardiac-Related Factors		
Unstable angina	Rest angina requiring intravenous administration of nitrates until arrival in the anesthetic room	2
Left ventricular dysfunction	Moderate or LVEF 30%–50%	1
	Poor or LVEF >30%	3
Recent myocardial infarct	(<90% days)	2
Pulmonary hypertension	Systolic pulmonary artery pressure >60 mmHg	2
Surgery-Related Factors		
Emergency	Carried out on referral before the beginning of the next working day	2
Other than isolated CABG	Major cardiac procedure other than or in addition to CABG	2
Surgery on thoracic aorta	For disorder of ascending aorta, arch, or descending aorta	3
Postinfarct septal rupture		4

CABG = coronary artery bypass graft surgery; LVEF = left ventricular ejection fraction.
From Nashef SA, Roques F, Michel P, et al: European system for cardiac operative risk evaluation (EuroSCORE). Eur J Cardiothorac Surg 16:9, 1999.

up to 50% in those with a prior history of myocardial infarction or an abnormal resting ECG. The mean sensitivity and specificity are 68% and 77%, respectively, for detection of single-vessel disease; 81% and 66% for detection of multivessel disease; and 86% and 53% for detection of three-vessel or left main coronary artery disease.[12]

The level at which ischemia is evident on the exercise ECG can be used to estimate an "ischemic threshold" for a patient to guide perioperative medical management,

Table 1-3 Application of EuroSCORE Scoring System

EuroSCORE	Patients (n)	Died (n)	95% Confidence Limits for Mortality	
			Observed	Expected
0-2 (low risk)	4529	36 (0.8%)	0.56-1.10	1.27-1.29
3-5 (medium risk)	5977	182 (3.0%)	2.62-3.51	2.90-2.94
6 plus (high risk)	4293	480 (11.2%)	10.25-12.16	10.93-11.54
Total	14,799	698 (4.7%)	4.37-5.06	4.72-4.95

From Nashef SA, Roques F, Michel P, et al: European system for cardiac operative risk evaluation (EuroSCORE). Eur J Cardiothorac Surg 16:9, 1999.

Table 1-4 Cardiac Anesthesia Risk Evaluation Score

Score	Description
1	Patient with stable cardiac disease and no other medical problem. A noncomplex surgery is undertaken.
2	Patient with stable cardiac disease and one or more controlled medical problems.* A noncomplex surgery is undertaken.
3	Patient with any uncontrolled medical problem[†] or patient in whom a complex surgery is undertaken.[‡]
4	Patient with any uncontrolled medical problem *and* in whom a complex surgery is undertaken.
5	Patient with chronic or advanced cardiac disease for whom cardiac surgery is undertaken as a last hope to save or improve life.
E	Emergency: surgery as soon as diagnosis is made and operating room is available.

*Examples: controlled hypertension, diabetes mellitus, peripheral vascular disease, chronic obstructive pulmonary disease, controlled systemic diseases, others as judged by clinicians.

†Examples: unstable angina treated with intravenous heparin or nitroglycerin, preoperative intra-aortic balloon pump, heart failure with pulmonary or peripheral edema, uncontrolled hypertension, renal insufficiency (creatinine level > 140 μmol/L, debilitating systemic diseases, others as judged by clinicians.)

‡Examples: reoperation, combined valve and coronary artery surgery, multiple valve surgery, left ventricular aneurysmectomy, repair of ventricular septal detect after myocardial infarction, coronary artery bypass of diffuse or heavily calcified vessels, others as judged by clinicians.

From Dupuis JY, Wang F, Nathan H, et al: The cardiac anesthesia risk evaluation score: A clinically useful predictor of mortality and morbidity after cardiac surgery. Anesthesiology 94:194, 2001.

particularly in the prebypass period. This may support further intensification of perioperative medical therapy in high-risk patients, which may have an impact on perioperative cardiovascular events.

Nonexercise (Pharmacologic) Stress Testing

Pharmacologic stress testing has been advocated for patients in whom exercise tolerance is limited, both by comorbid diseases and by symptomatic peripheral vascular disease. Often, these patients may not stress themselves sufficiently during daily life to

Table 1-5 **Significant Independent Risk Factors for In-Hospital Mortality for Isolated Aortic Valve Replacement and for Aortic Valvuloplasty or Valve Replacement Plus Coronary Artery Bypass Grafting**

Risk Factor	Isolated Aortic Valve Replacement (C=0.809)		Aortic Valvuloplasty or Valve Replacement Plus CABG (C=0.727)	
	Odds Ratio	95% CI for Odds Ratio	Odds Ratio	95% CI for Odds Ratio
Age ≥ 55 years	1.06	1.04, 1.08	1.04	1.02, 1.06
Hemodynamic instability	3.97	1.85, 8.51	NS	
Shock	8.68	2.76, 27.33	9.09	3.82, 21.62
Congestive heart failure in same admission	2.26	1.54, 3.30	NS	
Extensively calcified ascending aorta	1.96	1.22, 3.15	1.56	1.16, 2.08
Diabetes	2.52	1.67, 3.81	NS	
Dialysis-dependent renal failure	5.51	2.58, 11.73	3.17	1.70, 5.90
Pulmonary artery systolic pressure ≥50 mmHg	2.35	1.61, 3.41	2.28	1.75, 2.96
Body surface area	NS		0.28	0.16, 0.50
Previous cardiac operation	NS		2.13	1.54, 2.96
Renal failure, no dialysis	NS		2.36	1.32, 4.21
Aortoiliac disease	NS		1.88	1.26, 2.82

From Hannan EL, Racz MJ, Jones RH, et al: Predictors of mortality for patients undergoing cardiac valve replacements in New York State. Ann Thorac Surg 70:1212, 2000, with permission from The Society of Thoracic Surgeons.

1

BOX 1-2 *Preoperative Cardiovascular Testing*

- Coronary angiography
- Exercise electrocardiography
- Nonexercise (pharmacologic) stress testing
- Dipyridamole thallium scintigraphy
- Dobutamine stress echocardiography

BOX 1-3 *Indications for Myocardial Perfusion Imaging*

- Risk stratification
- Myocardial viability assessment
- Preoperative evaluation
- Evaluation after percutaneous coronary intervention or coronary artery bypass grafting
- Monitoring medical therapy in coronary artery disease

provoke symptoms of myocardial ischemia or congestive heart failure. Pharmacologic stress testing techniques either increase myocardial oxygen demand (dobutamine) or produce coronary vasodilatation leading to coronary flow redistribution (dipyridamole/adenosine).[13] Echocardiographic or nuclear scintigraphic imaging (SPECT) is used in conjunction with the pharmacologic therapy to perform myocardial perfusion imaging for risk stratification and myocardial viability assessment (Box 1-3).

Dipyridamole-Thallium Scintigraphy

Dipyridamole works by blocking adenosine reuptake and increasing adenosine concentration in the coronary vessels. Adenosine is a direct coronary vasodilator. After infusion of the vasodilator, flow is preferentially distributed to areas distal to normal coronary arteries, with minimal flow to areas distal to a coronary stenosis.[14] A radioisotope, such as thallium or technetium-99m sestamibi, is then injected. Normal myocardium will show up on initial imaging, whereas areas of either myocardial necrosis or ischemia distal to a significant coronary stenosis will demonstrate a defect. After a delay of several hours, or after infusion of a second dose of technetium-99m sestamibi, the myocardium is again imaged. Those initial defects that remain as defects are consistent with old scar, whereas those defects that demonstrate normal activity on subsequent imaging are consistent with areas at risk for myocardial ischemia.

Dobutamine Stress Echocardiography

Dobutamine stress echocardiography (DSE) involves the identification of new or worsening regional wall motion abnormalities using two-dimensional echocardiography during intravenous infusion of dobutamine. It has been shown to have the same accuracy as dipyridamole thallium scintigraphy for the detection of coronary artery disease. There are several advantages to DSE compared with dipyridamole thallium scintigraphy: the DSE study also can assess left ventricular function and valvular abnormalities; the cost of the procedure is significantly lower; there is no radiation exposure; the duration of the study is significantly shorter; and results are immediately available.

SOURCES OF PERIOPERATIVE MYOCARDIAL INJURY IN CARDIAC SURGERY

Myocardial injury, manifested as transient cardiac contractile dysfunction ("stunning") and/or acute myocardial infarction, is the most frequent complication after cardiac surgery and is the single most important cause of hospital complications and death. Furthermore, patients who have a perioperative myocardial infarction have poor long-term prognosis: only 51% of such patients remain free from adverse cardiac events after 2 years compared with 96% of patients without myocardial infarction.

Myocardial necrosis is the result of progressive pathologic ischemic changes that start to occur in the myocardium within minutes after the interruption of its blood flow, as seen in cardiac surgery (Box 1-4). The duration of the interruption of blood

> **BOX 1-4** *Determinants of Perioperative Myocardial Injury*
>
> • Disruption of blood flow
> • Reperfusion of ischemic myocardium
> • Adverse systemic effects of cardiopulmonary bypass

flow, either partial or complete, determines the extent of myocardial necrosis. This is consistent with the finding that both the duration of the period of aortic cross-clamping and the duration of cardiopulmonary bypass consistently have been shown to be the main determinants of postoperative outcomes in virtually all studies.

Reperfusion of an Ischemic Myocardium

Surgical interventions requiring interruption of blood flow to the heart must, out of necessity, be followed by restoration of perfusion. Numerous experimental studies have provided compelling evidence that reperfusion, although essential for tissue and/or organ survival, is not without risk, owing to the extension of cell damage as a result of reperfusion itself. Myocardial ischemia of limited duration (<20 minutes), followed by reperfusion, are accompanied by functional recovery without evidence of structural injury or biochemical evidence of tissue injury.[15]

Paradoxically, reperfusion of cardiac tissue, which has been subjected to an extended period of ischemia, results in a phenomenon known as "myocardial reperfusion injury." Thus, there exists a paradox in that tissue viability can be maintained only if reperfusion is instituted within a reasonable time period but only at the risk of extending the injury beyond that due to the ischemic insult itself. This is supported by the observation that ventricular fibrillation is prominent when the regionally ischemic canine heart is subjected to reperfusion.

Adverse Systemic Effects of Cardiopulmonary Bypass

In addition to the effects of disruption and restoration of myocardial blood flow, cardiac morbidity may result from many of the components used to perform cardiovascular operations, which lead to systemic insults that result from cardiopulmonary bypass circuit-induced contact activation. Inflammation in cardiac surgical patients is produced by complex humoral and cellular interactions, including activation, generation, or expression of thrombin, complement, cytokines, neutrophils, adhesion molecules, mast cells, and multiple inflammatory mediators.[16] Because of the redundancy of the inflammatory cascades, profound amplification occurs to produce multiorgan system dysfunction that can manifest as coagulopathy, respiratory failure, myocardial dysfunction, renal insufficiency, and neurocognitive defects.

ASSESSMENT OF PERIOPERATIVE MYOCARDIAL INJURY IN CARDIAC SURGERY

There is a lack of consensus regarding how to measure myocardial injury in cardiac surgery because of the continuum of cardiac injury. ECG changes, biomarker elevations, and measures of cardiac function all have been used, but all assessment modalities are affected by the direct myocardial trauma of surgery.

> ### BOX 1-5 *Assessment of Perioperative Myocardial Injury*
>
> - Assessment of cardiac function
>   - Echocardiography
>   - Nuclear imaging
>   - Electrocardiography: Q waves, ST-T segment changes
> - Serum biomarkers
>   - Myoglobin
>   - Creatine kinase
>   - CK-MB (creatine kinase-myocardial band)
>   - Troponin
>   - Lactate dehydrogenase

Traditionally, acute myocardial infarction was determined electrocardiographically. Cardiac biomarkers are elevated postoperatively and can be used for postoperative risk stratification, in addition to being used to diagnose acute morbidity (Box 1-5).

Assessment of Cardiac Function

Cardiac contractile dysfunction is the most prominent feature of myocardial injury, despite the fact that there are virtually no perfect measures of postoperative cardiac function. The need for inotropic support, thermodilution cardiac output measurements, and transesophageal echocardiography may represent practical intraoperative options for cardiac contractility evaluation. Failure to wean from cardiopulmonary bypass, in the absence of systemic factors such as hyperkalemia and acidosis, is the best evidence of intraoperative myocardial injury or cardiac dysfunction.

Regional wall motion abnormalities follow the onset of ischemia in 10 to 15 seconds. Echocardiography can therefore be a very sensitive and rapid monitor for cardiac ischemia/injury. If the abnormality is irreversible, this indicates irreversible myocardial necrosis. The importance of transesophageal echocardiographic assessment of cardiac function is further enhanced by its value as a predictor of long-term survival. In patients undergoing CABG, a postoperative decrease in left ventricular ejection fraction compared with preoperative baseline predicts decreased long-term survival.[17]

Electrocardiography

The presence of new persistent Q waves of at least 0.03-second duration, broadening of preexisting Q waves, or new QS deflections on the postoperative ECG have been considered evidence of perioperative acute myocardial infarction. However, new Q waves may also be due to unmasking of an old myocardial infarction. Crescenzi and colleagues[18] demonstrated that the association of a new Q wave and high levels of biomarkers was strongly associated with postoperative cardiac events; whereas the isolated appearance of a new Q wave had no impact on the postoperative cardiac outcome.

Serum Biochemical Markers to Detect Myocardial Injury

Serum biomarkers have become the primary means of assessing the presence and extent of acute myocardial infarction after cardiac surgery. Serum biomarkers that indicate myocardial damage include the following (with postinsult peak time given in parentheses): myoglobin (4 hours), total creatine kinase (16 hours), CK-MB isoenzyme (24 hours), troponins I and T (24 hours), and lactate dehydrogenase (LDH) (76 hours). The CK-MB isoenzyme has been most widely used, but studies have suggested that troponin I is the most sensitive and specific in depicting myocardial ischemia and infarction[19] (Fig. 1-1). Recently, a universal definition of myocardial infarction has been published, and following CABG it includes an elevation of biomarkers to 5 times baseline levels plus either new Q waves or a new LBBB, or evidence of new loss of viable myocardium by imaging techniques.[20]

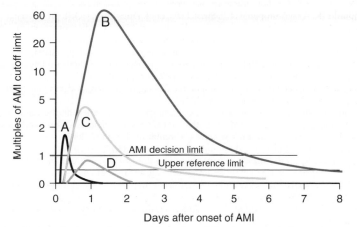

Figure 1-1   Timing of release of various biomarkers following acute, ischemic myocardial infarction. Peak A, early release of myoglobin or creatine kinase (CK)-MB isoforms after AMI (acute myocardial infarction); peak B, cardiac troponin after AMI; peak C, CK-MB after AMI; peak D, cardiac troponin after unstable angina. Data are plotted on a relative scale, where 1.0 is set at the AMI cutoff concentration. (From Apple FS, Gibler WB: National Academy of Clinical Biochemistry Standards of Laboratory Practice: Recommendations for the use of cardiac markers in coronary artery disease. Clin Chem 45:1104, 1999.)

SUMMARY

1

- Multivariate modeling has been used to develop risk indices, which focus on preoperative variables, intraoperative variables, or both.
- Key predictors of perioperative risk are dependent on the type of cardiac operation and the outcome of interest.
- New risk models have become available for valvular heart surgery or combined coronary and valvular cardiac procedures.
- Perioperative cardiac morbidity is multifactorial, and understanding these factors helps define individual risk factors.
- Assessment of myocardial injury is based on the integration of information from myocardial imaging (eg, echocardiography), electrocardiography, and serum biomarkers, with significant variability in the diagnosis based on the criteria selected.

REFERENCES

1. Kouchoukos NT, Ebert PA, Grover FL, et al: Report of the Ad Hoc Committee on Risk Factors for Coronary Artery Bypass Surgery. Ann Thorac Surg 45:348, 1988
2. Paiement B, Pelletier C, Dyrda I, et al: A simple classification of the risk in cardiac surgery. Can Anaesth Soc J 30:61, 1983

3. Smith PK, Smith LR, Muhlbaier LH: Risk stratification for adverse economic outcomes in cardiac surgery. Ann Thorac Surg 64:S61, 1997; discussion S80, 1997
4. Parsonnet V, Dean D, Bernstein A: A method of uniform stratification of risk for evaluating the results of surgery in acquired adult heart disease. Circulation 79:I-3, 1989
5. Higgins T, Estafanous F, Loop F, et al: Stratification of morbidity and mortality outcome by preoperative risk factors in coronary artery bypass patients. JAMA 267:2344, 1992
6. Hannan EL, Kilburn H Jr, O'Donnell JF, et al: Adult open heart surgery in New York State: An analysis of risk factors and hospital mortality rates. JAMA 264:2768, 1990
7. Shroyer AL, Grover FL, Edwards FH: 1995 Coronary artery bypass risk model: The Society of Thoracic Surgeons Adult Cardiac National Database. Ann Thorac Surg 65:879, 1998
8. Nashef SA, Roques F, Michel P, et al: European system for cardiac operative risk evaluation (EuroSCORE). Eur J Cardiothorac Surg 16:9, 1999
9. Toumpoulis IK, Anagnostopoulos CE, Swistel DG, et al: Does EuroSCORE predict length of stay and specific postoperative complications after cardiac surgery? Eur J Cardiothorac Surg 27:128, 2005
10. Dupuis JY, Wang F, Nathan H, et al: The cardiac anesthesia risk evaluation score: A clinically useful predictor of mortality and morbidity after cardiac surgery. Anesthesiology 94:194, 2001
11. Hannan EL, Racz MJ, Jones RH, et al: Predictors of mortality for patients undergoing cardiac valve replacements in New York State. Ann Thorac Surg 70:1212, 2000
12. Horacek BM, Wagner GS: Electrocardiographic ST-segment changes during acute myocardial ischemia, Cardiol Electrophysiol Rev 6:196, 2002
13. Grossman GB, Alazraki N: Myocardial perfusion imaging in coronary artery disease. Cardiology 10:1, 2004
14. Klocke FJ, Baird MG, Bateman TM, et al: ACC/AHA/ASNC guidelines for the clinical use of cardiac radionucleotide imaging: Executive summary. Circulation 108:1404, 2003
15. Bolli R: Mechanism of myocardial "stunning." Circulation 82:723, 1990
16. Levy JH, Tanaka KA: Inflammatory response to cardiopulmonary bypass. Ann Thorac Surg 75:S715, 2003
17. Jacobson A, Lapsley D, Tow DE, et al: Prognostic significance of change in resting left ventricular ejection fraction early after successful coronary artery bypass surgery: A long-term follow-up study. J Am Coll Cardiol 184A, 1995
18. Crescenzi G, Bove T, Pappalardo F, et al: Clinical significance of a new Q wave after cardiac surgery, Eur J Cardiothorac Surg 25:1001, 2004
19. Greenson N, Macoviak J, Krishnaswamy P, et al: Usefulness of cardiac troponin I in patients undergoing open heart surgery. Am Heart J 141:447, 2001
20. Thygesen K, Alpert JS, White HD, et al: Universal definition of myocardial infarction. J Am Coll Cardiol 50:2173, 2007

I

Chapter 2

The Cardiac Catheterization Laboratory

Mark Kozak, MD • Bryan Robertson, MD • Charles E. Chambers, MD

From its inception until recently, the cardiac catheterization laboratory was primarily a diagnostic unit. In the 21st century, its focus has changed to therapy. As the noninvasive modalities of echocardiography, computed tomography, and magnetic resonance imaging improve in resolution, sensitivity, and specificity, the role of the diagnostic cardiac catheterization will likely decline in the next decade. The diagnosis and treatment of peripheral and cerebral vascular disease are now commonly performed in catheterization laboratories previously restricted to cardiac work. Newer coronary stents, as well as patent foramen ovale (PFO)/atrial septal defect (ASD)/ventricular septal defect (VSD) closure devices, are emerging as alternatives to cardiac surgery for many patients. Percutaneous valve replacement/repair is in development as well. In this arena, the need for more "routine" involvement of anesthesiologists in the catheterization laboratory will be important.

Diagnostic catheterization led to interventional therapy in 1977 when Andreas Gruentzig performed his first percutaneous transluminal coronary angioplasty (PTCA). Refinements in both diagnostic and interventional equipment occurred during the decade of the 1980s, with the 1990s seeing advances in both new device technologies for coronary artery disease (CAD) and the entry of cardiologists into the diagnosis and treatment of peripheral vascular disease. The 2000s will see advances in all of these interventional areas as well as the emergence of percutaneous valve replacement/repair.

This brief historical background serves as an introduction to the discussion of diagnostic and therapeutic procedures in the adult catheterization laboratory. The reader must realize the dynamic nature of this field. Whereas failed percutaneous coronary interventions (PCIs) once occurred in up to 5% of coronary interventions, most centers now report procedural failure rates under 1%. Simultaneously, the impact on the anesthesiologist has changed. The high complication rates of years past required holding an operating room (OR) open for all PCIs, and many almost expected to see the patient in the OR. Current low complication rates lead to complacency, along with amazement and perhaps confusion when a PCI patient comes emergently to the OR. Additionally, the anesthesiologist may find the information in this chapter useful in planning the preoperative management of a patient undergoing a cardiac or a noncardiac surgical procedure based on diagnostic information obtained in the catheterization laboratory. Finally, it is the goal of these authors to provide a current overview of this field so that the collaboration between the anesthesiologist and the interventional cardiologist will be mutually gratifying.

CATHETERIZATION LABORATORY FACILITIES

Room Setup/Design/Equipment

The setup and design for the cardiac catheterization laboratory vary from a single room, as seen in a mobile catheterization laboratory or a small community hospital, to a multilaboratory facility, as is found in large tertiary care centers (Box 2-1). In these facilities with multiple laboratories, a central work area is needed to coordinate patient flow to each of the surrounding laboratories and for centralized equipment storage. Patient holding areas are used for observation and evaluation of patients before and after the procedure.

Facility Case Load

All catheterization facilities must maintain appropriate patient volume to assure competence. American College of Cardiology/American Heart Association (ACC/AHA) guidelines recommend that a minimum of 300 adult diagnostic cases and 75 pediatric cases per facility per year be performed to provide adequate care. A case load of at least 200 percutaneous coronary interventions (PCIs) per year, with an ideal volume of 400 cases annually, is recommended.

BOX 2-1 *Components of a Catheterization Laboratory*
• Imaging equipment • Monitoring equipment • Emergency equipment • Radiation safety • Shielding • Lead aprons

Facilities performing PCIs without in-house surgical backup are becoming more prevalent. Despite this, national guidelines still recommend that both elective and emergent PCIs be performed in centers with surgical capabilities. Although emergent CABG is infrequent in the stent era, when emergent CABG is required the delays inherent in the transfer of patients to another hospital would compromise the outcomes of these patients.

Although minimal volumes are recommended, no regulatory control currently exists. In a study of volume-outcome relationships published for New York State, a clear inverse relationship between laboratory case volume and procedural mortality and coronary artery bypass graft (CABG) rates was identified. In a nationwide study of Medicare patients, low-volume centers had a 4.2% 30-day mortality, whereas the mortality in high-volume centers was 2.7%. Centers of excellence, based on physician and facility volume as well as overall services provided, may well be the model for cardiovascular care in the future.

Physician Credentialing

The more experience an operator has with a particular procedure, the more likely this procedure will have a good outcome. The American College of Cardiology Task Force has established guidelines for the volume of individual operators in addition to the facility volumes mentioned earlier. The current recommendations for competence in diagnostic cardiac catheterization require a fellow perform a minimum of 300 angiographic procedures, with at least 200 catheterizations as the primary operator, during his or her training.[1]

In 1999, the American Board of Internal Medicine established board certification for interventional cardiology. To be eligible, a physician has to complete 3 years of a cardiology fellowship, complete a (minimum) of a 1-year fellowship in interventional cardiology, and obtain board certification in general cardiology. In addition to the diagnostic catheterization experience discussed earlier, a trainee must perform at least 250 coronary interventional procedures. Board certification requires renewal every 10 years and initially was offered to practicing interventionalists with or without formal training in intervention. In 2004, the "grandfather" pathway ended, and a formal interventional fellowship is required for board certification in interventional cardiology. After board certification, the physician should perform at least 75 PCIs as a primary operator annually.

The performance of peripheral interventions in the cardiac catheterization laboratory is increasing. Vascular surgeons, interventional radiologists, and interventional cardiologists all compete in this area. The claim of each subspecialty to this group of patients has merits and limitations. Renal artery interventions are the most common peripheral intervention performed by interventional cardiologists, but distal peripheral vascular interventions are performed in many laboratories. Stenting of the carotid arteries looks favorable when compared with carotid endarterectomy. Guidelines are being developed with input from all subspecialties. These guidelines and oversight by individual hospitals will be needed to ensure that the promise of clinical trials is translated into quality patient care.

PATIENT SELECTION FOR CATHETERIZATION

Indications for Cardiac Catheterization in the Adult Patient

Table 2-1 lists generally agreed on indications for cardiac catheterization. With respect to CAD, approximately 15% of the adult population studied will have normal coronary arteries. Coronary angiography is, for the moment, still considered

2

Table 2-1 Indications for Diagnostic Catheterization in the Adult Patient

Coronary Artery Disease

Symptoms

Unstable angina
Postinfarction angina
Angina refractory to medications
Typical chest pain with negative diagnostic testing
History of sudden death

Diagnostic Testing

Strongly positive exercise tolerance test
Early positive, ischemia in > 5 leads, hypotension, ischemia present
   for > 6 minutes of recovery
Positive exercise testing following after myocardial infarction
Strongly positive nuclear myocardial perfusion test
Increased lung uptake or ventricular dilation after stress
Large single or multiple areas of ischemic myocardium
Strongly positive stress echocardiographic study
Decrease in overall ejection fraction or ventricular dilation with stress
Large single area or multiple or large areas of new wall motion abnormalities

Valvular Disease

Symptoms

Aortic stenosis with syncope, chest pain, or congestive heart failure
Aortic insufficiency with progressive heart failure
Mitral insufficiency or stenosis with progressive congestive heart failure symptoms
Acute orthopnea/pulmonary edema after infarction with suspected acute
   mitral insufficiency

Diagnostic Testing

Progressive resting LV dysfunction with regurgitant lesion
Decreased LV function and/or chamber dilation with exercise

Adult Congenital Heart Disease

Atrial Septal Defect

Age > 50 with evidence of coronary artery disease
Septum primum or sinus venosus defects

Ventricular Septal Defect

Catheterization for definition of coronary anatomy

Coarctation of the Aorta

Detection of collateral vessels
Coronary arteriography if increased age and/or risk factors are present

Other

Acute myocardial infarction therapy—consider primary PCI
Mechanical complication after infarction
Malignant cardiac arrhythmias
Cardiac transplantation
Pretransplant donor evaluation
Post-transplant annual coronary artery graft rejection evaluation
Unexplained congestive heart failure
Research studies with institutional review board review and patient consent

LV = left ventricular.

I

the gold standard for defining CAD. With advances in magnetic resonance imaging and multislice computed tomography, the next decade may well see a further evolution of the catheterization laboratory to an interventional suite with fewer diagnostic responsibilities.

Patient Evaluation before Cardiac Catheterization

Diagnostic cardiac catheterization in the 21st century is universally considered an outpatient procedure except for the patient at high risk. Therefore, the precatheterization evaluation is essential for quality patient care. Evaluation before cardiac catheterization includes diagnostic tests that are necessary to identify the high-risk patient. An ECG must be performed on all patients shortly before catheterization. Necessary laboratory studies before catheterization include a coagulation profile (prothrombin time [PT], partial thromboplastin time [PTT], and platelet count), hemoglobin, and hematocrit. Electrolytes are obtained along with a baseline determination of blood urea nitrogen (BUN) and creatinine to assess renal function. Urinalysis and chest radiograph may provide useful information but are no longer routinely obtained by all operators. Prior catheterization reports should be available. If the patient had prior PCI or coronary artery bypass surgery, this information must also be available.

Patient medications must be addressed. On the morning of the catheterization, antianginal and antihypertensive medications are routinely continued while diuretic therapy is held. Diabetic patients are scheduled early, if possible. Because breakfast is held, no short-acting insulin is given. Patients on oral anticoagulation should stop warfarin sodium (Coumadin) therapy 48 to 72 hours before catheterization (INR ≤ 1.8). In patients who are anticoagulated for mechanical prosthetic valves, the patient may best be managed with intravenous heparin before and after the procedure, when the warfarin effect is not therapeutic. Low-molecular-weight heparins (LMWHs) are used in this setting, but this is controversial. LMWHs vary in their duration of action, and their effect cannot be monitored by routine tests. This effect needs to be considered, particularly with regard to hemostasis at the vascular access site. Intravenous heparin is routinely discontinued 2 to 4 hours before catheterization, except in the unstable angina patient. Aspirin therapy for angina patients or in patients with prior CABG is often continued, particularly in patients with unstable angina.

CARDIAC CATHETERIZATION PROCEDURE

Whether the procedure is elective or emergent, diagnostic or interventional, coronary or peripheral, certain basic components are relatively constant in all circumstances.

Patient Preparation

Patients with previous allergic reactions to iodinated contrast agents require adequate prophylaxis. Greenberger and colleagues studied 857 patients with a prior history of an allergic reaction to contrast media. In this study, 50 mg of prednisone was administered 13, 7, and 1 hour before the procedure. Diphenhydramine, 50 mg, was also administered intramuscularly 1 hour before the procedure. Although no severe anaphylactic reactions occurred, the overall incidence of urticarial reactions in known high-risk patients was 10%. The use of nonionic contrast agents may further decrease reactions in patients with known contrast allergies. The administration

2

of histamine-2 blockers (cimetidine, 300 mg) is less well studied. For patients undergoing emergent cardiac catheterization with known contrast allergies, 200 mg of hydrocortisone is administered intravenously immediately and repeated every 4 hours until the procedure is completed. Diphenhydramine, 50 mg, given intravenously, is recommended 1 hour before the procedure.

Patient Monitoring and Sedation

Standard limb leads with one chest lead are used for ECG monitoring during cardiac catheterization. One inferior and one anterior ECG lead are monitored during diagnostic catheterization. During an interventional procedure, two ECG leads are monitored in the same coronary artery distribution as the vessel undergoing PTCA. Radiolucent ECG leads improve monitoring without interfering with angiographic data.

Cardiac catheterization laboratories routinely monitor arterial oxygen saturation by pulse oximetry (SpO_2) on all patients. Utilizing pulse oximetry, Dodson and associates demonstrated that 38% of 26 patients undergoing catheterization had episodes of hypoxemia ($SpO_2 < 90\%$) with a mean duration of 53 seconds. Variable amounts of premedication were administered to the patients.

Sedation in the catheterization laboratory, either from preprocedure administration or subsequent intravenous administration during the procedure, may lead to hypoventilation and hypoxemia. The intravenous administration of midazolam, 1 to 5 mg, with fentanyl, 25 to 100 μg, is common practice. Institutional guidelines for conscious sedation typically govern these practices. Light to moderate sedation is beneficial to the patient, particularly for angiographic imaging and interventional procedures. Deep sedation, in addition to its widely recognized potential to cause respiratory problems, poses distinct problems in the catheterization laboratory. Deep sedation often requires supplemental oxygen, and this complicates the interpretation of oximetry data and may alter hemodynamics. Furthermore, deep sedation may exacerbate respiratory variation, altering hemodynamic measurements.

Sparse data exist regarding the effect of sedation on hemodynamic variables and respiratory parameters in the cardiac catheterization laboratory. One study examined the cardiorespiratory effects of diazepam sedation and flumazenil reversal of sedation in patients in the cardiac catheterization laboratory. A sleep-inducing dose of diazepam was administered intravenously in the catheterization laboratory; this produced only slight decreases in mean arterial pressure (MAP), pulmonary capillary wedge pressure, and left ventricular (LV) end-diastolic pressure (LVEDP), with no significant changes in intermittently sampled arterial blood gases. Flumazenil awakened the patient without significant alterations in either hemodynamic or respiratory variables.

More complex interventions have resulted in longer procedures. Although hospitals require conscious sedation policies, individual variation in the type and degree of sedation is common. Although general anesthesia is rarely required for adult patients, it is needed more frequently for pediatric procedures. In the future, more complex adult interventions may well require the presence of an anesthesiologist in the catheterization laboratory, similar to the early days of adult coronary intervention.

Left-Sided Heart Catheterization

Left-sided heart catheterization has traditionally been performed by either the brachial or femoral artery approach. In the 1950s, the brachial approach was first introduced utilizing a cutdown with brachial arteriotomy. The brachial arteriotomy is often time consuming, can seldom be performed more than three times in the same patient, and has higher complication rates. This led operators to adopt the femoral approach.

Introduced more than 15 years ago, the percutaneous radial artery approach is an alternative that is increasingly used. The percutaneous radial approach is also more time consuming than the femoral approach but may have fewer complications. This approach may be preferred in patients with significant peripheral vascular disease or recent (<6 months) femoral/abdominal aortic surgeries and those with significant hypertension, on oral anticoagulants with a PT greater than 1.8, or who are morbidly obese. With increasing utilization of the radial artery as a conduit for CABG, care must be taken if this vessel has been used for radial access during catheterization.

Right-Sided Heart Catheterization

Clinical applications of right-sided heart hemodynamic monitoring changed greatly in 1970 with the flow-directed, balloon-tipped, pulmonary artery (PA) catheter developed by Swan and Ganz. This balloon flotation catheter allowed the clinician to measure PA pressure (PAP) and pulmonary capillary wedge pressure (PCWP) without fluoroscopic guidance. It also incorporated a thermistor, making the repeated measurement of cardiac output feasible. With this development, the PA catheter left the cardiac catheterization laboratory and entered both the operating room and intensive care unit.

In the cardiac catheterization laboratory, right-sided heart catheterization is performed for diagnostic purposes. The routine use of right-sided heart catheterization during standard left-sided heart catheterization was studied by Hill and coworkers. Two hundred patients referred for only left-sided heart catheterization for suspected CAD underwent right-sided heart catheterization. This resulted in an additional 6 minutes of procedure time and 90 seconds of fluoroscopy. Abnormalities were detected in 35% of the patients. However, management was altered in only 1.5% of the patients. With this in mind, routine right-sided heart catheterization cannot be recommended. Box 2-2 outlines acceptable indications for right-sided heart catheterization during left-sided heart catheterization.

Diagnostic Catheterization Complications

Complications are related to multiple factors, but severity of disease is important. Mortality rates are shown in Table 2-2. Complications are specific for both right- and left-heart catheterization (Table 2-3). Although advances in technology continue, these complication rates are still present today, most likely due to the higher risk patient undergoing catheterization.

BOX 2-2 *Indications for Diagnostic Right-Sided Heart Catheterization during Left-Sided Heart Catheterization*

- Significant valvular pathology
- Suspected intracardiac shunting
- Acute infarct: differentiation of free wall versus septal rupture
- Evaluation of right- and/or left-sided heart failure
- Evaluation of pulmonary hypertension
- Severe pulmonary disease
- Evaluation of pericardial disease
- Constrictive pericarditis
- Restrictive cardiomyopathy
- Pericardial effusion
- Pretransplant assessment of pulmonary vascular resistance and response to vasodilators

---

Table 2-2 Cardiac Catheterization Mortality Data

Patient Characteristics*	Mortality Rate (%)
Overall mortality from cardiac catheterization	0.14
Age-related mortality	
<1 yr	1.75
>60 yr	0.25
Coronary artery disease	
One-vessel disease	0.03
Three-vessel disease	0.16
Left main disease	0.86
Congestive heart failure	
NYHA functional class I or II	0.02
NYHA functional class III	0.12
NYHA functional class IV	0.67
Valvular heart disease	
All valvular disease patients	0.28
Mitral valve disease	0.34
Aortic valve disease	0.19

NYHA = New York Heart Association.

From Pepine CJ, Allen HD, Bashore TM, et al: ACC/AHA guidelines for cardiac catheterization and cardiac catheterization laboratories. Circulation Nov, 84(5): 2213–2247

*Other reported high-risk characteristics: unstable angina, acute myocardial infarction, renal insufficiency, ventricular arrhythmias, cyanotic congenital heart disease (including arterial desaturation and pulmonary hypertension). Detailed data from large-scale studies on these characteristics are unavailable.

Table 2-3 Complications of Diagnostic Catheterization

Left Heart		Right Heart	
Cardiac	Noncardiac	Cardiac	Noncardiac
Death	Stroke	Conduction abnormality	Pulmonary artery rupture
Myocardial infarction	Peripheral embolization	RBBB	Pulmonary infarction
Ventricular fibrillation	Air thrombus	Complete heart block (RBBB superimposed on LBBB)	Balloon rupture
Ventricular tachycardia	Cholesterol	Arrhythmias	Paradoxical (systemic) air embolus
Cardiac perforation	Vascular surgical repair	Valvular damage	
	Pseudoaneurysm	Perforation	
	AV fistula		
	Embolectomy		
	Repair of brachial arteriotomy		
	Evacuation of hematomas		
	Contrast related		
	Renal insufficiency		
	Anaphylaxis		

AV = arteriovenous; RBBB = right bundle-branch block; LBBB = left bundle-branch block.

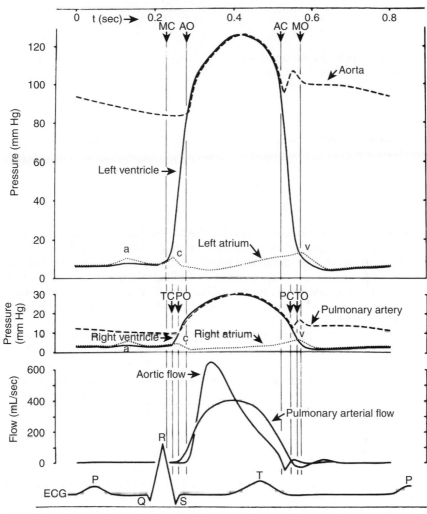

Figure 2-1 The cardiac cycle, demonstrating simultaneous left ventricular, aortic, and left atrial pressures (*top*); right ventricular, pulmonary arterial, and right atrial pressures (*middle*); and electrocardiogram (ECG) and aortic and pulmonary flows (*bottom*). Also displayed are the temporal relationships of mitral valve opening (MO) and closure (MC), aortic valve opening (AO) and closure (AC), tricuspid opening (TO) and closure (TC), and pulmonic valve opening (PO) and closure (PC). (From Milnor WR: Hemodynamics, 2nd ed. Baltimore, Williams & Wilkins, 1989, p 145.)

Definition of Pressure Waveforms— Cardiac Cycle

Right-Sided Heart Pressures

The right-sided heart pressures, as measured in the cardiac catheterization laboratory, consist of the central venous pressure (CVP) or right atrial (RA) pressure (RAP), right ventricular (RV) pressure (RVP), PAP, and PCWP. The CVP consists of three waves and two descents (Fig. 2-1, Box 2-3). The A wave occurs synchronously with the Q wave of the ECG and accompanies atrial contraction. Next, a smaller C wave

---

BOX 2-3 *Hemodynamics and Valvular Pathology*

- Primary data
  - Pressures (PCW, PA, RV, RA, LV)
  - Thermodilution cardiac output
  - Oxygen saturation of blood
  - Oxygen consumption
- Calculated values
  - Valve areas
  - Vascular resistance
  - Shunt ratio
  - Fick cardiac output

---

appears, which results from tricuspid valve closure and bulging of the valve into the right atrium as the right ventricle begins to contract. After this, with the tricuspid valve in the closed position, the atrium relaxes, resulting in the X descent. This is followed by the V wave, which corresponds to RA filling that occurs during RV systole with a closed tricuspid valve. As the RV relaxes, the RVP then becomes less than the RAP, the tricuspid valve opens, and the atrial blood rapidly empties into the ventricle. This is signified by the Y descent.

Beginning in early diastole, the RV waveform reaches its minimum pressure shortly before or as the tricuspid valve opens. During the rapid filling phase of diastole, the ventricular pressure rises slowly and usually an A wave, which signifies atrial contraction, is seen just before the onset of ventricular systole. As ventricular contraction occurs, peak systolic pressure is rapidly reached. Just before the onset of contraction, and after the A wave, the RV end-diastolic pressure (RVEDP) can be determined.

The PAP is usually greater than the RVP during the time the pulmonic valve is closed, during ventricular relaxation and filling. During systole, RVP crosses over PAP by a small margin, causing the pulmonic valve to open, and the ventricle ejects blood into the PA. It is not uncommon for a 5-mm gradient to exist between the RV and PA during peak systolic contraction. The minimal PA diastolic pressure can also be measured just before the onset of contraction, as an estimate of the PCWP; however, the presence of increased pulmonary vascular resistance will invalidate this correlation. With an inflated balloon, the tip of the PA catheter is protected from pulsatile pressures and "looks forward" to the pressure in the pulmonary venous system and the left atrium. This "wedge" pressure shows many of the characteristics of the left atrial (LA) pressure (LAP). The differences between these two waves are considered in the discussion of LAP below.

Left-Sided Heart Pressures

The LA, LV, aortic, and peripheral pressures are commonly measured in the cardiac catheterization laboratory. The LAP can be measured directly if a transseptal catheter is placed. Because this is not commonly done, the PCWP is used to estimate LAP. The LAP has a very similar appearance (A, C, V waves; X, Y descent) to that in the RA, although the pressures seen are about 5 mm Hg higher. The A wave in the RA tracing is normally larger than the V wave whereas the opposite is true in the LA (or PCWP). The PCWP provides reasonable estimations of the LAP, although the waveform is often damped and also delayed in time compared with the LAP (Fig. 2-2).

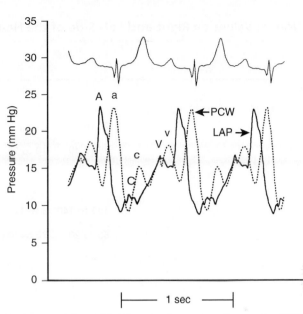

Figure 2-2   Simultaneous left atrial (LAP) and pulmonary capillary wedge (PCW) pressures, demonstrating the accuracy of the PCW in replicating the A, C, and V waves seen in the LAP (corresponding to a, c, and v waves in the PCW). Also shown is the time delay seen in the PCW trace, which results from the pressure wave traveling back through the compliant pulmonary venous system to the pulmonary artery catheter. (Modified from Grossman W, Barry WH: Cardiac catheterization. In Braunwald E [ed]: Heart Disease: A Textbook of Cardiovascular Medicine, 3rd ed. Philadelphia, WB Saunders, 1988, p 252.)

LV pressure also has many similar characteristics to the RVP, although because this is a thick-walled chamber, the generated pressures are higher than those reached in the RV. The central aortic pressure displays a higher diastolic pressure than that seen in the ventricle due to the properties of resistance in the arterial tree and the presence of a competent aortic valve. The dicrotic notch, which signifies the aortic valve closure, is a prominent feature of the aortic pressure wave in the central aorta. As the site of pressure measurement moves more distally in the arterial tree, there is a progressive distortion of the arterial waveform, usually demonstrated as an increase in systolic pressure. This is thought to be due to the addition of the pressure wave of reflected waves from the elastic arterial wall. Summation of reflected pressure waves has been postulated as a contributing factor in aneurysm formation. Additionally, the rapid propagation of reflected waves along stiff arteries has been advanced as an explanation of the systolic hypertension seen in the elderly. Table 2-4 displays the range of normal pressures on the right and left side of the heart.

Cardiac Output Measurements

The techniques of measuring an average CO remain important means to a complete assessment of the patient in the cardiac catheterization laboratory. The measurement of CO along with other information allows the physician to estimate whether the metabolic needs of the patient are being met, that is, whether the oxygen supply or oxygen delivery is matching the oxygen demand. In addition, quantitating the CO also allows the calculation of shunt flows,

Table 2-4 Normal Values on Right and Left Side of the Heart

	a Wave	v Wave	Mean	Systolic	End-Diastolic	Mean
Pressure (mm Hg)						
Right atrium	2 to 10	2 to 10	0 to 8			
Right ventricle				20 to 30	0 to 8	
Pulmonary artery				20 to 30	10 to 15	15 to 20
Pulmonary artery "wedge"	3 to 15	3 to 12	1 to 10			
Left ventricle				100 to 140	3 to 12	
Peripheral artery or aorta				60 to 90	70 to 105	100 to 140
Flow						
Cardiac output (L/min)	4.5 to 7.0					
Cardiac index (L/min/m²)	2.5 to 4.2					
Oxygen consumption index (mL/min/m²)	100 to 150					
A–VO$_2$ difference (mL O$_2$/100 mL blood)	3.0 to 5.0					

Resistance	Wood's Unit (mmHg/min/μL)	Metric Units (dynes·s·cm^{-5})
Systemic vascular resistance (SVR)	12 to 18 WU	900 to 1500 U
Systemic vascular resistance index	20 to 32 WU/m²	1700 to 2600 U/m²
Pulmonary vascular resistance (PVR)	0.5 to 1.5 WU	40 to 100 U
Pulmonary vascular resistance index	0.8 to 2.3 WU/m²	70 to 180 U/m²
Resistance ratio (PVR/SVR)	<0.15	<0.15

A–VO$_2$ = arterial-venous oxygen difference.

regurgitant fractions, systemic vascular resistance (SVR), and pulmonary vascular resistance (PVR).

Valvular Pathology

Each type of valvular pathology has its own particular hemodynamic "fingerprint," the character of which depends on the severity of the pathology, as well as its duration.

Stenotic Lesions

To assess the severity of stenotic lesions, the transvalvular gradient as well as the transvalvular flow must be quantified. For a given amount of stenosis, hydraulic principles state that as flow increases, so also will the pressure drop across the orifice. Both the CO and the HR determine flow; it is during the systolic ejection period that flow occurs through the semilunar valves and during the diastolic filling period for the atrioventricular (AV) valves.

Gorlin and Gorlin derived a formula from fluid physics to relate valve area with blood flow and blood velocity:

$$\text{Valve area} \propto \text{Blood flow/Blood velocity}$$

In general, as a valve orifice becomes increasingly stenotic, the velocity of flow must progressively increase if total flow across the valve is to be maintained. To estimate valve area, flow velocity can be measured by the Doppler principle; however, in the catheterization laboratory, this is not as practical as measuring blood *pressures* on either side of the valve.

As described by Gorlin, the velocity of blood flow is related to the square root of the pressure drop across the valve:

$$P_1 - P_2 \propto (\text{Blood velocity})^2$$

Stated another way, for any given orifice size, *the transvalvular pressure gradient is a function of the square of the transvalvular flow rate.* For example, with mitral stenosis, as the valve area progressively decreases, a modest increase in the rate of flow across the valve causes progressively larger increases in the pressure gradient across the valve (Fig. 2-3).

ANGIOGRAPHY

Ventriculography

Determination of Ejection Fraction

Ventriculography is routinely performed in the single-plane 30-degree right anterior oblique (RAO) or biplane 60-degree left anterior oblique (LAO) and 30-degree RAO projections using 20 to 45 mL of contrast agent with injection rates of 10 to 15 mL/s (Box 2-4). Complete opacification of the ventricle without inducing ventricular extrasystole is necessary for accurate assessment during ventriculography. These premature contractions not only alter the interpretation of mitral regurgitation (MR) but also result in a false increase in the global ejection fraction (EF).

The EF is a global assessment of ventricular function and is calculated as follows:

$$EF = [EDV - ESV]/EDV = SV/EDV$$

where EF is ejection fraction, EDV is end-diastolic volume, ESV is end-systolic volume, and SV is stroke volume.

Abnormalities in Regional Wall Motion

Segmental wall motion abnormalities (SWMAs) are defined in both the RAO and LAO projections. A 0 to 5 grading scale may be used with hypokinesis (decreased motion), akinesis (no motion), and dyskinesis (paradoxical or aneurysmal motion):

0 = normal
1 = mild hypokinesis
2 = moderate hypokinesis

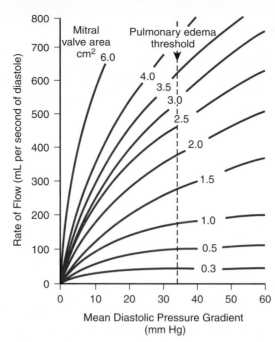

Figure 2-3   Rate of flow in diastole versus mean pressure gradient for several degrees of mitral stenosis. The pressure gradient is directly proportional to the square of the flow rate, such that as the degree of stenosis progresses, modest increases in flow (as with light exercise) will require large increases in the pressure gradient. As an example, a cardiac output (CO) of 5.2 L/min, heart rate (HR) of 60 beats per minute, and diastolic filling time of 0.5 second results in a 200 mL/s flow during diastole (see text for details). For mild mitral stenosis (valve area = 2.0 cm²), the required pressure gradient remains small (<10 mm Hg). In the case of severe stenosis (valve area < 1.0 cm²), the resultant gradient is high enough to place the patient past the threshold for pulmonary edema. (From Wallace AG: Pathophysiology of cardiovascular disease. In Smith LH Jr, Thier SO [eds]: The International Textbook of Medicine, Vol 1, Pathophysiology: The Biological Principles of Disease. Philadelphia, WB Saunders, 1981, p 1192.)

3 = severe hypokinesis
4 = akinesis
5 = dyskinesis (aneurysmal)

Each wall segment is identified as outlined in Figure 2-4 for both the LAO and RAO projections. These segments correspond roughly to vascular territories.

Assessment of Mitral Regurgitation

The qualitative assessment of the degree of MR can be made with LV angiography. It is dependent on proper catheter placement outside the mitral apparatus in the setting of no ventricular ectopy. The assessment is, by convention, done on a scale of 1+ to 4+, with 1+ being mild and 4+ being severe MR. As defined by ventriculography, 1+ regurgitation is that in which the contrast agent clears from the LA with each beat, never causing complete opacification of the LA. Moderate or 2+ MR is present when the opacification does not clear with one beat, leading to complete opacification of the LA after several beats. In 3+ MR (moderately severe), the LA becomes completely opacified, becoming equal in opacification to the LV after several beats. In 4+ or severe regurgitation, the LA densely opacifies with one beat and the contrast agent refluxes into the pulmonary veins.

By combining data from left ventriculography and right-sided heart catheterization, a more quantitative assessment of MR can be made by calculating the regurgitant

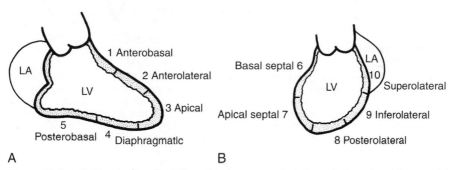

Figure 2-4   A, Terminology for left ventricular segments 1 through 5 analyzed from a right anterior oblique ventriculogram. **B,** Terminology for left ventricular segments 6 through 10 analyzed from left anterior oblique ventriculogram. LV = left ventricle; LA = left atrium. (From Principal Investigators of CASS and their Associates: National Heart, Lung, and Blood Institute Coronary Artery Surgery Study. Circulation 63[suppl II]:1, 1981.)

fraction. This can be effectively calculated by measuring the following: LVEDV, LVESV, and the difference between these two, or the total LV stroke volume (TSV). The TSV (stroke volume calculated from angiography) may be quite high, but it must be remembered that a significant portion of this volume will be ejected backward into the LA. The forward stroke volume (FSV) must be calculated from a measurement of forward CO by the Fick or thermodilution method. The regurgitant stroke volume (RSV) can then be calculated by subtracting the FSV from the TSV (TSV − FSV). The regurgitant fraction (RF) is then calculated as the RSV divided by the TSV:

$$RF = (RSV)/(TSV)$$

A regurgitant fraction less than 20% is considered mild, 20% to 40% is considered moderate, 40% to 60% is considered moderately severe, and greater than 60% is considered severe MR.

Coronary Arteriography

Description of Coronary Anatomy

The left main coronary artery is 1 to 2.5 cm in length (Fig. 2-5). It bifurcates into the circumflex (CX) and left anterior descending (LAD) arteries. Occasionally, the CX and LAD arteries may arise from separate ostia or the left main artery may trifurcate, giving rise to a middle branch, the ramus intermedius, which supplies the high lateral

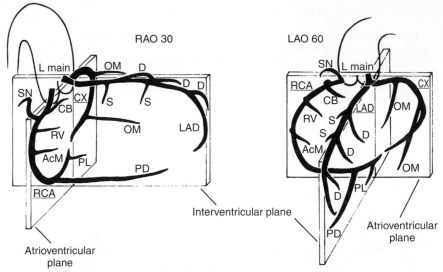

Figure 2-5 Representation of coronary anatomy relative to the interventricular and atrioventricular valve planes. RAO = right anterior oblique; LAO = left anterior oblique. Coronary branches are as indicated: L main = left main; LAD = left anterior descending; D = diagonal; S = septal; CX = circumflex; OM = obtuse marginal; RCA = right coronary; CB = conus branch; SN = sinus node; RV = right ventricle; AcM = acute marginal; PD = posterior descending; PL = posterolateral left ventricular. (From Baim DS, Grossman W: Coronary angiography. In Grossman W, Baim DS [eds]: Cardiac Catheterization, Angiography, and Intervention, 4th ed. Philadelphia, Lea & Febiger, 1991, p 200.)

ventricular wall. Both septal perforators and diagonal branch vessels arise from the LAD artery, which is described as proximal, mid, and distal based on the location of these branch vessels. The proximal LAD artery is before the first septal and first diagonal branch; the mid LAD artery is between the first and second septal and diagonal branches; and the distal LAD artery is beyond the major septal and large diagonal vessels. The distal LAD artery provides the apical blood supply in two thirds of patients, with the distal right coronary artery (RCA) supplying the apex in the remaining one third.

The CX artery is located in the AV groove and is angiographically identified by its location next to the coronary sinus. The latter is seen as a large structure that opacifies during delayed venous filling after left coronary injections. Marginal branches arise from the CX artery and are the vessels in this coronary artery system that are usually bypassed. The CX artery in the AV groove is often not surgically approachable.

The dominance of a coronary system is defined by the origin of the posterior descending artery (PDA), which through septal perforators supplies the inferior one third of the ventricular septum. The origin of the AV nodal artery is often near the origin of the PDA. In 85% to 90% of patients, the PDA originates from the RCA. In the remaining 10% to 15% of patients, the CX artery gives rise to the PDA. Codominance, or a contribution from both the CX artery and RCA, can occur and is defined when septal perforators from both vessels arise and supply the posteroinferior aspect of the left ventricle. Surgical bypass of this region may be difficult when this anatomy exists.

Assessing the Degree of Stenosis

By convention, the severity of a coronary stenosis is quantified as percent diameter reduction. Multiple views of each vessel are recorded, and the worst narrowing is recorded and used to make clinical decisions. This diameter reduction corresponds

Table 2-5   Collateral Vessels

Left Anterior Descending Coronary Artery (LAD)

Right-to-Left

Conus to proximal LAD
Right ventricular branch to mid LAD
Posterior descending septal branches at mid vessel and apex

Left-to-Left

Septal to septal within LAD
Circumflex-OM to mid-distal LAD

Circumflex Artery (Cx)

Right-to-Left

Posterior descending artery to septal perforator
Posterior lateral branch to OM

Left-to-Left

Cx to Cx in AV groove (left atrial circumflex)
OM to OM
LAD to OM via septal perforators

Right Coronary (RCA)

Right-to-Right

Kugels—proximal RCA to AV nodal artery
RV branch to RV branch
RV branch to posterior descending
Conus to posterior lateral

Left-to-Right

Proximal mid and distal septal perforators from distal LAD OM to posterior lateral
OM to AV nodal
AV groove Cx to posterior lateral

AV = atrioventricular; OM = obtuse marginal; RV = right ventricular.

to cross-sectional area reduction; a 50% and 75% diameter reduction results in a 75% and 90% cross-sectional area reduction, respectively. Using the reduction in diameter as a measure of lesion severity is difficult when diffuse CAD creates difficulty in defining "normal" coronary diameter. This is particularly true in insulin-dependent diabetic patients as well as in individuals with severe lipid disorders.

Coronary Collaterals

Common angiographically defined coronary collaterals are described in Table 2-5. Although present at birth, these vessels become functional and enlarge only if an area of myocardium becomes hypoperfused by the primary coronary supply. Angiographic identification of collateral circulation requires both the knowledge of potential collateral source as well as prolonged imaging to allow for coronary collateral opacification.

The increased flow from the collateral vessels may be sufficient to prevent ongoing ischemia. To recruit collateral vessels for an ischemic area, a stenosis in a main coronary or branch vessel must reduce the luminal diameter by 80% to 90%. Clinical studies suggest that collateral flow can double within 24 hours during an episode of acute ischemia. However, well-developed collateral vessels require time to develop and only these respond to nitroglycerin (NTG). The RCA is a better collateralized vessel than the left coronary artery. Areas that are supplied by good collateral vessels are less likely to be dyskinetic or akinetic.

INTERPRETING THE CATHETERIZATION REPORT

Information obtained in the cardiac catheterization laboratory is representative of the patient's pathophysiologic process at only one point in time. Therefore, these data are static and not dynamic. In addition, alterations in fluid and medication management before catheterization can influence the results obtained. The hemodynamic information is usually obtained after the patient has fasted for 8 hours. Particularly in patients with dilated, poorly contractile hearts, the diminished filling pressures seen in the fasted state may lower the CO. In other circumstances fluid status will be altered in the opposite direction. Patients with known renal insufficiency are hydrated overnight before administration of a contrast agent. In these instances, the right- and left-sided heart hemodynamics may not reflect the patient's usual status. Additionally, medications may be held before catheterization, particularly diuretics. Acute β-adrenergic blocker withdrawal can produce a rebound tachycardia, altering hemodynamics and potentially inducing ischemia. These should be noted in interpreting the catheterization data.

Sedation may falsely alter blood gas and hemodynamic measurements if hypoxia occurs. Patients with chronic lung disease may be particularly sensitive to sedatives, and respiratory depression may result in hypercapnia and hypoxia. Careful notations in the catheterization report must be made of medications administered as well as the patient's symptoms. Ischemic events during catheterization may dramatically affect hemodynamic data. Additionally, therapy for ischemia (e.g., NTG) may affect both angiographic and hemodynamic results.

Technical factors may influence coronary arteriography and ventriculography. The table in the catheterization laboratory may not hold very heavy patients. Patient size may limit x-ray tissue penetration and adequate visualization and may prevent proper angulations. Stenosis at vessel bifurcations may not be identified in the hypertensive patient with tortuous vessels. Catheter-induced coronary spasm, most commonly seen proximally in the RCA, must be recognized, treated with NTG, and not reported as a fixed stenosis. Myocardial bridging results in a dynamic stenosis seen most commonly in the mid-LAD artery during systole. This is seldom of clinical significance and should not be confused with a fixed stenosis present throughout the cardiac cycle. With ventriculography, frequent ventricular ectopy or catheter placement in the mitral apparatus may result in nonpathologic (artificial) MR. This must be recognized to avoid inappropriate therapy.

Finally, catheterization reports are often unique to institutions and are often purely computer generated, including valve area calculations. Familiarity with the catheterization report at each institution and discussions with cardiologists are essential to allow for a thorough understanding of the information and its location in the report and the potential limitations inherent in any reporting process.

INTERVENTIONAL CARDIOLOGY: PERCUTANEOUS CORONARY INTERVENTION

This section is designed to present the current practice of interventional cardiology (Box 2-5). Although begun by Andreas Gruentzig in September 1977 as percutaneous transluminal coronary angioplasty (PTCA), catheter-based interventions have dramatically expanded beyond the balloon to include a variety of percutaneous coronary interventions (PCIs). Worldwide, this field has expanded to include approximately 900,000 PCI procedures annually.

The interventional cardiology section is divided in two subsections. The first subsection consists of a general discussion of issues that relate to all catheter-based

BOX 2-5	*Interventional Cardiology–Timeline*
1977	Percutaneous transluminal coronary angioplasty
1991	Directional atherectomy
1993	Rotational atherectomy
1994	Stents with extensive antithrombotic regimen
1995	Abciximab approved
1996	Simplified antiplatelet regimen after stenting
2001	Distal protection
2003	Drug-eluting stents

interventions. This includes a general discussion of indications, operator experience, equipment and procedures, restenosis, and complications. Anticoagulation and controversial issues in interventional cardiology are also reviewed. The second subsection is devoted to a discussion of the various catheter-based systems for PCI. Beginning with the first, PTCA, most devices are presented, including current technology and devices in development. With this review, the cardiac anesthesiologist may better understand the current practice and future direction of interventional cardiology.

General Topics for All Interventional Devices

Indications

Box 2-6 provides a summary of current clinical indications for PCI. Although initially reserved only for patients who were also suitable candidates for CABG, PCI is routinely performed in patients who are not candidates for CABG. In considering both the indications as well as the appropriateness of PCI, the physician must review the patient's historical presentation, including functional class, treadmill results with or without perfusion data, and wall motion assessment.

Equipment and Procedure

Significant advances have been and will continue to be made with all aspects of PCI. Although the femoral artery is still the most commonly utilized access site, the radial artery is utilized more frequently for coronary interventions. Despite numerous advances, all percutaneous coronary interventions still involve sequential placement of the following: guide catheter in the ostium of the vessel, guidewire across the lesion and in the distal vessel, and device(s) of choice at the lesion site.

Guide catheters are available in multiple shapes and sizes for coronary and graft access, device support, and radial artery entry. Guidewires offer more flexible tips for placement in tortuous vessels as well as stiffer shafts to allow for the support of the newer devices during passage within the vessel. Separate guidewire placement within branch vessels may be required for coronary lesions at vessel bifurcations (Fig. 2-6). In selecting the appropriate device for the lesion, quantitative angiography and/or intravascular ultrasound (IVUS) may be used to determine the size of the vessel and composition of the lesion.

Restenosis

Once PTCA/PCI became an established therapeutic option for treating patients with CAD, it was soon realized that there were two major limitations: acute closure and restenosis. Stents and antiplatelet therapy significantly decreased the incidence of

---

BOX 2-6 *Clinical Indications for Percutaneous Coronary Interventional Procedures*

Cardiac Symptoms

- Unstable angina pectoris/non–ST-segment myocardial infarction
- Angina refractory to antianginal medications
- Post–myocardial infarction angina
- Sudden cardiac death

Diagnostic Testing

- Early positive exercise tolerance testing
- Positive exercise tolerance test despite maximal antianginal therapy
- Large areas of ischemic myocardium on perfusion or wall motion studies
- Positive preoperative dipyridamole or adenosine perfusion study
- Electrophysiologic studies suggestive of arrhythmia related to ischemia

Acute Myocardial Infarction

- Cardiogenic shock
- Unsuccessful thrombolytic therapy in unstable patient with large areas of myocardium at risk
- Contraindication to thrombolytic therapy
- Cerebrovascular event
- Intracranial neoplasm
- Uncontrollable hypertension
- Major surgery < 14 days
- Potential for uncontrolled hemorrhage

---

acute closure. Before stents were available, restenosis occurred in 30% to 40% of PTCA procedures. With stent use, this figure decreased to about 20%. Thus, restenosis remained the Achilles heel of intracoronary intervention until the current drug-eluting stent era.

Restenosis usually occurs within the first 6 months after an intervention and has three major mechanisms: vessel recoil, negative remodeling, and neointimal hyperplasia. Vessel recoil is caused by the elastic tissue in the vessel and occurs early after balloon dilation. It is no longer a significant contributor to restenosis because metal stents are nearly 100% effective in preventing any recoil. Negative remodeling refers to late narrowing of the external elastic lamina and adjacent tissue. This accounted for up to 75% of lumen loss in the past. This process is also prevented by metal stents and no longer contributes to restenosis. Neointimal hyperplasia is the major component of in-stent restenosis. Neointimal hyperplasia is exuberant in the diabetic patient, and this serves to explain the increased incidence of restenosis in this population.

The major gains in combating restenosis have been in the area of stenting. Intracoronary stents maximize the increase in lumen area during the PCI procedure and decrease late lumen loss by preventing recoil and negative remodeling. However, neointimal hyperplasia is enhanced owing to a "foreign body–like reaction" to the stents. Different stent designs as well as varying strut thickness lead to different restenosis rates. Systemic administration of antiproliferate drugs decreases restenosis but causes significant systemic side effects. Drug-eluting stents, with a polymer utilized to attach the antiproliferative drug to the stent, have shown the best results to date for decreasing restenosis.[2]

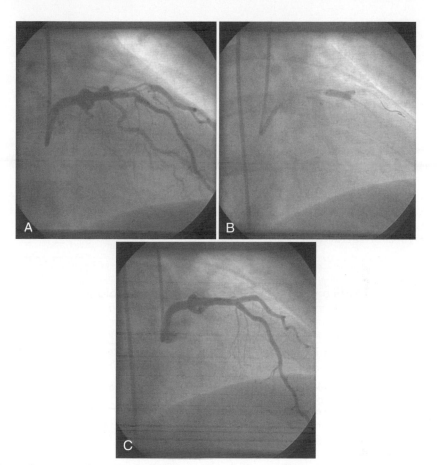

Figure 2-6 Complex coronary angioplasty. **A,** Lesion in the left anterior descending (LAD) artery at its bifurcation as well as a severe ostial diagonal stenosis. **B,** "Kissing balloon" inflation performed simultaneously within both the deployed LAD and diagonal stents. **C,** After dilation with patent LAD artery and diagonal branch.

2

Anticoagulation

Thrombosis is a major component in acute coronary syndromes as well as acute complications during PCI; its management is in constant evolution (Box 2-7). During interventional procedures, the guide catheter, guidewire, and device in the coronary artery serve as nidi for thrombus. Additionally, most catheter interventions disrupt the vessel wall, exposing thrombogenic substances to blood. Table 2-6 summarizes the current anticoagulation agents utilized in the setting of PCI.

Outcomes: Success and Complications

In the 20 years of catheter-based interventional procedures, the marked improvement in success rates with simultaneous decreases in adverse events clearly reflects both the significant technologic advancement as well as increased operator experience. PCI was once considered successful with the luminal narrowing reduced to less than 50% residual stenosis. In current practice with stent placement, seldom is a residual stenosis greater than 20% accepted, and excellent stent expansion without edge dissection is required before termination of the procedure. The initial National Heart, Lung,

BOX 2-7 *Anticoagulation*

Antithrombin Agents

- Heparin (IV during PCI)
- Enoxaparin (SQ before, IV during PCI)
- Bivalirudin (IV during PCI)
- Argatroban (IV during PCI)
- Warfarin (PO after PCI—rarely)

Antiplatelet Agents

- Aspirin (PO before and after PCI)
- Ticlopidine (PO before and after PCI)
- Clopidogrel (PO before and after PCI-preferred)
- Abciximab (IV during PCI; bolus + 12-hour infusion)
- Tifibatide (IV during PCI; bolus + 18-hour infusion)
- Tirofiban (IV before, during, and after PCI)

Table 2-6 Anticoagulation in Interventional Cardiology

Antiplatelet Agents	Dose	Mechanism of Action	Duration of Treatment	Binding
Aspirin	75-325 mg	Acetylates cyclooxy-genase	Indefinite	Irreversible
Thienopyridines (clopidogrel)	300-600 mg Load 75 mg/day	Binds platelet ADR	1 to 9 mo	Irreversible
Glycoprotein IIB/IIIA inhibitors	Agent specific	Platelet IIB/IIIA Receptor	12 to 18 hr post PTCI	Receptor
Anticoagulants				
Heparin	ACT specific	Indirect inhibition of thrombin	During PCI	60 to 90 min post-infusion
Low-molecular-weight heparin	Agent specific	Inhibition of factor Xa	During PCI	8 to 12 hr
Direct thrombin inhibitors	Agent specific	Direct inhibition of thrombin	During PCI	Slowly reversible

and Blood Institute (NHLBI) PTCA registry from 1979 to 1983 reported a success rate of 61% and a major coronary event rate of 13.6%. The 1985 to 1986 NHLBI registry reported a success rate of 78%, with the incidence of acute myocardial infarction as 4.3% and the emergency CABG rate as 3.4%. In the stent era, success rates are over 90% and emergent surgery rates less than 1% in laboratories performing more than 400 PCIs.[3]

Operating Room Backup

When PTCA was introduced, all patients were considered candidates for CABG. The physicians' learning curve in the early 1980s was considered 25 to 50 cases; increased complications were seen during these initial cases. All PCI procedures had immediate operating room availability, with the anesthesiologist often in the catheterization laboratory. In the 1990s, operating room backup was needed less often. Perfusion

I

BOX 2-8   *Failed Intervention*

- Perform "usual" preoperative evaluation for emergent procedure
- Inventory of vascular access sites: pulmonary artery catheter, intra-arterial balloon pump
- Defer removal of sheaths
- Review medicines administered
  - Boluses may linger even if infusion stopped (e.g., abciximab)
  - Check medicines before catheterization laboratory (e.g., enoxaparin, clopidogrel)
- Confirm availability of blood products

---

catheter technology developed to allow for longer inflation times with less ischemia. The role for perfusion balloons and operating room backup has diminished with the use of stents. With the current low incidence of emergent CABG, few institutions maintain a cardiac room on standby for routine coronary interventions.

Infrequently, high-risk interventional cases may still require a cardiac room on immediate standby. Preoperative anesthetic evaluation, which allows for preoperative assessment of the overall medical condition, past anesthetic history, current drug therapy, allergic history, and a physical examination concentrating on airway management considerations, is reserved for these high-risk cases.

As a less stringent policy for operating room backup is required, PCI procedures are now performed in hospitals with no in-house cardiac surgery, although this is not standard practice and remains controversial. Regardless of the location of the interventional procedure, when an emergency CABG is required, it is important to provide enough "lead" time to adequately prepare an operating room. Additionally, because this happens infrequently, cooperation among the interventionalist, surgeon, and anesthesiologist is essential for optimal patient care in this critically ill population.

General Management for Failed Percutaneous Coronary Intervention

Several possible scenarios may result from a failed PCI (Box 2-8). First, the interventional procedure may not successfully open the vessel but no coronary injury has occurred; the patient often remains in the hospital until a CABG can be scheduled. The second type of patient has a patent vessel with an unstable lesion. This most often occurs when a dissection cannot be contained by stents but the vessel remains open. The third patient type has an occluded coronary vessel after a failed PCI with stenting either not an option or unsuccessful. In this instance, myocardial ischemia/infarction ensues dependent on the degree of collateralization. This patient most commonly requires emergent surgical intervention.

In preparation for the operating room, a perfusion catheter, intra-aortic balloon pump, pacemaker, and/or PA catheter may be inserted dependent on patient stability, operating room availability, and patient assessment by the cardiologist, cardiothoracic surgeon, and anesthesiologist. Although designed to better stabilize the patient, these procedures are at the expense of ischemic time. Once in the operating room, decisions on the placement of catheters for monitoring should take several details into consideration. If perfusion has been reestablished, and the degree of coronary insufficiency is mild (no ECG changes, absence of angina), time can be taken to place an arterial catheter and a PA catheter. *It must be remembered, however, that these patients have usually received significant anticoagulation with heparin and often glycoprotein IIb/IIIa platelet receptor inhibitors; attempts at catheter placement should not be undertaken when direct pressure cannot be applied to a vessel.* The most experienced individual should perform these procedures.

BOX 2-9 *Coronary Intervention in Acute Myocardial Infarction (Primary Percutaneous Coronary Intervention [PCI] Versus Coronary Artery Bypass Graft [CABG] Surgery)*

Thrombolytics Preferred

- Symptoms < 3 hours
- No contraindications
- Would take > 90 minutes until PCI (actual balloon inflation)

Primary PCI Preferred

- Contraindications to thrombolytics (e.g., postoperatively)
- Cardiogenic shock
- PCI (balloon inflation) < 90 minutes
- Late presentations (probably)
- Elderly (possibly)

The worst scenario is the patient who arrives in the operating room in either profound circulatory shock or full cardiopulmonary arrest. In these patients, cardiopulmonary bypass (CPB) should be established as quickly as possible. No attempt should be made to establish access for monitoring that would delay the start of surgery. The only real requirement to start a case such as this is to have good intravenous access, a five-lead ECG, airway control, a functioning blood pressure cuff, and arterial access from the PCI procedure.

In many cases of emergency surgery, the cardiologist has placed femoral artery sheaths for access during the PCI. *These should not be removed,* again because of heparin, and possibly glycoprotein IIb/IIIa inhibitor therapy during the PCI. A femoral artery sheath will provide extremely accurate pressures, which closely reflect central aortic pressure. Also, a PA catheter may have been placed in the catheterization laboratory, and this can be adapted for use in the operating room.

Several surgical series have looked for associations with mortality in patients who present for emergency CABG after failed PCI. The presence of complete occlusion, urgent PCI, and multivessel disease has been associated with an increased mortality.

In addition, long delays due to not having a rapid surgical alternative will lead to increases in morbidity and mortality. The paradigm shift in cardiovascular medicine toward PCIs and away from surgery will be slowed if significant numbers of serious complications occur due to prolonged delays in moving the patient to surgery.[4,5]

Controversies in Interventional Cardiology

Therapy for Acute Myocardial Infarction: Primary Percutaneous Coronary Intervention Versus Thrombolysis

Thrombolytic therapy was introduced for patients with acute myocardial infarction in the 1970s (Box 2-9). The decades of the 1980s and 1990s have seen extensive multicenter trials comparing the benefits of (1) thrombolytic therapy versus no thrombolytic therapy, (2) one thrombolytic agent compared with another, (3) different adjunctive medications given with thrombolytic therapy (platelet glycoprotein inhibitors, LMWHs, direct thrombin inhibitors), and (4) thrombolytic therapy

Table 2-7	Current Thrombolytic Therapy			
	Streptokinase	Alteplase	Reteplase	Tenecteplase
Abbreviation	SK	tPA	rPA	TNKase
Dose (>90 kg)	1.5 million U	100 mg	20 units	50 mg
Half-life	23 min	<5 min	13 to 16 min	20 to 24 min
Infusion time	60 min	1.5 hr (double bolus)	30 min (double bolus)	Single bolus
Fibrin specificity	+	++	++	+++
Antigenicity	Yes	No	No	No
Concomitant heparin	No	Yes	Yes	Yes

Source: Lexi-Comp Online.

versus primary PCI (bringing the patient directly to the catheterization laboratory). Table 2-7 lists the currently available drugs used for thrombolytic therapy in patients with acute myocardial infarction.

The recently published guidelines by the ACC/AHA on management of patients with ST-segment elevation myocardial infarction emphasize early reperfusion and discuss the choice between thrombolytic therapy and primary PCI.[6] If a patient presents within 3 hours of symptom onset, the guidelines express no preference for either strategy with the following caveats: Primary PCI is preferred if (1) door-to-balloon time is less than 90 minutes and is performed by skilled personnel (operator annual volume > 75 cases with 11 primary PCI, and laboratory volume > 200 cases with 36 primary PCI); (2) thrombolytic therapy is contraindicated; and (3) the patient is in cardiogenic shock. Thrombolytic therapy should be considered if symptom onset is less than 3 hours and door to balloon time is more than 90 minutes. Patients older than age 75 years should be individually assessed, because they have a higher mortality from the myocardial infarction but a higher risk of complications, particularly intracranial bleeding, with thrombolytic therapy.

Therapy for acute myocardial infarction is evolving. With encouraging results from PCI in experienced hands when a facility is immediately available, more centers are considering acute primary PCI as standard of care, some in catheterization laboratories without operating room backup.[7] Many patients present late or undergo thrombolytic therapy. If such patients are hemodynamically or electrically unstable, or if they have recurrent symptoms, a consensus would favor catheterization and revascularization. If such patients are stable, their management is controversial, although many cardiologists in the United States would recommend catheterization and revascularization.

PCI VERSUS CABG

The choice of therapy for multivessel CAD must be made by comparing PCI with CABG. In the mid 1980s, when PCI consisted only of balloon PTCA, the first comparisons of catheter intervention to CABG were begun. By the early to mid 1990s, nine randomized clinical trials had been published comparing PTCA with CABG in patients with significant CAD. Only the Bypass Angioplasty Revascularization

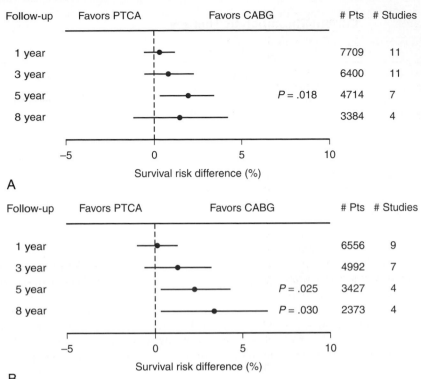

Follow-up	Favors PTCA	Favors CABG	# Pts	# Studies
1 year			7709	11
3 year			6400	11
5 year		$P = .018$	4714	7
8 year			3384	4

Survival risk difference (%)

A

Follow-up	Favors PTCA	Favors CABG	# Pts	# Studies
1 year			6556	9
3 year			4992	7
5 year		$P = .025$	3427	4
8 year		$P = .030$	2373	4

Survival risk difference (%)

B

Figure 2-7   Randomized trials of coronary artery bypass graft surgery (CABG) versus percutaneous transluminal coronary angioplasty (PTCA) in patients with multivessel coronary disease showing risk difference for all-cause mortality for years 1, 3, 5, and 8 after initial revascularization. **A,** All trials. **B,** Multivessel trials. (Redrawn from Hoffman SN, TenBrook JA, Wolf MP, et al: A meta-analysis of randomized controlled trials comparing coronary artery bypass graft with percutaneous transluminal coronary angioplasty: One- to eight-year outcomes. J Am Coll Cardiol 41:1293, 2003. Copyright 2003, with permission from The American College of Cardiology Foundation.)

Investigation (BARI) trial was statistically appropriate for assessing mortality. These results are summarized in Figure 2-7. The conclusions of these studies included similarities between the two approaches with respect to relief of angina and 5-year mortality. Costs were initially lower in the PCI group, but by 5 years they had converged because of repeat PCI procedures precipitated by restenosis, which occurred in 20% to 40% of the PCI group.[8]

The only clear difference between PCI and CABG for patients with multivessel disease was identified in the diabetic patient subset of the BARI trial. A difference in mortality was seen in a subgroup analysis of the BARI trial in which both insulin-dependent and non–insulin-dependent diabetic patients with multivessel disease had a lower 5-year mortality with CABG (19.4%) than with PCI (34.5%).

Regretfully, these trials were outdated by the time of their publication. For the patient undergoing PCI, stents had become the norm with a significant decrease in emergent CABG, due to reduced acute closure, as well as a decrease in repeat procedures, due to less restenosis. For the patient undergoing CABG, off-pump bypass (OPCAB) became more common during this time period with its potential to decrease complications. Additionally, the importance of arterial grafting with its favorable impact on long-term graft patency was recognized.

I

To address the changes in PCI and CABG therapy, four more randomized trials were undertaken, and these are included in Figure 2-7. The results of these newer studies were similar to the results of the earlier ones. In the arterial revascularization therapy study (ARTS) trial, diabetic patients had poorer outcomes with PCI. Repeat procedures, although higher in the PCI group at 20%, were significantly lower than with the earlier trials. CABG patients also had improved outcomes; for instance, cognitive impairment occurred in fewer patients in the recent studies. A meta-analysis of all 13 randomized trials identified a 1.9% absolute survival advantage at 5 years in the CABG patients, but no significant difference at 1, 3, or 8 years.[9] As with the first generation of PCI versus CABG trials, the second-generation trials were outdated before publication due to the advent of the drug-eluting stents. The ARTS II and BARI II trials are now in progress and will address this issue.

Other contentious issues exist in the management of CAD. The roles of staged PCI procedures in patients with multivessel disease, ad hoc PCI, and combination procedures [left internal mammary artery (LIMA) to LAD and PCI of other vessels] have generated debate within the interventional and surgical communities.

In conclusion, the physician must weigh the data and explain the advantages and disadvantages of both techniques to each patient. CABG offers a more complete revascularization with survival advantages in selective groups and a decreased need for repeat procedures. The disadvantages of a CABG are the higher early risk, longer hospitalization and recovery, initial expense, increased difficulty of second procedures, morbidity associated with leg incisions, and limited durability of venous grafts. The current high cost of drug-eluting stents will negate the initial cost advantage of PCI if multiple stents are used. From the perspective of a hospital administrator in the United States, current reimbursement policies favor CABG over the placement of multiple drug-eluting stents.[10]

SPECIFIC INTERVENTIONAL DEVICES

Interventional Diagnostic Devices

Three intravascular diagnostic tools for the interventionalist are currently available. Angioscopy, the least applied of the three, offers the most accurate assessment of intravascular thrombus. Cineangiography and IVUS are often inadequate for visualization of thrombus. Although useful as an investigative technique, angioscopy has not entered into routine interventional practice.

IVUS is the only method by which the vessel wall of the coronary artery can be visualized in vivo. A miniature transducer mounted on the tip of a 3-Fr catheter is advanced over the standard guidewire into the coronary artery. The IVUS transducer is about 1 mm in diameter with frequencies of about 30 MHz. These high frequencies allow for excellent resolution of the vessel wall. By comparison, contrast angiography images only the lumen, with the status of the vessel wall inferred from the image of the lumen.[11] IVUS is useful in evaluating equivocal left main lesions, ostial stenoses, and vessels overlapping angiographically (Fig. 2-8). IVUS is superior to angiography in the early detection of the diffuse, immune-mediated arteriopathy of cardiac transplant allografts.

Atherectomy Devices: Directional and Rotational

Atherectomy devices are designed to remove some amount of plaque or other material from an atherosclerotic vessel. Of these devices, directional coronary atherectomy (DCA; Guidant Corporation, Indianapolis, IN) became the first nonballoon

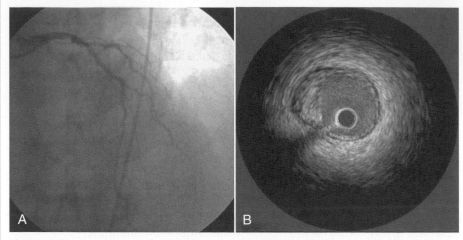

Figure 2-8   A, Diagnostic angiography reveals a borderline occlusive lesion of 50% stenosis (by diameter) in the distal left main artery. **B,** Intravascular ultrasound reveals an eccentric plaque to the left of the ultrasonographic catheter (central lucency) that is nonocclusive by both diameter and cross-sectional area.

technology to gain U.S. Food and Drug Administration (FDA) approval, in 1991. DCA removes tissue from the coronary artery, thus "debulking" the area of stenosis utilizing a low-pressure balloon located on one side of the metal housing, which, when inflated, forces tissue into an elliptical opening on the opposite side of the housing. A cylindrical cutting blade shaves the tissue and stores it in the distal nose cone of the device. Although tissue removal is an attractive concept, application of DCA was limited by the need for large (9.5 to 11 Fr) guiding catheters with early devices. Trials comparing DCA with PTCA did not show improved angiographic restenosis rates, and higher rates of acute complications were seen with DCA. Newer iterations of the device can be used with smaller (7 to 8 Fr) guide catheters. DCA is used infrequently in most institutions because its clinical benefit is inconclusive.[12]

The FDA approved rotational coronary atherectomy in 1993. The Rotablator catheter (Boston Scientific Corp, Natick, MA) is designed to differentially remove nonelastic tissue, utilizing a diamond-studded bur rotating at 140,000 to 170,000 rpm. Designed to alter lesion compliance, particularly in heavily calcified vessels, rotational atherectomy is often used before balloon dilation to permit full expansion of the vessel. The ablated material is emulsified into 5-μm particles, which pass through the distal capillary bed. Heavily calcified lesions are commonly chosen for rotational atherectomy.

Intracoronary Laser

Excimer laser coronary angioplasty (ELCA) (Spectranetics, Colorado Springs, CO) uses xenon chloride (XeCl) and operates in the ultraviolet range (308 nm) to photochemically ablate tissue. Currently, ELCA is indicated for use in lesions that are long (>2 mm in length), ostial, in saphenous vein bypass grafts, and unresponsive to PTCA. With the development of the eccentric directional laser, treatment of eccentric or bifurcation lesions can be approached with increased success. Also, in-stent restenosis can be effectively treated with the excimer laser.[13] The Prima FX laser wire (Spectranetics, Colorado Springs, CO) is a 0.018-inch wire with the ability to deliver excimer laser energy to areas of chronic, total occlusion. With conventional equipment, failure to cross such lesions with a guidewire is frequent.

BOX 2-10 *Stents*

Antiplatelet Therapy after Stent Placement—Indefinite Aspirin Therapy plus:

- Bare metal stent, clopidogrel 3 months
- Cypher (sirolimus) stent, clopidogrel 1 year
- Taxus (paclitaxel) stent, clopidogrel 1 year
- With bare metal stents, thienopyridines reduce subacute thrombosis from 3% to < 1%.
- DES never tested without clopidogrel.
- Concern with DES is delay in endothelial coverage of stent, similar to brachytherapy.
- With clopidogrel, subacute thrombosis rates of drug-eluting and bare metal stents are identical.

Stents and Elective Surgery

- Delay until clopidogrel completed: recommended.
- Perform during clopidogrel therapy: accept bleeding risk.
- Discontinue clopidogrel early: not recommended.

The Prima FX has CE mark approval in Europe but is investigational in the United States. The optimal wavelength for the treatment of coronary atheroma has yet to be determined.

Intracoronary Stent

The term *stent* was used first in reference to a dental mold developed by an English dentist, Charles Thomas Stent, in the mid-19th century. The word evolved to describe various supportive devices used in medicine. To date, the introduction of intracoronary stents has had a larger impact on the practice of interventional cardiology than any other development.

The use of intracoronary stents exploded during the mid 1990s (Box 2-10). Receiving FDA approval in April 1993, the Gianturco-Roubin (Cook Flex stent), a coiled balloon-expandable stent was approved for the treatment of acute closure after PCI. Use of the Gianturco-Roubin stent was limited by difficulties with its delivery and high rates of restenosis. The first stent to receive widespread clinical application was the Palmaz-Schatz (Johnson and Johnson, New Brunswick, NJ) tubular slotted stent approved for the treatment of de novo coronary stenosis in 1994. Throughout the 1990s, multiple stents were introduced with improved support and flexibility and thinner struts, resulting in improved delivery and decreased restenosis rates.

As discussed earlier, the major limitations of catheter-based interventions had been acute vessel closure and restenosis. Stents offered an option for stabilizing intimal dissections while limiting late lumen loss, which are major components of acute closure and restenosis, respectively. Clinical trials have demonstrated the ability of stents not only to salvage a failed PTCA (thus avoiding emergent CABG) but also to reduce restenosis. Multiple studies demonstrated the benefit of stenting compared with PTCA alone in a variety of circumstances, including long lesions, vein grafts, chronic occlusions, and the thrombotic occlusions of AMI. Only in small vessels did stenting not demonstrate a restenosis benefit when compared with balloon angioplasty. Clinical restenosis rates fell from 30% to 40% with PTCA to less than 20% with bare metal stents.

With the realization that restenosis involves poorly regulated cellular proliferation, researchers focused on medicines that had antiproliferative effects. Many of these medicines are toxic when given systemically, a tolerable situation in oncology but not for a relatively benign condition such as restenosis. For such medicines, local delivery was attractive, and the stent provided a vehicle.

Rapamycin, a macrolide antibiotic, is a natural fermentation product produced by *Streptomyces hygroscopicus,* which was originally isolated in a soil sample from Rapa Nui (Easter Island). Rapamycin was soon discovered to have potent immunosuppressant activities, making it unacceptable as an antibiotic but attractive for prevention of transplant rejection. Rapamycin works through inhibition of a protein kinase called the mammalian target of rapamycin (mTOR), a mechanism that is distinct from other classes of immunosuppressants. Because mTOR is central to cellular proliferation as well as immune responses, this agent was an inspired choice for a stent coating. The terms *rapamycin* and *sirolimus* are often used interchangeably. A metal stent does not hold drugs well and permits little control over their release. These limitations required that polymers be developed to attach a drug to the stent and to allow the drug to slowly diffuse into the wall of the blood vessel, while eliciting no inflammatory response.[14] The development of drug-eluting stents would not have been possible without these (proprietary) polymers. This led to the true revolution in PCI, which occurred with the approval in April 2003 of the first drug-eluting stent. Johnson and Johnson/Cordis introduced their Cypher stent. This is their Velocity stent and polymer, which elutes rapamycin over 14 days; the drug is completely gone by 30 days post implantation.

The RAVEL trial randomized 238 patients to receive either a sirolimus-eluting stent (SES) or a bare metal stent. Remarkably, there was no restenosis in the group that received a sirolimus-eluting stent. The SIRIUS trial randomized 1058 patients to a sirolimus-eluting stent or a bare metal stent. At 9 months, restenosis rates were 8.9% in the sirolimus-eluting stent group and 36.3% in the bare metal stent group, with no difference in adverse events. Clinically driven repeat procedures were required in 3.9% and 16.6%, respectively. This benefit was sustained, if not slightly improved, at 12 months. Although initially approved only for use in de novo lesions in native vessels of stable patients, subsequent publications have shown similar benefits in every clinical scenario that has been studied.[15] Initial concerns regarding subacute stent thrombosis have proved unjustified with the rate of thrombosis approximately 1%, equal to that seen in bare metal stent patients.

The next drug-eluting stent to receive FDA approval in March 2004 was the Taxus stent (Boston Scientific Corp, Natick, MA). The Taxus stent uses a polymer coating to deliver paclitaxel, a drug that also has many uses in oncology. This is a lipophilic molecule, derived from the Pacific yew tree *Taxus brevifolia*. It interferes with microtubular function, affecting mitosis and extracellular secretion, thereby interrupting the restenotic process at multiple levels. The Taxus IV study randomized 1314 patients to the Taxus stent or a bare metal stent. Angiographic restenosis was reduced from 26.6% in the BMS group to 7.9% in the Taxus group with no significant difference in adverse events. Clinically driven repeat procedures were required in 12.0% and 4.7%, respectively.

When first introduced, stents were sparingly used, primarily owing to the initial aggressive anticoagulation regimens recommended. These regimens included intravenous heparin and dextran along with oral aspirin, dipyridamole, and warfarin. This required long hospitalizations and led to bleeding problems at vascular access sites. These complicated combinations of medicines were used in the clinical trials that led to the approval of the stents and were chosen based on the fear of thrombosis and limited animal data. Despite the use of these drugs, stent thrombosis still occurred in 3% to 5% of patients. The use of intracoronary ultrasound improved stent deployment by revealing incomplete expansion with conventional deployment techniques. This led to high-pressure balloon inflations, complete stent expansion, and simplified pharmacologic therapy.

Initially aspirin and ticlopidine (Ticlid) were used instead of warfarin, but clopidogrel (Plavix) replaced ticlopidine because it has a better side-effect profile. The combination of a thienopyridine and aspirin has markedly reduced thrombotic events and vascular complications. The timing and dosing of clopidogrel therapy are still evolving with doses of 300 to 600 mg given at least 2 to 4 hours before PCI. Given that PCI is often performed immediately after a diagnostic study, some cardiologists begin clopidogrel before diagnostic studies. PCI can be performed immediately after the diagnostic study with a reduction in adverse events that is comparable to that seen with glycoprotein inhibitors but at a fraction of the cost. However, if the diagnostic study indicates a need for CABG, bleeding complications will be increased if clopidogrel has been given during the 5 days before CABG.

Currently, stents are placed at the time of most PCI procedures, if the size and anatomy of the vessel permit. There are several reasons not to use a drug-eluting stent in every procedure. First, drug-eluting stents are available in fewer sizes. Second, a longer course of thienopyridine is required, and this may not be desirable if, for instance, a surgical procedure is urgently needed. Stent thromboses, myocardial infarctions, and deaths have been reported when antiplatelet therapy is interrupted. Finally, the cost of a drug-eluting stent is about three times that of a bare metal stent, and this increment is not fully reflected in reimbursement. As additional drug-eluting stents reach the market, prices may decline. With the significant reduction in restenosis, the drug-eluting stent may give PCI an advantage over CABG in multivessel disease. The consequences of this may be dramatic, as hospitals (and cardiac surgeons and cardiac anesthesiologists) see reduced CABG volumes and reduced volumes of repeat PCI in restenotic vessels. If these profitable procedures are replaced by money-losing ones, as placement of multiple drug-eluting stents currently is, many hospitals will suffer.[16]

Intravascular Brachytherapy

Brachytherapy was first introduced and developed for the treatment of malignant disease. In an attempt to decrease the neointimal proliferative process associated with restenosis, brachytherapy has been applied to the coronary artery. Two types of radiation are utilized in the coronary arteries: gamma and beta. Gamma radiation, such as that from iridium-192, has no mass, only energy; therefore, there is limited tissue attenuation. Beta-emitters, such as phosphorus-32 and yttrium-90, lose an orbiting electron or positron; the mass of this particle permits significant tissue attenuation.

Radiation safety for the patient, staff, and operator is essential for intravascular brachytherapy. For the staff and the operator, radiation exposure is related to both the energy of the isotope and the type of emission. Staff exposure is much higher with gamma emitters than with beta emitters, owing to its insignificant tissue attenuation. From the patient's perspective, brachytherapy is prescribed to provide a specific dose to the target vessel. Total body exposure is higher with gamma radiation, again because attenuation is minimal. Because gamma radiation requires significant extra shielding and requires the staff to leave the room during delivery of therapy, beta radiation is used more commonly. Additionally, the long-term effects from patient exposure need to be considered. Finally, significant expertise is required for intracoronary brachytherapy. In addition to the interventionalist, a radiation oncologist, medical physicist, and radiation safety officer must participate in these procedures.

Brachytherapy, using either a gamma or beta emitter, has proved effective for the treatment of in-stent restenosis. After brachytherapy, clopidogrel must be continued for at least 6 to 12 months to prevent late stent thrombosis that occurs due to delayed endothelialization of the stent. The future for brachytherapy in the era of drug-eluting stents is unknown.[17] The drug-eluting stent has significantly decreased in-stent restenosis. If restenosis does occur with drug-eluting stents, whether brachytherapy should be undertaken or a repeat drug-eluting stent placement performed is unclear. Because of the complexity of brachytherapy, unless it is truly proved superior to other modalities, its use in the interventional suite will be limited.

OTHER CATHETER-BASED PERCUTANEOUS THERAPIES

Percutaneous Valvular Therapy

Mitral Balloon Valvuloplasty

Percutaneous mitral valvuloplasty (PMC) was first performed in 1982 as an alternative to surgery for patients with rheumatic mitral stenosis. The procedure is usually performed via an antegrade approach and requires expertise in transseptal puncture. During the early years of PMC, the simultaneous inflation of two balloons in the mitral apparatus was required to obtain an adequate result. The development of the Inoue balloon (Toray, Inc., Houston, TX) in the 1990s simplified this procedure. This single balloon, with a central waist for placement at the valve, does not require wire placement across the aortic valve.

The key to mitral valvuloplasty is patient selection. Absolute contraindications to mitral valvuloplasty include a known LA thrombus or recent embolic event of less than 2 months and severe cardiothoracic deformity or bleeding abnormality preventing transseptal catheterization. Relative contraindications include significant MR, pregnancy, concomitant significant aortic valve disease, or significant CAD.

All patients must undergo transesophageal echocardiography to exclude LA thrombus as well as transthoracic echocardiography to classify the patient by anatomic groups. The most widely used classification, the Wilkins score, addresses leaflet mobility, valve thickening, subvalvular thickening, and valvular calcification. These scoring systems, as well as operator experience, predict outcomes. In experienced hands, the procedure is successful in 85% to 99% of cases. Risks of PMC include a procedural mortality of 0% to 3%, hemopericardium in 0.5% to 12%, and embolism in 0.5% to 5%. Severe MR occurs in 2% to 10% of procedures and often requires emergent surgery.[18] Although peripheral embolization occurs in up to 4% of patients, long-term sequelae are rare.

The procedure requires a large puncture in the interatrial septum, and this does not close completely in all patients. However, a clinically significant atrial septal defect with Q_p/Q_s of 1.5 or greater occurs in 10% or fewer of cases; surgical repair is seldom necessary. Advances in patient selection, operator experience, and equipment have significantly reduced procedural complications. Restenosis rates are dependent on the degree of commissural calcium. Transesophageal echocardiography or intracardiac echocardiography is helpful during balloon mitral valvuloplasty. These imaging modalities offer guidance with the transseptal catheter placement, verification of balloon positioning across the valve, and assessment of procedural success. Long-term results have been good.

Aortic Balloon Valvuloplasty

Percutaneous aortic balloon valvuloplasty was introduced in the 1980s. This procedure is usually performed via a femoral artery, using an 11-Fr sheath and 18- to 23-mm balloons. Some advocate the double-balloon technique for aortic valvuloplasty to decrease restenosis with a balloon placed through each femoral artery and inflated simultaneously.

Symptomatic improvement does occur with at least a 50% reduction in gradient in more than 80% of cases. Complications include femoral artery repair in up to 10% of patients, a 1% incidence of stroke, and a less than 1% incidence of cardiac fatality. Contraindications to aortic balloon valvuloplasty are significant peripheral vascular disease and moderate-to-severe aortic insufficiency. Aortic insufficiency usually increases at least one grade during valvuloplasty. The development of severe aortic regurgitation acutely leads to pulmonary congestion and possibly death, because the hypertrophied ventricle is unable to dilate.

Initial success rates are acceptable, but restenosis occurs as early as 6 months after the procedure and nearly all patients will have restenosis by 2 years. Therefore, the use of aortic valvuloplasty has waned. Current indications include the following: inoperable patient willing to accept the restenosis rate for temporary reduction in symptoms; noncardiac surgery patient hoping to decrease the surgical risk; and patient with poor LV function, in an attempt to improve ventricular function for further consideration of aortic valve replacement.

Percutaneous Valve Replacement

Surgical valve replacement is widely performed for regurgitant and stenotic valves. Although surgical morbidity and mortality continue to improve, the risks remain prohibitive for some patients. Catheter-based alternatives to surgical valve replacement have been explored since the 1960s but were not successful until 2000, when percutaneous pulmonic valve replacement was performed. The first procedures were performed in patients who had had prior cardiac surgery and were not considered good candidates for reoperation. The procedures are performed with the use of general anesthesia with intracardiac echocardiographic guidance. A biologic valve is sutured onto a platinum stent and delivered on a balloon. The stent compresses the native valve against the wall of the annulus. Large 18- to 20-Fr delivery systems are used. The results in high-risk patients have been promising, and the device is now being tested in a lower risk group, that is, as a true alternative to surgery. The success of percutaneous pulmonic valve replacement prompted interest in the aortic and mitral valves.

The first percutaneous aortic valve replacement in humans was performed in France in 2002. This valve is created by shaping bovine pericardium into leaflets and mounting them within a balloon-expandable stent. Both retrograde and antegrade approaches have been used. Early results are encouraging, as improvements in symptoms and ventricular function are seen after percutaneous aortic valve replacement.[19]

The percutaneous approach for MR includes both attempts to replace as well as to repair the mitral valve. Preliminary work has included two approaches. The first approach involves placement of a device composed of a distal and proximal anchor within the coronary sinus. This device can then be shortened to decrease the size of the mitral annulus and decrease MR, similar to a surgically placed annuloplasty ring. The second approach involves percutaneous stitching of the mitral valve, similar to the surgical Alfieri operation. Finally, both temporary and permanent mitral valve implantations have been attempted but are early in the experimental process.

Although still experimental, percutaneous valve replacement and repair are exciting and offer a new dimension in catheter-based therapy. Experience is limited compared with the years of work and thousands of patients with surgical intervention. Although promising, enthusiasm may best be tempered at this stage. However, as this field expands, the role of the cardiac anesthesiologist in the catheterization laboratory for these complex procedures will likely expand.

2

THE CATHETERIZATION LABORATORY AND THE ANESTHESIOLOGIST

The objective of this chapter has been to provide a broad overview of the catheterization laboratory for the anesthesiologist. As success rates for coronary interventions have increased and complication rates have decreased, there have been fewer opportunities for the cardiologist and the anesthesiologist to interact in the catheterization suite. However, in the 21st century, the role of the anesthesiologist in the catheterization laboratory is destined to change. In this dynamic field of interventional cardiology, more complex and prolonged procedures, such as percutaneous valvular therapy, may well require the renewed collaboration of the interventional cardiologist and the cardiac anesthesiologist.[20]

SUMMARY

- The cardiac catheterization laboratory has evolved from a diagnostic facility to a therapeutic one.
- Guidelines for diagnostic cardiac catheterization have established indications and contraindications, as well as criteria to identify high-risk patients. Careful evaluation of the patient before the procedure is necessary to minimize risks.
- A general overview of hemodynamics is presented, including waveform generation and analysis, cardiac output measurement, and assessment of valvular pathology. Basic angiography is also reviewed, including ventriculography, aortography, and coronary cineangiography.
- Interventional cardiology began in the late 1970s as balloon angioplasty with a success rate of 80% and emergent coronary artery bypass graft surgery (CABG) rates of 3% to 5%. Although current success rates exceed 95% with CABG rates less than 1%, the failed percutaneous coronary intervention (PCI) patient presents a challenge for the anesthesiologist because of hemodynamic problems, concomitant medications, and the underlying cardiac disease.
- Thrombosis is a major cause of complications during PCI, and platelets are primary in this process.
- In the stent era, acute closure from coronary dissection has diminished significantly. Restenosis rates have fallen precipitously since the introduction of the drug-eluting stents.
- For patients presenting with acute myocardial infarction, both primary PCI and thrombolytic therapy are effective. In multivessel disease, the advantage of CABG over PCI is narrowing, and drug-eluting stents may reverse this advantage.
- Extensive thrombus, heavy calcification, degenerated saphenous vein grafts, and chronic total occlusions present specific challenges in PCI. Various specialty devices have been developed to address these problems with varying degrees of success.
- The reach of the interventional cardiologist is extending beyond the coronary vessels, and now includes closure of congenital defects and percutaneous treatment of valvular disease. These long and complex procedures are more likely to require general anesthesia.

I

REFERENCES

1. Hirshfeld JW, Balter S Jr, Brunker JA, et al: ACC Clinical Competence Statement. Recommendations for the assessment and maintenance of proficiency in coronary interventional procedures. Statement of the American College of Cardiology. J Am Coll Cardiol 31:722, 1998
2. Sousa JE, Serruys PW, Costa MA: New frontiers in cardiology: Drug-eluting stents: I. Circulation 107:2274, 2003
3. Williams DO, Holubkov R, Yeh W, et al: Percutaneous coronary intervention in the current era compared with 1985. The National Heart, Lung, and Blood Institute Registries. Circulation 102:2945, 2000
4. Holmes DR, Firth BG, Wood DL: Paradigm shifts in cardiovascular medicine. J Am Coll Cardiol 43:507, 2004
5. Lotfi M, Mackie K, Dzavik V, Seidelin PH: Impact of delays to cardiac surgery after failed angioplasty and stenting. J Am Coll Cardiol 43:337, 2004
6. Antman EM, Anbe DT, Armstrong PW, et al: ACC/AHA guidelines for the management of patients with ST-elevation myocardial infarction: executive summary. Circulation 110:588, 2004.
7. Waters RE, Singh KP, Roe MT, et al: Rationale and strategies for implementing community-based transfer protocols for primary percutaneous coronary intervention for acute ST-segment elevation myocardial infarction. J Am Coll Cardiol 43:2153, 2004
8. Casey C, Faxon DP: Multi-vessel coronary disease and percutaneous coronary intervention. Heart 90:341, 2004
9. Hoffman SN, TenBrook JA, Wolf MP, et al: A meta-analysis of randomized controlled trials comparing coronary artery bypass graft surgery with percutaneous transluminal coronary angioplasty: One- to eight-year outcomes. J Am Coll Cardiol 41:1293, 2003
10. Holmes DR: Stenting small coronary arteries: Works in progress. JAMA 292:2777, 2004.
11. vonBirgelen C, Hartmann M, Mintz GS, et al: Relationship between cardiovascular risk as predicted by established risk scores versus plaque progression as measured by serial intravascular ultrasound in left main coronary arteries. Circulation 110:1579, 2004
12. Tsuchikane E, Sumitsuji S, Awata N, et al: Final results of the Stent versus Directional Coronary Atherectomy Randomized Trial (START). J Am Coll Cardiol 34:1050, 1999
13. Mehran R, Dangas G, Mintz GS, et al: Treatment of in-stent restenosis with excimer laser coronary angioplasty versus rotational atherectomy: Comparative mechanisms and results. Circulation 101:2484, 2000
14. Serruys P, Kutryk M, Ong A: Coronary artery stents. N Engl J Med 354:486, 2006.
15. Lemos PA, Saia F, Hofma SH, et al: Short- and long-term clinical benefit of sirolimus-eluting stents compared with conventional bare stents for patients with acute myocardial infarction. J Am Coll Cardiol 43:704, 2004
16. Lemos PA, Serruys PW, Sousa JE: Drug-eluting stents: Cost versus clinical benefit. Circulation 107:3003, 2003
17. Teirstein PS, King S: Vascular radiation in a drug-eluting stent world: It's not over til it's over. Circulation 108:384, 2003
18. Vahanian A, Palacios IF: Percutaneous approaches to valvular disease. Circulation 109:1572, 2004
19. Bauer F, Eltchaninoff H, Tron C, et al: Acute improvement in global and regional left ventricular systolic function after percutaneous heart valve implantation in patients with symptomatic aortic stenosis. Circulation 110:1473, 2004
20. O'Neill W, Dixon S, Grimes C: The year in interventional cardiology. J Am Coll Cardiol 45:1017, 2005

2

Section II

Cardiovascular Physiology, Pharmacology, and Molecular Biology

Chapter 3

Cardiac Physiology

Brian Johnson, MD • Maher Adi, MD • Michael G. Licina, MD •
Zak Hillel, MD • Daniel Thys, MD • Roberta L. Hines, MD •
Joel A. Kaplan, MD

A thorough knowledge of the principles of cardiovascular physiology is the foundation for the practice of cardiovascular anesthesia. It serves as the basis of understanding the pathophysiologic mechanisms of cardiac disease as well as the patient's pharmacologic and surgical management.

To assess the physiologic basis for cardiac dysfunction, a systematic inspection of the elements that determine cardiac output (CO) is required. These intrinsic factors—heart rate (HR)/rhythm, preload, contractility, and afterload—are codependent such that abnormality in one often results in altered function in the others. This complex interaction is intrinsically designed to regulate beat-to-beat changes in the cardiovascular system, thereby adapting to changes in physiologic demands.

Heart rate, preload, afterload, and contractility determine CO, which, in turn, when combined with peripheral arterial resistance, determines arterial pressure for organ perfusion. Similarly, the arterial system contributes to ventricular afterload, and these interactions influence mechanoreceptors in the carotid artery and aortic arch, providing feedback signals to higher levels in the central nervous system (medullary and vasomotor center). These centers then modulate venous return, HR, contractility, and arterial resistance (Fig. 3-1).

The heart's primary function is to deliver sufficient oxygenated blood to meet the metabolic requirements of the peripheral tissues. Under normal circumstances, the heart acts as a servant by varying the CO in accordance with total tissue needs. Tissue needs may vary with exercise, heart disease, trauma, surgery, or administration of drugs. Although tissue needs regulate circulatory requirements, the heart can become a limiting factor, particularly in patients with cardiac disease. In this regard, it is important to differentiate circulatory function from cardiac and myocardial function.

The focus of this chapter is on the heart's function as a pump. The various determinants of its pumping function are reviewed and, where applicable, newer clinical measurements of ventricular function are discussed.

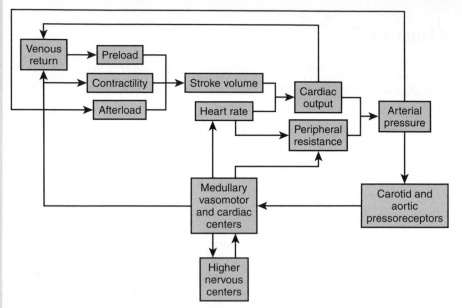

Figure 3-1   Interactions controlling the intact circulation. Changes in one or more of the determinants of cardiovascular performance directly affect the integrity of the circulation. Such interdependence must be considered when analyzing or treating hemodynamic disturbances. (Modified from Braunwald E: Regulation of the Circulation, NEJM 290 (20): 1124–1129, 1974.)

CARDIAC CYCLE

The cardiac cycle of the left ventricle (LV) begins as excitation of the myocardium, which results in a sequence of mechanical events that lead to a pressure gradient being developed, ejection of the stroke volume (SV), and forward flow of blood through the body. These phases can be discussed based on the electrical activity, intracardiac pressures, intracardiac volumes, opening and closing of the cardiac valves, or the flow of blood into the peripheral circulation. Most practical of these is the relationship of pressure to volume over the course of the cycle. In this regard, systole represents the rapid increase in intracardiac pressure followed by the rapid decrease in volume. Diastole, on the other hand, represents first a rapid decrease in pressure followed by an increase in volume. An alternative to this approach is to exclude any temporal element and to study the relation of pressure to volume in the framework of a pressure-volume diagram (Fig. 3-2). In this diagram, the pressure is typically displayed on the vertical axis and the volume on the horizontal axis. This yields a pressure-volume loop of four distinct phases over the course of one contraction: isovolumic contraction, ventricular ejection (rapid and slow), isovolumic relaxation, and filling (rapid and diastasis).

Phases of the Cardiac Cycle

Isovolumic Contraction Phase

This phase represents the first portion of systolic activity of the myocardial muscle. It occurs just after the QRS complex on the ECG, when individual myocardial fibers begin to shorten. As the contraction continues, the ventricular pressure increases

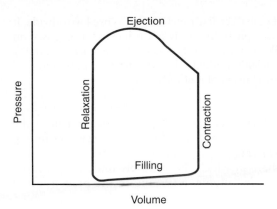

Figure 3-2 Phases of the cardiac cycle displayed in a pressure-volume diagram.

rapidly, exceeding atrial pressure and forcing the atrioventricular (AV) valve to close due to the reversed pressure gradient. While the AV valve closes, it also balloons up into the atrium and causes the chordal apparatus to tense, holding the coaptation point at its optimal position, thus preventing regurgitation. This now forms a sealed chamber (ventricle) because the AV valve has closed and the semilunar valves have yet to open. The ventricle continues to alter shape without changing its volume, thereby resulting in increased pressure. In awake canine hearts, the ventricle has been shown to change into an ellipse. This shape seems to be volume dependent, and at lower volumes the shape during contraction is spherical.[1]

Early work by Frank has shown that tension (T) developed by cardiac muscle is determined by the initial length (L) or stretch of the muscle. In isolated muscles, the optimal tension developed is known as Lmax. At muscle lengths below or above Lmax, the developed tension is less than maximal.

Ejection Phase

As soon as the developed pressure exceeds that of the resting pressure of the aorta or pulmonary artery, the semilunar valves open and the ejection phase begins. The actual opening of the valves is due to the movement of blood across the valve leaflets caused by the pressure gradient. The ejection phase leads to a marked decrease in ventricular volume and a slight increase in pressure initially that rapidly decreases to the dicrotic notch pressure. The equalization of the pressure gradient between the ventricular and aortic pressures signals the end of the ejection phase and allows closure of the semilunar valves. This is the point of smallest ventricular size and volume, also known as the end-systolic volume (ESV). This ESV is greatly dependent on the contractile state of the ventricle and the properties of the vascular system.

The relationship among muscle force, velocity, and length is not readily applied to the clinical setting, owing to the extreme difficulty of obtaining measurements in intact hearts. In clinical practice, these difficulties lead to use of the end-diastolic volume (EDV) and ESV, which are relatively easy to measure. The difference between these two is the SV:

$$SV = EDV - ESV$$

In addition, by using the SV equation divided by the EDV, ejection fraction (EF) can be obtained:

$$EF = (EDV - ESV)/EDV$$
$$EF = SV/EDV$$

EF is a well-known estimation of global cardiac function that is used worldwide. It allows application of the Starling principle in the study of cardiac function based on changes in EDV as they relate to SV. The use of transesophageal echocardiography (TEE) has greatly enhanced the clinician's ability to directly visualize EDV and ESV using biplane apical and single-plane ellipsoidal methods.[2]

Isovolumic Relaxation Phase

The biochemical process of isovolumic relaxation begins to occur before the blood has even stopped flowing out of the ventricle and is an energy-consuming process. The term *relaxation phase* refers to the period immediately after closure of the semilunar valves. It is a phase in which the ventricle undergoes a rapid decrease in pressure and no change in volume, returning to the precontractile configuration.

Filling Phase (Diastolic Filling)

As the relaxation phase continues, the ventricular pressure continues to drop. At the same time, the atria are receiving blood flow from the pulmonary veins (left atrium [LA]) or the superior and inferior vena cava (right atrium [RA]), thus experiencing rises in pressure and volume. As the atrial pressure rises and ventricular pressure drops, a crossover point is reached where the AV valves open and blood flows down the pressure gradient into the ventricle. There are two phases to this flow: (1) a rapid phase based solely on the pressure gradient, and (2) a slower active phase based on the contraction of the atria (atrial kick). During this filling, the ventricular volume increases rapidly and yet the ventricular pressure changes very little, if at all, in the normal heart. This is measured by the end-diastolic pressure-volume relation (EDPVR), which describes ventricular distensibility and has a strong relationship to the compliance of the ventricle, extrinsic factors, and the determinants of ventricular relaxation. This process continues until the next electrical signal, which starts the contraction phase again.

DIASTOLIC FUNCTION

Diastology, or the study of diastolic function, has become the most important focus of cardiac physiology in the past few years. Diastolic dysfunction has been seen in 40% to 50% of patients with congestive heart failure (CHF) despite normal systolic function.[3] This led to a shift in thinking about cardiac function not only as the typical systolic factors of contractile force, ejection of SV, and generation of CO but also as diastolic factors. The use of transthoracic echocardiography (TTE) and TEE has greatly improved this knowledge of diastole by showing the actual real-time activities in the heart, as related to filling pressures, shape, and relaxation. It is now possible to relate diastolic dysfunction, which is increased impedance to ventricular filling, to structural and pathologic causes of CHF (Table 3-1).

Determinants of Diastolic Function

Myocardial Relaxation

Relaxation of the myocardium is the first step in the physiologic process of diastole. It begins during the end of the previous systolic contraction and is intimately related to systolic forces. It is also key in the determination of the length and amount of early

Table 3-1 Conditions Involving Diastolic Heart Failure*

Conditions	Mechanisms of Diastolic Dysfunction
Mitral or tricuspid stenosis	Increased resistance to atrial emptying
Constrictive pericarditis	Increased resistance to ventricular inflow, with decreased ventricular diastolic capacity
Restrictive cardiomyopathies (amyloidosis, hemochromatosis, diffuse fibrosis)	Increased resistance to ventricular inflow
Obliterative cardiomyopathy (endocardial fibroelastosis, Loeffler's syndrome)	Increased resistance to ventricular inflow
Ischemic heart disease	Postinfarction scarring and hypertrophy (remodeling)
Flash pulmonary edema, dyspnea during angina	Diastolic calcium overload
Impaired myocardial relaxation	Increased resistance to ventricular inflow
Hypertrophic heart disease (hypertrophic cardiomyopathy, chronic hypertension, aortic stenosis)	Impaired myocardial relaxation Diastolic calcium overload Increased resistance to ventricular inflow due to thick chamber walls, altered collagen matrix Activation of renin-angiotensin system
Volume overload (aortic or mitral regurgitation, arteriovenous fistula)	Increased diastolic volume relative to ventricular capacity Myocardial hypertrophy, fibrosis
Dilated cardiomyopathy	Impaired myocardial relaxation Diastolic calcium overload Myocardial fibrosis or scar

*Diastolic heart failure is increased resistance to filling of one or both cardiac ventricles.
From Grossmvan W: Diastolic dysfunction in congestive heart failure. N Engl J Med 325:1557, 1991.

passive ventricular filling. Relaxation relies heavily on the use of energy and adenosine triphosphate (ATP) to drive the calcium from the cell into the sarcoplasmic reticulum. This energy-dependent process is controlled by myriad regulatory proteins and by numerous clinical factors. Failure of relaxation leads to rapid Ca^{2+} overload, particularly at increased levels of stimulating frequency.

PASSIVE VENTRICULAR FILLING

The first phase of filling starts with the opening of the mitral valve and the flow of blood down the newly generated pressure gradient from the LA into the LV. The rate of flow has both a rapid rate and slow rate as the pressure gradient approaches equilibration. Diastasis is the period of no flow across the mitral valve after the conclusion of passive filling and immediately before atrial systole. The main determinants of transmitral flow are the LV compliance (stiffness) and the rate of rise of the transmitral gradient. Many disease states can contribute to increasing stiffness of the ventricle and thus affect the amount of passive filling that can occur during the early phase of diastole. In aging, angina, coronary artery disease, and hypertrophic obstructive cardiomyopathy, myocardial stiffness is greatly increased, thus impairing inflow into the ventricle.[4] Numerous drugs and cardiac revascularization can all improve dysfunction or reduce exercise-induced stiffness.

ATRIAL OR ACTIVE FILLING

Atrial contraction, or "atrial kick," occurs at the end of diastole just before the closing of the mitral valve and after passive flow has reached the diastasis. Normally, greater than 75% of flow occurs during the passive portion of diastole. In the presence of severe diastolic dysfunction, this normal relationship cannot take place and the atrial kick becomes essential to maintain SV and cardiac output. The atrial kick continues to compensate for decreased LV compliance (increase in LVEDP), and LV filling is initially maintained. Eventually, the increased pressures overcome the capacity of the LA to contribute to the total LV volume, and the atrium assumes a very passive role and becomes dilated. If normal sinus rhythm is not maintained, the atrial kick cannot function in its supportive role, and further CHF occurs rapidly. Reestablishment of normal sinus rhythm by cardioversion or sequential pacing can reverse the CHF symptoms.

Relating Echocardiography to Diastolic Function

The relationship between the stages of diastolic function and findings on both TEE and TTE has greatly enhanced the study and importance of diastolic function (Box 3-1). Using TTE and TEE in combination with Doppler techniques has made it possible via indirect means to obtain LV filling patterns.[5] The most commonly accepted means of analyzing the flow patterns are via the Doppler transmitral flow and the pulmonary vein flow. Newer modes of measurement using tissue Doppler and color M-mode are leading to further insights into diastolic function.

Transmitral flow patterns are the first method, which is performed by placing a pulsed-wave Doppler signal in the area between the leaflet tips of the mitral valve. Two waves are obtained: first the E wave, which represents the early passive flow across the mitral valve; and second, the A wave, which represents atrial systole (Fig. 3-3). The small area of no flow between the E and A waves represents the diastasis.

BOX 3-1 *Diastolic Function Can Be Measured Clinically by Use of*

- Transmitral pulsed-wave Doppler flow patterns
- Pulmonary vein two-dimensional Doppler flow patterns
- Color M-mode Doppler echocardiography
- Tissue Doppler echocardiography

QUANTITATION OF TRANSMITRAL FLOW VELOCITY PROFILES

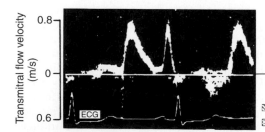
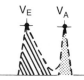

------- Area under broken line = SD
FVI$_E$ V$_E$ = Peak early filling velocity
FVI$_A$ V$_A$ = Peak atrial filling velocity

Figure 3-3 Transmitral flow-velocity profile and diagrammatic representation of its quantification.

By comparing the ratios of these two waves it is possible to form a view of diastolic function. The ratios change with disease and age to yield several patterns, which represent different stages of failure. In early diastolic failure, the E/A wave ratio becomes less than 1, and the waves reverse with the E wave being shorter than the A wave; this is known as the delayed relaxation pattern. As failure progresses, the waves become pseudonormalized; that is, the E/A ratio reverts to the normal pattern of greater than 1. The final stage of failure as seen via the mitral valve shows a high, rapidly decelerating E wave with a small A wave; this pattern is known as the restrictive pattern. The use of these patterns on Doppler imaging allows for the staging of diastolic failure from a mild form to a more severe form.[6,7]

SYSTOLIC FUNCTION

Systolic function is the period existing between closure of the mitral valve and the start of contraction to the end of ejection of blood from the heart. The primary purpose of systole is the ejection of blood into the circulation via the generation of a pressure gradient. Systolic function has been used to determine outcome and therapeutic effectiveness for years.

Cardiac Output

Cardiac output is the amount of blood flowing into the circulation per minute. It reflects not only the condition of the heart but also the entire vascular system and is subject to the autoregulatory systems of the vasculature and tissues. The equation for CO is listed below and involves HR and SV.

$$CO = SV \times HR$$

The primary determinants for CO are the HR and the SV. It is also dependent on many other secondary factors, including venous return, systemic vascular resistance, peripheral oxygen use, total blood volume, respiration, and body position. Normal range of CO is between 5 and 6 L/min in a 70-kg man, with an SV of 60 to 90 mL per beat and an HR of 80 beats per minute. CO is highly variable in the normal healthy individual, being able to increase up to 25 to 30 L/min during situations of high metabolic demand.

The cardiac index (CI) is used to compare different sizes of individuals and is now part of routine clinical practice. This is done by correcting the standard CO equation for body surface area (BSA).

$$CI = (SV \times HR)/BSA$$

$$CI = CO/BSA$$

Normal values are 2.5 to 3.5 L/min/m^2 for the normal 70-kg man. By correcting for BSA, it is then possible to compare patients at a common level of function, despite differences in body habitus.

Stroke Volume

The SV is the amount of blood ejected by the ventricle with each single contraction. The determinants of SV are preload, afterload, and contractility. Although these variables have a very clear meaning in reference to isolated muscles, their exact significance is much more ambiguous in the intact heart.

3

59

Preload

DEFINITION

Preload is equal to the ventricular wall stress at end-diastole. It is determined by ventricular EDV, end-diastolic pressure (EDP), and wall thickness. To apply the preload principle to clinical practice, the following adjustments can be made:

1. *Substituting ventricular volumes for preload stress.* In clinical practice, ventricular volumes appear to most closely approximate muscle fiber length. In normal humans, a straight-line relationship has been demonstrated between EDV and SV.
2. *Substituting ventricular pressures for ventricular volumes.* Ventricular pressures are often substituted for ventricular volumes when assessing the filling conditions of the ventricle. Clinically, left atrial pressure (LAP), pulmonary artery occlusion or capillary wedge pressure (PAOP or PCWP), pulmonary artery diastolic pressure (PADP), right atrial pressure (RAP), and central venous pressure (CVP) are often used as substitutes for LVEDP and LVEDV. Their accuracy in predicting LV preload is determined by the distensibility properties of the ventricle, the integrity of the mitral valve, the presence of normal pulmonary conditions, the integrity of the pulmonic and tricuspid valves, and RV function.

The assumption that ventricular distensibility is normal is not a valid assumption in many patients with cardiac disease. With coronary artery disease or aortic disease, diastolic function is often altered so that small increases in ventricular volume can produce large changes in ventricular pressure.

DETERMINANTS

Factors affecting the preload of the heart include the total blood volume, body position, intrathoracic pressure, intrapericardial pressure, venous tone, pumping action of skeletal muscles, and the atrial contribution to ventricular filling.

MEASUREMENT

The LVEDV is difficult to measure clinically, and measurements have only recently become possible with techniques such as echocardiography. TEE has been extensively used to measure LV areas as an approximation of LV volumes. Some studies have found a good correlation between areas and volumes and have also shown that in surgical patients EDV derived from a single plane is a significant determinant of SV.[8]

The LVEDP can be measured with placement of a catheter into the LA. The LA catheter is commonly inserted surgically through one of the pulmonary veins. The LAP provides a good approximation of LVEDP, provided the mitral valve is normal (Fig. 3-4). The most common technique for the estimation of LVEDP during cardiac surgery is the placement of a pulmonary artery (PA) catheter. The PCWP usually provides a good approximation of LVEDP. Marked alterations in airway pressure, such as occur during the use of high levels of positive end-expiratory pressure (PEEP), may disturb the relationship between the PCWP and LAP. Depending on the compliance of the pulmonary parenchyma, either part or all of the airway pressure may be transmitted to the PA catheter. This must be considered when evaluating LV filling pressure with the PA catheter in patients receiving mechanical ventilation and PEEP. When the catheter cannot be advanced into the wedge position, the PADP may be used to estimate the LVEDP. It is usually quite accurate unless the pulmonary vascular resistance (PVR) is markedly elevated. The CVP provides the poorest estimate

II

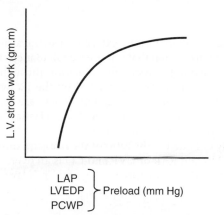

Figure 3-4   The Frank-Starling relation of chamber diastolic length (represented as left ventricular end-diastolic pressure [LVEDP], pulmonary capillary wedge pressure [PCWP], or left atrial pressure [LAP]) and ventricular performance (cardiac output [CO], stroke volume [SV], cardiac index [CI], left ventricular [LV] stroke work). With increasing diastolic muscle fiber length, that is, preload, both left and right ventricular performance can increase steadily. However, once the limit of preload reserve is reached, myocardial performance cannot be enhanced further by augmenting SV.

BOX 3-2   *Measurements of Afterload*

- Wall stress
- Impedance
- Effective arterial elastance
- Systolic intraventricular pressure
- Systemic vascular resistance
- Pulmonary vascular resistance

---

of LVEDP, although it is frequently used in patients with good function of the RV and LV. When cardiac disease is characterized by disparate RV and LV functions, the CVP may be misleading as an indicator of LVEDP.

Afterload

DEFINITION

Afterload is the second major determinant of the mechanical properties of cardiac muscle fibers and performance of the intact heart (Box 3-2). Afterload can be considered either as the stress imposed on the ventricular wall during systole or as the arterial impedance to the ejection of SV.

WALL STRESS

Afterload defined as systolic ventricular wall stress is the burden that the RV or LV wall has to shoulder for ejecting its SV. This stress can be expressed and quantified by the Laplace equation:

$$\sigma = (P \cdot r)/2h$$

where σ is the stress (dynes·cm^{-2}), P is the pressure generated by the LV throughout systole, and r and h are the corresponding radius and thickness of the RV or LV wall.

IMPEDANCE

Afterload can also be considered as the external or extracardiac forces (impedance) present in the systemic circulation that oppose ventricular ejection and pulsatile flow. Because the LV is coupled to the systemic circulation through the open aortic valve, the pulsatile flow (SV) and pressure generated by the LV will be hindered by the compliance and resistance of the arterial system. These are determined by the physical properties of the aorta and its side branches (viscoelastic properties and diameter) and by the properties of their content (blood).

The SVR clinically obtained as the ratio of the pressure differential between mean arterial pressure (MAP) and RAP or CVP and CO is an oversimplified version of the resistance. It is based on the circulatory analog of Ohm's law:

$$Q = P/R$$

or

$$P = Q \times R$$

which determines that the pressure (P) generated during the ejection of a given flow (Q) is proportional to that flow and to the resistance (R) encountered by that flow. This resistance is mainly determined by arteriolar resistance (SVR) so that

$$SVR = [MAP - RAP]/CO$$

Contractility

DEFINITION

The third determinant of SV is contractility. *Contractility* is an intrinsic property of the cardiac cell that defines the amount of work that the heart can perform at a given load. It is primarily determined by the availability of intracellular Ca^{2+}. With depolarization of the cardiac cell, a small amount of Ca^{2+} enters the cell and triggers the release of additional Ca^{2+} from intracellular storage sites (sarcoplasmic reticulum). The Ca^{2+} binds to troponin, tropomyosin is displaced from the active binding site on actin, and actin-myosin crossbridges are formed. All agents with positive inotropic properties, such as the catecholamines, have in common that they increase intracellular Ca^{2+}, whereas negative inotropes have the opposite effect (Table 3-2).[9]

DETERMINANTS

The large number of methods developed to measure contractility in the intact heart suggests that it is difficult to measure. Indices of contractility can be classified according to the phase of the cardiac cycle during which they are obtained.

Isovolumic Contraction Phase Indices. Isovolumic phase indices are obtained during the isovolumic phase of the contraction before the opening of the aortic valve. The prototype of such indices is dP/dt. It is obtained by placing a catheter with a micromanometer at its tip into the LV. The LV pressure is continuously sampled while an electronic differentiator calculates the first derivative of pressures, or dP/dt (mm Hg/s). The highest value of dP/dt, or peak dP/dt, is considered proportional to contractility. Because the heart's developed tension, or pressure, is dependent on the initial length of the cardiac muscle, it is predictable that dP/dt will be preload dependent.

Ejection Phase Indices. The standard ejection phase index of contractility is the EF:

$$EF = SV/EDV$$

II

Table 3-2 Factors Affecting Contractility

Factors Increasing Contractility
- Sympathetic stimulation—direct increases of the force of contraction, as well as indirect increases due to increased heart rate (rate treppe effect or Bowditch phenomenon)
- Parasympathetic inhibition producing increased heart rate
- Administration of positive inotropic drugs such as digitalis

Factors Decreasing Contractility
- Parasympathetic stimulation—decreased rate effect
- Sympathetic inhibition via withdrawal of catecholamines or blockade of adrenergic receptors
- Administration of β-adrenergic–blocking drugs, slow calcium channel blockers, or other myocardial depressants
- Myocardial ischemia and infarction
- Intrinsic myocardial diseases such as cardiomyopathies
- Hypoxia and acidosis

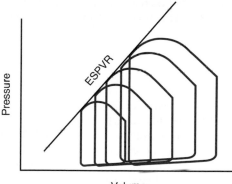

Figure 3-5 The end-systolic pressure-volume relationship (ESPVR) is obtained by connecting all the end-systolic points measured during a rapid decrease in preload.

3

With the increasing availability of noninvasive cardiac imaging techniques, ejection phase indices are widely used in clinical practice. One of the reasons for their widespread use is that a clear association between EF and prognosis has been found.

Load-Independent Indices. Because traditional indices of contractility are load dependent, different approaches to the quantification of the contractile properties of the heart have been explored. In one such approach, Suga and colleagues[10,11] studied instantaneous pressure and volume in the canine heart. The ratio of ventricular pressure over volume is the ventricular elastance, which varies throughout the cardiac cycle. For each cardiac cycle, these researchers defined the maximal value of this ratio as the end-systolic elastance (E_{ES}) and the point at which it was reached as the end-systolic point. They further noted that with rapid decreases in preload all consecutive end-systolic points were positioned on a single straight line, known as the end-systolic pressure-volume relation (ESPVR) (Fig. 3-5). The slope of this line (E_{ES}) is proportional to contractility; it is steeper at higher contractility and flatter at lower contractility.

BOX 3-3   *In Comparison to the Left Ventricle, the Right Ventricle Is*

- More complex with phases of contraction
- Better suited to eject large volumes of blood
- More sensitive to afterload
- Less sensitive to preload

Heart Rate

The second major determinate of CO is HR. It is one of the most variable determinants of overall cardiac function. It also has great importance to all portions of the cardiac cycle. The HR is controlled by multiple systems, such as the cardiac conduction system, central nervous system, and autonomic nervous system, which respond via complex pathways to changes in the internal and external conditions. Besides the neural and hormonal factors, many pharmacologic controls are available as well.

An interesting relationship is the fact that HR itself can increase the contractility of the heart. This is known as the treppe or step (Bowditch) phenomenon, which shows that at increased HRs, the slope of the ESPVR increases in a stepwise fashion related to the increased rate. This increase is thought to be due to increases in the level of intracellular calcium.

RIGHT VENTRICULAR FUNCTION

The contractile pattern, as well as the afterload presented to each ventricle (i.e., RV vs. LV), results in marked physiologic differences between the ventricles (Box 3-3). In contrast to the LV, which has a relatively simple and unified mechanism of contraction (by coaxial shortening), RV contraction occurs in three distinct phases. Initially, the spiral muscles contract, resulting in a downward movement of the tricuspid valve and shortening of the longitudinal axis of the RV chamber. This is followed by movement of the RV free wall inward toward the intraventricular septum. Because the RV free wall has limited muscular power, alterations in or failure of the intraventricular septum to contract normally will disturb the systolic function of the RV to a *much greater* degree than does a loss of RV free wall contractility. Finally, the third phase of RV contraction occurs when LV contraction imposes a "wringer" action, further augmenting overall RV contraction.

Global RV function is exquisitely sensitive to the impedance offered by the pulmonary vasculature.[12] In comparison with the LV, which maintains a constant output over a relatively wide range of afterloads, the RV output abruptly decreases with even small increases in afterload (Fig. 3-6). Under normal conditions of RV function, any increase in afterload is accompanied by a substantial decrease in RVEF. However, normal RV contractile function is usually maintained until the mean PAP is 40 mm Hg or greater. Conversely, the RV appears to be less preload dependent than the LV (i.e., for a given preload, a smaller increase in SV is seen in the RV).

VENTRICULAR INTERACTION

Ventricular interaction is a process that is vital to the integration of heart and lung function. This relationship occurs both during systole and diastole and is a result of an intimate anatomic association between the RV and LV. The major physiologic impact

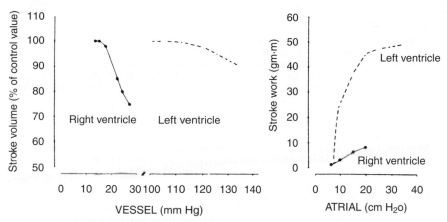

Figure 3-6 Varying effects of afterload and preload seen in ventricular function curves from the right and left ventricles. The RV output is more afterload dependent and less preload dependent than the LV output. (From McFadden ER, Braunwald E: Cor pulmonale and pulmonary thromboembolism. In Braunwald E [ed]: Textbook of Cardiovascular Medicine. Philadelphia, WB Saunders, 1980, pp 1643–1680.)

of this ventricular interaction relates to (1) the effect of the distention of one ventricle on the other, and (2) the contribution of LV contraction to the development of RV systolic pressure. Factors that contribute to normal ventricular interaction include the intraventricular septum, pericardium, and shared coronary blood flow.[13-16]

The importance of alterations in RV function has been demonstrated in a variety of clinical settings. Abnormalities of RV performance may occur (1) as a primary event, (2) secondary to LV failure, or (3) secondary to alterations in the mechanisms of ventricular interaction.

SUMMARY

- Heart rate, preload, afterload, and contractility determine the cardiac output. Alterations in one or more of the determinants of cardiovascular performance directly affect the integrity of the circulation.
- Phases of the cardiac cycle are best displayed in a pressure-volume diagram/loop.
- Diastology has recently become the most important focus of cardiac physiology.
- Diastole consists of isovolumic relaxation, passive ventricular filling, and active or atrial filling.
- The stroke volume is the difference between the end-diastolic volume and the end-systolic volume. The ejection fraction is the stroke volume divided by the end-diastolic volume.
- The end-diastolic pressure-volume relation is the preferred load-independent measurement of myocardial contractility.
- The heart rate affects cardiac output, stroke volume, coronary artery filling, and myocardial contractility.
- There are marked physiologic differences between the right and left ventricles.
- Pressure-volume loops can be used to demonstrate the differences between systolic and diastolic failure.
- The Frank-Starling relationship and the pressure-volume loop are both clinically useful physiologic tools.

3

REFERENCES

1. Grayzel J: The cardiac cycle, J Cardiothorac Vasc Anesth 5:649, 1991
2. Schiller NB: Ejection fraction by echocardiography. Am Heart J 146:380, 2003
3. Groban L: Diastolic dysfunction in the elderly. J Cardiothorac Vasc Anesth 19:228, 2005
4. Redfield MM: Understanding diastolic heart failure. N Engl J Med 350:1930, 2004
5. Maurer MS, Spevack D, Birkhoff D, et al: Diastolic dysfunction diagnosed by Doppler echocardiography, J Am Coll Cardiol 44:1543, 2004
6. Zile MR, Brutsaert DL: New concepts in diastolic dysfunction and diastolic heart failure: I. Diagnosis, prognosis, and measurements of diastolic function. Circulation 105:1387, 2002
7. Weyman AE: The year in echocardiography. J Am Coll Cardiol 45:448, 2005
8. Thys DM, Hillel Z, Goldman ME, et al: Comparison of hemodynamic indices derived by invasive monitoring and two-dimensional echocardiography, Anesthesiology 67:630, 1987
9. Krueger JW: Fundamental mechanisms that govern cardiac function: A short review of sarcomere mechanics, Heart Failure 4:137, 1988
10. Suga H, Sagawa K, Shoukas AA: Load independence of the instantaneous pressure-volume ratio of the canine left ventricle and effects of epinephrine and heart rate on the ratio. Circ Res 32:314, 1973
11. Suga H, Sagawa K: Instantaneous pressure-volume relationships and their ratio in the excised supported canine left ventricle. Circ Res 35:117, 1974
12. Stein PD, Sabbath HH, Auler DT, et al: Performance of the failing and non-failing right ventricle of patients with pulmonary hypertension, Am J Cardiol 44:1050, 1979
13. Dell'Italia LJ, Walsh RA: Right ventricular diastolic pressure-volume relations and regional dimensions during acute alterations in loading conditions. Circulation 77:1276, 1988
14. Dell'Italia L: The right ventricle: Anatomy, physiology and clinical implications, Curr Probl Cardiol 16:659, 1991
15. Katz A: Ernest Henry Starling: His predecessors and the "law of the heart". Circulation 106:2986, 2002
16. Carabello B: Evolution of the study of left ventricular function: Everything old is new again. Circulation 105:2701, 2002

Chapter 4

Coronary Physiology and Atherosclerosis

Edward R.M. O'Brien, MD • Howard J. Nathan, MD

When caring for patients with coronary artery disease (CAD), the anesthesiologist must prevent or minimize myocardial ischemia by maintaining optimal conditions for perfusion of the heart. This goal can be achieved only with an understanding of the many factors that determine myocardial blood flow in both health and disease.

ANATOMY AND PHYSIOLOGY OF BLOOD VESSELS

The coronary vasculature has been traditionally divided into three functional groups: large conductance vessels visible on coronary angiography, which offer little resistance to blood flow; small resistance vessels ranging in size from about 250 to 10 μm in diameter; and veins. Although it has been taught that arterioles (precapillary vessels < 50 μm) account for most of the coronary resistance, studies indicate that, under resting conditions, 45% to 50% of total coronary vascular resistance resides in vessels larger than 100 μm in diameter. This may be due, in part, to the relatively great length of the small arteries.

Normal Artery Wall

The arterial lumen is lined by a monolayer of endothelial cells that overlies smooth muscle cells (Fig. 4-1). The inner layer of smooth muscle cells, known as the intima, is circumscribed by the internal elastic lamina. Between the internal elastic lamina

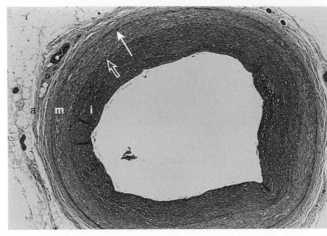

Figure 4-1 Normal human coronary artery of a 32-year-old woman. The intima (i) and media (m) are composed of smooth muscle cells. The adventitia (a) consists of a loose collection of adipocytes, fibroblasts, vasa vasorum, and nerves. The media is separated from the intima by the internal elastic lamina (*open arrow*) and the adventitia by the external elastic lamina (*solid arrow*). (Movat's pentachrome-stained slide, original magnification ×6.6.)

and external elastic lamina is another layer of smooth muscle cells, the media. Outside the external elastic lamina is an adventitia that is sparsely populated by cells and microvessels of the vasa vasorum.

Endothelium

Although the vascular endothelium was once thought of as an inert lining for blood vessels, it is more accurately characterized as a very active, distributed organ with many biologic functions. It has synthetic and metabolic capabilities and contains receptors for a variety of vasoactive substances.

Endothelium-Derived Relaxing Factors

The first vasoactive endothelial substance to be discovered was prostacyclin (PGI_2), a product of the cyclooxygenase pathway of arachidonic acid metabolism (Box 4-1). The production of PGI_2 is activated by shear stress, pulsatility of flow, hypoxia, and a variety of vasoactive mediators. Upon production it leaves the endothelial cell and acts in the local environment to cause relaxation of the underlying smooth muscle or to inhibit platelet aggregation. Both actions are mediated by the stimulation of adenylyl cyclase in the target cell to produce cyclic adenosine monophosphate (cAMP).

It has been shown that many physiologic stimuli cause vasodilation by stimulating the release of a labile, diffusible, nonprostanoid molecule termed *endothelium-derived relaxing factor* (EDRF), now known to be nitric oxide (NO). NO is the basis of a widespread paracrine signal transduction mechanism whereby one cell type can modulate the behavior of adjacent cells of a different type.[1,2] NO is a very small lipophilic molecule that can readily diffuse across biologic membranes and into the cytosol of nearby cells. The half-life of the molecule is less than 5 seconds so that only the local environment can be affected. NO is synthesized from the amino acid l-arginine by NO synthase (NOS). When NO diffuses into the cytosol of the target cell, it binds with the heme group of soluble guanylate

---

BOX 4-1   *Endothelium-Derived Relaxing and Contracting Factors*

Healthy endothelial cells have an important role in modulating coronary tone by producing:

Vascular Muscle-Relaxing Factors

- Prostacyclin
- Nitric oxide
- Hyperpolarizing factor

Vascular Muscle-Contracting Factors

- Prostaglandin H_2
- Thromboxane A_2
- Endothelin

BOX 4-2   *Endothelial Inhibition of Platelets*

Healthy endothelial cells have a role in maintaining the fluidity of blood by producing:

- Anticoagulant factors: protein C and thrombomodulin
- Fibrinolytic factor: tissue-type plasminogen activator
- Platelet inhibitory substances: prostacyclin and nitric oxide

---

cyclase, resulting in a 50- to 200-fold increase in production of cyclic guanosine monophosphate (cGMP), its second messenger. If the target cells are vascular smooth muscle cells, vasodilation occurs; if the target cells are platelets, adhesion and aggregation are inhibited.

It is likely that NO is the final common effector molecule of nitrovasodilators (including sodium nitroprusside and organic nitrates such as nitroglycerin). The cardiovascular system is in a constant state of active vasodilation that is dependent on the generation of NO. The molecule is more important in controlling vascular tone in veins and arteries compared with arterioles. Abnormalities in the ability of the endothelium to produce NO likely play a role in diseases such as diabetes, atherosclerosis, and hypertension. The venous circulation of humans seems to have a lower basal release of NO and an increased sensitivity to nitrovasodilators compared with the arterial side of the circulation.[3]

Endothelium-Derived Contracting Factors

Contracting factors produced by the endothelium include prostaglandin H_2, thromboxane A_2 (via cyclooxygenase), and the peptide endothelin. Endothelin is a potent vasoconstrictor peptide (100-fold more potent than norepinephrine).[4]

Endothelial Inhibition of Platelets

A primary function of endothelium is to maintain the fluidity of blood. This is achieved by the synthesis and release of anticoagulant (e.g., thrombomodulin, protein C), fibrinolytic (e.g., tissue-type plasminogen activator), and platelet inhibitory (e.g., PGI_2, NO) substances (Box 4-2). Mediators released from aggregating platelets stimulate the release of NO and PGI_2 from intact endothelium, which act together to increase blood flow and decrease platelet adhesion and

BOX 4-3 *Determinants of Coronary Blood Flow*
The primary determinants of coronary blood flow are: • Perfusion pressure   • Myocardial extravascular compression   • Myocardial metabolism   • Neurohumoral control

aggregation, thereby flushing away microthrombi and maintaining the patency of the vessel.

DETERMINANTS OF CORONARY BLOOD FLOW

Under normal conditions, there are four major determinants of coronary blood flow: perfusion pressure, myocardial extravascular compression, myocardial metabolism, and neurohumoral control.

Perfusion Pressure and Myocardial Compression

Coronary blood flow is proportional to the pressure gradient across the coronary circulation (Box 4-3). This gradient is calculated by subtracting downstream coronary pressure from the pressure in the root of the aorta.

During systole, the heart throttles its own blood supply. The force of systolic myocardial compression is greatest in the subendocardial layers, where it approximates intraventricular pressure. Resistance due to extravascular compression increases with blood pressure, heart rate, contractility, and preload.

Although the true downstream pressure of the coronary circulation is likely close to the coronary sinus pressure, other choices may be more appropriate in clinical circumstances. The most appropriate measure of the driving pressure for flow is the average pressure in the aortic root during diastole. This can be approximated by aortic diastolic or mean pressure.

Myocardial Metabolism

Myocardial blood flow, like flow in the brain and skeletal muscle, is primarily under metabolic control. Even when the heart is cut off from external control mechanisms (neural and humoral factors), its ability to match blood flow to its metabolic requirements is almost unaffected. Because coronary venous oxygen tension is normally 15 to 20 mm Hg, there is only a small amount of oxygen available through increased extraction. A major increase in cardiac oxygen consumption ($M\dot{V}O_2$), beyond the normal resting value of 80 to 100 mL O_2/100 g of myocardium, can occur only if oxygen delivery is increased by augmentation of coronary blood flow. Normally, flow and metabolism are closely matched so that over a wide range of oxygen consumption coronary sinus oxygen saturation changes little.[5]

Hypotheses of metabolic control propose that vascular tone is linked either to a substrate that is depleted, such as oxygen or adenosine triphosphate (ATP), or to the accumulation of a metabolite such as carbon dioxide (CO_2) or hydrogen ion (Box 4-4). Adenosine has been proposed in both categories.

II

> **BOX 4-4** *Myocardial Metabolism*
>
> Several molecules have been proposed as the link between myocardial metabolism and myocardial blood flow, including:
>
> - Oxygen
> - Carbon dioxide
> - Adenosine
>
> Current evidence suggests that a combination of local factors act together, each with differing importance during rest, exercise, and ischemia, to match myocardial oxygen delivery to demand.

Neural and Humoral Control

Coronary Innervation

The heart is supplied with branches of the sympathetic and parasympathetic divisions of the autonomic nervous system. Large and small coronary arteries and veins are richly innervated. The sympathetic nerves to the heart and coronary vessels arise from the superior, middle, and inferior cervical sympathetic ganglia and the first four thoracic ganglia. The stellate ganglion (formed when the inferior cervical and first thoracic ganglia merge) is a major source of cardiac sympathetic innervation. The vagi supply the heart with efferent cholinergic nerves.

Parasympathetic Control

Vagal stimulation causes bradycardia, decreased contractility, and lower blood pressure. The resultant fall in MVo_2 causes a metabolically-mediated coronary vasoconstriction. The direct effect of activation of cholinergic receptors on coronary vessels is vasodilation. These direct effects can be abolished by atropine.

β-Adrenergic Coronary Dilation

β-Receptor activation causes dilation of both large and small coronary vessels even in the absence of changes in blood flow.

α-Adrenergic Coronary Constriction

The direct effect of sympathetic stimulation is coronary vasoconstriction, which is in competition with the metabolically-mediated dilation of exercise or excitement. Whether adrenergic coronary constriction is powerful enough to further diminish blood flow in ischemic myocardium or if it can have some beneficial effect in the distribution of myocardial blood flow is controversial.

Coronary Pressure-Flow Relations

Autoregulation

Autoregulation is the tendency for organ blood flow to remain constant despite changes in arterial perfusion pressure. Autoregulation can maintain flow to myocardium served by stenotic coronary arteries despite low perfusion pressure distal to the obstruction. This is a local mechanism of control and can be observed in isolated, denervated hearts. If MVo_2 is fixed, coronary blood flow remains relatively constant between mean arterial pressures of 60 to 140 mm Hg.

4

Coronary Reserve

Myocardial ischemia causes intense coronary vasodilation. Following a 10- to 30-second coronary occlusion, restoration of perfusion pressure is accompanied by a marked increase in coronary flow. This large increase in flow, which can be five or six times resting flow in the dog, is termed *reactive hyperemia*. The repayment volume is greater than the debt volume. There is, however, no overpayment of the oxygen debt because oxygen extraction falls during the hyperemia. The presence of high coronary flows when coronary venous oxygen content is high suggests that mediators other than oxygen are responsible for this metabolically-induced vasodilation. The difference between resting coronary blood flow and peak flow during reactive hyperemia represents the autoregulatory coronary flow reserve: the further capacity of the arteriolar bed to dilate in response to ischemia.[6]

Transmural Blood Flow

It is well known that when coronary perfusion pressure is inadequate, the inner one third to one fourth of the left ventricular wall is the first region to become ischemic or necrotic.[7] This increased vulnerability of the subendocardium may be due to an increased demand for perfusion or a decreased supply, compared with the outer layers.

If coronary pressure is gradually reduced, autoregulation is exhausted and flow decreases in the inner layers of the left ventricle before it begins to decrease in the outer layers (Fig. 4-2). This indicates that there is less flow reserve in the subendocardium than in the subepicardium.

Three mechanisms have been proposed to explain the decreased coronary reserve in the subendocardium: differential systolic intramyocardial pressure, differential diastolic intramyocardial pressure, and interactions between systole and diastole.

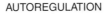

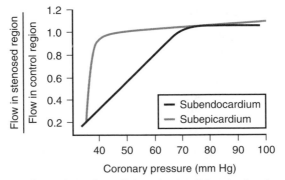

Figure 4-2   Pressure-flow relationships of the subepicardial and subendocardial thirds of the left ventricle in anesthetized dogs. In the subendocardium, autoregulation is exhausted and flow becomes pressure dependent when pressure distal to a stenosis falls below 70 mm Hg. In the subepicardium, autoregulation persists until perfusion pressure falls below 40 mm Hg. Autoregulatory coronary reserve is less in the subendocardium. (Redrawn from Guyton RA, McClenathan JH, Newman GE, Michaelis LL: Significance of subendocardial ST segment elevation caused by coronary stenosis in the dog. Am J Cardiol 40:373, 1977.)

ATHEROSCLEROSIS

The atherosclerotic lesion consists of an excessive accumulation of smooth muscle cells in the intima, with quantitative and qualitative changes in the noncellular connective tissue components of the artery wall and intracellular and extracellular deposition of lipoproteins and mineral components (e.g., calcium). By definition, *atherosclerosis* is a combination of "atherosis" and "sclerosis." The latter term, *sclerosis*, refers to the hard collagenous material that accumulates in lesions and is usually more voluminous than the pultaceous "gruel" of the atheroma (Fig. 4-3).

Stary noted that the earliest detectable change in the evolution of coronary atherosclerosis in young people was the accumulation of intracellular lipid in the subendothelial region, giving rise to lipid-filled macrophages or "foam cells."[8] Grossly, a collection of foam cells may give the artery wall the appearance of a "fatty streak." In general, fatty streaks are covered by a layer of intact endothelium and are not characterized by excessive smooth muscle cell accumulation. At later stages of atherogenesis, extracellular lipoproteins accumulate in the musculoelastic layer of the intima, eventually forming an avascular core of lipid-rich debris that is separated from the central arterial lumen by a fibrous cap of collagenous material. Foam cells are not usually seen deep within the atheromatous core but are frequently found at the periphery of the lipid core.

Arterial Wall Inflammation

A number of studies have demonstrated the presence of monocytes/macrophages and T lymphocytes in the arteries of not only advanced lesions but also early atherosclerotic lesions of young adults.[9] Moreover, in experimental atherosclerosis, leukocyte infiltration into the vascular wall is known to precede smooth muscle cell hyperplasia. Once inside the artery wall, mononuclear cells may play several important roles in lesion development. For example, monocytes may transform into macrophages

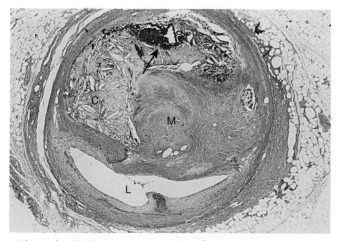

Figure 4-3   Atherosclerotic human coronary artery of an 80-year-old man. There is severe narrowing of the central arterial lumen (L). The intima consists of a complex collection of cells, extracellular matrix (M), and a necrotic core with cholesterol (C) deposits. Rupture of plaque microvessels has resulted in intraplaque hemorrhage (*arrow*) at the base of the necrotic core. (Movat's pentachrome-stained slide, original magnification ×40.)

and become involved in the local oxidation of low-density lipoproteins (LDLs) and accumulation of oxidized LDLs. Alternatively, macrophages in the artery wall may act as a rich source of factors that, for example, promote cell proliferation, migration, or the breakdown of local tissue barriers. The latter process of local tissue degradation may be very important for the initiation of acute coronary artery syndromes because loss of arterial wall integrity may lead to plaque fissuring or rupture.

Role of Lipoproteins in Lesion Formation

The clinical and experimental evidence linking dyslipidemias with atherogenesis is well established and need not be reviewed here. However, the exact mechanisms by which lipid moieties contribute to the pathogenesis of atherosclerosis remain elusive. Although the simple concept of cholesterol accumulating in artery walls until flow is obstructed may be correct in certain animal models, this theory is not correct for human arteries.

One of the major consequences of cholesterol accumulation in the artery wall is thought to be the impairment of endothelial function. The endothelium is more than a physical barrier between the bloodstream and the artery wall. Under normal conditions, the endothelium is capable of modulating vascular tone (e.g., via NO), thrombogenicity, fibrinolysis, platelet function, and inflammation. In the presence of traditional risk factors, particularly dyslipidemias, these protective endothelial functions are reduced or lost. A number of clinical studies demonstrate dramatic improvements in endothelial function, as well as cardiovascular morbidity and mortality, with the use of inhibitors of 3-hydroxy-3-methylglutaryl coenzyme A (HMG-CoA) reductase, or "statins."[10]

PATHOPHYSIOLOGY OF CORONARY BLOOD FLOW

Coronary Artery Stenoses and Plaque Rupture

Coronary atherosclerosis is a chronic disease that develops over decades, remaining clinically silent for prolonged periods of time (Box 4-5). Clinical manifestations of CAD occur when the atherosclerotic plaque mass encroaches on the vessel lumen and obstructs coronary blood flow, causing angina. Alternatively, cracks or fissures may develop in the atherosclerotic lesions and result in acute thromboses that cause unstable angina or myocardial infarction.

Patients with stable angina typically have lesions with smooth borders on angiography. Only a minority of coronary lesions are concentric, with most having a complex geometry varying in shape over their length. Eccentric stenoses, with a remaining pliable, musculoelastic arc of normal wall, can vary in diameter and resistance

---

> **BOX 4-5** *Pathophysiology of Coronary Blood Flow*
>
> - In the majority of patients experiencing a myocardial infarction, the coronary occlusion occurs at the site of less than 50% stenosis.
> - Plaque rupture leads to incremental growth of coronary stenoses and can cause coronary events.
> - Plaque rupture occurs at the shoulder of the plaque where inflammatory cells are found.

in response to changes in vasomotor tone or intraluminal pressure. The majority of human coronary stenoses are compliant. The intima of the normal portion of the vessel wall is often thickened, making endothelial dysfunction probable. In contrast, patients with unstable angina usually have lesions characterized by overhanging edges, scalloped or irregular borders, or multiple irregularities. These complicated stenoses likely represent ruptured plaque or partially occlusive thrombus or both.[11] Superficial intimal injury (plaque erosions) and intimal tears of variable depth (plaque fissures) with overlying microscopic mural thrombosis are commonly found in atherosclerotic plaques. In the absence of obstructive luminal thrombosis, these intimal injuries do not cause clinical events. However, disruption of the fibrous cap, or plaque rupture, is a more serious event that typically results in the formation of clinically significant arterial thromboses. From autopsy studies it is known that rupture-prone plaques tend to have a thin, friable fibrous cap. The site of plaque rupture is thought to be the shoulder of the plaque, where substantial numbers of mononuclear inflammatory cells are commonly found.[12] The mechanisms responsible for the local accumulation of these cells at this location in the plaque are unknown; presumably, monocyte chemotactic factors, the expression of leukocyte cell adhesion molecules, and specific cytokines are involved. Moreover, macrophages in plaques have been shown to express factors such as stromelysin, which promote the breakdown of the extracellular matrix and thereby weaken the structural integrity of the plaque.

Coronary Collateral Vessels

Coronary collateral vessels are anastomotic connections, without an intervening capillary bed, between different coronary arteries or between branches of the same artery. In the normal human heart, these vessels are small and have little or no functional role. In patients with CAD, well-developed coronary collateral vessels may play a critical role in preventing death and myocardial infarction. Individual differences in the capability of developing a sufficient collateral circulation is a determinant of the vulnerability of the myocardium to coronary occlusive disease.[13]

It has been estimated that, in humans, perfusion via collateral vessels can equal perfusion via a vessel with a 90% diameter obstruction. Although coronary collateral flow can be sufficient to preserve structure and resting myocardial function, muscle dependent on collateral flow usually becomes ischemic when oxygen demand rises above resting levels. It is possible that evidence from patients with angina underestimates collateral function of the population of all patients with CAD.[14]

Pathogenesis of Myocardial Ischemia

Ischemia is the condition of oxygen deprivation accompanied by inadequate removal of metabolites consequent to reduced perfusion. Clinically, myocardial ischemia is a decrease in the blood flow supply/demand ratio resulting in impaired function. There is no universally accepted "gold standard" for the presence of myocardial ischemia. In practice, symptoms, anatomic findings, and evidence of myocardial dysfunction must be combined before concluding that myocardial ischemia is present.

Determinants of Myocardial Oxygen Supply/Demand Ratio

An increase in myocardial oxygen requirement beyond the capacity of the coronary circulation to deliver oxygen results in myocardial ischemia (Box 4-6). This is the most common mechanism leading to ischemic episodes in chronic stable angina

4

BOX 4-6 *Determinants of Myocardial Oxygen Supply/ Demand Ratio*

The major determinants of myocardial oxygen consumption are:

- Heart rate
- Myocardial contractility
- Wall stress (chamber pressure × radius/wall thickness)

---

and during exercise testing. Intraoperatively, the anesthesiologist must measure and control the determinants of myocardial oxygen consumption and protect the patient from "demand" ischemia. The major determinants of myocardial oxygen consumption are heart rate, myocardial contractility, and wall stress (chamber pressure × radius/wall thickness).

An increase in heart rate can reduce subendocardial perfusion by shortening diastole. Coronary perfusion pressure may fall due to reduced systemic pressure or increased left ventricular end-diastolic pressure. With the onset of ischemia, perfusion may be further compromised by delayed ventricular relaxation (decreased subendocardial perfusion time) and decreased diastolic compliance (increased left ventricular end-diastolic pressure). Anemia and hypoxia can also compromise delivery of oxygen to the myocardium.

Dynamic Stenosis

Patients with CAD can have variable exercise tolerance during the day and between days. Ambulatory monitoring of the ECG has demonstrated that ST-segment changes indicative of myocardial ischemia, in the absence of changes in oxygen demand, are common.[15] These findings are explained by variations over time in the severity of the obstruction to blood flow imposed by coronary stenoses.

Although the term *hardening of the arteries* suggests rigid, narrowed vessels, in fact most stenoses are eccentric and have a remaining arc of compliant tissue. A modest amount (10%) of shortening of the muscle in the compliant region of the vessel can cause dramatic changes in lumen caliber. This was part of Prinzmetal's original proposal to explain coronary spasm. Maseri and associates[16] suggest that the term *spasm* be reserved for "situations where coronary constriction is both focal, is sufficiently profound to cause transient coronary occlusion, and is responsible for reversible attacks of angina at rest" (i.e., variant angina).

Coronary Steal

Steal occurs when the perfusion pressure for a vasodilated vascular bed (in which flow is pressure dependent) is lowered by vasodilation in a parallel vascular bed, both beds usually being distal to a stenosis.[17] Two kinds of coronary steal are illustrated: collateral and transmural (Fig. 4-4).

Collateral steal in which one vascular bed (R_3), distal to an occluded vessel, is dependent on collateral flow from a vascular bed (R_2) supplied by a stenotic artery is diagrammed in Figure 4-4A. Because collateral resistance is high, the R_3 arterioles are dilated to maintain flow in the resting condition (autoregulation). Dilation of the R_2 arterioles increases flow across the stenosis R_1 and decreases pressure P_2. If R_3 resistance cannot further decrease sufficiently, flow there decreases, producing or worsening ischemia in the collateral-dependent bed.

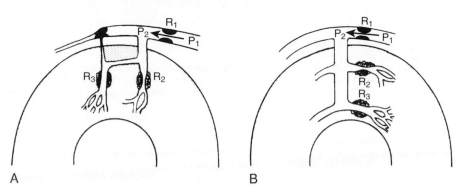

Figure 4-4 Conditions for coronary steal between different areas of the heart (collateral steal [**A**]) and between the subendocardial and the subepicardial layers of the left ventricle (transmural steal [**B**]). See text for detailed description. R_1 = stenosis resistance; P_1 = aortic pressure; P_2 = pressure distal to the stenosis; R_2 and R_3 = resistance of autoregulating and pressure-dependent vascular beds, respectively. (From Epstein SE, Cannon RO, Talbot TL: Hemodynamic principles in the control of coronary blood flow. Am J Cardiol 56:4E, 1985.)

Transmural steal is illustrated in Figure 4-4B. Normally, vasodilator reserve is less in the subendocardium. In the presence of a stenosis, flow may become pressure dependent in the subendocardium while autoregulation is maintained in the subepicardium.

SUMMARY

- To safely care for patients with coronary artery disease in the perioperative period, the clinician must understand how the coronary circulation functions in health and disease.
- Coronary endothelium modulates myocardial blood flow by producing factors that relax or contract the underlying vascular smooth muscle.
- Vascular endothelial cells help maintain the fluidity of blood by elaborating anticoagulant, fibrinolytic, and antiplatelet substances.
- One of the earliest changes in coronary artery disease, preceding the appearance of stenoses, is the loss of the vasoregulatory and antithrombotic functions of the endothelium.
- The mean systemic arterial pressure and not the diastolic pressure may be the most useful and reliable measure of coronary perfusion pressure in the clinical setting.
- Although sympathetic activation increases myocardial oxygen demand, activation of α-adrenergic receptors causes coronary vasoconstriction.
- It is unlikely that one substance alone (e.g., adenosine) provides the link between myocardial metabolism and myocardial blood flow under a variety of conditions.
- As coronary perfusion pressure decreases, the inner layers of myocardium nearest the left ventricular cavity are the first to become ischemic and display impaired relaxation and contraction.
- The progression of an atherosclerotic lesion is similar to the process of wound healing.
- Lipid-lowering therapy can help restore endothelial function and prevent coronary events.

4

REFERENCES

1. Ignarro LJ: Nitric oxide: A novel signal transduction mechanism for transcellular communication. Hypertension 16:477, 1990
2. Lincoln TM, Dey N, Sellak H: Invited review: cGMP-dependent protein kinase signaling mechanisms in smooth muscle: From the regulation of tone to gene expression. J Appl Physiol 91:1421, 2001
3. Harrison DG, Cai H: Endothelial control of vasomotion and nitric oxide production. Cardiol Clin 21:289, 2003
4. Goodwin AT, Yacoub MH: Role of endogenous endothelin on coronary flow in health and disease. Coron Artery Dis 12:517, 2001
5. Feigl EO: Coronary physiology. Physiol Rev 63:1, 1983
6. Kern MJ: Coronary physiology revisited: Practical insights from the cardiac catheterization laboratory. Circulation 101:1344, 2000
7. Hoffman JIE: Transmural myocardial perfusion. Prog Cardiovasc Dis 29:429, 1987
8. Stary HC: Evolution and progression of atherosclerotic lesions in coronary arteries of children and young adults. Arteriosclerosis 9(suppl 1):I-19, 1989
9. Katsuda S, Boyd HC, Fligner C, et al: Human atherosclerosis: Immunocytochemical analysis of the cell composition of lesions of young adults. Am J Pathol 140:907, 1992
10. Treasure CB, Klein JL, Weintraub WS: Beneficial effects of cholesterol-lowering therapy on the coronary endothelium in patients with coronary artery disease. N Engl J Med 332:481, 1995
11. Pasterkamp G, de Kleijn D, Borst C: Arterial remodeling in atherosclerosis, restenosis and after alteration of blood flow: Potential mechanisms and clinical implications. Cardiovasc Res 45:843, 2000
12. Van der Wal AC, Becker AE, van der Loos CM, et al: Site of intimal rupture or erosion of thrombosed coronary atherosclerotic plaque is characterized by an inflammatory process irrespective of the dominant plaque morphology. Circulation 89:36, 1994
13. Koerselman J, van der Graf Y, De Jaegere PP, et al: Coronary collaterals: An important and underexposed aspect of coronary artery disease. Circulation 107:2507, 2003
14. Fujita M, Tambara K: Recent insights into human coronary collateral development. Heart 90:246, 2004
15. Stone PH: Mechanisms of silent myocardial ischemia: Implications for selection of optimal therapy. Adv Cardiol 37:328, 1990
16. Maseri A, Newman C, Davies G: Coronary vasomotor tone: A heterogeneous entity. Eur Heart J 10(suppl F):2, 1989
17. Konidala S, Gutterman DD: Coronary vasospasm and the regulation of coronary blood flow. Prog Cardiovasc Dis 46:349, 2004

II

Chapter 5

Molecular Cardiovascular Medicine

Marcel E. Durieux, MD, PhD • J. Paul Mounsey, MD

In the past decades we have witnessed what may well be termed a revolution in the biomedical sciences, as molecular methodologies have suddenly become more evident on the clinical scene. Molecular biology originated in the 1950s, its birth most commonly identified with the description of the structure of deoxyribonucleic acid (DNA) by Watson and Crick.[1]

Not generally appreciated was the rapidity with which molecular biology would advance. Now, five decades since the discovery of the structure of DNA, the human genome has been sequenced completely. Techniques for manipulating nucleic acids have been simplified enormously, and for many routine procedures kits are now available. The development of the polymerase chain reaction (PCR), a technique of remarkable simplicity and flexibility, has dramatically increased the speed with which many molecular biology procedures can be performed.

Cardiovascular medicine has been a major beneficiary of these advances. Not only have the electrophysiologic and pump functions of the heart been placed on a firm molecular footing, but for a number of disease states the pathophysiology has been determined, allowing progress in therapeutic development. Importantly, there is no indication that the pace of progress in molecular biology has slowed. If anything, the opposite is the case, and more dramatic advances may be expected in the years to come. Thus, techniques such as gene therapy may become available as therapeutic options in cardiac disease.

In this chapter, the most important aspects of molecular cardiovascular medicine are surveyed, with specific emphasis on medical issues relevant to the anesthesiologist. The myocyte membrane signaling proteins are of primary importance in this respect, and the two major classes—membrane channels and membrane receptors—are discussed. Simply stated, the channels form the machinery behind the cardiac rhythm, whereas the receptors are involved in regulation of cardiac function.

MACHINERY BEHIND THE CARDIAC RHYTHM: ION CHANNELS

The cardiac action potential results from the flow of ions through ion channels, which are the membrane-bound proteins that form the structural basis of cardiac electrical excitability. In response to changes in electrical potential across the cell membrane, ion channels open to allow the passive flux of ions into or out of the cell along their electrochemical gradients. Ion flux results in a flow of current, which displaces the cell membrane potential toward the potential at which the electrochemical gradient for the ion is zero, called the equilibrium potential (E) for the ion. Depolarization of the cell could, in principle, result from an inward cation current or an outward anion current; for repolarization the reverse is true. In excitable cells, action potentials are mainly caused by the flow of cation currents. Membrane depolarization results principally from the flow of Na^+ down its electrochemical gradient (E_{Na} is around +50 mV), whereas repolarization results from the outward flux of K^+ down its electrochemical gradient (E_K is around −90 mV). Opening and closing of multiple ion channels of a single type result in an individual ionic current. The integrated activity of many different ionic currents, each activated over precisely regulated potential ranges and at different times in the cardiac cycle, results in the cardiac action potential (Box 5-1).

Phase 0: The Rapid Upstroke of the Cardiac Action Potential

The rapid upstroke of the cardiac action potential (phase 0) is caused by the flow of a large inward Na^+ current (I_{Na}) (Box 5-2). I_{Na} is activated by depolarization of the sarcolemma to a threshold potential of −65 to −70 mV. I_{Na} activation, and hence the action potential, is an all-or-nothing response. Subthreshold depolarizations have only local effects on the membrane. After the threshold for activation of fast Na^+ channels is exceeded, Na^+ channels open (i.e., I_{Na} activates) and Na^+ ions enter the cell down their electrochemical gradient. This results in displacement of the membrane potential toward the equilibrium potential for Na^+ ions, around +50 mV. I_{Na} activation is transient, lasting at most 1 to 2 ms because, simultaneous with activation, a second, slightly slower conformational change in the channel molecule occurs (inactivation), which closes the ion pore in the face of continued membrane depolarization. The channel cannot open again until it has recovered from inactivation (i.e., regained its

---

BOX 5-1 *Properties of Ion Channels*

- Ion selectivity
- Rectification (passing current more easily in one direction than the other)
- Gating (mechanism for opening and closing the channel):
  - Activation (opening)
  - Inactivation (closing)

BOX 5-2 *Cardiac Action Potential*

- Phase 0 (rapid upstroke): primarily Na^+ channel opening
- Phase 1 (early rapid repolarization): inactivation of Na^+ current, opening of K^+ channels
- Phase 2 (plateau phase): balance between K^+ currents and Ca^{2+} currents
- Phase 3 (final rapid repolarizations): activation of Ca^{2+} channels
- Phase 4 (diastolic depolarization): balance between Na^+ and K^+ currents

resting conformation), a process that requires repolarization to the resting potential for a defined period of time. The channels cycle through three states: *resting* (and available for activation), *open,* and *inactivated.* While the channel is inactivated, it is absolutely refractory to repeated stimulation.

Phase 1: Early Rapid Repolarization

The early rapid repolarization phase of the action potential, which follows immediately after phase 0, results both from rapid inactivation of the majority of the Na^+ current and from activation of a transient outward current (I_{TO}), carried mainly by K^+ ions.

Phases 2 and 3: The Plateau Phase and Final Rapid Repolarization

The action potential plateau and final rapid repolarization are mediated by a balance between the slow inward current and outward, predominantly K^+, currents. During the plateau phase, membrane conductance to all ions falls and very little current flows. Phase 3, regenerative rapid repolarization, results from time-dependent inactivation of L-type Ca^{2+} current and increasing outward current through delayed rectifier K^+ channels. The net membrane current becomes outward and the cell repolarizes.

Phase 4: Diastolic Depolarization and I_f

Phase 4 diastolic depolarization, or normal automaticity, is a normal feature of cardiac cells in the sinus and atrioventricular (AV) nodes, but subsidiary pacemaker activity is also observed in the His-Purkinje system and in some specialized atrial and ventricular myocardial cells. Pacemaker discharge from the sinus node normally predominates because the rate of diastolic depolarization in the sinoatrial (SA) node is faster than in other pacemaker tissues. Pacemaker activity results from a slow net gain of positive charge, which depolarizes the cell from its maximal diastolic potential to threshold.

Molecular Biology of Ion Channels

The preceding sections have focused on the electrical events that underlie cardiac electrical excitability and on the identification of cardiac ionic currents on the basis of their biophysical properties. Subsequent sections examine the molecular physiology of these electrical phenomena. The first step in understanding the molecular physiology of cardiac electrical excitability is to identify the ion channel proteins responsible for the ionic currents.

Ion Channel Pore and Selectivity Filter

The presence of four homologous domains in voltage-gated Na^+ and Ca^{2+} channels suggests that basic ion channel architecture consists of a transmembrane pore surrounded by the four homologous domains arranged symmetrically (Fig. 5-1).

Clinical Correlates

Ion Channels and Antiarrhythmic Drugs

The prototype antiarrhythmic agents, such as disopyramide and quinidine, have diverse effects on cardiac excitability, and these, along with agents introduced more recently, frequently exhibit significant proarrhythmia with potentially fatal consequences. In the Cardiac Arrhythmia Suppression Trial (CAST), mortality among asymptomatic post–myocardial infarction patients was approximately doubled by treatment with the potent Na^+ channel-blocking agents encainide and flecainide, an effect that is likely attributable to slowing of conduction velocity with a consequent increase in fatal reentrant arrhythmias.[2,3] The only drugs currently available that definitely prolong life by reducing fatal arrhythmias are β-blockers, and these agents have no channel-blocking effects.

Ion Channels in Disease

Elucidation of the molecular mechanisms of the cardiac action potential is beginning to directly affect patient management, particularly in patients with inherited genetic abnormalities of ion channels leading to cardiac sudden death. Two groups of diseases serve to illustrate this point—the LQT syndrome and the Brugada

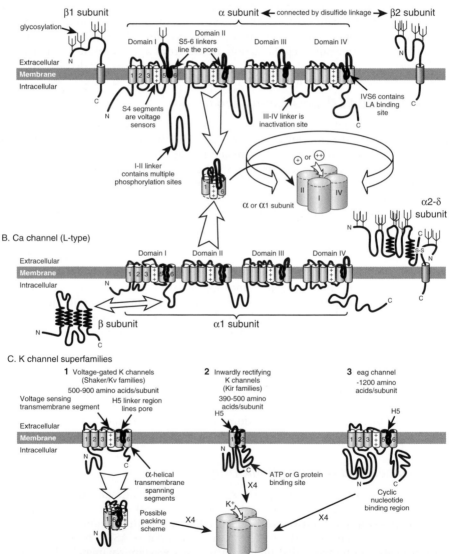

Figure 5-1   Diagrams of ion channel molecular structure. **A,** Na⁺ channel. **B,** Ca²⁺ channel. **C,** K⁺ channels. ATP = adenosine triphosphate. For further discussion, see text.

syndrome. An understanding of the molecular mechanism of cardiac electrical excitability is also leading to the emergence of gene therapies and stem cell therapies that may in the future allow manipulation of cardiac rhythm and function.[4,5]

CONTROLLING CARDIAC FUNCTIONING: RECEPTORS

Receptors are membrane proteins that transduce signals from the outside to the inside of the cell. When a *ligand*—a hormone carried in blood, a neurotransmitter released from a nerve ending, or a local messenger released from neighboring cells—binds to the receptor, it induces a conformational change in the receptor molecule. The configuration of the intracellular segment of the receptor changes and results in activation of intracellular systems, with a variety of effects, ranging from enhanced phosphorylation and changes in intracellular (second) messenger concentrations to activation of ion channels.

Receptors

Receptors are grouped into several broad classes, the *protein tyrosine kinase receptors* and the *G protein–coupled receptors* (GPCRs) being the most important ones. The protein tyrosine kinase receptors are large molecular complexes. Ligand binding induces activation of a phosphorylating enzyme activity in the intracellular segment of the molecule. Because phosphorylation is one of the major mechanisms of cellular regulation, such receptors can have a variety of cellular effects (Box 5-3). In contrast, GPCRs are much smaller. Ligand binding results in activation of an associated protein (*G protein*) that subsequently influences cellular processes.

The heart and blood vessels express a variety of GPCRs. The β-adrenergic and muscarinic acetylcholine receptors are those most important for regulation of cardiac functioning, but a number of others play relevant modulatory roles. These include the α-adrenergic, adenosine A_1, adenosine triphosphate (ATP), histamine-2 (H_2), vasoactive intestinal peptide (VIP), and angiotensin II receptors (Fig. 5-2).

Adrenergic Receptors and Signaling Pathways

Adrenergic Receptors

Main control over cardiac contractility is provided by the β-adrenergic signaling pathways, which can be activated by circulating catecholamines or those released locally from adrenergic nerve endings on the myocardium.

BOX 5-3   *G Protein–Coupled Receptors*

- β-Adrenergic receptors
- α-Adrenergic receptors
- Muscarinic acetylcholine receptors
- Adenosine A_1 receptors
- Adenosine triphosphate receptors
- Histamine-2 receptors
- Vasoactive intestinal peptide receptors
- Angiotensin II receptors

5

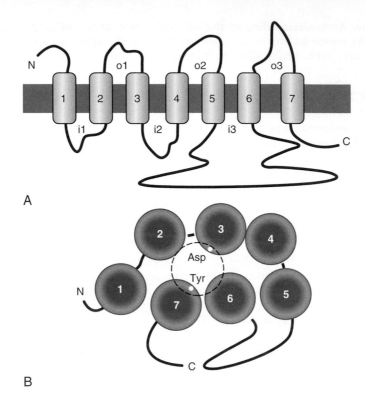

Figure 5-2 Model of G protein–coupled receptor. **A,** Linear model. Seven hydrophobic stretches of approximately 20 amino acids are present, presumably forming α helices that pass through the cell membrane, thus forming seven-transmembrane domains (t1 through t7). Extracellularly the N terminus (N) and three outside loops (o1 through o3) are found; intracellularly there are similarly three loops (i1 through i3) and the C terminus (C). **B,** Top-down view. Although in **A** the molecule is pictured as a linear complex, the transmembrane domains are thought to be in close proximity, forming an ellipse with a central ligand-binding cavity (indicated by a *dashed circle*). Asp and Tyr refer to two amino acids important for ligand interaction. G protein binding takes place at the i3 loop and the C terminus.

The two main subtypes of β-adrenergic receptors are the β_1 and β_2 subclasses. A β_3 subtype exists as well, but its role in the cardiovascular system is unclear; its most important role is in fat cells. Both β_1 and β_2 receptors are present in heart, and both contribute to the increased contractility induced by catecholamine stimulation (this is different from the situation in vascular muscle, where β-adrenergic stimulation induces relaxation). Under normal conditions, the relative ratio of β_1 to β_2 receptors in heart is approximately 70:30, but, as discussed later, this ratio can be changed dramatically by cardiac disease.

Structurally, as well as functionally, the various β-adrenergic receptors are closely related. Both couple to G_s proteins and thereby activate adenylate cyclase, leading to increased intracellular levels of cyclic adenosine monophosphate (cAMP). There may, however, be differences in some details of their intracellular signaling. For example, it has been suggested that β_2 receptors couple more effectively than β_1 receptors and induce greater changes in cAMP levels. In addition to their effect on cAMP signaling, β-adrenergic receptors may couple to myocardial Ca^{2+} channels.

The inotropic and electrophysiologic effects of β-adrenergic signaling are an indirect result of increases in intracellular cAMP levels. cAMP activates a specific protein kinase (PKA) that in turn is able to phosphorylate a number of important cardiac ion channels (including L-type Ca^{2+} channels, Na^+ channels, voltage-dependent K^+ channels, and Cl^- channels). Phosphorylation alters channel functioning, and it is these changes in membrane electrophysiologic events that modify myocardial behavior.

The α-adrenergic receptors, like their β-receptor counterparts, can be divided into several molecular groups: the α_1- and α_2-receptors. Both of these groups consist of several closely related subtypes, with different tissue distributions and functions that are as yet not very well differentiated. In general, α_1-receptors couple to G_q proteins, thereby activating phospholipase C, which increases intracellular Ca^{2+} concentrations. α_2-Receptors couple to G_i, which inhibits adenylate cyclase, thereby lowering intracellular cAMP concentrations.

Regulation of β-Receptor Functioning

Although β-receptor stimulation allows the dramatic increases in cardiac output of which the human heart is capable, it is clearly intended to be a temporary measure. Prolonged adrenergic stimulation has highly detrimental effects on the myocardium: The pronounced increases in cAMP levels are followed by increases in intracellular Ca^{2+} concentration, reductions in RNA and protein synthesis, and finally cell death. Thus, β-receptor modulation is best viewed as part of the "fight or flight" response—beneficial in the short term but detrimental if depended on too long. Cardiac failure, in particular, has been shown to be associated with prolonged increases in adrenergic stimulation, even to the extent that norepinephrine "spillover" from cardiac nerve endings can be detected in the blood of patients in heart failure.[6]

One mechanism for decreasing β-receptor functioning is the *downregulation* (i.e., decrease in density) of receptors. In cardiac failure, receptor levels are reduced up to 50%. β_1-Receptors downregulate more than do β_2-receptors, resulting in a change in the β_1:β_2 ratio. As mentioned earlier, the normal ratio is approximately 70:30; in the failing heart, it is approximately 3:2. Various molecular mechanisms exist for this downregulation. Some of them, particularly in the longer term, are degradation and permanent removal of receptors from the cell surface. In the short term, receptors can be temporarily removed from the cell membrane and "stored" in intracellular vesicles, where they are not accessible to agonists. These receptors are, however, fully functional and can be recycled to the membrane when adrenergic overstimulation has ceased.[7]

Muscarinic Receptors and Signaling Pathways

Muscarinic Acetylcholine Receptors

The second major receptor type involved in cardiac regulation is the muscarinic receptor. Although five subtypes of muscarinic receptors exist, only one of these (m2) is present in cardiac tissue. Most of these muscarinic receptors are present on the atria. Indeed, it was thought until recently that there was no vagal innervation of the ventricles, but this view turns out to be incorrect. The ventricles are innervated by the vagus, and muscarinic receptors are, in fact, present in the ventricles, albeit at lower concentrations than in the atria; the amount of muscarinic receptor protein in atrium is approximately twofold greater than in ventricle (200 to 250 vs. 70 to 100 fmol/mg protein). Thus, although the primary function of cardiac muscarinic signaling is heart rate control through actions at the atrial level, vagal stimulation is, in fact, able to directly influence ventricular functioning.[8]

Clinical Correlate: Adenosine Signaling and Cardiac Function

Understanding of the role of adenosine in cardiac regulation has expanded significantly over the past years. Its established use as an antiarrhythmic compound and its probable role in cardiac preconditioning are two examples of clinical advances resulting from this increase in understanding. Adenosine acts through a GPCR, activating several intracellular signaling systems.[9-11]

Adenosine Signaling

Although adenosine can be generated by several pathways, in the heart it is usually found as a dephosphorylation product of AMP.[12] Because AMP accumulation is a sign of a low cellular energy charge, an increased adenosine concentration is a marker of unbalanced energy demand and supply; thus, ischemia, hypoxemia, and increased catecholamine concentrations are all associated with increased adenosine release. Adenosine is rapidly degraded by various pathways, both intracellularly and extracellularly. As a result, its half-life is extremely short, on the order of 1 second. Therefore, it is not only a marker of a cardiac "energy crisis" but its concentrations will fluctuate virtually instantly with the energy balance of the heart; it provides a real-time indication of the cellular energy situation.

Adenosine signals through GPCRs of the purinergic receptor family. Two subclasses of purinoceptors exist: P_1 (high affinity for adenosine and AMP) and P_2 (high affinity for ATP and ADP). The P_1-receptor class can be divided into (at least) two receptor subtypes: A_1 and A_2. A_1-receptors are present mostly in the heart, and, when activated, inhibit adenylate cyclase; A_2-receptors are present in the vasculature and, when activated, stimulate adenylate cyclase. The A_2-receptors mediate the vasodilatory actions of adenosine. The A_1-receptors mediate its complex cardiac effects.

Antiarrhythmic Actions of Adenosine

From these molecular actions of adenosine, its clinical effects can easily be deduced. The antiarrhythmic actions are largely a result of its activation of K_{ACh}. Remembering the tissue distribution of K_{ACh}, it could be anticipated that adenosine will be much more effective in the treatment of supraventricular arrhythmias than ventricular arrhythmias, and such is indeed the case. Because of its negative chronotropic effects on the atrial conduction system, the compound is most effective in treating supraventricular tachycardias that contain a reentrant pathway involving the atrioventricular node. The efficacy of adenosine in terminating such tachycardias has been reported as greater than 90%. In contrast, it is consistently ineffective in tachycardias not involving the atrioventricular node.[13,14]

ANESTHETIC ACTIONS

Interactions with Channels: Ca^{2+} Channels

Of the variety of ion channels present in the heart, those most likely to be significantly affected by anesthetics in the clinical setting are the voltage-gated Ca^{2+} channels.

Anesthetic actions on cardiac Ca^{2+} channels have been studied in a variety of models. The original observations that halothane blocked Ca^{2+} flux into heart cells date back to the 1970s, and much specific information has been gained since then.[15]

Almost all volatile anesthetics inhibit L-type Ca^{2+} channels.[16] Inhibition is modest (25% to 30% at 1 MAC anesthetic) but certainly sufficient to account for the physiologic changes induced by the anesthetics. Volatile anesthetics decrease peak current and, in addition, tend to increase the rate of inactivation. Hence, maximal Ca^{2+} current is depressed and duration of Ca^{2+} current is shortened. Together, these actions significantly limit the Ca^{2+} influx into the cardiac myocyte.

Not only volatile, but also injected, anesthetics have been reported to inhibit cardiac L-type Ca^{2+} channels in some models. However, the concentrations used generally exceed those used in clinical practice. Thiopental and methohexital block L-type Ca^{2+} currents. Similarly, propofol has been reported to inhibit these channels, but at concentrations well beyond the clinical range.[17]

SUMMARY

- The rapid development of molecular biology techniques has greatly expanded the understanding of cardiac functioning and is beginning to be applied clinically.
- Cardiac ion channels form the machinery behind the cardiac rhythm; cardiac membrane receptors regulate cardiac function.
- Sodium, potassium, and calcium channels are the main types involved in the cardiac action potential. Many subtypes exist, and their molecular structures are known in some detail, allowing a molecular explanation for such phenomena as voltage sensing, ion selectivity, and inactivation.
- Muscarinic and adrenergic receptors, both of the G protein–coupled receptor class, are the main regulators of cardiac function.
- Adenosine plays important roles in myocardial preconditioning through an action on ATP-regulated K^+ channels and is an effective antiarrhythmic drug by its action on G protein–coupled adenosine receptors.
- Volatile anesthetics significantly affect calcium channels and muscarinic receptors.
- Cardiovascular diagnosis through molecular techniques and treatment through gene therapy have not yet become standard practice but offer potential for future clinical options.

5

REFERENCES

1. Watson JA, Crick FHC: Molecular structure of nucleic acids: A structure for deoxyribose nucleic acid. Nature 171:737, 1953
2. Kaupp UB, Seifert R: Molecular diversity of pacemaker ion channels. Annu Rev Physiol 63:235, 2001
3. Echt DS, Liebson PR, Mitchell LB, et al: Mortality and morbidity in patients receiving encainide, flecainide, or placebo. The Cardiac Arrhythmia Suppression Trial. N Engl J Med 324:781, 1991
4. Mohler PJ, Schott JJ, Gramolini AO, et al: Ankyrin-B mutation causes type 4 long-QT cardiac arrhythmia and sudden cardiac death. Nature 421:634, 2003
5. Antzelevitch C, Brugada P, Brugada J, et al: Brugada syndrome: A decade of progress. Circ Res 91:1114, 2002
6. Hasking GJ, Esler MD, Jennings GL, et al: Norepinephrine spillover to plasma in patients with congestive heart failure: Evidence of increased overall and cardiorenal sympathetic nervous activity. Circulation 73:615, 1986
7. Harding SE, Brown LA, Wynne DG, et al: Mechanisms of beta-adrenoceptor desensitisation in the failing human heart. Cardiovasc Res 28:1451, 1994

8. Deighton NM, Motomura S, Borquez D, et al: Muscarinic cholinoceptors in the human heart: Demonstration, subclassification, and distribution. Naunyn Schmiedebergs Arch Pharmacol 341:14, 1990
9. Belardinelli L, Shryock JC, Song Y, et al: Ionic basis of the electrophysiological actions of adenosine on cardiomyocytes. FASEB J 9:359, 1995
10. Shen WK, Kurachi Y: Mechanisms of adenosine-mediated actions on cellular and clinical cardiac electrophysiology. Mayo Clin Proc 70:274, 1995
11. Murphy E: Primary and secondary signaling pathways in early preconditioning that converge on the mitochondria to produce cardioprotection. Circ Res 94:7, 2004
12. Schutz W, Schrader J, Gerlach E: Different sites of adenosine formation in the heart. Am J Physiol 240:H963, 1981
13. Rankin AC, Brooks R, Ruskin JN, McGovern BA: Adenosine and the treatment of supraventricular tachycardia. Am J Med 92:655, 1992
14. diMarco JP, Sellers TD, Lerman BB, et al: Diagnostic and therapeutic use of adenosine in patients with supraventricular tachyarrhythmias. J Am Coll Cardiol 6:417, 1985
15. Bosnjak ZJ, Supan FD, Rusch NJ: The effects of halothane, enflurane, and isoflurane on calcium current in isolated canine ventricular cells. Anesthesiology 74:340, 1991
16. Fassl J, Halaszovich CR, Huneke R, et al: Effects of inhalational anesthetics on L-type Ca^{2+} currents in human atrial cardiomyocytes during beta-adrenergic stimulation. Anesthesiology 99:90, 2003
17. Ikemoto Y, Yatani A, Arimura H, Yoshitake J: Reduction of the slow inward current of isolated rat ventricular cells by thiamylal and halothane. Acta Anaesthesiol Scand 29:583, 1985

II

Chapter 6

Systemic Inflammation

Elliott Bennett-Guerrero, MD

Numerous advances in perioperative care have allowed increasingly high-risk patients to safely undergo cardiac surgery. Although mortality rates of 1% are quoted for "low-risk" cardiac surgery, results from large series of patients older than 65 years suggest that mortality rates are actually more substantial.[1] Postoperative morbidity is common and complications include atrial fibrillation, poor ventricular function requiring inotropic agents, and non–cardiac-related causes such as infection, gastrointestinal dysfunction, acute lung injury, stroke, and renal dysfunction.[2]

Many postoperative complications appear to be caused by an exaggerated systemic proinflammatory response to surgical trauma.[3] The most severe form of this inflammatory response leads to multiple organ dysfunction syndrome and death. Milder forms of a proinflammatory response cause less severe organ dysfunction, which does not lead to admission to an intensive care unit but nevertheless causes suffering, increased hospital length of stay, and increased cost. The etiology and the clinical relevance of systemic inflammation after cardiac surgery are poorly understood. Systemic inflammation is a multifactorial process and has profound secondary effects on both injured and normal tissues. Proinflammatory mediators can have beneficial as well as deleterious effects on multiple organ systems. According to most theories, tissue injury, endotoxemia, and contact of blood with the foreign surface of the cardiopulmonary bypass (CPB) circuit are some of the major factors postulated to initiate a systemic inflammatory response. Nevertheless, there is controversy surrounding the etiology as well as pathogenesis of inflammation in the perioperative period.

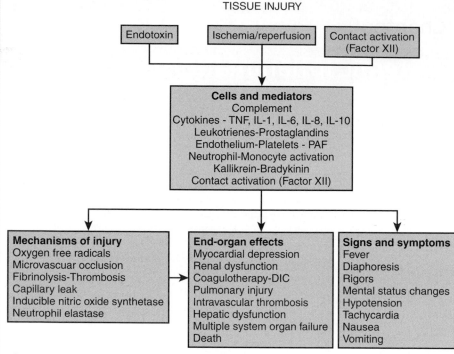

Figure 6-1   Overview of inflammation. TNF = tumor necrosis factor; IL = interleukin; PAF = platelet-activating factor; DIC = disseminated intravascular coagulation.

SYSTEMIC INFLAMMATION AND CARDIAC SURGERY

The systemic inflammatory response after cardiac surgery is multifactorial. A schematic of the inflammatory process is depicted in Figure 6-1. There does not appear to be much disagreement with the statement that all of these processes may happen and may be responsible for causing complications in cardiac surgical patients. Tissue injury, endotoxemia, and contact of blood with the foreign surface of the CPB circuit are thought to initiate a systemic inflammatory response after cardiac surgery. What is least understood and most controversial is the issue of which of these many processes is the most clinically relevant. It appears as if major surgery is an important cause of systemic inflammation and that CPB further exacerbates the elaboration of proinflammatory mediators.

Mechanisms of Inflammation-Mediated Injury

Activation of neutrophils and other leukocytes is central to most theories regarding inflammation-induced injury.[4] Neutrophil activation leads to the release of oxygen radicals, intracellular proteases, and fatty acid (e.g., arachidonic acid) metabolites. These products, as well as those from activated macrophages and platelets, can cause or exacerbate tissue injury.

In localized areas of infection, oxygen free radicals liberated by activated neutrophils aid in the destruction of pathogens.[5] Complement, in particular C5a, results in activation of leukocytes and oxygen free radical formation. These activated neutrophils liberate toxic amounts of oxygen free radicals such as hydrogen peroxide, hydroxyl radicals, and superoxide anion. Oxygen free radicals are thought to cause cellular injury ultimately through damage to the lipid membrane.

A related mechanism of injury results from the degranulation of neutrophils. Activated neutrophils release granules containing myeloperoxidase, as well as other toxic digestive enzymes such as neutrophil elastase, lactoferrin, β-glucuronidase, and N-acetyl-β-glucosaminidase.[6] Release of these intracellular enzymes not only causes tissue damage but also reduces the number of cells that can participate in bacterial destruction.

Another mechanism of inflammation-mediated injury involves microvascular occlusion. Activation of neutrophils leads to adhesion of leukocytes to endothelium and formation of clumps of inflammatory cells as microaggregates.

Finally, activated leukocytes release leukotrienes such as leukotriene B_4. Leukotrienes are arachidonic acid metabolites generated by the lipoxygenase pathway. They markedly increase vascular permeability and are potent arteriolar vasoconstrictors. These leukotriene-mediated effects account for some of the clinical signs of systemic inflammation, in particular generalized edema as well as "third-space losses." Prostaglandins, generated from arachidonic acid via the cyclooxygenase pathway, also act as mediators of the inflammatory process.

Physiologic Mediators of Inflammation

Cytokines

Cytokines are believed to play a pivotal role in the pathophysiology of acute inflammation associated with cardiac surgery.[7] Cytokines are proteins released from activated macrophages, monocytes, fibroblasts, and endothelial cells that have far-reaching regulatory effects on cells. They are small proteins that exert their effects by binding to specific cell surface receptors. Many of these proteins are called *interleukins* because they aid in the communication between white blood cells (leukocytes).

Cytokines are an important component of the acute-phase response to injury or infection. The acute-phase response is the host's physiologic response to tissue injury or infection and is intended to fight infection as well as contain areas of diseased or injured tissue. Cytokines mediate this attraction of immune system cells to local areas of injury or infection. They also help the host through activation of the immune system, thus providing for an improved defense against pathogens. Most cytokines are proinflammatory, whereas others appear to exert an anti-inflammatory effect, suggesting a complex feedback system designed to limit the amount of inflammation. Excessive levels of cytokines, however, may result in an exaggerated degree of systemic inflammation, which may lead to greater secondary injury. Numerous cytokines (e.g., tumor necrosis factor [TNF], interleukin [IL]-1 to IL-16) and other protein mediators have been described and may play an important role in the pathogenesis of postoperative systemic inflammation (Box 6-1).[8,9]

Complement System

The complement system describes at least 20 plasma proteins and is involved in the chemoattraction, activation, opsonization, and lysis of cells. Complement is also involved in blood clotting, fibrinolysis, and kinin formation. These proteins are found in the plasma as well as in the interstitial spaces, mostly in the form of enzymatic precursors.

6

91

> **BOX 6-1** *Most Commonly Measured Biochemical Markers of Inflammation*
>
> - Tumor necrosis factor-α
> - Interleukin-8
> - Interleukin-6
> - C-reactive protein

The complement cascade is illustrated in Figure 6-2. The complement cascade can be triggered by either the *classical pathway* or the *alternate pathway.* In the alternate pathway, C3 is activated by contact of complement factors B and D with complex polysaccharides, endotoxin, or exposure of blood to foreign substances such as the CPB circuit. *Contact activation* (Fig. 6-3) describes contact of blood with a foreign surface with resulting adherence of platelets and activation of factor XII (Hageman factor). Activated factor XII has numerous effects, including initiation of the coagulation cascade through factor XI and conversion of prekallikrein to kallikrein. Kallikrein leads to generation of plasmin, which is known to activate the complement as well as the fibrinolytic systems. Kallikrein generation also activates the kinin-bradykinin system.

The classical pathway involves the activation of C1 by antibody-antigen complexes. In the case of cardiac surgery, there are two likely mechanisms for the activation of the classical pathway. Endotoxin can be detected in the serum of almost all patients undergoing cardiac surgery. Endotoxin forms an antigen-antibody complex with antiendotoxin antibodies normally found in serum, which can then activate C1. The administration of protamine after separation from CPB has been reported to result in heparin/protamine complexes, which can also activate the classical pathway[10] Contact activation leads to activation of factor XII, which results in the generation of plasmin. Plasmin is capable of activating complement factors C1 and C3.

Activated C3, as well as other complement factors downstream in the cascade, has several actions. The effects of activated complement fragments on mast cells and their circulating counterparts, the basophil cells, may be relevant to the development of postoperative complications potentially attributable to complement activation. Fragments C3a and C5a (also called "anaphylatoxins") lead to the release of numerous mediators, including histamine, leukotriene B_4, platelet-activating factor, prostaglandins, thromboxanes, and TNF. These mediators, when released from mast cells, result in endothelial leak, interstitial edema, and elevated tissue blood flow. Complement factors such as C5a and C3b complexed to microbes stimulate macrophages to secrete inflammatory mediators such as TNF. C3b activates neutrophils and macrophages and enhances their ability to phagocytose bacteria. The lytic complex or membrane attack complex, composed of complement factors C5b, C6, C7, C8, and C9, is capable of directly lysing cells. Activated complement factors make invading cells "sticky" such that they bind to one another (i.e., agglutinate). The complement-mediated processes of capillary dilation, leakage of plasma proteins and fluid, and accumulation and activation of neutrophils make up part of the acute inflammatory response.

Endotoxin

Endotoxin, also called lipopolysaccharide (LPS), is a component of the cell membrane of gram-negative bacteria. It is a potent activator of complement and cytokines and appears to be one of the initial triggers of systemic inflammation.

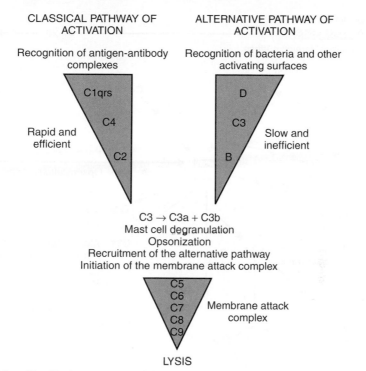

CLASSICAL PATHWAY OF
ACTIVATION

Recognition of antigen-antibody
complexes

C1qrs

C4

Rapid and
efficient

C2

ALTERNATIVE PATHWAY OF
ACTIVATION

Recognition of bacteria and other
activating surfaces

D

C3

Slow and
inefficient

B

C3 → C3a + C3b
Mast cell degranulation
Opsonization
Recruitment of the alternative pathway
Initiation of the membrane attack complex

C5
C6
C7   Membrane attack
C8   complex
C9

LYSIS

Figure 6-2 Simplified components of the complement system. (Paul WE: Introduction to the immune system IN Paul WE: Fundamental Immunology. New York, Roven, 1989.)

ENDOTOXEMIA

Endotoxemia refers to the presence of endotoxin in the blood. It is common in cardiac surgical patients.[11,12] It is not surprising that some investigators have failed to detect endotoxemia during cardiac surgery given its transient and intermittent nature, although differences in endotoxin-assaying techniques used may also contribute to this discrepancy.

Normally, intestinal flora contain a large amount of endotoxin from gram-negative microorganisms. The average human colon contains approximately 25 billion ng of endotoxin, which is an enormous quantity when 300 ng of endotoxin is considered toxic to humans. The leakage of live bacterial cells into the bloodstream can result in infection as these viable bacteria multiply. However, many of the bacteria in the intestine are dead, and thus endotoxin can also enter the bloodstream contained within cell membrane fragments of dead bacteria. In this case, infection per se does not develop. Instead, endotoxin may initiate a systemic inflammatory response through potent activation of macrophages and other proinflammatory cells. A plasma endotoxin concentration of only 1 ng/mL has been reported to be lethal in humans.

On entry into the bloodstream, endotoxin forms complexes with numerous intravascular compounds, including high-density lipoprotein, lipopolysaccharide-binding protein, and endotoxin-specific immunoglobulins. Endotoxin has been

6

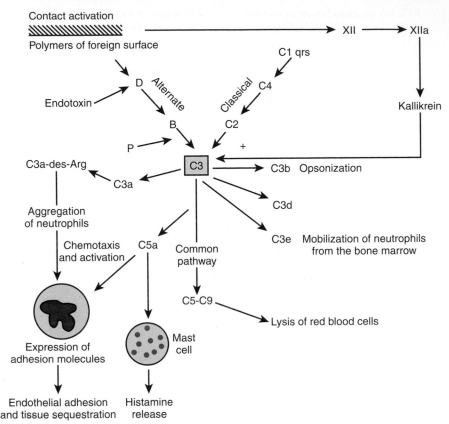

Figure 6-3 Contact activation of the complement cascade during cardiopulmonary bypass. Activation of complement occurs primarily through the alternate pathway. (From Ohri SK: The effects of cardiopulmonary bypass on the immune system. Perfusion 8:121, 1993.)

linked to dysfunction in every organ system of the body and may be the key initiating factor in the development of systemic inflammation.

Normal Host Defenses against Endotoxemia

Early Tolerance

If endotoxemia is deleterious to patients, it would be logical to assume that patients have defense mechanisms against this ubiquitous toxin. Two distinct types of tolerance to endotoxin exist and are classified as *early tolerance* and *late tolerance*. Early tolerance to endotoxin represents a reduction in the proinflammatory effects of LPS when administered several hours after a prior infusion of LPS. It appears to be due to an LPS-induced refractory state of macrophages in which they release less TNF in response to endotoxin. This early refractive state shows no LPS specificity and can be overcome with increased doses of endotoxin. The degree of this tolerance is directly proportional to the dose and, hence, intensity of the initial LPS-induced inflammatory state. Early tolerance begins within hours of LPS exposure and decreases almost to baseline within 2 days. It cannot be transferred with plasma. Early tolerance may protect the host from lethal systemic inflammation after an overwhelming exposure of LPS.

Late Tolerance

Late tolerance to endotoxin is due to the synthesis of immunoglobulins, that is, antibodies, directed against the offending LPS. Late tolerance begins approximately 72 hours after exposure to LPS, which correlates with the appearance of the early-appearing IgM class of antibodies. This form of tolerance persists for at least 2 weeks and correlates with the presence of serum immunoglobulins.

Antiendotoxin Antibodies

There is a growing body of evidence that suggests that antibodies to endotoxin may be an important determinant of adverse outcome after cardiac surgery. According to this theory, the presence of protective antiendotoxin antibodies *preoperatively* reduces the incidence of complications caused by LPS-induced systemic inflammation. Only antibodies that are present preoperatively can buffer the effects of perioperative endotoxemia, because a minimum of 72 hours is required for the synthesis of new antibodies after exposure to endotoxin encountered during surgery. It is also known that CPB results in denaturation of antibodies, which decreases the number of protective antibodies even further. Moreover, there is evidence that antibody production by B lymphocytes (plasma cells) is depressed after cardiac surgery, which reduces the effectiveness of the humoral immune response to toxins encountered during surgery.

SPLANCHNIC PERFUSION

Splanchnic hypoperfusion appears to be an important cause of systemic inflammation. The gut is one of the most susceptible organs to hypoperfusion during conditions of trauma or stress.[13,14] Studies suggest that during periods of hypovolemia, the gut vasoconstricts, thus shunting blood toward "more vital organs" such as the heart and brain. In addition to hypovolemia, endogenously released vasoconstrictors during CPB, such as angiotensin II, thromboxane A_2, and vasopressin, may also result in decreased splanchnic perfusion. Vasoconstrictors such as phenylephrine are routinely administered by anesthesiologists and perfusionists to increase blood pressure and are likely to further reduce gut perfusion.

Gastric Tonometry

A U.S. Food and Drug Administration–approved monitor (the gastrointestinal tonometer) exists that can detect gut hypoperfusion. The tonometer is a naso/orogastric tube that has been modified to include a silicone balloon into which air or saline is introduced (Trip Catheter; Datex-Engstrom, Tewksbury, MA). The gastric mucosal bed is similar to the overall splanchnic mucosa in its propensity to become hypoperfused during periods of physiologic stress. Hypoperfused areas of tissue develop regional hypercapnia (elevated Pco_2), which diffuses into the tonometer balloon allowing for an indirect measurement of gastric mucosal Pco_2. Hypoperfusion is manifested by a positive gap (gastric mucosal Pco_2 > arterial Pco_2) between the gastric mucosal Pco_2 and the arterial Pco_2. A gap greater than 8 to 10 mm Hg is considered by many investigators to reflect splanchnic hypoperfusion.

Gastric Mucosal Hypoperfusion during Cardiac Surgery

Gut hypoperfusion can progress to ischemia, which may result in complications that take place many hours and days after an episode of hypovolemia. Many of the complications seen after major surgery are consistent with a toxic exposure to endotoxemia, which presumably arises from translocation through an impaired gut mucosa.

Several studies have observed a high incidence of splanchnic hypoperfusion during cardiac surgery, with some showing an association between abnormal gut perfusion during cardiac surgery and postoperative complications.[15,16]

POSTOPERATIVE COMPLICATIONS ATTRIBUTABLE TO INFLAMMATION

Types of Complications

Many postoperative complications appear to be caused by an exaggerated systemic proinflammatory response to surgical trauma. A common misunderstanding relates to the types of postoperative complications that may be attributable to systemic inflammation and, in particular, splanchnic hypoperfusion. Many of the complications that are thought to be linked to splanchnic hypoperfusion do not involve the gastrointestinal system. Because splanchnic hypoperfusion may cause injury through endotoxemia and resulting systemic inflammation, it would be expected that every organ system of the body would be potentially involved. Endotoxin has been reported to have adverse effects on the pulmonary, renal, cardiac, and vascular systems. Endotoxin affects the coagulation system and may be both antihemostatic, potentially explaining bleeding, and prothrombotic. Prothrombotic effects may account for some cases of postoperative stroke, deep venous thrombosis, and pulmonary emboli. There is also circumstantial evidence that systemic inflammation may worsen neurologic injury.

Potential Therapies for the Prevention of Inflammation-Related Complications

Numerous strategies and pharmacologic agents have been postulated to reduce the severity and incidence of systemic inflammation. Many studies have demonstrated reductions in intermediate endpoints, such as laboratory indices of complement activation and cytokinemia. At the present time, there are no therapies in widespread clinical use for the prevention or treatment of organ dysfunction resulting from systemic inflammation, although several approaches have been studied (Box 6-2).

Corticosteroid Administration

Several attempts have been made to prevent elevations in proinflammatory cytokines and complement activation during cardiac surgery with corticosteroid administration.[17] The overall data suggest that corticosteroids are probably of limited benefit and may, in fact, be harmful.[18]

Role of Cardiopulmonary Bypass Technique

Although heparin-coated circuits have many theoretic advantages, there is little evidence that their use during cardiac surgery results in fewer clinically significant adverse complications.

II

BOX 6-2 *Previously Studied Interventions*

- Corticosteroids
- Cardiopulmonary bypass technique
- Complement inhibition
- Ultrafiltration
- Leukocyte depletion
- Aprotinin administration
- Endotoxin immune-related strategies
- E5564
- Pentoxifylline
- Anesthetic agents
- Selective digestive decontamination

The role of membrane oxygenators as a means of reducing systemic inflammation-related complications is also controversial. Less complement activation has been observed with the use of membrane oxygenators, although other studies have found no difference.[19] There is also controversy as to whether hypothermia during CPB worsens systemic inflammation. Hypothermia has been shown to reduce markers of complement activation. Finally, current data suggest that the use of CPB for cardiac surgery may not in and of itself be more deleterious than cardiac surgery without the use of CPB. Results from randomized clinical trials do not suggest that outcomes are substantially different in patients undergoing on-pump versus off-pump CABG.[20-22]

Complement Inhibition

The results from several large randomized clinical trials in which complement activation is selectively blocked have become available. These studies indicate that attenuation of complement activation results in less myocardial injury; however, there did not appear to be an impact on complications such as pulmonary and renal dysfunction and severe vasodilation. These results suggest that complement activation may not play as great a role in the development of systemic inflammation–mediated morbidity as previously thought.

Ultrafiltration

Removal of excess fluid with ultrafiltration has been proposed as a method for removing proinflammatory mediators during cardiac surgery, particularly in the pediatric population. It is unclear in studies performed thus far whether beneficial effects of ultrafiltration are due to one or some combination of the following factors: prevention of initiation of inflammation, removal of inflammatory mediators, or removal of excessive fluid alone.

Aprotinin Administration

Aprotinin, a 58-amino-acid serine protease inhibitor isolated from bovine lung, has been shown in numerous studies to decrease bleeding associated with cardiac surgery. It antagonizes numerous proteolytic enzymes, including plasmin and kallikrein, and may have some anti-inflammatory effects. The blood-sparing effects of aprotinin were apparently discovered serendipitously while it was being evaluated as an anti-inflammatory agent in cardiac surgical patients. Despite more than 45 randomized clinical trials conducted to date, there are few data to support the hypothesis that aprotinin administration reduces postoperative complications attributable to excessive systemic inflammation. In these trials, numerous surrogate markers of postoperative morbidity, such as the duration of postoperative tracheal intubation, intensive care unit stay, and hospital length of stay, were not reported to be improved in aprotinin-treated patients.

ROLE OF ANESTHETIC AGENTS AND VASOACTIVE AGENTS

Anesthetic agents, defined here as drugs that induce hypnosis, amnesia, muscle relaxation, or regional anesthesia, have not been shown to result in clinically meaningful reductions in systemic inflammation after cardiac surgery. Numerous studies have evaluated the effect of these agents on the immune system with varied results, but no studies have reported a difference in outcome with one technique versus another.

There is evidence that splanchnic hypoperfusion and endotoxin-induced inflammation can be prevented in the operating room by strategies familiar to clinicians. Strategies involve the use of fluid loading to maximize stroke volume as well as the use of adequate levels of vasodilating volatile anesthetics. Inodilating agents, such as milrinone, amrinone, dopexamine, and dobutamine, may be more protective of splanchnic perfusion than inoconstricting agents such as epinephrine, norepinephrine, and dopamine.

SUMMARY

- Mortality and morbidity are relatively common after major surgery.
- Postoperative morbidity often involves multiple organ systems, which implicates a systemic process.
- A large body of evidence suggests that excessive systemic inflammation is a cause of postoperative organ dysfunction.
- No interventions have been proved in large randomized clinical trials to protect patients from systemic inflammation–mediated morbidity.

REFERENCES

1. Hammermeister KE, Burchfiel C, Johnson R, Grover FL: Identification of patients at greatest risk for developing major complications at cardiac surgery. Circulation 82:IV-380, 1990
2. Rady MY, Ryan T, Starr NJ: Perioperative determinants of morbidity and mortality in elderly patients undergoing cardiac surgery. Crit Care Med 26:225, 1998
3. Bone RC, Balk RA, Cerra FB, et al: Definitions for sepsis and organ failure and guidelines for the use of innovative therapies in sepsis. The ACCP/SCCM Consensus Conference Committee. American College of Chest Physicians/Society of Critical Care Medicine. Chest 101:1644, 1992
4. Miller BE, Levy JH: The inflammatory response to cardiopulmonary bypass. J Cardiothorac Vasc Anesth 11:355, 1997
5. Weiss SJ: Tissue destruction by neutrophils. N Engl J Med 320:365, 1989
6. Royston D, Fleming JS, Desai JB, et al: Increased production of peroxidation products associated with cardiac operations: Evidence for free radical generation. J Thorac Cardiovasc Surg 91:759, 1986
7. Tonnesen E, Christensen VB, Toft P: The role of cytokines in cardiac surgery. Int J Cardiol 53(suppl):S1, 1996
8. Rothenburger M, Soeparwata R, Deng MC, et al: Prediction of clinical outcome after cardiac surgery: The role of cytokines, endotoxin, and antiendotoxin core antibodies. Shock 16(suppl 1):44, 2001
9. Rothenburger M, Tjan TD, Schneider M, et al: The impact of the pro- and anti-inflammatory immune response on ventilation time after cardiac surgery. Cytometry 53B:70, 2003
10. Kirklin JK, Chenoweth DE, Naftel DC, et al: Effects of protamine administration after cardiopulmonary bypass on complement, blood elements, and the hemodynamic state. Ann Thorac Surg 41:193, 1986
11. Oudemans-van Straaten HM, Jansen PG, Hoek FJ, et al: Intestinal permeability, circulating endotoxin, and postoperative systemic responses in cardiac surgery patients. J Cardiothorac Vasc Anesth 10:187, 1996
12. Watarida S, Mori A, Onoe M, et al: A clinical study on the effects of pulsatile cardiopulmonary bypass on the blood endotoxin levels. J Thorac Cardiovasc Surg 108:620, 1994
13. Deitch EA: Bacterial translocation of the gut flora. J Trauma 30:S184, 1990

14. Mythen MG, Webb AR: The role of gut mucosal hypoperfusion in the pathogenesis of postoperative organ dysfunction. Intensive Care Med 20:203, 1994
15. Mythen MG, Webb AR: Intraoperative gut mucosal hypoperfusion is associated with increased postoperative complications and cost. Intensive Care Med 20:99, 1994
16. Mythen MG, Webb AR: Perioperative plasma volume expansion reduces the incidence of gut mucosal hypoperfusion during cardiac surgery. Arch Surg 130:423, 1995
17. Tabardel Y, Duchateau J, Schmartz D, et al: Corticosteroids increase blood interleukin-10 levels during cardiopulmonary bypass in men. Surgery 119:76, 1996
18. Chaney MA: Corticosteroids and cardiopulmonary bypass: A review of clinical investigations. Chest 121:921, 2002
19. Videm V, Fosse E, Mollnes TE, et al: Complement activation with bubble and membrane oxygenators in aortocoronary bypass grafting. Ann Thorac Surg 50:387, 1990
20. Puskas JD, Williams WH, Mahoney EM, et al: Off-pump vs conventional coronary artery bypass grafting: Early and 1-year graft patency, cost, and quality-of-life outcomes: A randomized trial. JAMA 291:1841, 2004
21. Khan NE, De Souza A, Mister R, et al: A randomized comparison of off-pump and on-pump multivessel coronary-artery bypass surgery. N Engl J Med 350:21, 2004
22. Racz MJ, Hannan EL, Isom OW, et al: A comparison of short- and long-term outcomes after off-pump and on-pump coronary artery bypass graft surgery with sternotomy. J Am Coll Cardiol 43:557, 2004

6

Chapter 7

Pharmacology of Anesthetic Drugs

Kelly Grogan, MD • Daniel Nyhan, MD •
Dan E. Berkowitz, MD

An enormous body of literature has accumulated describing the effects of the different anesthetic agents on the heart and the regional vascular beds. Recently, this has been due to the great interest in anesthesia-induced preconditioning (APC).

VOLATILE AGENTS

Acute Effects

Myocardial Function

The influence of volatile anesthetics on contractile function has been investigated extensively, and it is now widely agreed that volatile agents cause dose-dependent depression of contractile function (Box 7-1). Moreover, different volatile agents are not identical in this regard and the preponderance of information indicates that halothane and enflurane exert equal but more potent myocardial depression than do isoflurane, desflurane, or sevoflurane.[1] This reflects in part reflex sympathetic activation with the latter agents. It is also widely accepted that in the setting of preexisting myocardial depression, volatile agents have a greater effect than in normal myocardium. At the cellular level, volatile anesthetics exert their negative inotropic effects mainly by modulating sarcolemmal (SL) L-type Ca^{2+} channels, the sarcoplasmic reticulum (SR), and the contractile proteins. However, the mechanisms whereby anesthetic agents modify ion channels are not completely understood.

> **BOX 7-1** *Volatile Anesthetic Agents*
>
> - All volatile anesthetic agents cause dose-dependent decreases in systemic blood pressure, which for halothane and enflurane are predominantly due to attenuation of myocardial contractile function and which for isoflurane, desflurane, and sevoflurane are predominantly due to decreases in systemic vascular resistance. Moreover, volatile agents obtund all components of the baroreceptor reflex arc.
> - The effects of volatile agents on myocardial diastolic function are not yet well characterized and await the application of "bedside" emerging technologies that have the sensitivity to quantitate indices of diastolic function.
> - Volatile anesthetics lower the arrhythmogenic threshold to catecholamines. However, the underlying molecular mechanisms are not well understood.
> - When confounding variables are controlled (e.g., systemic blood pressure), isoflurane does not cause "coronary steal" by a direct effect on coronary vasculature.
> - The effects of volatile agents on systemic regional vascular beds and on the pulmonary vasculature are complex and depend on variables that include, but are not confined to, the specific anesthetic under study, the specific vascular bed, the vessel size, and whether endothelial-dependent or endothelial-independent mechanisms are being investigated.

Cardiac Electrophysiology

Volatile anesthetic agents lower the arrhythmogenic threshold for epinephrine. Moreover, not all volatile agents are similar, with the order of sensitization being halothane > enflurane > sevoflurane > isoflurane = desflurane. The molecular mechanisms underlying this effect of volatile anesthetics are poorly understood.

Coronary Vasoregulation

Volatile anesthetic agents modulate several determinants of both myocardial oxygen supply and demand. Moreover, it is now established that volatile agents also directly modulate the response of myocytes to ischemia.

The effect of isoflurane on coronary vessels was controversial and dominated much of the literature in this area in the 1980s and early 1990s. The current assessments of the effects of isoflurane have been succinctly detailed by Tanaka and associates.[2] Several reports had indicated that it caused direct coronary arteriolar vasodilatation in vessels of 100 μm or less and that isoflurane could cause "coronary steal" in patients with "steal-prone" coronary anatomy. Several studies in which potential confounding variables were controlled indicated clearly that isoflurane did not cause coronary steal. Studies of sevoflurane and desflurane showed similar results and are consistent with a mild direct coronary vasodilator effect of these agents.

Systemic Vascular Effects

All volatile anesthetic agents decrease systemic blood pressure (BP) in a dose-dependent manner. With halothane and enflurane, the decrease in systemic BP is primarily due to decreases in stroke volume (SV) and cardiac output (CO) whereas isoflurane, sevoflurane, and desflurane decrease overall systemic vascular resistance (SVR) while maintaining CO.

Baroreceptor Reflex

All volatile agents attenuate the baroreceptor reflex. Baroreceptor reflex inhibition by halothane and enflurane is more potent than that observed with isoflurane, desflurane, or sevoflurane, each of which has a similar effect. Each component of the

---

BOX 7-2 *Volatile Agents and Myocardial Ischemia*

- Volatile anesthetic agents have been demonstrated to attenuate the effects of myocardial ischemia (acute coronary syndromes).
- Nonacute manifestations of myocardial ischemia include hibernating myocardium, stunning, and preconditioning.
- Halothane and isoflurane facilitate the recovery of stunned myocardium.
- Preconditioning, a profoundly important adaptive protective mechanism in biologic tissues, can be provoked by protean nonlethal stresses, including but not confined to ischemia.
- Volatile anesthetic agents can mimic preconditioning (anesthetic preconditioning), an observation that could have important clinical implications, as well as providing insight into the cellular mechanisms of action of volatile agents.

---

baroreceptor reflex arc (afferent nerve activity, central processing, efferent nerve activity) is inhibited by volatile agents.

Delayed Effects

Reversible Myocardial Ischemia

Prolonged ischemia results in irreversible myocardial damage and necrosis (Box 7-2). Shorter durations of myocardial ischemia can, depending on the duration and sequence of ischemic insults, lead to either preconditioning or myocardial stunning (Fig. 7-1). Stunning, first described in 1975, occurs after brief ischemia and is characterized by myocardial dysfunction in the setting of normal restored blood flow and by an absence of myocardial necrosis. Ischemic preconditioning (IPC) was first described by Murray and colleagues in 1986 and is characterized by an attenuation in infarct size after sustained ischemia, if this period of sustained ischemia is preceded by a period of brief ischemia. Moreover, this effect is independent of collateral flow. Thus, short periods of ischemia followed by reperfusion can lead to either stunning or preconditioning with a reduction in infarct size (Fig. 7-2).[3]

Anesthetic Preconditioning

Volatile agents can elicit delayed (late), as well as classic (early), preconditioning. Moreover, APC is dose dependent, exhibits synergy with ischemia in affording protection, and, perhaps not surprisingly in view of differential uptake and distribution of volatile agents, has been demonstrated to require different time intervals between exposure and the maintenance of a subsequent benefit that is agent dependent. Volatile agents that exhibit APC activate mitochondrial K^+_{ATP} channels, and this effect is blocked by specific mitochondrial K^+_{ATP} channel antagonists. However, the precise relative contributions of SL versus mitochondrial K^+_{ATP} channel activation to APC remain to be elucidated (Fig. 7-3).

INTRAVENOUS INDUCTION AGENTS

The drugs discussed in this section are all induction agents and hypnotics. These drugs belong to different classes (barbiturates, benzodiazepines, N-methyl-D-aspartate [NMDA] receptor antagonists, and α_2-adrenergic receptor agonists). Their effects on the cardiovascular system are therefore dependent on the class to which they belong.

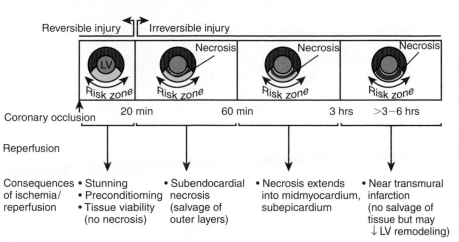

Reversible injury | Irreversible injury

	Necrosis	Necrosis	Necrosis
LV			
Risk zone	Risk zone	Risk zone	Risk zone

Coronary occlusion

| 20 min | 60 min | 3 hrs | >3−6 hrs |

Reperfusion

Consequences of ischemia/ reperfusion	• Stunning • Preconditioming • Tissue viability (no necrosis)	• Subendocardial necrosis (salvage of outer layers)	• Necrosis extends into midmyocardium, subepicardium	• Near transmural infarction (no salvage of tissue but may ↓ LV remodeling)

Figure 7-1 Effects of ischemia and reperfusion on the heart based on studies in anesthetized canine model of proximal coronary artery occlusion. Brief periods of ischemia of less than 20 minutes followed by reperfusion are not associated with development of necrosis (reversible injury). Brief ischemia/reperfusion results in the phenomenon of stunning and preconditioning. If duration of coronary occlusion is extended beyond 20 minutes, a wavefront of necrosis marches from subendocardium to subepicardium over time. Reperfusion before 3 hours of ischemia salvages ischemic but viable tissue. (This salvaged tissue may demonstrate stunning.) Reperfusion beyond 3 to 6 hours in this model does not reduce myocardial infarct size. Late reperfusion may still have a beneficial effect on reducing or preventing myocardial infarct expansion and left ventricular (LV) remodeling. (From Kloner RA, Jennings RB: Consequences of brief ischemia: Stunning, preconditioning, and their clinical implications: I. Circulation 104:2981, 2001.)

Acute Cardiac Effects

Myocardial Contractility

With regard to propofol, the studies remain controversial as to whether there is a direct effect on myocardial contractile function at clinically relevant concentrations. However, the weight of evidence suggests that the drug has a modest negative inotropic effect, which may be mediated by inhibition of L-type Ca^{2+} channels or modulation of Ca^{2+} release from the sarcoplasmic reticulum.

In one of the few human studies using isolated atrial muscle tissue, no inhibition of myocardial contractility was found in the clinical concentration ranges of propofol, midazolam, and etomidate. In contrast, thiopental showed strong negative inotropic properties whereas ketamine showed slight negative inotropic properties. Thus, negative inotropic effects may explain in part the cardiovascular depression on induction of anesthesia with thiopental but not with propofol, midazolam, and etomidate. Improvement of hemodynamics after induction of anesthesia with ketamine is a function of sympathoexcitation.

The effect of drugs such as propofol may also be markedly affected by the underlying myocardial pathology. For instance, Sprung and coworkers determined the direct effects of propofol on the contractility of human nonfailing atrial and failing atrial and ventricular muscles obtained from the failing human hearts of transplant patients or from nonfailing hearts of patients undergoing coronary artery bypass graft (CABG) surgery.[4] They concluded that propofol exerts a direct negative inotropic effect in nonfailing and failing human myocardium but only at concentrations larger than typical clinical concentrations. Negative inotropic effects are reversible with β-adrenergic stimulation, suggesting that propofol does not alter the contractile reserve but may shift the dose responsiveness to adrenergic stimulation.

7

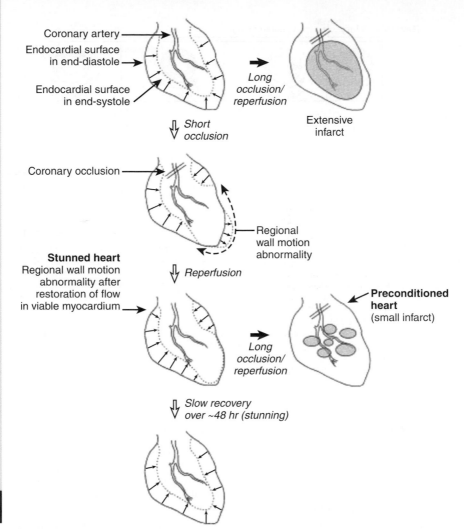

Figure 7-2 Schematic of stunning and preconditioning. Short coronary artery occlusions result in stunning, in which there is prolonged regional wall motion abnormality, despite presence of reperfusion and viable myocardial cells. Brief episodes of ischemia/reperfusion also precondition the heart. When the heart is then exposed to a longer duration of ischemia and reperfusion, myocardial infarct size is reduced. (From Kloner RA, Jennings RB: Consequences of brief ischemia: Stunning, preconditioning, and their clinical implications: I. Circulation 104:2981, 2001.)

Vasculature

As with the heart, the cumulative physiologic effects in the vasculature represent a summation of the effects of the agents on the central autonomic nervous system, as well as the direct effects of these agents on the vascular smooth muscle, and the modulating effects on the underlying endothelium. It is now well established that propofol decreases SVR in humans. This was demonstrated in a patient with an artificial heart in whom the CO remained fixed. The effect is predominantly mediated by alterations in sympathetic tone; however, in isolated arteries, propofol decreases vascular tone and agonist-induced contraction. The mechanism by which propofol

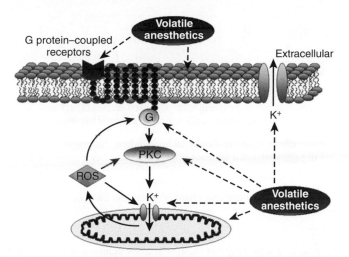

Figure 7-3   Multiple endogenous signaling pathways mediate volatile anesthetic-induced myocardial activation of an end-effector that promotes resistance against ischemic injury. Mitochondrial K^+_{ATP} channels have been implicated as the end-effector in this protective scheme, but sarcolemmal K^+_{ATP} channels may also be involved in this mechanism of protection. A trigger initiates a cascade of signal transduction events, resulting in the protection. Volatile anesthetics signal through adenosine and opioid receptors, modulate G proteins, stimulate protein kinase C (PKC) and other intracellular kinases, or have direct effects on mitochondria to generate reactive oxygen species (ROS) that ultimately enhance K^+_{ATP} channel activity. Volatile anesthetics may also directly facilitate K^+_{ATP} channel opening. *Dotted arrows* delineate the intracellular targets that may be regulated by volatile anesthetics; *solid arrows* represent potential signaling cascades. (From Tanaka K, Ludwig LM, Kersten JR, et al: Mechanisms of cardioprotection by volatile anesthetics. Anesthesiology 100:707, 2004.)

mediates these effects has been attributed in part to inhibition of Ca^{2+} influx through voltage or receptor-gated Ca^{2+} channels, as well as inhibition of Ca^{2+} release from intracellular Ca^{2+} stores.

INDIVIDUAL AGENTS

7

Thiopental

Thiopental has survived the test of time as an intravenous anesthetic drug (Box 7-3). Since Lundy introduced it in 1934, thiopental was the most widely used induction agent because of the rapid hypnotic effect (one arm-to-brain circulation time), highly predictable effect, lack of vascular irritation, and general overall safety. The induction dose of thiopental is lower for older than for younger healthy patients. Pharmacokinetic analyses confirm that the awakening from thiopental is due to rapid redistribution. Thiopental has a distribution half-life ($t\frac{1}{2}\alpha$) of 2.5 to 8.5 minutes, and the total body clearance varies, according to sampling times and techniques, from 0.15 to 0.26 L/kg/hr. The elimination half-life ($t\frac{1}{2}\beta$) varies from 5 to 12 hours. Barbiturates and propofol have increased volumes of distribution (Vd) when used during cardiopulmonary bypass (CPB).

Cardiovascular Effects

The hemodynamic changes produced by thiopental have been studied in normal patients and in patients with cardiac disease (Table 7-1). The principal effect is a decrease in contractility, which results from reduced availability of calcium to the

BOX 7-3 *Intravenous Anesthetics*

Thiopental

Thiopental decreases cardiac output by:

- A direct negative inotropic action
- Decreased ventricular filling, resulting from increased venous capacitance
- Transiently decreasing sympathetic outflow from the central nervous system

Because of these effects, caution should be used when thiopental is given to patients who have left or right ventricular failure, cardiac tamponade, or hypovolemia.

Midazolam

There are only small hemodynamic changes after the intravenous administration of midazolam.

Etomidate

Etomidate is described as the drug that changes hemodynamic variables the least. Studies in noncardiac patients and those who have heart disease document the remarkable hemodynamic stability after administration of etomidate.
Patients who have hypovolemia, cardiac tamponade, or low cardiac output probably represent the population for whom etomidate is better than other induction drugs, with the possible exception of ketamine.

Ketamine

A unique feature of ketamine is stimulation of the cardiovascular system, with the most prominent hemodynamic changes including significant increases in HR, CI, SVR, PAP, and systemic artery pressure. These circulatory changes cause an increase in MVo_2 with an appropriate increase in coronary blood flow.
Studies have demonstrated the safety and efficacy of induction with ketamine in hemodynamically unstable patients. It is the induction drug of choice for patients with cardiac tamponade physiology.

Dexmedetomidine

Dexmedetomidine is a highly selective, specific, and potent adrenoreceptor agonist.
α_2-Adrenergic agonists can safely reduce anesthetic requirements and improve hemodynamic stability. These agents may enhance sedation and analgesia without producing respiratory depression or prolonging recovery period.

myofibrils. There is also an increase in HR. The cardiac index (CI) is unchanged or reduced, and the mean aortic pressure (MAP) is maintained or slightly reduced. In the dose range studied, no relationship between plasma thiopental and hemodynamic effect has been found.

Mechanisms for the decrease in CO include (1) direct negative inotropic action, (2) decreased ventricular filling, resulting from increased venous capacitance, and (3) transiently decreased sympathetic outflow from the central nervous system. The increase in HR (10% to 36%) that accompanies thiopental administration probably results from the baroreceptor-mediated sympathetic reflex stimulation of the heart. Thiopental produces dose-related negative inotropic effects that appear to result from a decrease in calcium influx into the cells with a resultant diminished amount of calcium at sarcolemma sites. Patients who had compensated heart disease and received 4 mg/kg of thiopental had a greater (18%) BP drop than did other patients. The increase in HR (11% to 36%) encountered in patients with coronary artery disease (CAD), anesthetized with thiopental

Table 7-1 Induction Agents and Hemodynamic Changes

Parameter	Thiopental	Midazolam	Etomidate	Propofol	Ketamine
Heart rate	0% to +36%	−14% to +21%	0% to +22%	−6% to +12%	0% to +59%
MAP	−18% to +8%	−12% to −26%	0% to −20%	0% to −47%	0% to +40%
SVR	0% to +19%	0% to −20%	0% to −17%	−9% to −25%	0% to +33%
PAP	Unchanged	Unchanged	0% to −17%	−4% to +8%	+44% to +47%
PVR	Unchanged	Unchanged	0% to +27%	—	0% to +33%
LAP/PCWP	Unchanged	0% to −25%	—	—	—
LVEDP/PCWP	—	—	0% to −11%	+13%	Unchanged
RAP	0% to +33%	Unchanged	Unchanged	−8% to −21%	+15% to +33%
CI	0% to −24%	0% to −25%	0% to +14%	−6% to −26%	0% to +42%
SV	−12% to −35%	0% to −18%	0% to −15%	−8% to −18%	0% to −21%
LVSWI	0% to −26%	−28% to −42%	0% to −27%	−15% to −40%	0% to +27%
RVSWI	NR	−41% to −57%	—	—	—
dP/dt	−14%	0% to −12%	0% to −18%	—	Unchanged
1/PEP^2	−18% to −28%	—	—	—	—
STI	—	—	Unchanged	—	NR

(1 to 4 mg/kg), is potentially deleterious because of the obligatory increase in myocardial oxygen consumption (MVo_2).

Despite the well-known potential for cardiovascular depression when thiopental is given rapidly in large doses, this drug has minimal hemodynamic effects in normal patients and in those who have heart disease when it is given slowly or by infusion. Significant reductions in cardiovascular parameters occur in patients who have impaired ventricular function. When thiopental is given to hypovolemic patients, there is a significant reduction in CO (69%), as well as a large decrease in BP, which indicate that patients without adequate compensatory mechanisms may have serious hemodynamic depression with a thiopental induction. Clearly, thiopental produces greater changes in BP and HR than does midazolam when used for induction of ASA Class III and IV patients.

Uses in Cardiac Anesthesia

Thiopental can be used safely for the induction of anesthesia in normal patients and in those who have compensated cardiac disease. Because of the negative inotropic effects, increase in venous capacitance, and dose-related decrease in CO, caution should be used when thiopental is given to patients who have left or right ventricular failure, cardiac tamponade, or hypovolemia. The development of tachycardia is a potential problem in patients with ischemic heart disease.

An additional use for thiopental infusion is cerebral protection during CPB in patients undergoing selected cardiac operations. However, the cerebral protective effect of thiopental during CPB has been challenged by Zaidan and associates,[5] who demonstrated no differences in outcome between thiopental and control patients undergoing hypothermic CPB for CABG. Although the administration of a barbiturate during CPB may result in myocardial depression, necessitating additional inotropic support, a study by Ito and colleagues suggested beneficial effects of a thiopental infusion during CPB in maintaining peripheral perfusion, which allowed more uniform warming, decreased base deficit, and decreased requirements for postoperative pressor support.

Midazolam

Midazolam (Versed), a water-soluble benzodiazepine, was synthesized in the United States in 1975. It is unique among benzodiazepines because of its rapid onset, short duration of action, and relatively rapid plasma clearance. The dose for induction of general anesthesia is between 0.05 and 0.2 mg/kg and depends on the premedication and speed of injection.

The pharmacokinetic variables of midazolam reveal that it is cleared significantly more rapidly than are diazepam and lorazepam. The rapid redistribution of midazolam, as well as high liver clearance, accounts for its relatively short hypnotic and hemodynamic effects. The t½β is about 2 hours, which is at least 10-fold less than for diazepam.

Cardiovascular Effects

The hemodynamic effects of midazolam have been investigated in normal subjects, in ASA Class III patients, and in patients who have ischemic and valvular heart disease (VHD). Table 7-1 summarizes the hemodynamic changes after induction of anesthesia with midazolam. In general, there are only small hemodynamic changes after the intravenous administration of midazolam (0.2 mg/kg) in premedicated patients who have coronary artery disease (CAD). Changes of potential importance include a decrease in MAP of 20% and an increase in HR of 15%. The CI is maintained. Filling pressures are either unchanged or decreased in patients who have normal ventricular function but are significantly decreased in patients who have an elevated PCWP

(18 mm Hg or higher). As in patients with ischemic heart disease, the induction of anesthesia in patients with VHD is associated with minimal changes in CI, HR, and MAP after midazolam. When intubation follows anesthesia induction with midazolam, significant increases in HR and BP occur, because midazolam is not an analgesic. Adjuvant analgesic drugs are required to block the response to noxious stimuli.

There is a suggestion that midazolam affects the capacitance vessels more than does diazepam, at least during CPB, when decreases in venous reservoir volume of the pump are greater with midazolam than with diazepam. In addition, diazepam decreases SVR more than midazolam during CPB.

Midazolam (0.15 mg/kg) and ketamine (1.5 mg/kg) have proved to be a safe and useful combination for a rapid-sequence induction for emergency surgery. This combination was superior to thiopental alone, because it caused less cardiovascular depression, more amnesia, and less postoperative somnolence. If midazolam is given to patients who have received fentanyl, significant hypotension may occur, as seen with diazepam and fentanyl. However, midazolam is routinely combined with fentanyl for induction and maintenance of general anesthesia during cardiac surgery without adverse hemodynamic sequelae.[6,7]

Uses

Midazolam is distinctly different from the other benzodiazepines because of its rapid onset, short duration, water solubility, and failure to produce significant thrombophlebitis; it is therefore one of the mainstays of anesthesia in the cardiac operating rooms.

Etomidate

Etomidate is a carboxylated imidazole derivative. It was found that etomidate has a safety margin four times greater than the safety margin for thiopental. The recommended induction dose of 0.3 mg/kg has pronounced hypnotic effects. Etomidate is moderately lipid soluble and has a rapid onset (10 to 12 seconds) and a brief duration of action. It is hydrolyzed primarily in the liver and in the blood as well.

Cardiovascular Effects

In comparative studies with other anesthetic drugs, etomidate is usually described as the drug that changes hemodynamic variables the least. Studies in noncardiac patients and those who have heart disease document the remarkable hemodynamic stability after administration of etomidate. In comparison with other anesthetics, etomidate produces the least change in the balance of myocardial oxygen demand and supply. Systemic BP remains unchanged but may be decreased 10% to 19% in patients who have VHD.

Etomidate (0.3 mg/kg IV), used to induce general anesthesia in patients with acute myocardial infarction undergoing percutaneous coronary angioplasty, did not alter HR, MAP, and rate-pressure product (RPP), demonstrating the remarkable hemodynamic stability of this agent.[8] However, the presence of VHD may influence the hemodynamic responses to etomidate. Whereas most patients can maintain their BP, patients with both aortic and mitral VHD had significant decreases of 17% to 19% in systolic and diastolic BP and decreases of 11% and 17% in PAP and PCWP, respectively. CI in patients who had VHD and received 0.3 mg/kg either remained unchanged or decreased 13%. There was no difference in response to etomidate between patients who had aortic valve disease and those who had mitral valve disease.

Uses

There are certain situations in which the advantages of etomidate outweigh the disadvantages. Emergency uses include situations in which rapid induction is essential. Patients who have hypovolemia, cardiac tamponade, or low CO probably represent the population for whom etomidate is better than other drugs, with the possible exception of ketamine. The fact that the hypnotic effect is brief means that additional analgesic and/or hypnotic drugs must be administered. Etomidate offers no real advantage over most other induction drugs for patients undergoing elective surgical procedures.

Ketamine

Although ketamine produces rapid hypnosis and profound analgesia, respiratory and cardiovascular functions are not depressed as much as with most other induction agents. Disturbing psychotomimetic activity (described as vivid dreams, hallucinations, or emergence phenomena) remains a problem.

Cardiovascular Effects

The hemodynamic effects of ketamine have been examined in noncardiac patients, critically ill patients, geriatric patients, and patients who have a variety of heart diseases. Table 7-1 contains the range of hemodynamic responses to ketamine. One unique feature of ketamine is stimulation of the cardiovascular system. The most prominent hemodynamic changes are significant increases in HR, CI, SVR, PAP, and MAP. These circulatory changes cause an increase in $M\dot{V}o_2$ with an apparently appropriate increase in coronary blood flow (CBF). A second dose of ketamine produces hemodynamic effects opposite to those of the first. Thus, the cardiovascular stimulation seen after ketamine induction of anesthesia (2 mg/kg) in a patient who has VHD is not observed with the second administration, which is accompanied instead by decreases in the BP, PCWP, and CI.

Ketamine produces similar hemodynamic changes in normal patients and in patients who have ischemic heart disease. In patients who have elevated PAP (as with mitral valvular disease), ketamine seems to cause a more pronounced increase in PVR than in SVR. The presence of marked tachycardia after administration of ketamine and pancuronium can also complicate the induction of anesthesia in patients who have CAD or VHD with atrial fibrillation.

One of the most common and successful approaches to blocking ketamine-induced hypertension and tachycardia is the prior administration of benzodiazepines. Diazepam, flunitrazepam, and midazolam all successfully attenuate the hemodynamic effects of ketamine. For example, in a study involving 16 patients with VHD, ketamine (2 mg/kg) did not produce significant hemodynamic changes when preceded by diazepam (0.4 mg/kg). Indeed, HR, MAP, and RPP were unchanged; however, there was a slight but significant decrease in CI. The combination of diazepam and ketamine rivals the high-dose fentanyl technique with regard to hemodynamic stability. No patient had hallucinations, although 2% had dreams and 1% had recall of events in the operating room.

Studies have demonstrated the safety and efficacy of induction with ketamine (2 mg/kg) in hemodynamically unstable patients who required emergency operations. Most of these patients were hypovolemic because of trauma or massive hemorrhage. Ketamine induction was accompanied in the majority of patients by the maintenance of BP and, presumably, of CO as well. In patients who have an accumulation of pericardial fluid, with or without constrictive pericarditis, induction with ketamine (2 mg/kg) maintains CI and increases BP, SVR, and RAP. The HR in this group of patients is unchanged by ketamine, probably because cardiac tamponade already produced a compensatory tachycardia.

Uses

In adults, ketamine is probably the safest and most efficacious drug for patients who have decreased blood volume or cardiac tamponade. Undesired tachycardia, hypertension, and emergence delirium may be attenuated with benzodiazepines.

Propofol

Propofol is the most recent intravenous anesthetic to be introduced into clinical practice, and is the most widely used drug for inductions.

Cardiovascular Effects

The hemodynamic effects of propofol have been investigated in healthy ASA Class I and II patients, elderly patients, patients with CAD and good left ventricular function, and in patients with impaired left ventricular function (see Table 7-1). Numerous studies have also compared the cardiovascular effects of propofol with other commonly used induction drugs, including the thiobarbiturates and etomidate. It is clear that with propofol, systolic arterial pressure falls 15% to 40% after intravenous induction with 2 mg/kg and maintenance infusion with 100 μg/kg/min. Similar changes are seen in both diastolic arterial pressure and MAP.

The effect of propofol on HR is variable. The majority of studies have demonstrated significant reductions in SVR (9% to 30%), CI, SV, and left ventricular stroke work index (LVSWI) after propofol. Although controversial, the evidence points to a dose-dependent decrease in myocardial contractility.[9,10]

OPIOIDS IN CARDIAC ANESTHESIA

Terminology and Classification

Various terms are commonly used to describe morphine-like drugs that are potent analgesics. The word *narcotic* is derived from the Greek word for "stupor" and refers to any drug that produces sleep. In legal terminology, it refers to any substance that produces addiction and physical dependence. Its use to describe morphine or morphine-like drugs is misleading and should be discouraged. Opiates refer to alkaloids and related synthetic and semisynthetic drugs that interact stereospecifically with one or more of the opioid receptors to produce a pharmacologic effect. The more encompassing term, *opioid*, also includes the endogenous opioids and is used. Opioids may be agonists, partial agonists, or antagonists.

Opioid Receptors

The existence of separate opioid receptors was shown by correlating analgesic activity to the chemical structure of many opioid compounds (Box 7-4). The idea of multiple opioid receptors is an accepted concept, and a number of subtypes for each class of opioid receptors have been identified. Through biochemical and pharmacologic methods, the μ-, δ-, and κ-receptors have been characterized. Pharmacologically, it is well known that δ-opioid receptors consist of two subtypes: δ_1 and δ_2.[11]

Opioid receptors involved in regulating the cardiovascular system have been localized centrally to the cardiovascular and respiratory centers of the hypothalamus and brainstem and peripherally to cardiac myocytes, blood vessels, nerve terminals, and the adrenal medulla. It is generally accepted that opioid receptors are differentially

7

BOX 7-4   *Opioids*

- The μ-, κ-, and δ-opioid receptors and endogenous opioid precursors have been identified in both cardiac and vascular tissue.
- The functional role of opioid precursors/opioid receptors in the cardiovascular system in physiologic and pathophysiologic conditions (e.g., congestive heart failure, arrhythmia development) are areas of ongoing investigation.
- The predominant cardiovascular effect of exogenously administered opioids is to attenuate central sympathetic outflow
- Endogenous opioids and opioid receptors, especially the delta-1 receptor, are likely important contributors in effecting both early and delayed preconditioning in the heart.
- Plasma drug concentrations are profoundly altered by cardiopulmonary bypass as a result of hemodilution, altered plasma protein binding, hypothermia, exclusion of the lungs from the circulation, and altered hemodynamics that likely modulate hepatic and renal blood flow. The specific effects are drug dependent.

distributed between atria and ventricles. The highest specific receptor density for binding of κ-agonists is in the right atrium and least in the left ventricle. As with the κ-opioid receptor, the distribution of the δ-opioid receptor favors atrial tissue and the right side of the heart more than the left.

Cardiac Effects of Opioids

At clinically relevant doses, the cardiovascular actions of opioids are limited. The actions opioids exhibit are mediated both by opioid receptors located centrally in specific areas of the brain and nuclei that regulate the control of cardiovascular function and peripherally by tissue-associated opioid receptors. The opioids in general exhibit a variety of complex pharmacologic actions on the cardiovascular system (Fig. 7-4).[12]

Most of the hemodynamic effects of opioids in humans can be related to their influence on the sympathetic outflow from the central nervous system. The pharmacologic modulation of sympathetic activity by centrally or peripherally acting drugs elicits cardioprotective effects.

All opioids, with the exception of meperidine, produce bradycardia, although morphine given to unpremedicated normal subjects may cause tachycardia. The mechanism of opioid-induced bradycardia is central vagal stimulation. Premedication with atropine can minimize but not totally eliminate opioid-induced bradycardia, especially in patients taking β-adrenoceptor antagonists. Although severe bradycardia should be avoided, moderate slowing of the HR may be beneficial in patients with CAD by decreasing myocardial oxygen consumption.

Hypotension can occur after even small doses of morphine and is primarily related to decreases in SVR. The most important mechanism responsible for these changes is probably histamine release. The amount of histamine release is reduced by slow administration (<10 mg/min). Pretreatment with an H_1 or H_2 antagonist does not block these reactions, but they are significantly attenuated by combined H_1 and H_2 antagonist pretreatment. Opioids may also have a direct action on vascular smooth muscle, independent of histamine release.[13]

Cardioprotective Effects of Exogenous Opioid Agonists

In 1996, Schultz and colleagues were the first to demonstrate that an opioid could attenuate ischemia-reperfusion damage in the heart. Morphine at the dose of 300 μg/kg was given before left anterior descending coronary artery occlusion

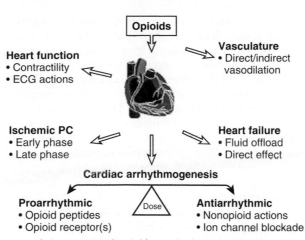

Figure 7-4 Some of the actions of opioids on the heart and cardiovascular system. Opioid actions may either involve direct opioid receptor-mediated actions, such as the involvement of the δ-opioid receptor in ischemic preconditioning (PC) or indirect, dose-dependent, non–opioid receptor–mediated actions such as ion channel blockade associated with the antiarrhythmic actions of opioids.

for 30 minutes in rats in vivo. Infarct area/area at risk was diminished from 54% to 12% by this treatment.[14] The infarct-reducing effect of morphine has been shown in hearts in situ, isolated hearts, and cardiomyocytes. Morphine also improved postischemic contractility. It is now well accepted that morphine provides protection against ischemia-reperfusion injury.[15] Fentanyl has been studied in a limited fashion and has had mixed results as far as its ability to protect the myocardium.[16] This may be due to differences in species studied and/or fentanyl concentrations.

Opioids in Cardiac Anesthesia

A technique of anesthesia for cardiac surgery involving high doses of morphine was developed in the late 1960s and early 1970s. This was based on the observation by Lowenstein and associates that patients requiring mechanical ventilation after surgery for end-stage VHD tolerated large doses of morphine for sedation without discernible circulatory effects. When they attempted to administer equivalent doses of morphine as the anesthetic for patients undergoing cardiac surgery, they discovered serious disadvantages, including inadequate anesthesia, even at doses of 8 to 11 mg/kg, episodes of hypotension related to histamine release, and increased intraoperative and postoperative blood and fluid requirements. Attempts to overcome these problems by combining lower doses of morphine with a variety of supplements (such as N_2O, halothane, or diazepam) proved unsatisfactory, resulting in significant myocardial depression, with decreases in CO and hypotension.

Because of these problems associated with the use of morphine, several other opioids were investigated in an attempt to find a suitable alternative. The use of fentanyl in cardiac anesthesia was first reported by Stanley and Webster in 1978. Since then there have been extensive investigations of fentanyl, as well as sufentanil and alfentanil, in cardiac surgery. The fentanyl group of opioids has proved to be the most reliable and effective for producing anesthesia both for patients with valvular disorders and CABG.

7

A major advantage of fentanyl and its analogs for patients undergoing cardiac surgery is their lack of cardiovascular depression.[17] This is of particular importance during the induction of anesthesia, when episodes of hypotension can be critical. Cardiovascular stability may be less evident during surgery; in particular, the period of sternotomy, pericardiectomy, and aortic root dissection may be associated with significant hypertension and tachycardia. During and after sternotomy, arterial hypertension, increases in SVR, and decreases in CO frequently occur. The variability in the hemodynamic responses to surgical stimulation, even with similar doses of fentanyl, is probably a reflection of differences in the patient populations studied by different authors. One factor is the influence of β-blocking agents. In patients undergoing CABG anesthetized with fentanyl, 86% of those not taking β-adrenergic blockers became hypertensive during sternal spread versus only 33% of those who were taking these agents.

The degree of myocardial impairment will also influence the response. Critically ill patients or patients with significant myocardial dysfunction appear to require lower doses of opioid for anesthesia. This may reflect altered pharmacokinetics in those patients. A decrease in liver blood flow consequent to decreased CO and congestive heart failure reduces plasma clearance. Thus, patients with poor left ventricular function may develop higher plasma and brain concentrations for a given loading dose or infusion rate than patients with good left ventricular function. Additionally, patients with depressed myocardial function may lack the ability to respond to surgical stress by increasing CO in the presence of progressive increases in SVR.

EFFECTS OF CARDIOPULMONARY BYPASS ON PHARMACOKINETICS AND PHARMACODYNAMICS

The institution of cardiopulmonary bypass has profound effects on the plasma concentration, distribution, and elimination of administered drugs. The major factors responsible for this are hemodilution and altered plasma protein binding, hypotension, hypothermia, pulsatile versus nonpulsatile flow, isolation of the lungs from the circulation, and uptake of anesthetic drugs by the bypass circuit. These changes result in altered blood concentrations, which are also dependent on particular pharmacokinetics of the drug in question.[18]

Hemodilution

At the onset of CPB, the circuit priming fluid is mixed with the patient's blood. In adults, the priming volume is 1.5 to 2 L and the prime may be crystalloid or may be crystalloid combined with blood or colloid. The overall result is a reduction in the patient's packed cell volume (PCV) to approximately 25% with an increase in plasma volume of 40% to 50%. This will decrease the total blood concentration of any free drug present in the blood. At the time of initiation of CPB, there is an immediate reduction in the levels of circulating proteins such as albumin and α_1-acid glycoprotein. This affects the protein binding of drugs due to alteration in the ratio of bound-to-free drug in the circulation.

In the blood, drugs exist as free (unbound) drug in equilibrium with bound (i.e., bound to plasma proteins) drug. It is the free drug that interacts with the receptor to produce the drug effect. Drugs are primarily bound to plasma protein albumin and α_1-acid glycoprotein. Changes in protein binding are of clinical significance only for drugs that are highly protein bound. The degree of drug-protein binding depends on the total drug concentration, the affinity of the protein for the drug, and the presence of other substances that may compete with the drug or alter the drug's binding site. If the drug in question has high plasma protein binding, then hemodilution results in a potentially relatively larger increase in free fraction than for a drug with low plasma protein binding.

Blood Flow

Hepatic, renal, cerebral, and skeletal perfusion have all been shown to be reduced during CPB, and the use of vasodilators and vasoconstrictor agents to regulate arterial pressure may further change regional blood flow. These alterations in regional blood flow distribution have implications for drug distribution and metabolism. The combination of hypotension, hypothermia, and nonpulsatile blood flow has significant impact on distribution of the circulation, with a marked reduction in peripheral flow and relative preservation of the central circulation.

CPB may be conducted with or without pulsatile perfusion. Nonpulsatile perfusion is associated with altered tissue perfusion. Nonpulsatile flow and decreased peripheral perfusion from CPB and hypothermia, as well as the administration of vasoconstrictors, may result in cellular hypoxia and probable intracellular acidosis. This may affect the tissue distribution of drugs whose tissue binding is sensitive to pH. On reperfusion, rewarming, and the reestablishment of normal cardiac (pulsatile) function, redistribution of drugs from poorly perfused tissue is likely to add to the systemic plasma concentration, as basic drugs will have been "trapped" in acidic tissue.

Hypothermia

Hypothermia is commonly used and has been shown to reduce hepatic and possibly renal enzyme function. Hypothermia depresses metabolism by inhibiting enzyme function and reduces tissue perfusion by increasing blood viscosity and activation of autonomic and endocrine reflexes to produce vasoconstriction. Hepatic enzymatic activity is decreased during hypothermia, and in addition there is marked intrahepatic redistribution of blood flow with the development of significant intrahepatic shunting. Hypothermia thus reduces metabolic drug clearance and has been shown to reduce the metabolism of propranolol and verapamil. Altered renal drug excretion occurs as a result of decreased renal perfusion, glomerular filtration rate, and tubular secretion. In dogs, glomerular filtration rate is decreased by 65% at 25°C.

Sequestration

When normothermia is reestablished, reperfusion of tissue might lead to washout of drug sequestered during the hypothermic CPB period. This may be one explanation for the increase in opioid plasma levels during the rewarming period.

Many drugs bind to components of the CPB circuit, and their distribution may be affected by changes in circuit design, for example, the use of membrane versus bubble oxygenators. In vitro, various oxygenators bind lipophilic agents such as volatile anesthetic agents, propofol, opioids, and barbiturates.[19,20]

During CPB, the lungs are isolated from the circulation with the pulmonary artery blood flow being interrupted. Basic drugs (lidocaine, propranolol, fentanyl) that are taken up by the lungs are therefore sequestered during CPB, and the lungs may serve as a reservoir for drug release when systemic reperfusion is established. Following the onset of CPB, plasma fentanyl concentrations decrease acutely and then plateau. However, when mechanical ventilation of the lungs is instituted before separation from CPB, plasma fentanyl concentrations increase. During CPB, pulmonary artery fentanyl concentrations exceed radial artery levels, but when mechanical ventilation resumes, the pulmonary artery/radial artery ratio is reversed, suggesting that fentanyl is being washed out from the lungs.

SUMMARY

- The observed acute effect of any specific anesthetic agent on the cardiovascular system represents the net effect on the myocardium, coronary blood flow, electrophysiologic behavior, vasculature, and neurohormonal reflex function.
- Volatile agents cause dose-dependent decreases in systemic blood pressure that for halothane and enflurane are mainly due to depression of contractile function and for isoflurane, desflurane, and sevoflurane are mainly due to decreases in systemic vascular resistance. Volatile anesthetic agents cause dose-dependent depression of contractile function mediated at a cellular level by attenuating calcium currents and decreasing calcium sensitivity. Decreases in systemic vascular responses reflect variable effects on both endothelium-dependent and endothelium-independent mechanisms.
- The net effect of volatile agents on coronary blood flow is determined by several variables, including anesthetic effects on systemic hemodynamics, myocardial metabolism, and direct effects on the coronary vasculature.
- Volatile anesthetic agents have been demonstrated to attenuate myocardial ischemia development by mechanisms that are independent of myocardial oxygen supply and demand and to facilitate functional recovery in stunned myocardium. Volatile agents can also simulate ischemic preconditioning, a phenomenon described as anesthetic preconditioning, and the underlying mechanisms are similar to those underlying ischemic preconditioning.
- The intravenous induction agents/hypnotics belong to different drug classes (barbiturates, benzodiazepines, N-methyl-D-aspartate receptor antagonists, and α_2-adrenergic receptor agonists). Although they all induce hypnosis, their sites of action and molecular targets differ based on their class.
- Induction agents inhibit cardiac contractility and relax vascular tone by inhibiting mechanisms that increase intracellular Ca^{2+}. The cumulative effects of the induction agents on contractility and vascular resistance and capacitance are mediated predominantly by their sympatholytic effects. These agents should be used with caution in patients with shock, heart failure, or other pathophysiologic circumstances in which the sympathetic nervous system is paramount in maintaining myocardial contractility and arterial and venous tone.
- Opioids exhibit diverse chemical structures, but all retain an essential T-shaped component necessary stereochemically for the activation of the different opioid receptors (the μ-, κ-, and δ-receptors).
- Acute exogenous opioid administration modulates multiple determinants of central and peripheral cardiovascular regulation. However, the predominant clinical effect is mediated by attenuation of central sympathetic outflow.
- Activation of the δ-opioid receptor can elicit preconditioning.

REFERENCES

1. Harkin CP, Pagel PS, Kersten JR, et al: Direct inotropic and lusitropic effects of sevoflurane. Anesthesiology 72:659, 1994
2. Tanaka K, Ludwig LM, Kersten JR, et al: Mechanisms of cardioprotection by volatile anesthetics. Anesthesiology 100:707, 2004
3. Kloner RA, Jennings RB: Consequences of brief ischemia: Stunning, preconditioning, and their clinical implications: I. Circulation 104:2981, 2001
4. Sprung J, Ogletree-Hughes ML, McConnell BK, et al: The effects of propofol on the contractility of failing and nonfailing human heart muscle. Anesth Analg 93:550, 2001

5. Zaidan J, Klochany A, Martin W, et al: Effect of thiopental on neurologic outcome following coronary artery bypass grafting. Anesthesiology 74:406, 1991
6. Newman M, Reves J: Pro: Midazolam is the sedative of choice to supplement narcotic anesthesia. J Cardiothorac Vasc Anesth 7:615, 1993
7. Theil D, Stanley T, White W, et al: Midazolam and fentanyl continuous infusion anesthesia for cardiac surgery: A comparison of computer-assisted versus manual infusion systems. J Cardiothorac Vasc Anesth 7:300, 1993
8. Kates R, Stack R, Hill R, et al: General anesthesia for patients undergoing percutaneous transluminal coronary angioplasty during acute myocardial infarction. Anesth Analg 65:815, 1986
9. de Hert S, Vermeyen K, Adriensen H: Influence of thiopental, etomidate and propofol on regional myocardial function in the normal and acute ischemic heart segments. Anesth Analg 70:600, 1990
10. Mulier J, Wouters P, van Aken H, et al: Cardiodynamic effects of propofol in comparison with thiopental: assessment with a transesophageal echocardiographic approach. Anesth Analg 72:28, 1991
11. McDonald J, Lambert D: Opioid receptors. Cont Educ. Anaesth Crit Care Pain 5:1, 2005
12. Barron BA: Opioid peptides and heart. Cardiovasc Res 43:13, 1999
13. White DA, Reitan JA, Kien ND, et al: Decrease in vascular resistance in the isolated canine hindlimb after graded doses of alfentanil, fentanyl, and sufentanil, Anesth Analg 71:29, 1990
14. Schultz JJ, Hsu AK, Gross GJ: Morphine mimics the cardioprotective effect of ischemic preconditioning via a glibenclamide-sensitive mechanism in the rat heart. Circ Res 78:1100, 1996
15. Benedict PE, Benedict MB, Su TP, et al: Opiate drugs and delta-receptor–mediated myocardial protection. Circulation 100(19 suppl):II-357, 1999
16. Kato R, Ross S, Foëx P: Fentanyl protects the heart against ischemic injury via opioid receptors, adenosine A1 receptors and KATP channel linked mechanism in rats, Br J Anaesth 84:204, 2000
17. Howie MB, Cheng D, Newman MF, et al: A randomized double-blinded multicenter comparison of remifentanil versus fentanyl when combined with isoflurane/propofol for early extubation in coronary artery bypass graft surgery. Anesth Analg 92:1084, 2001
18. Wood M: Pharmacokinetics and principles of drug infusions in cardiac patients. In Kaplan JA (ed): Cardiac Anesthesia, 4th ed. Philadelphia, WB Saunders, 1999, pp 657-685
19. Hickey S, Goylor JD, Kenny GN: In vitro uptake and elimination of isoflurane by different membrane oxygenators. J Cardiothorac Vasc Anesth 10:352, 1996
20. Rosen DA, Rosen KR: Elimination of drugs and toxins during cardiopulmonary bypass. J Cardiothorac Vasc Anesth 11:337, 1997

7

Chapter 8

Cardiovascular Pharmacology

Roger L. Royster, MD • John F. Butterworth IV, MD •
Leanne Groban, MD • Thomas F. Slaughter, MD •
David A. Zvara, MD

ANTI-ISCHEMIC DRUG THERAPY

Anti-ischemic drug therapy during anesthesia is indicated whenever evidence of myocardial ischemia exists. The treatment of ischemia during anesthesia is complicated by the ongoing stress of surgery, blood loss, concurrent organ ischemia, and the patient's inability to interact with the anesthesiologist. Nonetheless, the fundamental principles of treatment remain the same as in the unanesthetized state. All events of myocardial ischemia involve an alteration in the oxygen supply/demand balance (Table 8-1). The 2007 American College of Cardiology/American Heart Association (ACC/AHA) Guidelines on the Management and Treatment of Patients with Unstable Angina and Non–ST-Segment Elevation Myocardial Infarction provide an excellent framework for the treatment of patients with ongoing myocardial ischemia.[1]

Nitroglycerin

Nitroglycerin (NTG) is clinically indicated as initial therapy in nearly all types of myocardial ischemia. Chronic exertional angina, de novo angina, unstable angina, Prinzmetal's angina (vasospasm), and silent ischemia respond to NTG

Table 8-1	Myocardial Ischemia: Factors Governing O_2 Supply and Demand	
O_2 Supply		O_2 Demand
Heart rate*		Heart rate*
O_2 content		Contractility
Hemoglobin, percent oxygen saturation, Pao_2		Wall tension
Coronary blood flow		Afterload
CPP = DBP − LVEDP*		Preload (LVEDP)*
Coronary vascular resistance		

CPP = coronary perfusion pressure; DBP = diastolic blood pressure; LVEDP = left ventricular end-diastolic pressure.
*Affects both supply and demand.
Modified from Royster RL: Intraoperative administration of inotropes in cardiac surgery patients. J Cardiothorac Anesth 6(Suppl 5):17, 1990.

administration. During intravenous therapy with NTG, if blood pressure (BP) drops and ischemia is not relieved, the addition of phenylephrine will allow coronary perfusion pressure (CPP) to be maintained while allowing higher doses of NTG to be used for ischemia relief. If reflex increases in heart rate (HR) and contractility occur, combination therapy with β-adrenergic blockers may be indicated to blunt this undesired increase in HR. Combination therapy with nitrates and calcium channel blockers may be an effective anti-ischemic regimen in selected patients; however, excessive hypotension and reflex tachycardia may be a problem, especially when a dihydropyridine calcium antagonist is used.

Mechanism of Action

NTG enhances myocardial oxygen delivery and reduces myocardial oxygen demand. NTG is a smooth muscle relaxant that causes vasculature dilation.[2] Nitrate-mediated vasodilation occurs with or without intact vascular endothelium. Nitrites, organic nitrites, nitroso compounds, and other nitrogen oxide–containing substances (e.g., nitroprusside) enter the smooth muscle cell and are converted to reactive nitric oxide (NO) or S-nitrosothiols, which stimulate guanylate cyclase metabolism to produce cyclic guanosine monophosphate (cGMP) (Fig. 8-1). A cGMP-dependent protein kinase is stimulated with resultant protein phosphorylation in the smooth muscle. This leads to a dephosphorylation of the myosin light chain and smooth muscle relaxation. Vasodilation is also associated with a reduction of intracellular calcium. Sulfhydryl (SH) groups are required for formation of NO and the stimulation of guanylate cyclase. When excessive amounts of SH groups are metabolized by prolonged exposure to NTG, vascular tolerance occurs. The addition of N-acetylcysteine, an SH donor, reverses NTG tolerance. The mechanism by which NTG compounds are uniquely better venodilators, especially at lower serum concentrations, is unknown but may be related to increased uptake of NTG by veins compared with arteries.[3]

Physiologic Effects

Two important physiologic effects of NTG are systemic and regional venous dilation. Venodilation can markedly reduce venous pressure, venous return to the heart, and cardiac filling pressures. Prominent venodilation occurs at lower doses and does not increase further as the NTG dose increases. Venodilation results primarily in pooling

8

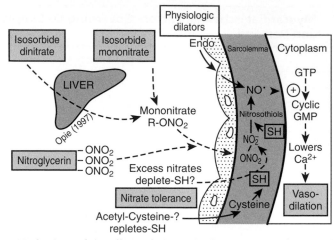

Figure 8-1 Mechanisms of the effects of nitrates in the generation of nitric oxide (NO•) and the stimulation of guanylate cyclase cyclic guanosine monophosphate (GMP), which mediates vasodilation. Sulfhydryl (SH) groups are required for the formation of NO• and the stimulation of guanylate cyclase. Isosorbide dinitrate is metabolized by the liver, whereas this route of metabolism is bypassed by the mononitrates. GTP=guanosine triphosphate. (Redrawn from Opie LH: Drugs for the Heart, 4th edition. Philadelphia, WB Saunders, 1995, p 33.)

of blood in the splanchnic capacitance system. Mesenteric blood volume increases as ventricular size, ventricular pressures, and intrapericardial pressure decrease.

NTG increases the distensibility and conductance of large arteries without changing systemic vascular resistance (SVR) at low doses. Improved compliance of the large arteries does not necessarily imply afterload reduction. At higher doses, NTG dilates smaller arterioles and resistance vessels, which reduces afterload and BP. Reductions in cardiac dimension and pressure reduce myocardial oxygen consumption (MVo_2) and improve myocardial ischemia. NTG may preferentially reduce cardiac preload while maintaining systemic perfusion pressure, an important hemodynamic effect in myocardial ischemia. However, in hypovolemic states, higher doses of NTG may markedly reduce systemic BP to dangerous levels. A reflex increase in HR may occur at arterial vasodilating doses.

NTG causes vasodilation of pulmonary arteries and veins and predictably decreases right atrial (RAP), pulmonary artery (PAP), and pulmonary capillary wedge pressures (PCWP). Pulmonary artery hypertension may be reduced in various disease states and in congenital heart disease with NTG.

NTG has several important effects on the coronary circulation (Box 8-1). NTG is a potent epicardial coronary artery vasodilator in both normal and diseased vessels. Stenotic lesions dilate with NTG, reducing the resistance to coronary blood flow (CBF) and improving myocardial ischemia. Smaller coronary arteries may dilate relatively more than larger coronary vessels; however, the degree of dilation may depend on the baseline tone of the vessel. NTG effectively reverses or prevents coronary artery vasospasm.

Total CBF may initially increase but eventually decreases with NTG despite coronary vasodilation. Autoregulatory mechanisms probably result in decreases in total flow as a result of reductions in wall tension and myocardial oxygen consumption. However, regional myocardial blood flow may improve by vasodilation of intercoronary collateral vessels or reduction of subendocardial compressive forces.

> ## BOX 8-1 *Effects of Nitroglycerin and Organic Nitrates on the Coronary Circulation*
>
> - Epicardial coronary artery dilation: small arteries dilate proportionately more than larger arteries
> - Increased coronary collateral vessel diameter and enhanced collateral flow
> - Improved subendocardial blood flow
> - Dilation of coronary atherosclerotic stenoses
> - Initial short-lived increase in coronary blood flow, later reduction in coronary blood flow as MV_{O_2} decreases
> - Reversal and prevention of coronary vasospasm and vasoconstriction
>
> Modified frgom Abrams J: Hemodynamic effects of nitroglycerin and long-acting nitrates. Am Heart J 110(part 2):216, 1985.

Coronary arteriographic studies in humans demonstrate that coronary collateral vessels increase in size after NTG administration. This effect may be especially important when epicardial vessels have subtotal or total occlusive disease. Improvement in collateral flow may also be protective in situations in which coronary artery steal may occur with other potent coronary vasodilator agents. The improvement in blood flow to the subendocardium, the most vulnerable area to the development of ischemia, is secondary to both improvement in collateral flow and reductions in left ventricular end-diastolic pressure (LVEDP), which reduce subendocardial resistance to blood flow. With the maintenance of an adequate CPP (e.g., with administration of phenylephrine), NTG can maximize subendocardial blood flow. The ratio of endocardial to epicardial blood in transmural segments is enhanced with NTG. Inhibition of platelet aggregation also occurs with NTG; however, the clinical significance of this action is unknown.

Intravenous Nitroglycerin

Nitroglycerin has been available since the early 1980s as an injectable drug with a stable shelf half-life in a 400-µg/mL solution of D_5W. Blood levels are achieved instantaneously, and arterial dilating doses with resulting hypotension may quickly occur. If the volume status of the patient is unknown, initial doses of 5 to 10 µg/min are recommended. The dose necessary for relieving myocardial ischemia may vary from patient to patient, but relief is usually achieved with 75 to 150 µg/min. In a clinical study of 20 patients with rest angina, a mean dose of 72 µg/min reduced or abolished ischemic episodes in 85% of patients. However, doses as high as 500 to 600 µg/min may be necessary for ischemic relief in some patients. Arterial dilation becomes clinically apparent at doses around 150 µg/min. Drug offset after discontinuation of an infusion is rapid (2 to 5 minutes). The dosage of NTG available is less when the drug is administered in plastic bags and polyvinylchloride tubing because of NTG absorption by the bag and tubing, although this is not a significant clinical problem because the drug is titrated to effect.

Summary

Nitroglycerin remains a first-line agent for the treatment of myocardial ischemia. Special care must be taken in patients with signs of hypovolemia or hypotension, because the vasodilating effects of the drug may worsen the clinical condition. Recommendations from the ACC/AHA on intraoperative use of NTG are given in Box 8-2.

BOX 8-2 *Recommendations for Intraoperative Nitroglycerin*

- Class I*   High-risk patients previously on nitroglycerin who have active signs of myocardial ischemia without hypotension.
- Class II†   As a prophylactic agent for high-risk patients to prevent myocardial ischemia and cardiac morbidity, particularly in those who have required nitrate therapy to control angina. The recommendation for prophylactic use of nitroglycerin must take into account the anesthetic plan and patient hemodynamics and must recognize that vasodilation and hypovolemia can readily occur during anesthesia and surgery.
- Class III‡ Patients with signs of hypovolemia or hypotension.

---

*Conditions for which there is evidence for and/or general agreement that a procedure be performed or a treatment is of benefit.

†Conditions for which there is a divergence of evidence and/or opinion about the treatment.

‡Conditions for which there is evidence and/or general agreement that the procedure is not necessary.

β-Adrenergic Blockers

β-Adrenergic blockers have multiple favorable effects in treating the ischemic heart during anesthesia (Box 8-3). They reduce oxygen consumption by decreasing HR, BP, and myocardial contractility. HR reduction increases diastolic CBF. Increased collateral blood flow and redistribution of blood to ischemic areas may occur with β-blockers. More free fatty acids may be available for substrate consumption by the myocardium. Microcirculatory oxygen delivery improves, and oxygen dissociates more easily from hemoglobin after β-adrenergic blockade. Platelet aggregation is inhibited. β-Blockers should be started early in ischemic patients in the absence of contraindications. Many patients at high risk of perioperative cardiac morbidity should be started on β-blocker therapy before surgery and continued on this therapy for up to 30 days after surgery.

Perioperative administration of β-adrenergic blockers reduces both mortality and morbidity when given to patients at high risk for coronary artery disease who must undergo noncardiac surgery.[4] These data suggest that intermediate- and high-risk patients presenting for noncardiac surgery should receive perioperative β-adrenergic blockade to reduce postoperative cardiac mortality and morbidity. Recommendations on the perioperative use of β-adrenergic blockade for noncardiac surgery are given in Box 8-4.

Physiologic Effects

ANTI-ISCHEMIC EFFECTS

β-Blockade on the ischemic heart may result in a favorable shift in the oxygen demand/ supply ratio.[5] The reductions in the force of contraction and HR reduce myocardial oxygen consumption and result in autoregulatory decreases in myocardial blood flow. Several studies have shown that blood flow to ischemic regions is maintained with propranolol.

ANTIHYPERTENSIVE EFFECTS

Both β_1- and β_2-receptor blockers inhibit myocardial contractility and reduce HR; both effects should reduce BP. No acute decrease in BP occurs during acute administration of propranolol. However, chronic BP reduction has been attributed to a chronic reduction in cardiac output (CO). Reductions in high levels of plasma renin have been suggested as effective therapy in controlling essential hypertension.

ELECTROPHYSIOLOGIC EFFECTS

Generalized slowing of cardiac depolarization results from reducing the rate of diastolic depolarization (phase 4). Action potential duration and the QT interval may

---

> **BOX 8-3** *Effects of β-Adrenergic Blockers on Myocardial Ischemia*
>
> - Reductions in myocardial oxygen consumption
> - Improvements in coronary blood flow
> - Prolonged diastolic perfusion period
> - Improved collateral flow
> - Increased flow to ischemic areas
> - Overall improvement in supply/demand ratio
> - Stabilization of cellular membranes
> - Improved oxygen dissociation from hemoglobin
> - Inhibition of platelet aggregation
> - Reduced mortality after myocardial infarction

> **BOX 8-4** *Recommendations for Perioperative Medical Therapy*
>
> - Class I   β-Blockers required in the recent past to control symptoms of angina or symptomatic arrhythmias or hypertension; β-blockers: patients at high cardiac risk, owing to the finding of ischemia on preoperative testing, who are undergoing vascular surgery
> - Class IIa   β-Blockers: preoperative assessment identifies untreated hypertension, known coronary disease, or major risk factors for coronary disease
> - Class III   β-Blockers: contraindication to β-blockade
>
> Adapted from Eagle KA, Berger PB, Calkins H, et al: ACC/AHA guideline update for perioperative cardiovascular evaluation for noncardiac surgery-executive summary: A report of the American College of Cardiology/American Heart Association Task Force on Practice Guidelines (Committee to Update the 1996 Guidelines on Perioperative Cardiovascular Evaluation for Noncardiac Surgery). J Am Coll Cardiol 39:542, 2002.

shorten with β-adrenergic blockers. The ventricular fibrillation threshold is increased with β-blockers. These antiarrhythmic actions of β-blockers are enhanced in settings of catecholamine excess, such as in pheochromocytoma, acute myocardial infarction, the perioperative period, and hyperthyroidism.

Pharmacology of Intravenous β-Adrenergic Blockers

PROPRANOLOL

Propranolol has an equal affinity for β_1- and β_2-receptors, lacks intrinsic sympathomimetic activity (ISA), and has no α-adrenergic receptor activity. It is the most lipid-soluble β-blocker and generally has the most central nervous system side effects. First-pass liver metabolism (90%) is very high, requiring much higher oral doses than intravenous doses for pharmacodynamic effect.

The usual intravenous dose of propranolol initially is 0.5 to 1.0 mg titrated to effect. A titrated dose resulting in maximum pharmacologic serum levels is 0.1 mg/kg. The use of continuous infusions of propranolol has been reported after noncardiac surgery in patients with cardiac disease. A continuous infusion of 1 to 3 mg/hr can prevent tachycardia and hypertension but must be used cautiously because of the potential of cumulative effects.

METOPROLOL

Metoprolol was the first clinically used cardioselective β-blocker (Table 8-2). Its affinity for β_1-receptors is 30 times higher than its affinity for β_2-receptors, as demonstrated by radioligand binding. Metoprolol is lipid soluble, with 50% of the drug metabolized during first-pass hepatic metabolism and with only 3%

123

excreted renally. Protein binding is less than 10%. Metoprolol's serum half-life is 3 to 4 hours.

As with any cardioselective β-blocker, higher serum levels may result in greater incidence of β_2-blocking effects. Metoprolol is administered intravenously in 1- to 2-mg doses, titrated to effect. The potency of metoprolol is approximately one half that of propranolol. Maximum β-blocker effect is achieved with 0.2 mg/kg given intravenously.

ESMOLOL

Esmolol's chemical structure is similar to that of metoprolol and propranolol, except it has a methylester group in the para position of the phenyl ring, making it susceptible to rapid hydrolysis by red blood cell esterases (9-minute half-life). Esmolol is not metabolized by plasma cholinesterase. Hydrolysis results in an acid metabolite and methanol with clinically insignificant levels. Ninety percent of the drug is eliminated in the form of the acid metabolite, normally within 24 hours. A loading dose of 500 µg/kg given intravenously, followed by a 50- to 300- µg/kg/min infusion, will reach steady-state concentrations within 5 minutes. Without the loading dose, steady-state concentrations are reached in 30 minutes.

Esmolol is cardioselective, blocking primarily β_1-receptors. It lacks ISA and membrane-stabilizing effects and is mildly lipid soluble. Esmolol produced significant reductions in BP, HR, and cardiac index after a loading dose of 500 µg/kg and an infusion of 300 µg/kg/min in patients with coronary artery disease, and the effects were completely reversed 30 minutes after discontinuation of the infusion. Initial therapy during anesthesia may require significant reductions in both the loading and infusion doses.

Hypotension is a common side effect of intravenous esmolol. The incidence of hypotension was higher with esmolol (36%) than with propranolol (6%) at equal therapeutic endpoints. The cardioselective drugs may cause more hypotension because of β_1-induced myocardial depression and the failure to block β_2 peripheral vasodilation. Esmolol appears safe in patients with bronchospastic disease. In another comparative study with propranolol, esmolol and placebo did not change airway resistance whereas 50% of patients treated with propranolol developed clinically significant bronchospasm.

LABETALOL

Labetalol provides selective α_1-receptor blockade and nonselective β_1- and β_2-blockade. The potency of β-adrenergic blockade is 5- to 10-fold greater than α_1-adrenergic blockade. Labetalol has partial β_2-agonist effects that promote vasodilation. Labetalol is moderately lipid soluble and is completely absorbed after oral administration. First-pass hepatic metabolism is significant with production of inactive metabolites. Renal excretion of the unchanged drug is minimal. Elimination half-life is approximately 6 hours.

In contrast to other β-blockers, clinically, labetalol should be considered a peripheral vasodilator that does not cause a reflex tachycardia. BP and systolic vascular resistance decrease after an intravenous dose. Stroke volume (SV) and CO remain unchanged, with HR decreasing slightly. The reduction in BP is dose related, and acutely hypertensive patients usually respond within 3 to 5 minutes after a bolus dose of 100 to 250 µg/kg. However, the more critically ill or anesthetized patients should have their BP titrated beginning with 5- to 10-mg intravenous increments. Reduction in BP may last as long as 6 hours after intravenous dosing.

Summary

β-Adrenergic blockers are first-line agents in the treatment of myocardial ischemia. These agents effectively reduce myocardial work and oxygen demand. There is growing evidence that β-adrenergic-blocking agents may play a significant role in reducing perioperative cardiac morbidity and mortality in noncardiac surgery.[6]

Table 8-2 Properties of β-Blockers in Clinical Use

Drug	Selectivity	Partial Agonist Activity	Usual Dose for Angina
Propranolol	None	No	20 to 80 mg twice daily
Metoprolol	β_1	No	50 to 200 mg twice daily
Atenolol	β_1	No	50 to 200 mg/d
Nadolol	None	No	40 to 80 mg/d
Timolol	None	No	10 mg twice daily
Acebutolol	β_1	Yes	200 to 600 mg twice daily
Betaxolol	β_1	No	10 to 20 mg/d
Bisoprolol	β_1	No	10 mg/d
Esmolol (intravenous)	β_1	No	50 to 300 µg/kg/min
Labetalol*	None	Yes	200 to 600 mg twice daily
Pindolol	None	Yes	2.5 to 7.5 mg 3 times daily

*Labetalol is a combined α- and β-blocker.
Adapted from Gibbons RJ, Chatterjee K, Daley J, et al: ACC/AHA/ACP-ASIM Guidelines for the Management of Patients with Chronic Stable Angina: A report of the American College of Cardiology/American Heart Association Task Force on Practice Guidelines (Committee on the Management of Patients with Chronic Stable Angina). J Am Coll Cardiol 33:2092, 1999.

Calcium Channel Blockers

Calcium channel blockers reduce myocardial oxygen demands by depression of contractility, HR, and/or decreased arterial BP.[7] Myocardial oxygen supply may be improved by dilation of coronary and collateral vessels. Calcium channel blockers are used primarily for symptom control in patients with stable angina pectoris. In an acute ischemic situation, calcium channel blockers (verapamil and diltiazem) may be used for rate control in situations when β-blockers cannot be used. The most important effects of calcium channel blockers, however, may be the treatment of variant angina. These drugs can attenuate ergonovine-induced coronary vasoconstriction in patients with variant angina, suggesting protection via coronary dilation. Most episodes of silent myocardial ischemia, which may account for 70% of all transient ischemic episodes, are not related to increases in myocardial oxygen demands (HR and BP) but, rather, intermittent obstruction of coronary flow likely caused by coronary vasoconstriction or spasm. All calcium channel blockers are effective at reversing coronary spasm, reducing ischemic episodes, and reducing NTG consumption in patients with variant or Prinzmetal's angina. Combinations of NTG and calcium channel blockers, which also effectively relieve and possibly prevent coronary spasm, are at present rational therapy for variant angina. β-Blockers may aggravate anginal episodes in some patients with vasospastic angina and should be used with caution. Preservation of CBF with calcium channel blockers is a significant difference from the predominant β-blocker anti-ischemic effects of reducing myocardial oxygen consumption.

Calcium channel blockers have proven effective in controlled trials of stable angina. However, rapid-acting dihydropyridines such as nifedipine may cause a reflex tachycardia, especially during initial therapy, and exacerbate anginal symptoms. Such proischemic effects probably explain why the short-acting dihydropyridine

8

nifedipine in high doses produced adverse effects in patients with unstable angina. The introduction of long-acting dihydropyridines such as extended-release nifedipine, amlodipine, felodipine, isradipine, nicardipine, and nisoldipine has led to fewer adverse events. These agents should be used in combination with β-blockers. Some patients may have symptomatic relief improved more with calcium channel blockers than with β-blocker therapy.

Calcium Channels

Calcium channels are functional pores in membranes through which calcium flows down an electrochemical gradient when the channels are open. Calcium channels exist in cardiac muscle, smooth muscle, and probably many other cellular membranes. These channels are also present in cellular organelle membranes such as the sarcoplasmic reticulum and mitochondria. Calcium functions as a primary generator of the cardiac action potential and an intracellular second messenger to regulate various intracellular events.

Calcium enters cellular membranes through voltage-dependent channels or receptor-operated channels. The voltage-dependent channels depend on a transmembrane potential for activation (opening). Receptor-operated channels either are linked to a voltage-dependent channel after receptor stimulation or directly allow calcium passage through cell or organelle membranes independent of transmembrane potentials.

There are three types of voltage-dependent channels: the T (transient), L (long-lasting), and N (neuronal) channels. The T and L channels are located in cardiac and smooth muscle tissue, whereas the N channels are located only in neural tissue. The T channel is activated at low voltages (−50 mV) in cardiac tissue, plays a major role in cardiac depolarization (phase 0), and is not blocked by calcium antagonists. The L channels are the classic "slow" channels, are activated at higher voltages (−30 mV), and are responsible for phase 2 of the cardiac action potential. These channels are blocked by calcium antagonists.

Calcium channel blockers interact with the L-type calcium channel and are composed of drugs from four different classes: (1) the 1,4-dihydropyridine (DHP) derivatives (nifedipine, nimodipine, nicardipine, isradipine, amlodipine, and felodipine); (2) the phenylalkyl amines (verapamil); (3) the benzothiazepines (diltiazem); and (4) a diarylaminopropylamine ether (bepridil). The L-type calcium channel has specific receptors, which bind to each of the different chemical classes of calcium channel blockers.

Physiologic Effects

HEMODYNAMIC EFFECTS

Systemic hemodynamic effects of calcium channel blockers represent a complex interaction among myocardial depression, vasodilation, and reflex activation of the autonomic nervous system (Table 8-3).

Nifedipine, like all dihydropyridines, is a potent arterial dilator with few veno-dilating effects. Reflex activation of the sympathetic nervous system may increase HR. The intrinsic negative inotropic effect of nifedipine is offset by potent arterial dilation, which results in lowering of BP and increase in CO in patients. Dihydropyridines are excellent antihypertensive agents, owing to their arterial vasodilatory effects. Antianginal effects result from reduced myocardial oxygen requirements secondary to the afterload-reducing effect and to coronary vascular dilation resulting in improved myocardial oxygen delivery.

Verapamil is a less potent arterial dilator than the dihydropyridines and results in less reflex sympathetic activation. In vivo, verapamil generally results in

II

Table 8-3 **Calcium Channel Blocker Vasodilator Potency and Inotropic, Chronotropic, and Dromotropic Effects on the Heart**

	Amlodipine	Diltiazem	Nifedipine	Verapamil
Heart rate	↑/0	↓	↑/0	↓
Sinoatrial node conduction	0	↓↓	0	↓
Atrioventricular node conduction	0	↓	0	↓
Myocardial contractility	↓/0	↓	↓/0	↓↓
Neurohormonal activation	↑/0	↑	↑	↑
Vascular dilatation	↑↑	↑	↑↑	↑
Coronary flow	↑	↑	↑	↑

From Eisenberg MJ, Brox A, Bestawros AN. Calcium channel blockers: An update. Am J Med 116:35, 2004.

moderate vasodilation without significant change in HR, CO, or SV. Verapamil can significantly depress myocardial function in patients with preexisting ventricular dysfunction.

Diltiazem is a less potent vasodilator and has fewer negative inotropic effects compared with verapamil. Studies in patients reveal reductions in SVR and BP, with increases in CO, pulmonary artery wedge pressure, and ejection fraction. Diltiazem attenuates baroreflex increases in HR secondary to NTG and decreases in HR secondary to phenylephrine. Regional blood flow to the brain and kidney increases, whereas skeletal muscle flow does not change. In contrast to verapamil, diltiazem is not as likely to aggravate congestive heart failure, although it should be used carefully in these patients.

Coronary Blood Flow

Coronary artery dilation occurs with the calcium channel blockers with increases in total CBF. Nifedipine is the most potent coronary vasodilator, especially in epicardial vessels, which are prone to coronary vasospasm. Diltiazem is effective in blocking coronary artery vasoconstriction caused by a variety of agents, including α-agonists, serotonin, prostaglandin, and acetylcholine.

Electrophysiologic Effects

Calcium channel blockers exert their primary electrophysiologic effects on tissue of the conducting system that is dependent on calcium for generation of the action potential, primarily at the sinoatrial (SA) and atrioventricular (AV) nodes. They do not alter the effective refractory period of atrial, ventricular, or His-Purkinje tissue. Diltiazem and verapamil exert these electrophysiologic effects in vivo and in vitro, whereas the electrophysiologic depression of the dihydropyridines (nifedipine) is completely attenuated by reflex sympathetic activation. Nifedipine actually can enhance SA and AV node conduction, whereas verapamil and diltiazem slow conduction velocity and prolong refractoriness of nodal tissue.

8

Pharmacology

NIFEDIPINE

Nifedipine was the first dihydropyridine derivative to be used clinically. Other dihydropyridines available for clinical use include nicardipine, isradipine, amlodipine, felodipine, and nimodipine. In contrast to the other calcium channel blockers, nimodipine is highly lipid soluble and penetrates the blood-brain barrier. It is indicated for vascular spasm after intracerebral bleeding.

Nifedipine's oral bioavailability is approximately 70%, with peak plasma levels occurring within 30 to 45 minutes. Protein binding is 95%, and elimination half-life is approximately 5 hours. Nifedipine is available for oral administration in capsular form. The compound degenerates in the presence of light and moisture, preventing commercially available intravenous preparations. Puncture of the capsule and sublingual administration provide an onset of effects in 2 to 3 minutes.

NICARDIPINE

Nicardipine is a dihydropyridine agent with a longer half-life than nifedipine and with vascular selectivity for coronary and cerebrovascular beds. Nicardipine may be the most potent overall relaxant of vascular smooth muscle among the dihydropyridines. Peak plasma levels are reached 1 hour after oral administration, with bioavailability of 35%. Plasma half-life is 8 to 9 hours. Although the drug undergoes extensive hepatic metabolism with less than 1% of the drug excreted renally, greater renal elimination occurs in some patients. Plasma levels may increase in patients with renal failure; reduction of the dose is recommended in these patients.

Verapamil

Verapamil's structure is similar to that of papaverine. Verapamil exhibits significant first-pass hepatic metabolism, with a bioavailability of only 10% to 20%. One hepatic metabolite, norverapamil, is active and has a potency approximately 20% of that of verapamil. Peak plasma levels are reached within 30 minutes. Bioavailability markedly increases in hepatic insufficiency, mandating reduced doses. Intravenous verapamil achieves hemodynamic and dromotropic effects within minutes, peaking at 15 minutes and lasting up to 6 hours. Accumulation of the drug occurs with prolonged half-life during long-term oral administration.

Diltiazem

After oral dosing, the bioavailability of diltiazem is greater than that of verapamil, varying between 25% and 50%. Peak plasma concentration is achieved between 30 and 60 minutes, and elimination half-life is 2 to 6 hours. Protein binding is approximately 80%. As with verapamil, hepatic clearance is flow dependent and major hepatic metabolism occurs with metabolites having 40% of the clinical activity of diltiazem. Hepatic disease may require decreased dosing, whereas renal failure does not affect dosing.

Significant Adverse Effects

Most significant adverse hemodynamic effects can be predicted from the calcium channel blockers' primary effects of vasodilation and negative inotropy, chronotropy, and dromotropy. Hypotension, heart failure, bradycardia and asystole, and AV nodal block have occurred with calcium channel blockers. These side effects are more likely to occur with combination therapy with β-blockers or digoxin, in the presence of hypokalemia.

Summary

Calcium antagonists provide excellent symptom control in patients with unstable angina. In the absence of β-adrenergic blockade, the short-acting dihydropyridine nifedipine may increase the risk of myocardial infarction or recurrent angina. When β-adrenergic blockers cannot be used, and HR slowing is indicated, verapamil and diltiazem may offer an alternative.[8]

DRUG THERAPY FOR SYSTEMIC HYPERTENSION

Systemic hypertension, long recognized as a leading cause of cardiovascular morbidity and mortality, accounts for enormous health-related expenditures. Nearly a fourth of the U.S. population has hypertensive vascular disease; however, 30% of these individuals are unaware of their condition and another 30% to 50% are inadequately treated. On a worldwide basis, nearly 1 billion individuals are hypertensive. Hypertension management comprises the most common reason underlying adult visits to primary care physicians, and antihypertensive drugs are the most prescribed medication class.

The Seventh Report of the Joint National Committee on Prevention, Detection, Evaluation, and Treatment of High Blood Pressure (JNC-7 Report) defined systolic BPs (Table 8-4) exceeding 140 mm Hg and diastolic BPs exceeding 90 mm Hg as stage 1 hypertension. BPs less than 120/80 mm Hg were defined as normal and those in between as consistent with "prehypertension."[9]

Risk for cardiovascular disease appears to increase at BPs exceeding 115/75 mm Hg, with a doubling in risk associated with each 20/10-mm Hg increment in systemic pressure. Thus, the most recent JNC-7 report recommends drug therapy for "prehypertensive" disease in patients with "compelling indications," such as chronic renal disease or diabetes. Antihypertensive therapy generally is targeted to achieve systemic BPs of less than 140/90 mm Hg; however, for high-risk patients such as those with diabetes or renal or cardiovascular disease, lower BP targets are suggested, typically less than 130/80 mm Hg.

Medical Treatment for Hypertension

More than 80 distinct medications are marketed for treatment of hypertension (Table 8-5). Often, combined therapy with two or more classes of antihypertensive medications may be needed to achieve treatment goals (Table 8-6). Although the specific drug selected for initial therapy now has been deemed less important than in the past, recognition that specific antihypertensive drug classes alleviate end-organ damage, beyond that simply associated with reductions in systemic BP, has led to targeted selection of antihypertensive drug combinations on the basis of coexisting risk factors such as recent myocardial infarction, chronic renal insufficiency, or diabetes.[10]

Management of Severe Hypertension

For purposes of characterizing treatment urgency, severe hypertension is characterized as either a hypertensive *emergency* with target organ injury (e.g., myocardial ischemia, stroke, pulmonary edema) or a hypertensive *urgency* with severe elevations in BP not yet associated with target organ damage. Chronic elevations in BP, even when of a severe nature, do not necessarily require urgent intervention and often may be managed with oral antihypertensive therapy on an outpatient basis. In contrast, a hypertensive emergency

Table 8-4 Classification and Management of Blood Pressure for Adults Aged 18 Years or Older

BP Classification	Systolic BP* (mm Hg)		Diastolic BP* (mm Hg)	Lifestyle Modification	Management* Initial Drug Therapy	
					Without Compelling Indication	With Compelling Indication
Normal	<120	and	<80	Encourage	No antihypertensive drug indicated	Drug(s) for the compelling indications†
Prehypertension	120 to 139	or	80 to 89	Yes		
Stage 1 hypertension	140 to 159	or	90 to 99	Yes	Thiazide-type diuretics for most; may consider ACE inhibitor, ARB, β-blocker, CCB, or combination	Drug(s) for the compelling indications Other antihypertensive drugs (diuretics, ACE inhibitor, ARB, β-blocker, CCB) as needed
Stage 2 hypertension	≥160	or	≥100	Yes	Two-drug combination for most (usually thiazide-type diuretic and ACE inhibitor or ARB or β-blocker or CCB)‡	Drug(s) for the compelling indications Other antihypertensive drugs (diuretics, ACE inhibitor, ARB, β-blocker, CCB) as needed

ACE = angiotensin-converting enzyme; ARB = angiotensin-receptor blocker; BP = blood pressure; CCB = calcium channel blocker.
*Treatment determined by highest BP category.
†Treat patients with chronic kidney disease or diabetes to BP goal or < 130/80 mm Hg.
‡Initial combination therapy should be used cautiously in those at risk for orthostatic hypotension.
Adapted with permission from Chobanian AV, Bakris GL, Black HR, et al. Seventh report of the Joint National Committee on Prevention, Detection, Evaluation, and Treatment of High Blood Pressure: The JNC-7 Report. JAMA 289:2560, 2003.

Table 8-5　Oral Antihypertensive Drugs

Drug (Trade Name)	Usual Dose Range (mg/d)	Usual Daily Frequency
Thiazide Diuretics		
Chlorothiazide (Diuril)	125 to 500	1 to 2
Chlorthalidone (generic)	12.5 to 25	1
Hydrochlorothiazide (Microzide, HydroDIURIL[†])	12.5 to 50	1
Polythiazide (Renese)	2 to 4	1
Indapamide (Lozol[†])	1.25 to 2.5	1
Metolazone (Mykrox)	0.5 to 1.0	1
Metolazone (Zaroxolyn)	2.5 to 5	1
Loop Diuretics		
Bumetanide (Bumex[†])	0.5 to 2	2
Furosemide (Lasix[†])	20 to 80	2
Torsemide (Demadex[†])	2.5 to 10	1
Potassium-Sparing Diuretics		
Amiloride (Midamor[†])	5 to 10	1 to 2
Triamterene (Dyrenium)	50 to 100	1 to 2
Aldosterone Receptor Blockers		
Eplerenone (Inspra)	50 to 100	1
Spironolactone (Aldactone[†])	25 to 50	1
β-Blockers		
Atenolol (Tenormin[†])	25 to 100	1
Betaxolol (Kerlone[†])	5 to 20	1
Bisoprolol (Zebeta[†])	2.5 to 10	1
Metoprolol (Lopressor[†])	50 to 100	1 to 2
Metoprolol extended release (Toprol XL)	50 to 100	1
Nadolol (Corgard[†])	40 to 120	1
Propranolol (Inderal[†])	40 to 160	2
Propranolol long-acting (Inderal LA[†])	60 to 180	1
Timolol (Blocadren[†])	20 to 40	2
β-Blockers with Intrinsic Sympathomimetic Activity		
Acebutolol (Sectral[†])	200 to 800	2
Penbutolol (Levatol)	10 to 40	1
Pindolol (generic)	10 to 40	2
Combined α-Blockers and β-Blockers		
Carvedilol (Coreg)	12.5 to 50	2
Labetalol (Normodyne, Trandate[†])	200 to 800	2
Angiotensin-Converting Enzyme Inhibitors		
Benazepril (Lotensin[†])	10 to 40	1
Captopril (Capoten[†])	25 to 100	2
Enalapril (Vasotec[†])	5 to 40	1 to 2
Fosinopril (Monopril)	10 to 40	1
Lisinopril (Prinivil, Zestril[†])	10 to 40	1
Moexipril (Univasc)	7.5 to 30	1
Perindopril (Aceon)	4 to 8	1
Quinapril (Accupril)	10 to 40	1

8

Table continued on following page

Table 8-5 Oral Antihypertensive Drugs (Continued)

Drug (Trade Name)	Usual Dose Range (mg/d)	Usual Daily Frequency
Ramipril (Altace)	2.5 to 20	1
Trandolapril (Mavik)	1 to 4	1
Angiotensin II Antagonists		
Candesartan (Atacand)	8 to 32	1
Eprosartan (Teveten)	400 to 800	1 to 2
Irbesartan (Avapro)	150 to 300	1
Losartan (Cozaar)	25 to 100	1 to 2
Olmesartan (Benicar)	20 to 40	1
Telmisartan (Micardis)	20 to 80	1
Valsartan (Diovan)	80 to 320	1 to 2
CCBs: Nondihydropyridines		
Diltiazem extended release (Cardizem CD, Dilacor XR, Tiazac†)	180 to 420	1
Diltiazem extended release (Cardizem LA)	120 to 540	1
Verapamil immediate release (Calan, Isoptin†)	80 to 320	2
Verapamil long-acting (Calan SR, Isoptin SR†)	120 to 480	1 to 2
Verapamil controlled onset, extended release (Covera HS, Verelan PM)	120 to 360	1
CCB: Dihydropyridines		
Amlodipine (Norvasc)	2.5 to 10	1
Felodipine (Plendil)	2.5 to 20	1
Isradipine (DynaCirc CR)	2.5 to 10	2
Nicardipine sustained release (Cardene SR)	60 to 120	2
Nifedipine long-acting (Adalat CC, Procardia XL)	30 to 60	1
Nisoldipine (Sular)	10 to 40	1
α_1-Blockers		
Doxazosin (Cardura)	1 to 16	1
Prazosin (Minipress†)	2 to 20	2 to 3
Terazosin (Hytrin)	1 to 20	1 to 2
Central α_2-Agonists and Other Centrally Acting Drugs		
Clonidine (Catapres†)	0.1 to 0.8	2
Clonidine patch (Catapres-TTS)	0.1 to 0.3	1 weekly
Methyldopa (Aldomet†)	250 to 1000	2
Reserpine (generic)	0.05 to 0.25	1
Guanfacine (Tenex†)	0.5 to 2	1
Direct Vasodilators		
Hydralazine (Apresoline†)	25 to 100	2
Minoxidil (Loniten†)	2.5 to 80	1 to 2

CCB = calcium channel blocker.

*In some patients treated once daily, the antihypertensive effect may diminish toward the end of the dosing interval (trough effect). BP should be measured just before dosing to determine if satisfactory BP control is obtained. Accordingly, an increase in dosage or frequency may need to be considered. These dosages may vary from those listed in the **Physicians' Drug Reference,** 51st ed.

†Available now or soon to become available in generic preparations.

Adapted with permission from Chobanian AV, Bakris GL, Black HR, et al: Seventh report of the Joint National Committee on Prevention, Detection, Evaluation, and Treatment of High Blood Pressure: The JNC-7 Report. JAMA 289:2560, 2003.

Table 8-6 Combination Drugs for Hypertension

Combination Type	Fixed-Dose Combination (mg)*	Trade Name
ACEIs and CCB	Amlodipine-benazepril hydrochloride (2.5/10, 5/10, 5/20, 10/20)	Lotrel
	Enalapril-felodipine (5/5)	Lexxel
	Trandolapril-verapamil (2/180, 1/240, 2/240, 4/240)	Tarka
ACEIs and diuretics	Benazepril-hydrochlorothiazide (5/6.25, 10/12.5, 20/12.5, 20/25)	Lotensin HCT
	Captopril-hydrochlorothiazide (25/15, 25/25, 50/15, 50/25)	Capozide
	Enalapril-hydrochlorothiazide (5/12.5, 10/25)	Vaseretic
	Fosinopril-hydrochlorothiazide (10/12.5, 20/12.5)	Monopril/HCT
	Lisinopril-hydrochlorothiazide (10/12.5, 20/12.5, 20/25)	Prinzide, Zestoretic
	Moexipril-hydrochlorothiazide (7.5/12.5, 15/25)	Uniretic
	Quinapril-hydrochlorothiazide (10/12.5, 20/12.5, 20/25)	Accuretic
ARBs and diuretics	Candesartan-hydrochlorothiazide (16/12.5, 32/12.5)	Atacand HCT
	Eprosartan-hydrochlorothiazide (600/12.5, 600/25)	Teveten-HCT
	Irbesartan-hydrochlorothiazide (150/12.5, 300/12.5)	Avalide
	Losartan-hydrochlorothiazide (50/12.5, 100/25)	Hyzaar
	Olmesartan medoxomil-hydrochlorothiazide (20/12.5, 40/12.5, 40/25)	Benicar HCT
	Telmisartan-hydrochlorothiazide (40/12.5, 80/12.5)	Micardis-HCT
	Valsartan-hydrochlorothiazide (80/12.5, 160/12.5, 160/25)	Diovan-HCT
BBs and diuretics	Atenolol-chlorthalidone (50/25, 100/25)	Tenoretic
	Bisoprolol-hydrochlorothiazide (2.5/6.25, 5/6.25, 10/6.25)	Ziac
	Metoprolol-hydrochlorothiazide (50/25, 100/25)	Lopressor HCT
	Nadolol-bendroflumethiazide (40/5, 80/5)	Corzide
	Propranolol LA-hydrochlorothiazide (40/25, 80/25)	Inderide LA
	Timolol-hydrochlorothiazide (10/25)	Timolide
Centrally acting drug and diuretic	Methyldopa-hydrochlorothiazide (250/15, 250/25, 500/30, 500/50)	Aldoril
	Reserpine-chlorthalidone (0.125/25, 0.25/50)	Demi-Regroton, Regroton

Table continued on following page

8

Table 8-6 Combination Drugs for Hypertension (Continued)

Combination Type	Fixed-Dose Combination (mg)*	Trade Name
Diuretic and diuretic	Reserpine-chlorothiazide (0.125/250, 0.25/500)	Diupres
	Reserpine-hydrochlorothiazide (0.125/25, 0.125/50)	Hydropres
	Amiloride-hydrochlorothiazide (5/50)	Moduretic
	Spironolactone-hydrochlorothiazide (25/25, 50/50)	Aldactazide
	Triamterene-hydrochlorothiazide (37.5/25, 75/50)	Dyazide, Maxzide

BB = β-blocker; ACEI = angiotensin-converting enzyme inhibitor; ARB = angiotensin-receptor blocker; CCB = calcium channel blocker.

*Some drug combinations are available in multiple fixed doses. Each drug dose is reported in milligrams.

Adapted with permission from Chobanian AV, Bakris GL, Black HR, et al. Seventh report of the Joint National Committee on Prevention, Detection, Evaluation, and Treatment of High Blood Pressure: The JNC-7 Report. JAMA 289:2560, 2003.

necessitates immediate therapeutic intervention, most often in an intensive care setting, with intravenous antihypertensive therapy and invasive arterial BP monitoring. In the most extreme cases of *malignant hypertension,* severe elevations in BP may be associated with retinal hemorrhages, papilledema, and evidence of encephalopathy, which may include headache, vomiting, seizure, and/or coma. Progressive renal failure and cardiac decompensation are additional clinical features characteristic of the most severe hypertensive emergencies.

The favored parenteral drug for rapid treatment of hypertensive emergencies remains sodium nitroprusside (Table 8-7). An NO donor, sodium nitroprusside induces arterial and venous dilation, providing rapid and predictable reductions in systemic BP. Prolonged administration of large doses may be associated with cyanide or thiocyanate toxicity; however, this is rarely a concern in the setting of acute hypertensive emergencies. Although less potent and predictable than sodium nitroprusside, NTG, another NO donor, may be preferable in the setting of myocardial ischemia or after coronary artery bypass grafting (CABG). NTG preferentially dilates venous capacitance beds as opposed to arterioles; however, rapid onset of tolerance limits the efficacy of sustained infusions to maintain BP control. Nicardipine, a parenteral dihydropyridine calcium channel blocker, and fenoldopam, a selective dopamine-1 (D_1)-receptor antagonist, have been utilized increasingly in select patient populations after CABG and in the setting of renal insufficiency, respectively.[11]

Several drugs remain available for intermittent parenteral administration in the setting of hypertensive emergencies or urgencies. Hydralazine, labetalol, and esmolol provide additional therapeutic options for intermittent parenteral injection for hypertensive control.

PHARMACOTHERAPY FOR ACUTE AND CHRONIC HEART FAILURE

Chronic heart failure is one major cardiovascular disorder that continues to increase in incidence and prevalence, both in the United States and worldwide. It affects nearly 5 million persons in the United States, and roughly 550,000 new cases are diagnosed each year.[12] Currently, 1% of those 50 to 59 years of age and 10% of individuals older than

80 have heart failure. Because heart failure is primarily a disease of the elderly, its prevalence is projected to increase twofold to threefold over the next decade, as the median age of the U.S. population continues to increase. The increasingly prolonged survival of patients with various cardiovascular disorders that culminate in ventricular dysfunction (e.g., patients with coronary artery disease are living longer rather than dying acutely with myocardial infarction) further compounds the heart failure epidemic. Despite improvements in the understanding of the neurohormonal mechanisms underlying its pathophysiology and remarkable advances made in pharmacologic therapy, heart failure continues to cost the United States an estimated $38 billion annually in medical expenditures, and it contributes to approximately 250,000 deaths per year. Given the public health impact of the disease and the rapid pace of therapeutic advances, it is essential that the perioperative physician remain aware of contemporary clinical practice for the benefit of those patients with chronic heart failure presenting to the operating room or intensive care unit.

Heart Failure Classification

The ACC/AHA updated guidelines for evaluating and managing heart failure include a new, four-stage classification system emphasizing both the evolution and progression of the disease (Box 8-5). It calls attention to patients with preclinical stages of heart failure to focus on halting disease progression. The staging system is meant to complement, not replace, the widely used New York Heart Association (NYHA) classification, a semiquantitative index of functional classification that categorizes patients with heart failure by the severity of their symptoms. The NYHA classification remains useful clinically because it reflects symptoms, which in turn correlate with quality of life and survival. The new classification system for heart failure, recognizing its progressive course and identifying those who are at risk, reinforces the importance of determining the optimal strategy for neurohormonal antagonism in an attempt to improve the natural history of the syndrome.

Heart failure remains the final common pathway for coronary artery disease, hypertension, valvular heart disease, and cardiomyopathy, in which the natural history results in symptomatic or asymptomatic left ventricular dysfunction. The neurohormonal responses to impaired cardiac performance (salt and water retention, vasoconstriction, sympathetic stimulation) are initially adaptive but, if sustained, become maladaptive, resulting in pulmonary congestion and excessive afterload. This, in turn, leads to a vicious cycle of increases in cardiac energy expenditure and worsening of pump function and tissue perfusion (Table 8-8). Although the cardiorenal and cardiocirculatory branches of this neurohormonal hypothesis of heart failure were the original foundation for the use of diuretics, vasodilators, and inotropes, respectively, seminal information in the early 1990s emerged from large, randomized clinical trials that showed angiotensin-converting enzyme (ACE) inhibitors and angiotensin receptor blockers, but not most other vasodilators, prolonged survival in patients with heart failure. In a similar fashion, the use of β-blockers, despite their negative inotropic effects, improved morbidity and mortality in randomized controlled trials.

The finding that low-dose aldosterone antagonists added to conventional therapy for heart failure reduced mortality in patients with severe heart failure suggests that there is more to the neurohormonal hypothesis of drug efficacy than cardiorenal and hemodynamic effects alone. Taken together with evidence from basic investigations showing that Ang II is a growth factor and a vasoconstrictor, the clinical data promoted a shift in focus from cardiorenal and cardiocirculatory processes toward cardiac remodeling as the central component in the progression of this neurohormone-mediated cardiac syndrome.[13] The renin-angiotensin-aldosterone system (RAAS), excess sympathetic activity, endothelin, and various cytokines all have been implicated as stimuli of proliferative signaling that contribute to maladaptive cardiac growth.

8

Table 8-7 Parenteral Drugs for Treatment of Hypertensive Emergencies*

Drug	Dose	Onset of Action	Duration of Action	Adverse Effects†	Special Indications
Vasodilators					
Sodium nitroprusside	0.25 to 10 µg/kg/min as IV infusion‡	Immediate	1 to 2 min	Nausea, vomiting, muscle twitching, sweating, thiocyanate and cyanide intoxication	Most hypertensive emergencies; caution with high intracranial pressure or azotemia
Nicardipine hydrochloride	5 to 15 mg/hr IV	5 to 10 min	15 to 30 min, may exceed 4 hr	Tachycardia, headache, flushing, local phlebitis	Most hypertensive emergencies except acute heart failure; caution with coronary ischemia
Fenoldopam mesylate	0.1 to 0.3 µg/kg/min IV infusion	<5 min	30 min	Tachycardia, headache, nausea, flushing	Most hypertensive emergencies; caution with glaucoma
Nitroglycerin	5 to 100 µg/min as IV infusion	2 to 5 min	5 to 10 min	Headache, vomiting, methemoglobinemia, tolerance with prolonged use	Coronary ischemia
Enalaprilat	1.25 to 5 mg every 6 hr IV	15 to 30 min	6 to 12 hr	Precipitous fall in pressure in high-renin states, variable response	Acute left ventricular failure; avoid in acute myocardial infarction

	Dose	Onset of Action	Duration of Action	Adverse Effects	Special Indications
Hydralazine hydrochloride	10 to 20 mg IV 10 to 40 mg IM	10 to 20 min IV 20 to 30 min IM	1 to 4 hr IV 4 to 6 hr IM	Tachycardia, flushing, headache, vomiting, aggravation of angina	Eclampsia
Adrenergic Inhibitors					
Labetalol hydrochloride	20 to 80 mg IV bolus every 10 min; 0.5 to 2.0 mg/min IV infusion	5 to 10 min	3 to 6 hr	Vomiting, scalp tingling, bronchoconstriction, dizziness, nausea, heart block, orthostatic hypotension	Most hypertensive emergencies except acute heart failure
Esmolol hydrochloride	250 to 500 µg/kg/min IV bolus, then 50 to 100 µg/kg/min by infusion; may repeat bolus after 5 min or increase infusion to 300 µg/min	1 to 2 min	10 to 30 min	Hypotension, nausea, asthma, first-degree heart block, heart failure	Aortic dissection, perioperative
Phentolamine	5 to 15 mg IV bolus	1 to 2 min	10 to 30 min	Tachycardia, flushing, headache	Catecholamine excess

*These doses may vary from those in the Physicians' Desk Reference, 51st ed.
†Hypotension may occur with all agents.
‡Requires special delivery system.
Reproduced with permission from Chobanian AV, Bakris GL, Black HR, et al. Seventh Report of the Joint National Committee on Prevention, Detection, Evaluation, and Treatment of High Blood Pressure. Hypertension 42:1206, 2003.

BOX 8-5 ACC/AHA Four-Stage Classification and Management Recommendations

Stage A High risk for developing heart failure. No structural or functional disorders of the heart. No symptoms of heart failure.

Examples Hypertension; coronary artery disease; diabetes mellitus; history of cardiotoxic therapy or alcohol abuse; history of rheumatic heart disease; family history of cardiomyopathy

Treatment Emphasize prevention: treat hypertension, encourage smoking cessation, treat dyslipidemia, encourage regular exercise; discourage excessive alcohol use or illicit drug use. Consider ACE inhibitor for patients with history of peripheral vascular disease, diabetes mellitus, or hypertension with associated risk factors.

Stage B Structural heart disease strongly associated with heart failure. No symptoms of heart failure.

Examples Patients with left ventricular hypertrophy or fibrosis, left ventricular dilatation or hypocontractility, asymptomatic valvular heart disease, or previous myocardial infarction.

Treatment Use all preventive measures listed under stage A. ACE inhibitors and/or β-blockers are recommended for patients with recent or remote history of myocardial infarction. Consider the same for patients with reduced ejection fraction, regardless of previous myocardial infarction history.

Stage C Structural heart disease with prior or current symptoms of heart failure.

Examples Patients with dyspnea or fatigue due to left ventricular systolic dysfunction; asymptomatic patients who are undergoing treatment for prior symptoms of heart failure.

Treatment Use all measures listed in stage A. Drugs recommended for routine use include loop diuretics, ACE inhibitors, β-blockers, and digitalis. Advise dietary salt restriction.

Stage D Advanced structural heart disease. Marked symptoms of heart failure at rest despite maximal medical therapy.

Examples Patients who are often hospitalized for heart failure and who cannot be safely discharged from the hospital; patients in the hospital awaiting heart transplantation; patients at home receiving continuous intravenous support for symptom relief or being supported with a mechanical circulatory assist device; patients in a hospice setting for the management of heart failure. Specialized interventions are required.

Treatment Use all measures listed under Stages A, B, and C. Specialized interventions include mechanical assist devices, heart transplantation, continuous intravenous inotropic infusions for palliation, hospice care.

ACE = angiotensin-converting enzyme; LV = left ventricular.
β-Blockers are relatively contraindicated in patients with bronchospastic pulmonary disease.
Adapted from permission from Clinical update: New guidelines for evaluating and managing heart failure. Women's Health in Primary Care 5(2):105, 2002.

Table 8-8 Neurohormonal Effects of Impaired Cardiac Performance on the Circulation

Response	Short-Term Effects	Long-Term Effects
Salt and water retention	Augments preload	Pulmonary congestion, edema
Vasoconstriction	Maintains blood pressure for perfusion of vital organs	Exacerbates pump dysfunction (excessive afterload), increases cardiac energy expenditure
Sympathetic stimulation	Increases heart rate and ejection	Increases energy expenditure

Modified from Katz AM: Heart failure. In Fozzard HA, Haber E, Jennings RB: The Heart and Cardiovascular System: Scientific Foundations, 2nd ed. New York, Raven, 1992, pp 333-353.

> ### BOX 8-6   *Mechanical Disadvantage Created by Left Ventricular Remodeling*
>
> - Increased wall stress (afterload)
> - Afterload mismatch
> - Episodic subendocardial hypoperfusion
> - Increased oxygen utilization
> - Sustained hemodynamic overloading
> - Worsening activation of compensatory mechanisms
>
> Adapted from Mann DL: Mechanisms and models in heart failure: an combinatorial approach. Circulation 100:999–1008, 1999.

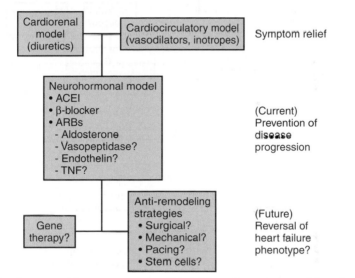

Figure 8-2   Current and future treatments of heart failure. Currently, heart failure therapies are focused on prevention of disease progression with drugs that antagonize neurohormonal systems. Future therapies may involve antagonists of other biologically active systems (e.g., endothelins, TNFα) and anti-remodeling strategies that may reverse the heart failure phenotype. ACEI=angiotensin-converting enzyme inhibitor; ARB=angiotensin-receptor blocker; NEP=neutral endopeptidase blocker. (Adapted from Mann DL. Mechanisms and model in heart failure: A combinatorial approach. Circulation 100:999, 1999.)

Accordingly, ventricular remodeling, or the structural alterations of the heart in the form of dilatation and hypertrophy (Box 8-6), in addition to the counterregulatory hemodynamic responses, lead to progressive ventricular dysfunction and represent the target of current therapeutic interventions (Fig. 8-2).

Pathophysiologic Role of the Renin-Angiotensin System in Heart Failure

The renin-angiotensin system (RAS) is one of several neuroendocrine systems that are activated in patients with heart failure. The RAS is also an important mediator in the progression of heart failure. In the short term, the juxtaglomerular cells of the kidney release the proteolytic enzyme renin in response to a decrease in BP or renal perfusion (e.g., hemorrhage) generating Ang I from circulating angiotensinogen. ACE cleavage of Ang II from Ang I in the lung produces circulating Ang II. Acutely, Ang II acts as a

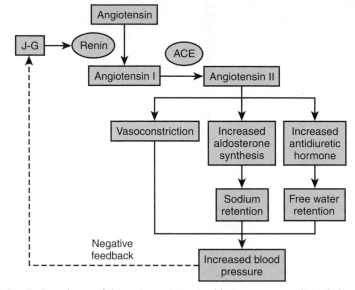

Figure 8-3 Basic pathway of the renin-angiotensin-aldosterone system (RAAS). (From Jaski BE: Basis of Heart Failure: A Problem Solving Approach. Boston, Kluwer Academic Publishers, 2000, with kind permission of Springer Science and Business Media.)

potent arteriolar and venous vasoconstrictor to return BP and filling pressure to baseline, respectively. Ang II also stimulates the release of aldosterone from the adrenal cortex and antidiuretic hormone from the posterior pituitary. Both contribute to increases in blood volume through their effects on the kidney to promote salt and water reabsorption, respectively. In the long term, elevations in Ang II lead to sodium and fluid retention and increases in systemic vascular resistance, which contribute to symptoms of heart failure, pulmonary congestion, and hemodynamic decompensation (Fig. 8-3).

In addition to these cardiorenal and cardiocirculatory effects, most of the hormones and receptors of the RAS are expressed in the myocardium, where they contribute to maladaptive growth or remodeling, a key factor in the progression of heart failure. Increased expression of mRNA for angiotensinogen, ACE, and Ang II has been identified in the failing human heart. Correspondingly, increased coronary sinus Ang II concentrations were measured in patients with dilated and ischemic cardiomyopathy, signifying a paracrine or autocrine action of the RAS. Moreover, progressive increases in coronary sinus Ang II production correlated with increases in NYHA functional classification of heart failure. Taken together, these data provide evidence that intracardiac RAS is involved in the evolution of the disease process.

The effects of Ang II on its receptors AT_1 and AT_2 are well appreciated. The AT_1 receptor is involved in several effects that lead to adverse cardiovascular outcomes. Activation of AT_1 receptors promotes aldosterone and vasopressin secretion with concomitant increases in salt and water reabsorption through the kidneys, vasoconstriction, catecholamine release, and cell growth and proliferation of cardiovascular tissue. Stimulation of AT_2 receptors, on the other hand, results in natriuresis, vasodilation, release of bradykinin and NO, and cell growth inhibition or apoptosis. The Ang II that is formed locally in the heart acts primarily through AT_1 receptors located on myocytes and fibroblasts where it participates in the regulation of cardiac remodeling. Through complex cascades of intracellular signal transduction that activate protein transcription factors within the nucleus initiating the creation of RNA transcripts, the long-term effects of intracardiac Ang II on the AT_1 receptor

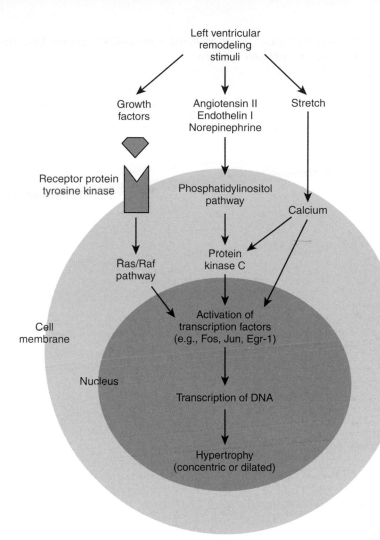

Figure 8-4   Left ventricular remodeling stimuli.

result in cardiomyocyte hypertrophy, fibroblast proliferation, and extracellular matrix deposition (Fig. 8-4). These processes contribute to progressive left ventricular remodeling and left ventricular dysfunction characteristic of heart failure.

Angiotensin-Converting Enzyme Inhibitors

CLINICAL EVIDENCE

Evidence supporting the beneficial use of ACE inhibitors in patients with heart failure comes from various randomized, placebo-controlled clinical trials (Table 8-9). Initially this class of drugs was evaluated for treatment of symptomatic heart failure (SOLVD, V-HeFT, CONSENSUS). Patients with NYHA class II to IV heart failure treated with ACE inhibitors had reductions in mortality ranging from 16% to 31%. Subsequently, ACE inhibitors were also found to improve outcome for asymptomatic patients with left ventricular systolic dysfunction in

Table 8-9   Selected Clinical Trials of Angiotensin-Converting Enzyme Inhibitors in Heart Failure

Patient Subset	Heart Failure Stage	Drug	Trial
Heart Failure			
NYHA Class II-III	C	Enalapril	SOLVD (treat); V-HeFT II
NYHA Class IV	D	Enalapril	CONSENSUS I
Asymptomatic Left Ventricular Dysfunction			
Ejection fraction < 35%	B	Enalapril	SOLVD (prevent)
Post–myocardial infarction (ejection fraction < 40%)	B	Captopril	SAVE
Acute myocardial infarction	B	Captopril	GISSI
		Lisinopril	ISIS-4
Asymptomatic High Risk (history of diabetes mellitus, pulmonary vascular disease, and coronary risk factors)	A	Ramipril	HOPE

the following categories: patients with ejection fractions less than 35% due to cardiomyopathy, patients within 2 weeks after myocardial infarction with ejection fractions less than 40%, and patients presenting within the first 24 hours of myocardial infarction regardless of ejection fraction. Results from the Heart Outcomes Prevention Evaluation (HOPE) study have further expanded the indications for this class of agents to include asymptomatic, high-risk patients to prevent new-onset heart failure.[14] In patients with diabetes or peripheral vascular disease and an additional atherosclerotic risk factor, but without clinical heart failure or systolic dysfunction, ramipril (10 mg/day) reduced the heart failure risk by 23%. Together, these data endorse the use of ACE inhibitors as first-line therapy for a broad spectrum of patients, including those with left ventricular systolic dysfunction, with or without symptoms, and in high-risk patients with vascular disease and/or diabetes, in addition to those with the traditional coronary risk factors. Since the beginning of these trials, the rationale for the use of ACE inhibitors has expanded from a reduction in the progression of clinical heart failure through ACE inhibitor–mediated vasodilatory action to acknowledgment that ACE inhibitors also directly affect the cellular mechanisms responsible for progressive myocardial pathology.

MECHANISMS OF ACTION

ACE inhibitors act by inhibiting one of several proteases responsible for cleaving the decapeptide, Ang I, to form the octapeptide Ang II. Because ACE is also the enzyme that degrades bradykinin, ACE inhibitors lead to increased circulating and tissue levels of bradykinin (Fig. 8-5). ACE inhibitors have several useful effects in chronic heart failure. They are potent vasodilators through decreasing Ang II and norepinephrine and increasing bradykinin, NO, and prostacyclin. By reducing the secretion of aldosterone and antidiuretic hormone (ADH), ACE inhibitors also reduce salt and water reabsorption

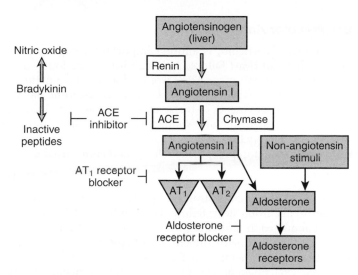

Figure 8-5   Activation of the renin-angiotensin-aldosterone system (RAAS). (Redrawn from Mann DL. Heart Therapy: A Companion to Braunwald's Heart Disease. Philadelphia: Saunders, 2004.)

from the kidney. ACE inhibitors reduce release of norepinephrine from sympathetic nerves by acting on AT_1 receptors at the nerve terminal. Within tissue, ACE inhibitors inhibit Ang II production and thus attenuate Ang II-mediated cardiomyocyte hypertrophy and fibroblast hyperplasia. Clinical evidence supporting an ACE inhibitor-mediated role in cardiac remodeling comes from comparative studies of enalapril versus placebo (SOLVD trial) and enalapril versus hydralazine isosorbide dinitrate (VHeft II trial).

ACE inhibitors attenuate insulin resistance, a common metabolic abnormality in heart failure patients, independent of Ang II activity. Ang II receptor antagonists do not attenuate insulin resistance. Both ACE inhibitors and angiotensin-receptor blockers have been shown to reduce proteinuria, and slow the progression to renal failure in hypertensives (and a common comorbidity in heart failure patients).

Angiotensin II Receptor Blockers for Heart Failure

PATHOPHYSIOLOGY/MECHANISM OF ACTION

Although ACE inhibitors reduce mortality, many patients will not tolerate their side effects. ACE inhibitors incompletely antagonize Ang II. These factors have prompted the development of specific Ang II receptor blockers in the pharmacologic treatment of heart failure. Non–ACE-generated Ang II within the myocardium contributes to left ventricular remodeling and progression of heart failure through AT_1 receptor effects. Selective AT_1 blockers prevent Ang II from acting on the cell, preventing vasoconstriction, sodium retention, and release of norepinephrine and delaying or preventing left ventricular hypertrophy and fibrosis. AT_2 receptors remain unaffected, and their actions, including NO release, remain intact.[15]

CLINICAL PRACTICE

Angiotensin-receptor blockers may be used as alternatives to ACE inhibitors for the treatment of patients with symptomatic heart failure if there are side effects to ACE inhibitors (e.g., persistent cough, angioedema, hyperkalemia, or worsening renal dysfunction) or persistent hypertension despite ACE inhibitors and β-blockers. Because ARBs do not affect bradykinin levels, cough and angioedema are rare side effects.

8

Aldosterone Receptor Antagonists

Aldosterone, a mineralocorticoid, is another important component of the neurohormonal hypothesis of heart failure. Although it was previously assumed that treatment with an ACE inhibitor (or ARB) would block the production of aldosterone in patients with heart failure, elevated levels of aldosterone have been measured despite inhibition of Ang II. Adverse effects of elevated aldosterone levels on the cardiovascular system include sodium retention, potassium and magnesium loss, ventricular remodeling (e.g., collagen production, myocyte growth, and hypertrophy), myocardial norepinephrine release, and endothelial dysfunction.

CLINICAL EVIDENCE

Two large-scale trials have demonstrated improved outcomes with aldosterone-receptor antagonism in chronic heart failure. The Randomized Aldactone Evaluation Study (RALES), conducted in more than 1600 symptomatic heart failure (e.g., stage C, NYHA III-IV) patients, showed the efficacy of spironolactone (26 mg/day) (in combination with standard therapy: ACE inhibitor, loop diuretic with or without digoxin and a β-blocker). Eplerenone is a new aldosterone antagonist that lacks some of spironolactone's common side effects. The Eplerenone Post-acute Myocardial Infarction Heart Failure Efficacy and Survival Study (EPHSUS), conducted in more than 6600 patients with symptomatic heart failure within 3 to 14 days after myocardial infarction, showed that eplerenone (25 to 50 mg/day) in combination with ACE inhibitor, loop diuretic, and β-blocker reduced all-cause mortality ($P = .008$), death from cardiovascular causes ($P = .0002$), and hospitalization for cardiovascular events.[16,17]

β-Adrenergic Receptor Antagonists

Sympathetic Nervous System Activation and Its Role in the Pathogenesis of Heart Failure

Activation of the sympathetic nervous system (SNS) (e.g., after myocardial infarction or with long-standing hypertension), much like increases in RAS activity, contributes to the pathophysiology of heart failure. In brief, SNS activation leads to pathologic left ventricular growth and remodeling. Myocytes thicken and elongate, with eccentric hypertrophy and increases in sphericity. Wall stress is increased by this architecture, promoting subendocardial ischemia, cell death, and contractile dysfunction. There is downregulation of calcium regulatory proteins, including sarcoplasmic reticulum calcium ATPase, and impairment of contractility and relaxation. The activated SNS can also be harmful to myocytes directly through programmed cell death. As myocytes are replaced by fibroblasts, the heart function deteriorates from this "remodeling." The threshold for arrhythmias may also be lowered, contributing in a vicious, deteriorating cycle.

How β-Adrenergic Receptor Blockers Influence the Pathophysiology of Heart Failure

In chronic heart failure, the beneficial effects of long-term β-blockade include improved systolic function and myocardial energetics and reversal of pathologic remodeling. A shift in substrate utilization from free fatty acids to glucose, a more efficient fuel in the face of myocardial ischemia, may partly explain the improved energetics and mechanics in the failing heart treated with β-blockade. Heart rate, a major determinant of myocardial oxygen consumption, is reduced by β_1-receptor blockade.

II

CLINICAL EVIDENCE

The use of β-blockers in patients with heart failure was initially accepted with skepticism related to the perceived risk of decompensation from transient negative inotropic effects. However, data from both human and animal studies have shown that β-blockers improve energetics and ventricular function and reverse pathologic chamber remodeling. Although this beneficial biologic process takes 3 months or more to manifest, it translates into improved outcomes (reduced deaths and hospitalizations) in patients with heart failure. The available randomized trials show that metoprolol CR/XL, bisoprolol, and carvedilol (in conjunction with ACE inhibitors) reduce morbidity (hospitalizations) in symptomatic, stage C and D (not in cardiogenic shock) heart failure patients (NYHA II-IV class).

β-Blockers are classified as being first-, second-, or third-generation drugs based on specific pharmacologic properties. First-generation agents, such as propranolol and timolol, block both β_1- and β_2-adrenoreceptors, are considered nonselective, and have no ancillary properties. Second-generation agents, such as metoprolol, bisoprolol, and atenolol, are specific for the β_1-adrenoreceptor subtype but lack additional mechanisms of cardiovascular activity. Third-generation agents, such as bucindolol, carvedilol, and labetalol, block both β_1- and β_2-adrenoreceptors as well as possessing vasodilatory and other ancillary properties. Specifically, labetalol and carvedilol produce vasodilation by α_1-adrenoreceptor antagonism.

CLINICAL PRACTICE

Current evidence suggests that β-blockers should be given to all heart failure patients with reduced ejection fraction (<0.40) who are stabilized on oral medications including ACE inhibitors and diuretics, unless there is a contraindication. This recommendation is endorsed by the ACC/AHA and the European Society of Cardiology. Specifically, long-term β-blockade is advocated in stage B-D heart failure patients in addition to ACE inhibition to limit disease progression and reduce mortality. Patients with ongoing decompensation (e.g., requiring intravenous inotropic or vasodilator therapy), overt fluid retention, or symptomatic hypotension should not receive β-blockers. There is no apparent decline in safety or efficacy when β-blockers are given to diabetics with heart failure. The long-term benefit of β-blocker therapy in patients with coexisting chronic obstructive pulmonary disease is uncertain, because these patients have been excluded from the major clinical trials.

The three agents with clinical trial evidence for improved morbidity and mortality in patients with heart failure are carvedilol, metoprolol CR/XL, and bisoprolol.[18] Starting doses of β-blockers should be small to minimize worsening of heart failure symptoms, hypotension, and bradycardia. The dose should be doubled every 1 to 2 weeks, as tolerated, until target doses shown to be effective in large trials are achieved. Although it is recommended that β-blocker therapy be continued indefinitely in patients with heart failure, if it is to be electively stopped, a slow downtitration is preferred. Acute withdrawal of β-blocker therapy in the face of high adrenergic tone may result in sudden cardiac death. The adverse effects of β-blocker therapy include fatigue, dizziness, hypotension, and bradycardia. Because the absolute risk of adverse events is small compared with the overall risk reduction of cardiovascular death, few patients have been withdrawn from β-blocker therapy.

Adjunctive Drugs

In addition to ACE inhibitors and β-blockers, diuretics and digoxin are often prescribed for patients with left ventricular systolic dysfunction and symptomatic heart failure.

Diuretics

For most patients, volume status should be optimized before introduction of β-blockers and ACE inhibitors. Patients with pulmonary congestion often will require a loop diuretic in addition to standard therapy. Diuretics relieve dyspnea, decrease heart size and wall stress, and correct hyponatremia of volume overload. However, overly aggressive and especially unmonitored diuretic therapy can lead to metabolic abnormalities, intravascular depletion, hypotension, and neurohormonal activation.

Digoxin

Digoxin continues to be useful for patients with symptomatic heart failure and left ventricular systolic dysfunction despite receiving ACE inhibitor, β-blocker, and diuretic therapy. Digoxin is the only positive inotropic drug approved for the management of chronic heart failure. Its indirect mechanism of positive inotropy begins with inhibition of the myocardial sarcolemmal Na^+-K^+ ATPase, resulting in increased intracellular Na^+. This, in turn, prompts the Na^+/Ca^{2+} exchanger to extrude Na^+ from the cell, increasing intracellular Ca^{2+}. The increased Ca^{2+} now available to the contractile proteins increases contractile function. Besides its inotropic effects, digoxin has important vagotonic and sympatholytic effects. In atrial fibrillation, digoxin slows the rate of conduction at the AV node. In heart failure patients it reduces sympathetic efferent nerve activity to the heart and peripheral circulation through direct effects on the carotid sinus baroreceptors. Digoxin increases HR variability, an additional beneficial action on autonomic function in the patient with heart failure. Although these properties are beneficial in controlling the ventricular rate in atrial fibrillation, digoxin has only a narrow therapeutic/toxicity ratio. Digoxin toxicity is dose dependent and modified by concurrent medications (non–potassium-sparing diuretics) or conditions (renal insufficiency, myocardial ischemia). Ventricular arrhythmias consequent to digoxin toxicity may be caused by calcium-dependent afterpotentials. In patients with intoxication and life-threatening arrhythmias, purified anti-digoxin FAB fragments from digoxin-specific antisera provide a specific antidote.

The efficacy of digoxin for symptomatic heart failure was shown in randomized, controlled trials. The Digitalis Investigators Group (DIG) trial, enrolling more than 6500 patients with an average follow-up of 37 months, showed that digoxin reduced the incidence of heart failure exacerbations. Although the study showed no difference in survival in patients with an ejection fraction less than 45% receiving either digoxin or placebo, the combined endpoint of death or hospitalization for heart failure was significantly reduced in patients who received digoxin (27% vs. 35%; relative risk, 0.72; 95% confidence interval, 0.66 to 0.79). Efficacy of digoxin in patients with mildly symptomatic heart failure was shown in pooled results from the Prospective Randomized Study of Ventricular Function (PROVED) and the Randomized Assessment of Digoxin and Inhibitors of Angiotensin-Converting Enzyme (RADIANCE) trials. Patients randomized to digoxin withdrawal had an increased likelihood of treatment failure compared with those who continued to receive digoxin, suggesting that patients with left ventricular systolic dysfunction benefit from digoxin (or, at least, do *not* benefit from digoxin withdrawal), even when they have only mild symptoms. Accordingly, digoxin is recommended for symptomatic heart failure unless contraindicated. Together with ACE inhibitors, β-blockers, and diuretics, digoxin should be added to the therapeutic armamentarium. Ideally, serum digoxin concentration should remain between 0.7 and 1.1 ng/mL. In the elderly patient with renal insufficiency, severe conduction abnormalities, or acute coronary syndromes, even a low dose of 0.125 mg/day should be used with extra caution.[19]

Future Therapy

Among the promising nonpharmacologic therapies for the management of heart failure are the implantable defibrillators and biventricular pacemakers. In the COMPANION trial (The Comparison of Medical Therapy, Pacing, and Defibrillation in Heart Failure), cardiac resynchronization therapy with a pacemaker combined with an implantable defibrillator significantly decreased the likelihood of death from or hospitalization for heart failure when compared with conventional pharmacologic therapy.[20]

Stem cell therapy is another potential treatment of heart failure. Stem cell therapy has shown promise in the treatment of ischemic heart disease both in the laboratory and in small clinical studies. Autologous bone marrow and peripheral blood stem cells transplanted in patients with acute myocardial infarction improved cardiac function. However, until double-blind, randomized controlled trials are performed, the true benefit of this innovative treatment remains unknown.

Management of Acute Exacerbations of Chronic Heart Failure

Patients with chronic heart failure, despite good medical management, may experience episodes of pulmonary edema or other signs of acute volume overload. These patients may require hospitalization for intensive management if diuretics fail to relieve their symptoms. Other patients may experience exacerbations of heart failure associated with acute myocardial ischemia or infarction, worsening valvular dysfunction, infections (including myocarditis), or failure to maintain an established drug regimen. Fonarow and associates described a risk stratification system for in-hospital mortality in acutely decompensated heart failure using data from a national registry. Low-, intermediate-, and high-risk patients with mortality ranging from 2.1% to 21.9% were identified using blood urea nitrogen, creatinine, and systolic BP on admission. These patients will require all the standard medications, as outlined in previous sections, and may also require infusions of vasodilators or positive inotropic drugs.[21]

Vasodilators

Intravenous vasodilators have long been used to treat the symptoms of low CO in patients with decompensated chronic heart failure. In general, vasodilators reduce ventricular filling pressures and SVR while increasing SV and CO. NTG is commonly used for this purpose and has been studied in numerous clinical trials. It is often initially effective at relatively small doses (20 to 40 µg/min) but frequently requires progressively increasing doses to counteract tachyphylaxis. NTG is associated with dose-dependent arterial hypotension.

Nesiritide

Brain natriuretic peptide (BNP) is a 32-amino acid peptide that is mainly secreted from the cardiac ventricles. Physiologically, BNP functions as a natriuretic and diuretic. It also serves as a counterregulatory hormone to Ang II, norepinephrine, and endothelin by decreasing the synthesis of these agents and by direct vasodilation.

As the clinical severity of heart failure increases, the concentrations of BNP in blood also increase. As a result, measurements of BNP in blood have been used to evaluate new onset of dyspnea (to distinguish between lung disease and heart failure). BNP concentrations in blood increase with decreasing left ventricular ejection fraction; therefore, measurements of this mediator have been used to estimate prognosis.

8

BNP concentrations decline in response to therapy with ACE inhibitors, Ang II antagonists, and aldosterone antagonists.

In addition, recombinant BNP has been released as a drug (nesiritide) indicated for patients with acute heart failure and dyspnea with minimal activity. Nesiritide produces arterial and venous dilatation through increasing cGMP. Nesiritide does not increase HR and has no effect on cardiac inotropy. It has a rapid onset of action and a short elimination half-life (15 minutes). In clinical studies, loading doses have ranged from 0.25 to 2 µg/kg and maintenance doses have ranged from 0.005 to 0.03 µg/kg/min. Studies have shown that nesiritide reduces symptoms of acute decompensated heart failure similarly to NTG, without development of acute tolerance. Patients receiving nesiritide experienced fewer adverse events than those receiving NTG. However, the mortality rate at 6 months was higher in the patients receiving nesiritide than in the NTG group.[22] Compared with dobutamine, nesiritide was associated with fewer instances of ventricular tachycardia or cardiac arrest.

Inotropes

Positive inotropic drugs, principally dobutamine or milrinone, have long been used to treat decompensated heart failure, despite the lack of data showing an outcome benefit to their use. In the past, some chronic heart failure patients would receive intermittent infusions of positive inotropic drugs as part of their maintenance therapy. Small studies consistently demonstrate improved hemodynamic values and reduced symptoms after administration of these agents to patients with heart failure. Studies comparing dobutamine to milrinone for advanced decompensated heart failure showed large differences in drug costs, favoring dobutamine, and only small hemodynamic differences, favoring milrinone.

Nevertheless, placebo-controlled studies suggest that there may be no role whatsoever for discretionary administration of positive inotropes to patients with chronic heart failure. In one study, 951 hospitalized patients with decompensated chronic heart failure who did not require intravenous inotropic support were assigned to receive a 48-hour infusion of either milrinone or saline. Meanwhile, all patients received ACE inhibitors and diuretics as deemed necessary. Total hospital days did not differ between groups; however, those receiving milrinone were significantly more likely to require intervention for hypotension or to have new atrial arrhythmias. A subanalysis of these results found that patients suffering from ischemic cardiomyopathy were particularly subject to adverse events from milrinone (a 42% incidence of death or rehospitalization versus 36% for placebo). At the present, positive inotropic drug support can be recommended only when there is no alternative. Thus, dobutamine and milrinone continue to be used to treat low CO in decompensated heart failure, but only in selected patients.[23]

Alternate Therapies

When drug treatment proves unsuccessful, heart failure patients may require invasive therapy, including ventricular assist devices, biventricular pacing, coronary artery bypass with or without surgical remodeling, or even cardiac orthotopic transplantation.

Low-Output Syndrome

Acute heart failure is a frequent concern of the cardiac anesthesiologist, particularly at the time of separation from cardiopulmonary bypass (CPB). The new onset of ventricular dysfunction and a low CO state after aortic clamping and reperfusion is a condition with more pathophysiologic similarity to cardiogenic shock than to

II

chronic heart failure and is typically treated with positive inotropic drugs, vasopressors (or vasodilators), if needed, and/or mechanical assistance. The latter more commonly takes the form of intra-aortic balloon counterpulsation and less commonly includes one of the several available ventricular assist devices.

Causes

Most patients undergoing cardiac surgery with CPB experience a temporary decline in ventricular function, with a recovery to normal function in a period of roughly 24 hours. Thus, pathophysiologic explanations must acknowledge the (usual) temporary nature of the low-output syndrome after CPB. Most likely, this results from one of three processes, all related to inadequate oxygen delivery to the myocardium: acute ischemia, hibernation, or stunning. All three processes would be expected to improve with adequate revascularization and moderate doses of positive inotropic drugs, consistent with the typical progress of the cardiac surgery patient. All three processes would be expected to be more troublesome in patients with preexisting chronic heart failure, pulmonary hypertension, or arrhythmias.

Risk Factors for the Low-Output Syndrome after Cardiopulmonary Bypass

The need for inotropic drug support after CPB can often be anticipated based on data available in the preoperative medical history, physical examination, and imaging studies. In a series of consecutive patients undergoing elective CABG, it was observed that increasing age, decreasing left ventricular ejection fraction, female sex, cardiac enlargement (on the chest radiograph), and prolonged duration of CPB were all associated with an increased likelihood that the patient would be receiving positive inotropic drugs on arrival in the intensive care unit. Similarly, in a study of patients undergoing cardiac valve surgery, it was found that increasing age, reduced left ventricular ejection fraction, and the presence of CAD all increased the likelihood that a patient would receive positive inotropic drug support.

Specific Drugs for Treating the Low-Output Syndrome

Whereas all positive inotropic drugs increase the strength of contraction in noninfarcted myocardium, mechanisms of action differ. These drugs can be divided into those that increase cyclic adenosine monophosphate (cAMP) (directly or indirectly) for their mechanisms of action and those that do not. The agents that do not depend on cAMP form a diverse group, including cardiac glycosides, calcium salts, calcium sensitizers, and thyroid hormone. In contrast to chronic heart failure, cardiac glycosides are not used for this indication, owing to their limited efficacy and narrow margin of safety. Calcium salts continue to be administered for ionized hypocalcemia and hyperkalemia, which are common occurrences during and after cardiac surgery. Increased Ca^{2+} in buffer solutions bathing cardiac muscle in vitro unquestionably increase inotropy. Calcium sensitizers, specifically levosimendan, function by binding to troponin C in a calcium-dependent fashion. Thus, levosimendan does not impair diastolic function because its affinity for troponin C declines with Ca^{2+} during diastole. Although several reports have described the successful use of levosimendan in patients recovering from CABG, clinical experience with this agent remains limited and there is no consensus as to how and when this agent should be used, relative to other, better established agents.[24]

Intravenous thyroid hormone (T_3, or liothyronine) has been studied extensively as a positive inotrope in cardiac surgery. There are multiple studies supporting the existence of euthyroid "sick" syndrome with persistent reduced concentrations of T_3 in blood after cardiac surgery in both children and adults. There are also data suggesting that after ischemia and reperfusion, T_3 increases inotropy faster than and as potently as isoproterenol. Nevertheless, randomized controlled clinical trials have failed to show efficacy of T_3 after CABG.

The cAMP-dependent agents form the mainstays of positive inotropic drug therapy after cardiac surgery. There are two main classes of agents: the phosphodiesterase (PDE) inhibitors and the β-adrenergic receptor agonists. There are many different phosphodiesterase inhibitors in clinical use around the world, including enoximone, inamrinone, milrinone, olprinone, and piroximone. Comparisons among the agents have failed to demonstrate important hemodynamic differences. Reported differences relate to pharmacokinetics and rare side effects, typically observed with chronic oral administrations during clinical trials. All members of the class produce rapid increases in contractile function and CO and decreases in SVR. The effect on BP is variable, depending on the pretreatment state of hydration and hemodynamics; nevertheless, the typical response is a small decrease in BP. There is either no effect on HR or a small increase. Inamrinone and milrinone have been shown to be effective, first-line agents in patients with reduced preoperative left ventricular function. Milrinone, the most commonly used member of the class, is most often dosed at a 50-µg/kg loading dose and 0.5-µg/kg/min maintenance infusion. It is often given in combination with a β-adrenergic receptor agonist.

Among the many β-adrenergic receptor agonists, the agents most often given to patients recovering from cardiac surgery are dopamine, dobutamine, and epinephrine. Dopamine has long been assumed to have dose-defined receptor specificity. At small doses (0.5 to 3 µg/kg/min), it is assumed to have an effect mostly on dopaminergic receptors. At intermediate doses, β-adrenergic effects are said to predominate; and at doses of 10 µg/kg/min or greater, α-adrenergic receptor effects predominate. Nevertheless, the relationship between dose and blood concentration is poorly predictable. Dopamine is a relatively weak inotrope that has a predominant effect on HR rather than on SV.

Dobutamine is a selective β-adrenergic receptor agonist. Most studies suggest that it causes less tachycardia and hypotension than isoproterenol. It has been frequently compared with dopamine, where dobutamine's greater tendency for pulmonary and systemic vasodilation is evident. Dobutamine has a predominant effect on HR, compared with SV, and as the dose is increased more than 10 µg/kg/min there are further increases in HR without changes in SV.

Epinephrine is a powerful adrenergic agonist, and, like dopamine, demonstrates differing effects depending on the dose. At small doses (10 to 30 ng/kg/min), despite an almost pure β-adrenergic receptor stimulus, there is almost no increase in HR. Clinicians have long assumed that epinephrine increases HR more than dobutamine administered at comparable doses. Nevertheless, in patients recovering from cardiac surgery, the opposite is true: dobutamine increases HR more than epinephrine.

Other β-adrenergic agonists are used in specific circumstances. For example, isoproterenol is often used after cardiac transplantation to exploit its powerful chronotropy and after correction of congenital heart defects to exploit its pulmonary vasodilatory effects. Norepinephrine is exploited to counteract profound vasodilation.

Pharmacologic Treatment of Diastolic Heart Failure

Abnormal diastolic ventricular function is a common cause of clinical heart failure. As many as one in three patients presenting with clinical signs of chronic heart failure has a normal or near-normal ejection fraction (≥40%). The risk of diastolic heart failure increases with age, approaching 50% in patients older than 70 years old. Diastolic heart failure is also more common in females and in patients with hypertension or diabetes mellitus. Although the prognosis of patients with diastolic heart failure is better than for systolic heart failure (5% to 8% vs. 10% to 15% annual mortality, respectively), the complication rate is the same. The 1-year readmission rate for patients with isolated diastolic heart failure approaches 50%.

In contrast to the large randomized trials that have led to the treatment guidelines for systolic heart failure, there are few randomized, double-blind, placebo-controlled, multicenter trials performed in patients with diastolic heart failure. Consequently, the guidelines are based on clinical experience, small clinical studies, and an understanding of the pathophysiologic mechanisms. The general approach to treating diastolic heart failure has three main components. First, treatment should reduce symptoms, primarily by lowering pulmonary venous pressure during rest and exercise by reducing left ventricular volume, maintaining AV synchrony, and increasing the duration of diastole by reducing HR. Second, treatment should target the underlying causes of diastolic heart failure. Specifically, ventricular remodeling should be reversed by controlling hypertension, replacing stenotic aortic valves, and treating ischemia. Third, treatment should target the underlying mechanisms that are altered by the disease processes, mainly neurohormonal activation. Drug treatment of diastolic heart failure with respect to these three goals is shown in Table 8-10.

Many of the drugs used to treat systolic heart failure are also used to treat diastolic heart failure. However, the reason for their use and the doses used may be different for diastolic heart failure. For instance, in diastolic heart failure β-blockers are used to increase the time of diastolic filling whereas in systolic heart failure, β-blockers are used to reverse heart remodeling (e.g., carvedilol). In fact, metoprolol-CR/XL may be a better β-blocker choice than carvedilol for diastolic heart failure because too low a BP (as a consequence of carvedilol) may be detrimental for the diastolic heart failure patient. Similarly, diuretic and NTG doses for diastolic heart failure are usually much smaller than for systolic heart failure, because the patient with diastolic heart failure is very sensitive to large reductions in preload. Calcium channel blockers are not a part of the armamentarium in the treatment of systolic heart failure but *may* be beneficial in treating diastolic heart failure through effects on rate control, specifically the long-acting dihydropyridine class of calcium channel blockers. With the exception of rate control in chronic atrial fibrillation, digoxin is not recommended for diastolic heart failure.

Except in the presence of acute diastolic heart failure, positive inotropic and chronotropic agents should be avoided because they may worsen diastolic function by increasing contractile force and HR, or by increasing calcium concentrations in diastole. However, in the short-term management of acute diastolic dysfunction or heart failure (e.g., post CPB), β-adrenergic agonists (e.g., epinephrine) and phosphodiesterase inhibitors (e.g., milrinone) enhance calcium sequestration by the sarcoplasmic reticulum and thereby promote a more rapid and complete myocardial relaxation between beats.[25,26]

Current Clinical Practice

The pharmacotherapy of heart failure begins with primary prevention of left ventricular dysfunction. Because hypertension and coronary artery disease are leading causes of left ventricular dysfunction, adequate treatment of both hypertension and hypercholesterolemia has been endorsed after encouraging results in prevention trials. Limitation of neurohormonal activation with ACE inhibitors, and possibly β-blockers, should be initiated in diabetic, hypertensive, and hypercholesterolemic

Table 8-10 Diastolic Heart Failure Treatments

Goal	Management Strategy	Drugs/Recommended Doses
Reduce the congestive state	Salt restriction	< 2 g of sodium/day
	Diuretics (avoid reductions in cardiac output)	Furosemide, 10 to 120 mg
	ACE inhibitors	Hydrochlorothiazide, 12.5 to 25 mg
	Angiotensin II receptor blockers	Enalapril, 2.5 to 40 mg
		Lisinopril, 10 to 40 mg
		Candesartan, 4 to 32 mg
		Losartan, 25 to 100 mg
Target underlying cause Control hypertension Restore sinus rhythm Prevent tachycardia Prevent/treat ischemia Treat aortic stenosis	Antihypertensive agents (<130/80) Cardioversion of atrial fibrillation Atrioventricular sequential pacing β-Blockers, calcium channel blockers Morphine, nitrates, oxygen, aspirin Angioplasty or revascularization? Aortic valve replacement (Theoretical)	β-Blockers, ACE inhibitors, all receptor blockers according to published guidelines Atenolol, 12.5 to 100 mg; metoprolol, 25 to 100 mg; diltiazem, 120 to 540 mg
Target underlying mechanisms Promote regression of hypertrophy and prevent myocardial fibrosis	Renin-angiotensin axis blockade	Enalapril, 2.5 to 40 mg Lisinopril, 10 to 40 mg Captopril, 25 to 150 mg Candesartan, 4 to 32 mg Losartan, 50 to 100 mg Spironolactone, 25 to 75 mg Eplerenone, 25 to 50 mg

ACE = angiotensin-converting enzyme.
Adapted from Aurigemma GP, Gaasch WH: Clinical practice. Diastolic heart failure. N Engl J Med 351:1097, 2004.

patients (AHA/ACC, stage A heart failure) who are at increased risk for cardiovascular events, despite normal contractile function, in order to reduce the onset of new heart failure (HOPE trial). In patients with asymptomatic left ventricular dysfunction (ejection fraction = 40%) (stage B), treatment with ACE inhibitors and β-blockers can blunt the disease progression. In the symptomatic patient with heart failure (stage C), diuretics are titrated to relieve symptoms of pulmonary congestion and peripheral edema and achieve a euvolemic state whereas ACE inhibitors and β-blockers are recommended to blunt disease progression. Although digoxin has no effect on patient survival, it may be considered in stage C if the patient remains symptomatic despite adequate doses of ACE inhibitors and diuretics. In general, the primary treatment objectives for stages A to C heart failure are to (1) improve quality of life, (2) reduce morbidity, and (3) reduce mortality. At this time, the most important factor affecting long-term outcome is blunting of neurohormonal stimulation, because this mediates disease progression. Pharmacologic therapy in stage D, or patients with severe, decompensated heart failure, is based on hemodynamic status to alleviate symptoms with diuretics, vasodilators, and, in palliative circumstances, intravenous inotropic infusions. ACE inhibitors and β-blockers are also incorporated in the treatment regimen to retard disease progression through reductions in ventricular enlargement, vascular hypertrophy, and ventricular arrhythmias[27] (Fig. 8-6).

PHARMACOTHERAPY FOR CARDIAC ARRHYTHMIAS

Perhaps the most widely used electrophysiologic and pharmacologic classification of antiarrhythmic drugs is that proposed by Vaughan Williams (Table 8-11). There is, however, substantial overlap in pharmacologic and electrophysiologic effects of specific agents among the classes, and the linkage between observed electrophysiologic effects and the clinical antiarrhythmic effect is often tenuous.[28]

Class I Antiarrhythmic Drugs: Sodium Channel Blockers

Class I drugs have the common property of inhibiting the fast inward depolarizing current carried by sodium ion. Because of the diversity of other effects of the class I drugs, a subgroup of the class has been proposed.

Class IA

PROCAINAMIDE

Electrophysiologic effects of procainamide include decreased Vmax and amplitude during phase 0, decreased rate of phase 4 depolarization, and prolonged effective refractory period (ERP) and action potential duration (APD). Clinically, procainamide prolongs conduction and increases the ERP in atrial and His-Purkinje portions of the conduction system, which may prolong PR interval and QRS complex durations.

Procainamide is used to treat ventricular arrhythmias and to suppress atrial premature beats to prevent the occurrence of atrial fibrillation and flutter. It has been very useful for chronic suppression of premature ventricular contractions.

Administered intravenously, procainamide is an effective emergency treatment for ventricular arrhythmias, especially after lidocaine failure, but, recently, amiodarone has become a more popular drug for intravenous suppression of ventricular arrhythmias.[29] Dosage is 100 mg, or approximately 1.5 mg/kg given at 5-minute intervals until the therapeutic effect is obtained or a total dose of 1 g or 15 mg/kg is given (Tables 8-12 and 8-13). Arterial pressure and the ECG should be monitored continuously during loading and administration stopped if significant hypotension occurs or if the QRS complex is prolonged by 50% or more. Maintenance infusion rates are 2 to 6 mg/min to maintain therapeutic plasma concentrations of 4 to 8 µg/mL.

Class IB

LIDOCAINE

First introduced as an antiarrhythmic drug in the 1950s, lidocaine has become the clinical standard for the acute intravenous treatment of ventricular arrhythmias except those precipitated by an abnormally prolonged QT interval. Lidocaine may, in fact, be one of the most useful drugs in clinical anesthesia because it has both local and general anesthetic properties, in addition to an antiarrhythmic effect.

8

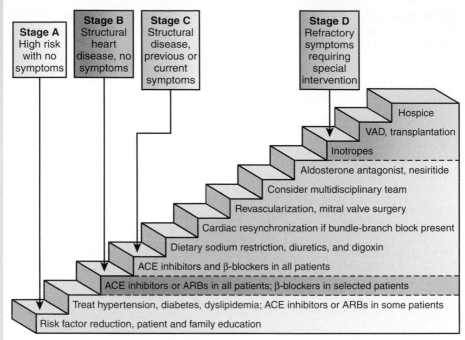

Stage A High risk with no symptoms

Stage B Structural heart disease, no symptoms

Stage C Structural disease, previous or current symptoms

Stage D Refractory symptoms requiring special intervention

Hospice

VAD, transplantation

Inotropes

Aldosterone antagonist, nesiritide

Consider multidisciplinary team

Revascularization, mitral valve surgery

Cardiac resynchronization if bundle-branch block present

Dietary sodium restriction, diuretics, and digoxin

ACE inhibitors and β-blockers in all patients

ACE inhibitors or ARBs in all patients; β-blockers in selected patients

Treat hypertension, diabetes, dyslipidemia; ACE inhibitors or ARBs in some patients

Risk factor reduction, patient and family education

Figure 8-6 Treatment options for the stages of heart failure. (Redrawn from Jessup M, Brozena S: Heart failure. N Engl J Med 348:2007, 2003.)

Table 8-11 Classification of Antiarrhythmic Drugs

Effect	Class			
	I (Membrane Stabilizers)	*II (β-Adrenergic Receptor Antagonists)*	*III (Drugs Prolonging Repolarization)*	*IV (Calcium Antagonists)*
Pharmacologic	Fast channel (Na⁺) blockade	β-Adrenergic receptor blockade	Uncertain: possible interference with Na⁺ and Ca²⁺ exchange	Decreased slow-channel calcium conductance
Electro-physiologic	Decreased rate of Vmax	Decreased Vmax, increased APD, increased ERP, and increased ERP/APD ratio	Increased APD, increased ERP, increased ERP/APD ratio	Decreased slow-channel depolarization; decreased APD

Vmax = maximal rate of depolarization; APD = action potential duration; ERP = effective refractory period.

The direct electrophysiologic effects of lidocaine produce virtually all of its antiarrhythmic action. Lidocaine depresses the slope of phase 4 diastolic depolarization in Purkinje fibers and increases the ventricular fibrillation threshold. Lidocaine may be ineffective in hypokalemic patients.

Therapeutic plasma levels of lidocaine range from 1.5 to 5 µg/mL; signs of toxicity are frequent with concentrations above 9 µg/mL. An initial bolus dose of 1 to 1.5 mg/kg

Table 8-12	**Intravenous Supraventricular Antiarrhythmic Therapy**
Class I	Procainamide (IA)—converts acute atrial fibrillation, suppresses PACs and precipitation of atrial fibrillation/flutter, converts accessory pathway SVT. 100 mg IV loading dose every 5 min until arrhythmia subsides or total dose of 15 mg/kg (rarely needed) with continuous infusion of 2 to 6 mg/min.
Class II	Esmolol—converts or maintains slow ventricular response in acute atrial fibrillation. 0.5 to 1 mg/kg loading dose with each 50 µg/kg/min increase in infusion, with infusions of 50 to 300 µg/kg/min. Hypotension and bradycardia are limiting factors.
Class III	Amiodarone—converts acute atrial fibrillation to sinus rhythm; 5 mg/kg IV over 15 min.
	Ibutilide (Convert)—converts acute atrial fibrillation and flutter. Adults (>60 kg): 1 mg given over 10 min IV, may be repeated once.
	Adults (<60 kg) and children: 0.01 mg/kg given over 10 min IV, may be repeated once.
Class IV	Verapamil—slow ventricular response to acute atrial fibrillation, converts AV node reentry SVT. 75 to 150 µg/kg IV bolus.
	Diltiazem—slow ventricular response in acute atrial fibrillation, converts AV node reentry SVT. 0.25 µg/kg bolus, then 100 to 300 µg/kg/hr infusion.
Others	Adenosine—converts AV node reentry SVT and accessory pathway SVT. Aids in diagnosis of atrial fibrillation and flutter. Adults: 3 to 6 mg IV bolus, repeat with 6- to 12-mg bolus. Children: 100 µg/kg bolus, repeat with 200-µg/kg bolus. Increased dosage required with methylxanthines, decreased use required with dipyridamole.
	Digoxin—maintenance IV therapy for atrial fibrillation and flutter, slows ventricular response. Adults: 0.25-mg IV bolus followed by 0.125 mg every 1 to 2 hr until rate controlled, not to exceed 10 µg/kg in 24 hr. Children (<10 years of age): 10- to 30-µg/kg load given in divided doses over 24 hours. Maintenance: 25% of loading dose.

should be followed immediately by a continuous infusion of 20 to 50 µg/kg/min to prevent the "therapeutic hiatus" produced by the rapid redistribution half-life of lidocaine.[30]

Class II: β-Adrenergic Receptor Antagonists

β-Adrenergic receptor blockers are very effective antiarrhythmics in patients during the perioperative period or who are critically ill because many arrhythmias in these patients are adrenergically mediated.

Propranolol

Propranolol was the first major β-receptor–blocking drug to be used clinically. Propranolol is very potent but is nonselective for β_1/β_2-receptor subtypes.

The electrophysiologic effects of β-receptor antagonism are decreased automaticity, increased APD, primarily in ventricular muscle, and a substantially increased ERP in the AV node. β-Blockade decreases the rate of spontaneous (phase 4) depolarization in the SA node; the magnitude of this effect depends on the background sympathetic tone. Although resting HR is decreased by β-blockade, the inhibition of

8

Table 8-13	**Intravenous Ventricular Antiarrhythmic Therapy**
Class I	Procainamide (IA)—100 mg IV loading dose every 5 min until arrhythmia subsides or total dose of 15 mg/kg (rarely needed) with continuous infusion of 2 to 6 mg/min Lidocaine (IB)—1.5 mg/kg in divided doses given twice over 20 min with continuous infusion of 1 to 4 mg/min
Class II	Propranolol—0.5 to 1 mg given slowly up to a total β-blocking dose of 0.1 mg/kg. Repeat bolus as needed. Metoprolol—2.5 mg given slowly up to a total β-blocking dose of 0.2 mg/kg. Repeat bolus as needed. Esmolol—0.5 to 1.0 mg/kg loading dose with each 50 μg/kg /min increase in infusion, with infusions of 50 to 300 μg/kg/min. Hypotension and bradycardia are limiting factors.
Class III	Bretylium—5 mg/kg loading dose given slowly with a continuous infusion of 1 to 5 mg/min. Hypotension may be a limiting factor with infusion. Amiodarone—150 mg IV over 10 min, then 1 mg/min for 6 hours, then 0.5 mg/min for the next 18 hr. Repeat bolus as needed.
Others	Magnesium—2 g MgSO$_4$ over 5 min, then continuous infusion of 1 g/hr for 6 to 10 hr to restore intracellular magnesium levels.

Adapted from Management of Cardiac Rhythm Disturbances. *46th Annual Refresher Course Lectures and Clinical Update Program*. Park Ridge, IL: American Society of Anesthesiologists; 1995: No. 255.

the increase of HR in response to exercise or emotional stress is much more marked. Automaticity in the AV node and more distal portions of the conduction system is also depressed. β-Blockade affects the ventricular fibrillation threshold variably, but it consistently reverses the fibrillation threshold-lowering effect of catecholamines.

An appropriate intravenous dose for acute control of arrhythmias is 0.5 to 1.0 mg titrated to therapeutic effect up to a total of 0.1 to 0.15 mg/kg. Stable therapeutic plasma concentrations of propranolol can be obtained with a continuous intravenous infusion. An effective level of β-blockade may be obtained with a continuous infusion approximating 3 mg/hr in adult postoperative patients previously receiving chronic treatment; however, with the availability of esmolol, the need for a propranolol infusion is no longer necessary.

Esmolol

Esmolol is a cardioselective (β$_1$) receptor antagonist with an extremely brief duration of action. In anesthetized dogs, esmolol infused at 50 μg/kg/min produced a steady-state β-blockade that was completely reversed 20 minutes after stopping the infusion. Esmolol has no effect on LVEDP, BP, HR, CO, or SVR; however, at 5 to 60 μg/kg/min, it does decrease left ventricular dP/dt. The decreased contractility, however, fully resolves by 20 minutes after the infusion.

Esmolol is rapidly metabolized in blood by hydrolysis of its methyl ester linkage. Its half-life in whole blood is 12.5 and 27.1 minutes in dogs and humans, respectively. The acid metabolite possesses a slight degree (1500 times less than esmolol) of β-antagonism. Esmolol is not affected by plasma cholinesterase; the esterase responsible is located in erythrocytes and is not inhibited by cholinesterase inhibitors, but it is deactivated by sodium fluoride. Of importance to clinical anesthesia, no metabolic interactions between esmolol and other ester molecules are known. Specifically, esmolol doses up to 500 μg/kg/min have not modified neuromuscular effects of succinylcholine.

Clinically, in asthmatic patients, esmolol (300 μg/kg/min) only slightly increases airway resistance. Also, in patients with chronic obstructive pulmonary disease who received esmolol, no adverse pulmonary effects occurred. In a multicenter trial, in a comparison with propranolol for the treatment of paroxysmal supraventricular tachycardia (PSVT), esmolol was equally efficacious and had the advantage of a much faster termination of the β-blockade. Esmolol has become a very useful agent in controlling sinus tachycardia in the perioperative period, a time when a titratable and brief β-blockade is highly desirable.

Dosing begins at 25 μg/kg/min and is titrated to effect up to 250 μg/kg/min. Doses higher than this may cause significant hypotension due to reduced CO in patients. Esmolol is especially effective in treating acute onset atrial fibrillation or flutter perioperatively and results in both acute control of the ventricular response and conversion of the arrhythmia back to sinus rhythm.[31]

Class III: Agents That Block Potassium Channels and Prolong Repolarization

Amiodarone

The drug has a wide spectrum of effectiveness, including supraventricular, ventricular, and preexcitation arrhythmias. It may also be effective against ventricular tachycardia and ventricular fibrillation refractory to other treatment. Amiodarone has been approved by the AHA as the first-line antiarrhythmic agent in cardiopulmonary resuscitation. Amiodarone may be effective prophylactically in preventing atrial fibrillation postoperatively. It also can decrease the number of shocks in patients who have implantable cardioverter defibrillators compared with other antiarrhythmic drugs.[32]

Amiodarone increases the amount of electric current required to elicit ventricular fibrillation (an increase in ventricular fibrillation threshold). In most patients, refractory ventricular tachycardia is suppressed by acute intravenous use of amiodarone. This effect has been attributed to a selectively increased activity in diseased tissue, as has been seen with lidocaine. Amiodarone also has an adrenergic-receptor (α and β) antagonistic effect produced by a noncompetitive mechanism; the contribution of this effect to the antiarrhythmic action of the drug is not known.

Hemodynamic effects of intravenously administered amiodarone include decreased left ventricular dP/dt, maximal negative dP/dt, mean aortic pressure, HR, and peak left ventricular pressure. A 5-mg/kg intravenous dose during cardiac catheterization decreased BP, LVEDP, and SVR and increased CO, but it did not affect HR. Chronic amiodarone therapy is not associated with clinically significant depression of ventricular function in patients without left ventricular failure. Hemodynamic deterioration may occur in some patients with compensated congestive heart failure, perhaps because of the antiadrenergic effects of the drug.

In acute situations with stable patients, a 150-mg intravenous bolus is followed by a 1.0-mg/min infusion for 6 hours and then 0.5 mg/min thereafter. In cardiopulmonary resuscitation, a 300-mg intravenous bolus is given and repeated with multiple boluses as needed if defibrillation is unsuccessful.

Despite relatively widespread use of amiodarone, anesthetic complications have infrequently been reported. In two case reports, bradycardia and hypotension were prominent. One of the reports described profound resistance to the vasoconstrictive effects of α-adrenergic agonists. The slow decay of amiodarone in plasma and tissue makes such adverse reactions possible long after discontinuing its administration. Because T_3 is reported

8

to reverse electrophysiologic effects of amiodarone, T_3 could possibly be used to reverse hemodynamic abnormalities, such as those described in these two case reports, although this theory has not been tested. Epinephrine has been shown to be more effective than dobutamine or isoproterenol in reversing amiodarone-induced cardiac depression.

Class IV: Calcium Channel Antagonists

Although the principal direct electrophysiologic effects of the three main chemical groups of calcium antagonists (verapamil, a benzoacetonitrite; nifedipine, a dihydropyridine; and diltiazem, a benzothiazepine) are similar, verapamil and diltiazem are the primary antiarrhythmic agents.

Verapamil and Diltiazem

Verapamil and diltiazem have been used extensively in the treatment of supraventricular arrhythmias, atrial fibrillation, and atrial flutter. They are especially effective at preventing or terminating PSVT by blocking impulse transmission through the AV node by prolonging AV nodal conduction and refractoriness. They are also useful in the treatment of atrial fibrillation and atrial flutter by slowing AV nodal conduction and decreasing the ventricular response. The effect on ventricular response is similar to that of the cardiac glycosides, although the onset is more rapid and acutely effective for control of tachycardia in patients.

In the perioperative period, verapamil is a useful antiarrhythmic agent. It successfully controlled a variety of supraventricular and ventricular arrhythmias. However, verapamil should be used cautiously intraoperatively because, in conjunction with inhalation anesthetics, significant cardiac depression may occur.

Verapamil dosage for acute intravenous treatment of PSVT is 0.07 to 0.15 mg/kg over 1 minute, with the same dose repeated after 30 minutes if the initial response is inadequate (10 mg maximum). Because the cardiovascular depressant effects of the inhalation anesthetics involve inhibition of calcium-related intracellular processes, the interaction of verapamil and these anesthetics is synergistic. In one large clinical series, verapamil given during steady-state halothane anesthesia transiently decreased BP and produced a 4% incidence of PR interval prolongation. In laboratory studies, verapamil interacts similarly with halothane, enflurane, and isoflurane to mildly depress ventricular function and to slow AV conduction (PR interval). AV block can occur, however, and may be refractory. In addition, AV block can occur when verapamil is combined with β-blockers.

Diltiazem in doses of 0.25 to 0.30 mg/kg administered intravenously followed by a titratable intravenous infusion of 10 to 20 mg/hr has been shown to be rapid acting and efficacious in controlling ventricular response rate in new-onset atrial fibrillation and atrial flutter. In addition, the prophylactic use of intravenous diltiazem has been shown to reduce the incidence of postoperative supraventricular arrhythmias after pneumonectomy and cardiac surgery. Diltiazem may also have a role in treating ventricular arrhythmias. In an experimental model, diltiazem has been shown to be protective against ventricular fibrillation with acute cocaine toxicity.

Other Antiarrhythmic Agents

Digoxin

The primary therapeutic use of digitalis drugs is to slow the ventricular response during atrial fibrillation or atrial flutter, which occurs because of a complex combination of direct and indirect actions on the AV node. The primary direct pharmacologic effect of digitalis is inhibition of the membrane-bound Na^+-K^+ ATPase.

The main preparation of cardiac glycosides available is digoxin. Digoxin reaches peak effects in 1.5 to 2 hours but has a significant effect within 5 to 30 minutes. For undigitalized patients, the initial dose is 0.5 to 0.75 mg of digoxin, with subsequent doses of 0.125 to 0.25 mg. The usual total digitalizing dose ranges from 0.75 to 1.0 mg by the intravenous route. Digoxin is approximately 25% protein bound, and the therapeutic range of plasma concentrations is 0.5 to 2.0 ng/mL.

Adenosine

The important cardiac electrophysiologic effects of adenosine are mediated by the A_1-receptor and consist of negative chronotropic, dromotropic, and inotropic actions. Adenosine decreases SA node activity, AV node conductivity, and ventricular automaticity. In many ways these effects mimic those of acetylcholine.

For clinical use, adenosine must be administered by a rapid intravenous bolus in a dose of 100 to 200 μg/kg, although continuous intravenous infusions of 150 to 300 μg/kg/min have been used to produce controlled hypotension. For practical purposes, in adults an intravenous dose of 3 to 6 mg is given by bolus followed by a second dose of 6 to 12 mg after 1 minute if the first dose was not effective. This therapy rapidly interrupts narrow-complex tachycardia caused by AV nodal reentry. Comparison with verapamil has shown adenosine to be equally effective as an antiarrhythmic agent but with the advantages of fewer adverse hemodynamic effects, a faster onset of action, and a more rapid elimination so that undesired effects are short-lived.[33]

Potassium

Because of the close relationship between extracellular pH and potassium, the primary mechanism of pH-induced arrhythmias may be alteration of potassium concentration. Both hypokalemia and hyperkalemia are associated with cardiac arrhythmias; however, hypokalemia is more common perioperatively in cardiac surgical patients and is more commonly associated with arrhythmias. Decreasing extracellular potassium concentration increases the peak negative diastolic potential, which would theoretically appear to decrease the likelihood of spontaneous depolarization. However, because the permeability of the myocardial cell membrane to potassium is directly related to extracellular potassium concentration, hypokalemia decreases cellular permeability to potassium. This prolongs the action potential by slowing repolarization, which in turn slows conduction and increases the dispersion of recovery of excitability and, thus, predisposes to the development of arrhythmias. ECG correlates of hypokalemia include appearance of a U wave and increased P-wave amplitude. The arrhythmias most commonly associated with hypokalemia are premature atrial contractions (PACs), atrial tachycardia, and supraventricular tachycardia (SVT). Hypokalemia also accentuates the toxicity of cardiac glycosides.

Moderate hyperkalemia, in contrast, increases membrane permeability to potassium, which increases the speed of repolarization and decreases APD, thereby decreasing the tendency to arrhythmias. An increased potassium concentration also affects pacemaker activity. The increased potassium permeability caused by hyperkalemia decreases the rate of spontaneous diastolic depolarization, which slows HR and, in the extreme case, can produce asystole. The repolarization abnormalities of hyperkalemia lead to the characteristic ECG findings of T-wave peaking, prolonged PR interval, decreased QRS amplitude, and a widened QRS complex. Both AV and intraventricular conduction abnormalities result from the slowed conduction and uneven repolarization.

Treatment of hyperkalemia is based on its magnitude and on the clinical presentation. For life-threatening, hyperkalemia-induced arrhythmias, the principle is rapid reduction of extracellular potassium concentration, a treatment that does not acutely decrease total body potassium content. Calcium chloride, 10 to 20 mg/kg, given by intravenous

8

infusion, will directly antagonize the effects of potassium on the cardiac cell membranes. Sodium bicarbonate, 1 to 2 mEq/kg, or a dose calculated from acid-base measurements to produce moderate alkalinity (pH approximately 7.45 to 7.50), will shift potassium intracellularly. A change in pH of 0.1 unit produces a 0.5 to 1.5 mEq/L change of potassium concentration in the opposite direction. An intravenous infusion of glucose and insulin has a similar effect; glucose at a dose of 0.5 to 2.0 g/kg with insulin in the ratio of 1 unit to 4 g of glucose is appropriate. Sequential measurement of serum potassium is important with this treatment because marked hypokalemia can result.

Acute hypokalemia frequently occurs after CPB as a result of hemodilution, urinary losses, and intracellular shifts, the latter perhaps relating to abnormalities of the glucose-insulin system seen with nonpulsatile hypothermic CPB. With frequent assessment of serum potassium concentrations and continuous ECG monitoring, potassium infusion at rates of up to 10 to 15 mEq/hr may be administered to treat serious hypokalemia.[34]

Magnesium

Magnesium deficiency is also a relatively common electrolyte abnormality in critically ill patients, especially in chronic situations. Hypomagnesemia is associated with a variety of cardiovascular disturbances, including arrhythmias. Sudden death from coronary artery disease, alcoholic cardiomyopathy, and congestive heart failure may involve magnesium deficiency. Functionally, magnesium is required for the membrane-bound Na^+/K^+ ATPase, which is the principal enzyme that maintains normal intracellular potassium concentration. Not surprisingly, the ECG findings seen with magnesium deficiency mimic those seen with hypokalemia: prolonged PR and QT intervals, increased QRS duration, and ST-segment abnormalities. In addition, as with hypokalemia, magnesium deficiency predisposes to the development of the arrhythmias produced by cardiac glycosides.

Arrhythmias induced by magnesium deficiency may be refractory to treatment with antiarrhythmic drugs and either electrical cardioversion or defibrillation. For this reason, adjunctive treatment of refractory arrhythmias with magnesium has been advocated even when magnesium deficiency has not been documented. Magnesium deficiency is common in cardiac surgery patients owing to the diuretic agents these patients are often receiving and because magnesium levels decrease with CPB because of hemodilution of the pump. Magnesium lacks a counterregulatory hormone to increase magnesium levels during CPB in contrast to the hypocalcemia that is corrected by parathyroid hormone. The results of magnesium administration trials involving CABG have been conflicting. Some studies have shown a benefit and others have not in regard to reducing the incidence of postoperative arrhythmias.[35]

SUMMARY

Anti-Ischemic Drug Therapy

- Ischemia during the perioperative period demands immediate attention by the anesthesiologist. The impact of ischemia may be both acute (impending infarction, hemodynamic compromise) and chronic (a marker of previously unknown cardiac disease, a prognostic indicator of poor outcome).
- Nitroglycerin is indicated in nearly all conditions of perioperative myocardial ischemia. Mechanisms of action include coronary vasodilation and favorable alterations in preload and afterload. Nitroglycerin is contraindicated when hypotension is present.

- Perioperative β-blockade may reduce the incidence of perioperative myocardial ischemia via a number of mechanisms. Favorable hemodynamic changes associated with β-blockade include a blunting of the stress response and reduced heart rate, blood pressure, and contractility. All of these conditions improve myocardial oxygen supply/demand ratios.
- Calcium channel blockers reduce myocardial oxygen demand by depression of contractility, heart rate, and/or decreased arterial blood pressure. Calcium channel blockers are often administered in the perioperative period for longer-term antianginal symptom control.

Drug Therapy for Systemic Hypertension

- Current guidelines suggest seeking a target blood pressure of less than 140/85 mm Hg to minimize long-term risk for adverse cardiovascular morbidity and mortality.
- For patients with diabetes, renal impairment, or established cardiovascular diseases, a lower target of less than 130/80 mm Hg is recommended.
- Mild-to-moderate hypertension does not represent an independent risk factor for perioperative complications; however, a diagnosis of hypertension necessitates preoperative assessment for target organ damage.
- Patients with poorly controlled preoperative hypertension experience more labile blood pressures in the perioperative setting with greater potential for hypertensive or hypotensive episodes or both.

Pharmacotherapy for Acute and Chronic Heart Failure

- The signs, symptoms, and treatment of chronic heart failure are as related to the neurohormonal response as they are to the underlying ventricular dysfunction.
- Current treatments of chronic heart failure are aimed at prolonging survival, not just relief of symptoms.
- The low cardiac output syndrome seen after cardiac surgery has a pathophysiology, treatment, and prognosis that differ from those of chronic heart failure, with which it is sometimes compared.

Pharmacotherapy for Cardiac Arrhythmias

- Physicians must be cautious in administering antiarrhythmic drugs because of the proarrhythmic effects that can increase mortality in certain subgroups of patients.
- Amiodarone has become a popular intravenous antiarrhythmic drug for use in the operating room and critical care areas because it has a broad range of effects for ventricular and supraventricular arrhythmias.
- β-Receptor antagonists are very effective but underused antiarrhythmic agents in the perioperative period because many arrhythmias are adrenergically mediated due to the stress of surgery and critical illness.
- Managing electrolyte abnormalities and treating underlying disease processes such as hypervolemia and myocardial ischemia are critical treatment steps before the administration of any antiarrhythmic agent.

REFERENCES

1. ACC/AHA 2007 Guideline Update for the Management of Patients with Unstable Angina and NonST-Segment Elevation Myocardial Infarction. A Report of the American College of Cardiology/American Heart Association Task Force on Practice Guidelines (Committee on Management of Patients with Unstable Angina). J Am Coll Cardiol 50:1-157, 2007
2. Abrams J: Mechanisms of action of the organic nitrates in the treatment of myocardial ischemia. Am J Cardiol 70:30B, 1992
3. Anderson TJ, Meredith IT, Ganz P, et al: Nitric oxide and nitrovasodilators: Similarities. differences, and potential interactions, J Am Coll Cardiol 24:555, 1994
4. London MJ, Zaugg M, Schaub MC, Spahn DR: Perioperative beta-adrenergic receptor blockade, Anesthesiology 100;170, 2004
5. ACC/AHA 2007 Guidelines on perioperative cardiovascular evaluation & care for noncardiac surgery. J Am Coll Cardiol 50:1707-1732, 2007
6. Giles J, Sear J, Foex P: Effect of chronic beta-blockage on perioperative outcome in patients undergoing noncardiac surgery. Anaesthesia 59:574, 2004
7. Eisenberg MJ, Brox A, Bestawros AN. Calcium channel blockers: An update. Am J Med 116:35, 2004
8. Wijeysundara DN, Deactie WS: Calcium Channel Blockers for reducing cardiac morbidity after noncardiac surgery: A meta-analysis. Anesth Analg 97:634-641, 2003.
9. Chobanian AV, Bakris GL, Black HR, et al: The Seventh Report of the Joint National Committee on Prevention, Detection, Evaluation, and Treatment of High Blood Pressure: the JNC 7 report. JAMA 289:2560, 2003
10. Psaty BM, Lumley T, Furberg CD, et al: Health outcomes associated with various antihypertensive therapies used as first-line agents: A network meta-analysis. JAMA 289:2534, 2003
11. Williams B: Recent hypertension trials. J Am Coll Cardiol 45:813, 2005
12. American Heart Association: Heart Disease and Stroke Statistics, 2004. Dallas, TX, American Heart Association. Available at: www.americanheart.org
13. Cohn JN, Ferrari R, Sharpe N: Cardiac remodeling-concepts and clinical implications: A consensus paper from an international forum on cardiac remodeling. J Am Coll Cardiol 35:569, 2000
14. Arnold JM, Yusuf S, Young J, et al: Prevention of Heart Failure in Patients in the Heart Outcomes Prevention Evaluation (HOPE) Study. Circulation 107:1284, 2003
15. Mann DL, Deswal A, Bozkurt B, Torre-Amione G: New therapeutics for chronic heart failure. Annu Rev Med 53:59, 2002
16. Pitt B, Remme W, Zannad F, et al: Eplerenone, a selective aldosterone blocker, in patients with left ventricular dysfunction after myocardial infarction. N Engl J Med 348:1309, 2003
17. Weber KT: Efficacy of aldosterone receptor antagonism in heart failure: Potential mechanisms. Current Heart Failure Reports I:51, 2004
18. Dulin B, Abraham WT. Pharmacology of carvedilol. Am J Cardiol 93:3B-6B, 2004
19. Rahimtoola SH: Digitalis therapy for patients in clinical heart failure. Circulation 109:2942, 2004
20. Bristow MR, Saxon LA, Boehmer J, et al: Cardiac-resynchronization therapy with or without an implantable defibrillator in advanced chronic heart failure. N Engl J Med 350:2140, 2004
21. Fonarow GC, Dams K, Abraham W, et al: Risk stratification for in-hospital mortality in acute decompensated heart failure. JAMA 293:572, 2005
22. Elkayam U, Akhter MW, Singh H, et al: Comparison of effects on left ventricular filling pressure of intravenous nesiritide and high-dose nitroglycerin in patients with decompensated heart failure. Am J Cardiol 93:237, 2004
23. DiDomenico RJ, Park HY, Southworth MR, et al: Guidelines for acute decompensated heart failure treatment. Ann Pharmacother 38:649, 2004
24. Lekmann A, Boldt J: New pharmacologic approaches for the perioperative treatment of ischemic cardiogenic shock. J Cardiothorac Vasc Anesth 19:97, 2005
25. Wang J, Kurrelmeyer KM, Torre-Amione G, Nagueh SF: Systolic and diastolic dyssynchony in patients with diastolic heart failure & the effect of medical treatment. J Am Coll Cardiol 49:88-96, 2007.
26. Lobato E, Willert J, Looke T, et al: Effects of milrinone versus epinephrine on left ventricular relaxation after cardiopulmonary bypass following myocardial revascularization. J Cardiothorac Vasc Anesth 19, 2005
27. Liu P, Konstam M, Force T: Highlights of the 2004 Scientific Sessions of the Heart Failure Society of America. J Am Coll Cardiol 45:617, 2005
28. Singh S, Patrick J: Antiarrhythmic drugs. Curr Treat Options Cardiovasc Med 6:357, 2004
29. Dimarco J, Gersh B, Opie L: Antiarrhythmic drugs and strategies. In Opie L, Horsh G, (eds): Drugs for the Heart. 6th ed. Philadelphia, Elsevier, 2005, pp 218-274
30. Dorian P, Cass D, Schwartz G, et al: Amiodarone compared with lidocaine for shock-resistant ventricular fibrillation. N Engl J Med 346:884, 2002

31. Kaplan JA: Role of ultrashort-acting beta-blockers in the perioperative period. J Cardiothorac Anesth 2:683, 1988
32. Dorian P, Mangat I: Role of amiodarone in the era of the implantable cardioverter defibrillator. J Cardiovasc Electrophysiol 14(9 Suppl):S78-S81, 2003
33. Hood MA, Smith WM: Adenosine versus verapamil in the treatment of supraventricular tachycardia: A randomized double-crossover trial. Am Heart J 123:1543, 1992
34. Mohnle P, Schwann N, Vaughn W, et al: Perturbations in laboratory values after coronary artery bypass surgery with cardiopulmonary bypass. J Cardiothorac Vasc Anesth 19:19, 2005
35. Geertman H, van der Starre P, Sie H, et al: Magnesium in addition to sotalol does not influence the incidence of postoperative atrial tachyarrhythmias after coronary artery bypass surgery. J Cardiothorac Vasc Anesth 18:309, 2004

8

Section III
Monitoring

Chapter 9

Monitoring of the Heart and Vascular System

David L. Reich, MD • Alexander J. Mittnacht, MD •
Martin J. London, MD • Joel A. Kaplan, MD

HEMODYNAMIC MONITORING

For patients with severe cardiovascular disease and those undergoing surgery associated with rapid hemodynamic changes, adequate hemodynamic monitoring should be available at all times. With the ability to measure and record almost all vital physiologic parameters, the development of acute hemodynamic changes may be observed and corrective action may be taken in an attempt to correct adverse hemodynamics and improve outcome. Although outcome changes are difficult to prove, it is a reasonable assumption that appropriate hemodynamic monitoring should reduce the incidence of major cardiovascular complications. This is based on the presumption that the data obtained from these monitors are interpreted correctly and that therapeutic decisions are implemented in a timely fashion.

Many devices are available to monitor the cardiovascular system. These devices range from those that are completely noninvasive, such as the blood pressure (BP) cuff and ECG, to those that are extremely invasive, such as the pulmonary artery (PA) catheter. To make the best use of invasive monitors, the potential benefits to be gained from the information must outweigh the potential complications. In many critically ill patients, the benefit obtained does seem to outweigh the risks, which

BOX 9-1   *Standard Monitoring for Cardiac Surgical Patients*

- (Invasive) blood pressure
- Electrocardiogram
- Pulse oximetry
- Capnometry
- Temperature
- Central venous pressure
- Urine output
- Intermittent arterial blood gas analysis

BOX 9-2   *Extended Monitoring for Patients Based on Case-Specific Factors*

- Pulmonary artery catheter
- Cardiac output measurements
- Transesophageal echocardiography
- Left atrial pressure
- Bispectral index monitoring
- Cerebral oximetry
- Jugular venous saturation or pressure
- Spinal drain (intrathecal) pressure

explains the widespread use of invasive monitoring. Transesophageal echocardiography (TEE), a minimally invasive technology, has gained in popularity as an alternative to the PA catheter and is considered a standard-of-care monitoring device in the perioperative management for certain procedures, such as mitral valvuloplasty or surgery for congenital heart defects.

Standard monitoring for cardiac surgical patients includes BP, ECG, central venous pressure (CVP), urine output, temperature, capnometry, pulse oximetry, and intermittent arterial blood gas analysis (Box 9-1). The next tier of monitoring includes PA catheters, left atrial pressure (LAP) catheters, thermodilution cardiac output (CO) measurements, TEE, and indices of tissue oxygen transport (Box 9-2). All of these measurements and their derivatives can be obtained and recorded. The interpretation of these complex data, however, requires an astute clinician who is aware of the patient's overall condition and the limitations of the monitors.[1]

ARTERIAL PRESSURE MONITORING

Blood pressure monitoring is the most commonly used method of assessing the cardiovascular system. The magnitude of the BP is directly related to the CO and the systemic vascular resistance (SVR). This is analogous to Ohm's law of electricity (voltage = current × resistance), in which BP is analogous to voltage, CO to flow, and SVR to resistance. An increase in the BP may reflect an increase in CO or SVR, or both. Although BP is one of the easiest cardiovascular variables to measure, it gives only indirect information about the patient's cardiovascular status.

Mean arterial pressure (MAP) is probably the most useful parameter to measure in assessing organ perfusion, except for the heart, in which the diastolic BP is the most important. MAP is measured directly by integrating the arterial waveform tracing over time, or using the formula:

$$MAP = (SBP + [2 \times DBP])/3$$

or

$$MAP = DBP + \left(\frac{SBP - DBP}{3} \right)$$

where SBP is systolic blood pressure and DBP is diastolic blood pressure. The pulse pressure is the difference between SBP and DBP.

Anesthesia for cardiac surgery is frequently complicated by rapid and sudden lability of the BP because of several factors, including direct compression of the heart, impaired venous return due to retraction and cannulation of the venae cavae and aorta, arrhythmias from mechanical stimulation of the heart, and manipulations that may impair right ventricular (RV) outflow and pulmonary venous return. Sudden losses of significant amounts of blood may induce hypovolemia at almost any time. The cardiac surgical population also includes many patients with labile hypertension and atherosclerotic heart disease. A safe and reliable method of measuring acute changes in the BP is required during cardiac surgery with cardiopulmonary bypass (CPB).

Continuous BP monitoring with noninvasive devices have not proven to be suitable for cardiac surgery. Intra-arterial monitoring provides a continuous, beat-to-beat indication of the arterial pressure and waveform, and having an indwelling arterial catheter enables frequent sampling of arterial blood for laboratory analyses. Direct intra-arterial monitoring remains the gold standard for cardiac surgical procedures.

Arterial Cannulation Sites

Factors that influence the site of arterial cannulation include the location of surgery, the possible compromise of arterial flow due to patient positioning or surgical manipulations, and any history of ischemia of or prior surgery on the limb to be cannulated. Another factor that may influence the cannulation site is the presence of a proximal arterial cutdown. The proximal cutdown may cause damped waveforms or falsely low BP readings due to stenosis or vascular thrombosis.

The radial artery is the most commonly used artery for continuous BP monitoring because it is easy to cannulate with a short (20-gauge) catheter. It is readily accessible during surgery, and the collateral circulation is usually adequate and easy to check. It is advisable to assess the adequacy of the collateral circulation and the absence of proximal obstructions before cannulating the radial artery for monitoring purposes.

The ulnar artery provides most blood flow to the hand in about 90% of patients. The radial and ulnar arteries are connected by a palmar arch, which provides collateral flow to the hand in the event of radial artery occlusion. It has been shown that if there is adequate ulnar collateral flow, circulatory perfusion pressure to the fingers is adequate after radial arterial catheterization. Many clinicians routinely perform Allen's test before radial artery cannulation to assess the adequacy of collateral circulation to the hand.

Allen's test is performed by compressing the radial and ulnar arteries and by exercising the hand until it is pale. The ulnar artery is then released (with the hand open loosely), and the time until the hand regains its normal color is noted. With a normal collateral circulation, the color returns to the hand in about 5 seconds. If, however, the hand takes longer than 15 seconds to return to its normal color, cannulation of the radial artery on that side is controversial. The hand may remain pale if the fingers are hyperextended or widely spread apart, even in the presence of a normal collateral circulation. Variations on Allen's test include using a Doppler probe or pulse oximeter to document collateral flow. If Allen's test demonstrates that the hand depends on the radial artery for adequate filling, and other cannulation sites are not available, the ulnar artery may be selected.[2]

Chest wall retractors, such as the Favaloro retractor, may impede radial arterial pressure monitoring in cardiothoracic procedures in some patients. The arm on the affected side may have diminished perfusion during extreme retraction of the chest wall. If the left internal mammary artery is used during myocardial revascularization, the right radial artery could be monitored to avoid this problem. Alternatively, a noninvasive BP cuff on the right side could be used to confirm the accuracy of the radial artery tracing during extreme chest wall retraction.

Monitoring of the radial artery distal to a brachial arterial cutdown site is not recommended. Acute thrombosis or residual stenosis of the brachial artery will lead to falsely low radial arterial pressure readings. Other considerations related to the choice of a radial arterial monitoring site include prior surgery of the hand, selection of the nondominant hand, and the preference of the surgeon, the anesthesiologist, or both.

The brachial artery lies medial to the bicipital tendon in the antecubital fossa, in close proximity to the median nerve. Brachial artery pressure tracings resemble those in the femoral artery, with less systolic augmentation than radial artery tracings. Brachial arterial pressures were found to more accurately reflect central aortic pressures than radial arterial pressures before and after CPB. The complications from percutaneous brachial artery catheter monitoring are lower than those after brachial artery cutdown for cardiac catheterization.[3] A few series of perioperative brachial arterial monitoring have documented the relative safety of this technique.

The femoral artery may be cannulated for monitoring purposes but is usually reserved for situations in which other sites are unable to be cannulated or it is specifically indicated (e.g., descending thoracic aortic aneurysm surgery for distal pressure monitoring). Peripheral artery cannulation for hemodynamic monitoring, including 3899 femoral artery cannulations, has been studied. Temporary occlusion was found in 10 patients (1.45%), whereas serious ischemic complications requiring extremity amputation were reported in 3 patients (0.18%). Other complications were pseudoaneurysm formation in 6 patients (0.3%), sepsis in 13 patients (0.44%), local infection (0.78%), bleeding (1.58%), and hematoma (6.1%). The femoral artery for hemodynamic monitoring purposes was as safe as radial artery cannulation.

In patients undergoing thoracic aortic surgery, distal aortic perfusion (using partial CPB, left-heart bypass, or a heparinized shunt) may be performed during aortic cross-clamping to preserve spinal cord and visceral organ blood flow. In these situations, it is useful to measure the distal aortic pressure at the femoral artery (or, dorsalis pedis or posterior tibial artery) to optimize the distal perfusion pressure. In repairs of aortic coarctation, simultaneous femoral and radial arterial monitoring may help determine the adequacy of the surgical repair by documenting the pressure gradient after the repair. It is necessary to consult with the surgeon before cannulating the femoral vessels because these vessels may be used for extracorporeal perfusion or placement of an intra-aortic balloon pump during the surgical procedure.

Indications

The indications for invasive arterial monitoring are provided in Box 9-3.

BOX 9-3 *Indications for Intra-Arterial Monitoring*

- Major surgical procedures involving large fluid shifts or blood loss
- Surgery requiring cardiopulmonary bypass
- Surgery of the aorta
- Patients with pulmonary disease requiring frequent arterial blood gases
- Patients with recent myocardial infarctions, unstable angina, or severe coronary artery disease
- Patients with decreased left ventricular function (congestive heart failure) or significant valvular heart disease
- Patients in hypovolemic, cardiogenic, or septic shock or with multiple organ failure
- Procedures involving the use of deliberate hypotension or deliberate hypothermia
- Massive trauma cases
- Patients with right-sided heart failure, chronic obstructive pulmonary disease, pulmonary hypertension, or pulmonary embolism
- Patients requiring inotropes or intra-aortic balloon counterpulsation
- Patients with electrolyte or metabolic disturbances requiring frequent blood samples
- Inability to measure arterial pressure noninvasively (e.g., morbid obesity)

Insertion Techniques

Direct Cannulation

Proper technique is helpful in obtaining a high degree of success in arterial catheterization. The wrist should be placed in a dorsiflexed position on an armboard and immobilized in a supinated position. It is helpful to draw the course of the artery for 1 inch and to be comfortably seated. Doppler devices and ultrasonic vessel finders may also be of value. Local anesthetic is injected intradermally over the artery, and a small skin nick may be made to allow passage of the catheter-over-needle assembly into the subcutaneous tissue without crimping secondary to penetration of the unit through the skin. A 20-gauge or smaller, 3- to 5-cm, nontapered Teflon catheter over needle is used, without a syringe attached, to make the puncture. If a syringe is used, the plunger should be removed to allow free flow of blood to detect when the artery has been punctured. The angle between the needle and the skin should be shallow (30 degrees or less), and the needle should be advanced parallel to the course of the artery. When the artery is entered, the angle between the needle and skin is reduced to 10 degrees, the needle is advanced another 1 to 2 mm to ensure that the tip of the catheter also lies within the lumen of the vessel, and the outer catheter is then threaded off the needle while watching that blood continues to flow out of the needle hub (Fig. 9-1). After insertion of the catheter, the wrist should be taken out of the dorsiflexed position, because continued extreme dorsiflexion can lead to median nerve damage by stretching of the nerve over the wrist. An armboard may still be used to prevent the wrist from flexing, which causes kinking of the catheter and damping of the arterial waveform.

Transfixation

If blood ceases flowing while the needle is being advanced, the needle has penetrated the back wall of the vessel. In this technique, the artery has been transfixed by passage of the catheter-over-needle assembly "through-and-through" the artery. The needle is then completely withdrawn. As the catheter is slowly withdrawn, pulsatile blood flow emerges from the catheter when its tip is within the lumen of the artery. The catheter is then slowly advanced into the artery. A guidewire may be helpful at this point if the catheter does not advance easily into the artery. Alternatively, the catheter-over-needle

9

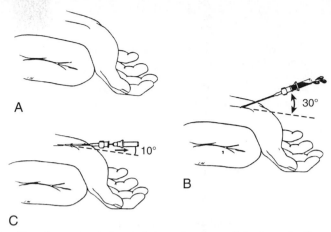

Figure 9-1 The direct-cannulation technique for the radial artery. **A,** The wrist is dorsi-flexed and loosely taped to a stable surface such as an armboard. **B,** The artery is directly can-nulated at a 30- to 40-degree angle to the plane of the wrist. Arterial blood flows steadily into the "flashback" chamber. **C,** The catheter-over-needle assembly is lowered until the an-gle is approximately 10 degrees to the plane of the wrist. The entire assembly is advanced an-other 1 to 2 mm, until the tip of the catheter lies within the lumen of the artery. The catheter is then advanced into the artery completely while the needle is held motionless. (From Lake CL: Cardiovascular Anesthesia. New York, Springer-Verlag, 1985, p 54.)

assembly may be withdrawn slowly as one unit until flow of blood has returned. As soon as this occurs, the needle and catheter are most likely in the lumen of the artery and the catheter may be gently threaded off the needle into the artery.

Seldinger Technique

The artery is localized with a needle, and a guidewire is passed through the needle into the artery. A catheter is then passed over the guidewire into the artery. Alternatively, a catheter-over-needle assembly may be inserted in the artery in a through-and-through fashion, the needle withdrawn, and the wire passed through the catheter after pulsatile flow is encountered. It is very important when using this technique to avoid withdrawal of guidewires through needles to prevent shearing of the wire and embolization.

CENTRAL VENOUS PRESSURE MONITORING

Central venous pressure catheters are used to measure the filling pressure of the right ventricle, give an estimate of the intravascular volume status, and assess RV function. For accurate pressure measurement, the distal end of the catheter must lie within one of the large intrathoracic veins or the right atrium. Although water manometers have been used in the past, an electronic system is preferred because it allows the observation of the right atrial (RA) waveform, which provides additional information. In any pressure monitoring system, it is necessary to have a reproducible landmark (e.g., the midaxillary line) as a zero reference. This is especially important in monitor-ing venous pressures, because small changes in the height of the zero reference point produce proportionally larger errors compared with arterial pressure monitoring.

The normal CVP waveform consists of three upward deflections (A, C, and V waves) and two downward deflections (X and Y descents) (Fig. 9-2). The A wave is produced by right atrial contraction and occurs just after the P wave on the ECG.

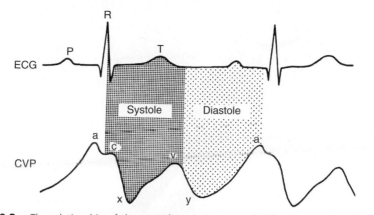

Figure 9-2 The relationship of the central venous pressure (CVP) tracing to the electrocardiogram (ECG) in normal sinus rhythm. The normal CVP waveform consists of three upward deflections (A, C, and V waves) and two downward deflections (X and Y descents). The A wave is produced by right atrial contraction and occurs just after the P wave on the ECG. The C wave occurs because of the isovolumic ventricular contraction forcing the tricuspid valve to bulge upward into the right atrium. The pressure within the right atrium then decreases as the tricuspid valve is pulled away from the atrium during right ventricular ejection, forming the X descent. The right atrium continues to fill during late ventricular systole, forming the V wave. The Y descent occurs when the tricuspid valve opens and blood from the right atrium empties rapidly into the right ventricle during early diastole. (Adapted from Mark JB: Central venous pressure monitoring: Clinical insights beyond the numbers. J Cardiothorac Vasc Anesth 5:163, 1991.)

The C wave occurs because of the isovolumic ventricular contraction forcing the tricuspid valve to bulge upward into the right atrium. The pressure within the right atrium then decreases as the tricuspid valve is pulled away from the atrium during RV ejection, forming the X descent. RA filling continues during late ventricular systole, forming the V wave. The Y descent occurs when the tricuspid valve opens and blood from the right atrium empties rapidly into the right ventricle during early diastole.

The CVP is a useful monitor if the factors affecting it are recognized and its limitations are understood. The CVP reflects the patient's blood volume, venous tone, and RV performance. Following serial measurements (trends) is more useful than individual numbers. The response of the CVP to a volume infusion is a useful test.

The CVP does not give a direct indication of left-heart filling pressure, but it may be used as an estimate of left-sided pressures in patients with good LV function. A good correlation has been shown between the CVP and left-sided filling pressures during a change in volume status in patients with coronary artery disease and left ventricular ejection fraction (LVEF) greater than 0.4.

Internal Jugular Vein

Cannulation of the internal jugular vein (IJV) was first described by English and coworkers in 1969. Its popularity among anesthesiologists has steadily increased since that time. Advantages of this technique include the high success rate as a result of the relatively predictable relationship of the anatomic structures; a short, straight course to the right atrium that almost always assures RA or superior vena cava (SVC) localization of the catheter tip; easy access from the head of the operating room table; and fewer complications than with subclavian vein catheterization. The IJV is located under the medial border of the lateral head of the sternocleidomastoid (SCM) muscle (Fig. 9-3). The carotid artery is usually deep and medial to the IJV. The right IJV is

9

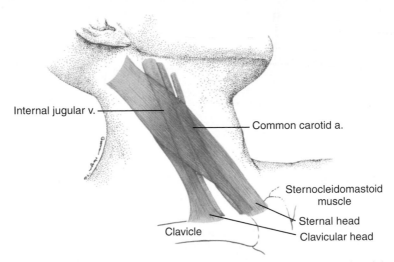

Internal jugular v.

Common carotid a.

Sternocleidomastoid muscle

Sternal head

Clavicle

Clavicular head

Figure 9-3 The internal jugular vein is usually located deep to the medial border of the lateral head of the sternocleidomastoid muscle, just lateral to the carotid pulse.

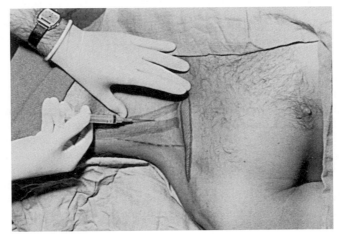

Figure 9-4 The preferred middle approach to the right internal jugular vein. The needle enters the skin at the apex of the triangle formed by the sternal and clavicular heads of the sternocleido-mastoid muscle. The needle is held at a 30- to 45-degree angle to the skin and directed toward the ipsilateral nipple.

preferred, because this vein takes the straightest course into the SVC, the right cupola of the lung may be lower than the left, and the thoracic duct is on the left side.

The preferred *middle approach* to the right IJV is shown in Figure 9-4. With the patient supine or in Trendelenburg position and the head turned toward the contralateral side, the fingers of the left hand are used to palpate the two heads of the SCM muscle and the carotid pulse. These fingers then hold the skin stable over the underlying structures while local anesthetic is infiltrated into the skin and sub-cutaneous tissues. A 22-gauge "finder" needle is placed at the apex of the triangle formed by the two heads of the SCM muscle at a 45-degree angle to the skin and directed toward the ipsilateral nipple. If venous blood return is not obtained, the needle is withdrawn to the subcutaneous tissue and then passed in a more lateral or medial direction until the vein is located. This needle reduces the risk of consequences related to inadvertent carotid arterial puncture and tissue trauma if localization of the vein is difficult. When venous blood is aspirated through the "finder" needle, the syringe and needle are withdrawn, leaving a small trail of blood on the drape to indicate the direction of the vein. Alternatively, the needle and syringe can be fixated and used as an identifying needle. Then, a syringe attached to an 18-gauge intravenous catheter-over-needle is inserted in an identical fashion. When venous return is present, the whole assembly is lowered to prevent the needle from going through the posterior wall of the central vein and advanced an additional 1 to 2 mm until the tip of the catheter is within the lumen of the vein. The catheter is then threaded into the vein.

Once the catheter is advanced into the vein, the needle is removed, and an empty syringe is attached to the cannula to withdraw a sample of blood. To confirm that an artery has not been inadvertently cannulated, comparison of the color of the blood sample to an arterial sample drawn simultaneously is recommended. If this is inconclusive or there is no arterial catheter in place, the cannula may be attached to a transducer by sterile tubing to observe the pressure waveform. Another option is to attach the cannula to sterile tubing and allow blood to flow retrograde into the tubing. The tubing is then held upright as a venous manometer, and the height of the blood column is observed. If the catheter is in a vein, it will stop rising at a level consistent with the CVP and demonstrate respiratory variation. A guidewire is then passed through the 18-gauge catheter, and the catheter is exchanged over the wire for a CVP catheter. The use of more than one technique to confirm the venous location of the catheter may provide additional reassurance of correct placement before cannulation of the vein with a larger cannula.

ULTRASONIC GUIDANCE OF INTERNAL JUGULAR VEIN CANNULATION

Ultrasound has been increasingly used to define the anatomic variations of the IJV. A review and meta-analysis of randomized controlled trials looking at ultrasound-guided central venous cannulation found that real-time two-dimensional ultrasound for IJV cannulation had a significantly higher success rate overall and on the first attempt compared with the landmark method in adults.[4] Most studies have demonstrated that two-dimensional ultrasonic guidance of IJV cannulation is helpful in locating the vein, permits more rapid cannulation, and decreases the incidence of arterial puncture.[5] Circumstances in which ultrasonic guidance of IJV cannulation can be advantageous include patients with difficult neck anatomy (e.g., short neck, obesity), prior neck surgery, anticoagulated patients, and infants.

Ultrasound has provided more precise data regarding the structural relationship between the IJV and the carotid artery (Fig. 9-5). Troianos and associates found that in more than 54% of patients, more than 75% of the IJV overlies the carotid artery. Patients who were older than 60 years were more likely to have this type of anatomy.[6] There was greater overlap of the IJV and the carotid artery when the head is rotated 80 degrees compared with head rotation of only 0 to 40 degrees. The data from 2 and 4 cm above the clavicle did not differ, and the percentage overlap was larger on the left side of the neck compared with the right. Excessive rotation of the head of the patient toward the contralateral side may distort the normal anatomy in a manner that increases the risk of inadvertent carotid artery puncture.[7] Doppler ultrasonography has also been used to demonstrate that the Valsalva maneuver increases IJV cross-sectional area by approximately 25% and that the Trendelenburg position increases it by approximately 37%.

9

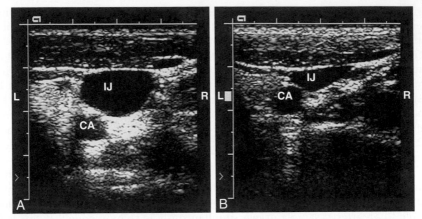

Figure 9-5 The ultrasound images depict the anatomic relationship of the right internal jugular (IJ) vein and the carotid artery (CA). **A,** With the Valsalva maneuver or in Trendelenburg position, the IJ is distended and circular. **B,** As gentle pressure is applied with the ultrasound probe, the IJ is partially compressed and flattened anteriorly and the CA size is unaffected. The compressibility of the IJ is its most characteristic feature during ultrasonic imaging.

External Jugular Vein

Although the EJV is another means of reaching the central circulation, the success rate with this approach is lower because of the tortuous path followed by the vein. A valve is usually present at the point where the EJV perforates the fascia to join with the subclavian vein. However, a success rate of 90% has been reported using a J-wire to manipulate past obstructions into the central circulation. The main advantage of this technique is that there is no need to advance a needle into the deeper structures of the neck.

For this approach, the patient is placed supine or in the Trendelenburg position until the EJV becomes distended. The vein is then cannulated with an intravenous catheter. A guidewire with curved tip (i.e., J-wire) is passed through the cannula and manipulated into the central circulation. The curved tip is necessary to negotiate the tortuous course between the EJV and the SVC. Manipulation of the shoulder and rotation of the guidewire between the operator's fingers may be useful maneuvers when difficulty is encountered in passing the wire into the superior vena cava.

Subclavian Vein

The subclavian vein is readily accessible from supraclavicular or infraclavicular approaches and has long been used for central venous access. The success rate is higher than the EJV approach but lower than the right IJV approach. Cannulation of the subclavian vein is associated with a higher incidence of complications than the IJV approach, especially pneumothorax. Other complications associated with subclavian vein cannulation are arterial punctures, misplacement of the catheter tip, aortic injury, cardiac tamponade, mediastinal hematoma, and hemothorax. This may be the cannulation site of choice, however, when CVP monitoring is indicated in patients undergoing carotid artery surgery. It is also useful for parenteral nutrition or for prolonged CVP access because the site is easier to maintain and well tolerated by patients.

The *infraclavicular approach* is performed with the patient supine or in the Trendelenburg position with a folded sheet between the scapulae and the shoulder lowered. The head is turned to the contralateral side. A thin-walled needle or intravenous catheter is inserted 1 cm below the midpoint of the clavicle and advanced toward the suprasternal notch under the posterior surface of the clavicle.

> **BOX 9-4** *Indications for Central Venous Catheter Placement*
>
> - Major operative procedures involving large fluid shifts or blood loss in patients with good heart function
> - Intravascular volume assessment when urine output is not reliable or unavailable (e.g., renal failure)
> - Major trauma
> - Surgical procedures with a high risk of air embolism, such as sitting-position cranioto-mies. The central venous pressure catheter also may be used to aspirate intracardiac air.
> - Frequent venous blood sampling
> - Venous access for vasoactive or irritating drugs
> - Chronic drug administration
> - Inadequate peripheral intravenous access
> - Rapid infusion of intravenous fluids (using large cannulae)
> - Total parenteral nutrition

When a free flow of venous blood is obtained, the guidewire is passed into the subclavian vessel and is exchanged for a CVP catheter.

Indications

Central venous pressure monitoring is often performed to obtain an indication of intravascular volume status. The accuracy and reliability of CVP monitoring depend on many factors, including the functional status of the right and left ventricles, the presence of pulmonary disease, and ventilatory factors, such as positive end-expiratory pressure (PEEP). The CVP may reflect left-sided heart filling pressures, but only in patients with good LV function. Elderly patients have a high incidence of coronary artery and pulmonary disease, and the CVP is therefore less likely to accurately reflect left-sided filling pressures in this population. Perioperative indications for the insertion of a central venous catheter are listed in Box 9-4.

The CVP should be monitored in all patients during CPB. When the catheter tip is in the SVC, it indicates RA pressure and cerebral venous pressure. Significant increases in CVP can produce critical decreases in cerebral perfusion pressure. This is occasionally caused by a malpositioned SVC cannula during CPB and must be corrected immediately by the surgeon to avoid cerebral edema and poor cerebral perfusion.

Complications

The complications of central venous cannulation can be roughly divided into three categories: complications of vascular access, complications of catheter insertion, or complications of catheter presence. These are summarized in Box 9-5.

Inadvertent arterial puncture during central venous cannulation is not uncommon. The two main reasons why this phenomenon occurs are that all veins commonly used for cannulation lie in close proximity to arteries and that the venous anatomy is quite variable. Localized hematoma formation is the usual consequence. This may be minimized if a small-gauge needle is initially used to localize the vein or ultrasonic guidance is employed.

If RA or RV perforation occurs during central venous cannulation, pericardial effusion or tamponade may result. The likelihood of this complication is increased when inflexible guidewires, long dilators, or catheter are used.

BOX 9-5 *Complications of Central Venous Catheterization*

Complications of Central Venous Cannulation

- Arterial puncture with hematoma
- Arteriovenous fistula
- Hemothorax
- Chylothorax
- Pneumothorax
- Nerve injury
- Brachial plexus
- Stellate ganglion (Horner's syndrome)
- Air emboli
- Catheter or wire shearing
- Right atrial or right ventricular perforation

Complications of Catheter Presence

- Thrombosis, thromboembolism
- Infection, sepsis, endocarditis
- Arrhythmias
- Hydrothorax

The dilators used in many of the central catheters kits may be a major cause of vessel perforation. The dilator may bend the guidewire, creating its own path, causing it to perforate a vessel wall. Several kits have dilators that are much longer than the catheters, and they constitute a further risk factor for possible perforation of the heart or vessels.

The physiology of fluid accumulation in the pericardial sac is such that sudden cardiovascular collapse occurs once a critical volume has been reached. This is explained by the compliance curve of the normal pericardium. The curve is flat until the critical volume is reached and then rises steeply with any further increment in volume. If pericardial tamponade is imminent, immediate pericardiocentesis is indicated. Withdrawal of small volumes of blood results in marked hemodynamic improvement because of the nature of pericardial compliance.

Transient atrial and ventricular arrhythmias commonly occur as the guidewire is passed into the right atrium or right ventricle during central venous cannulation using the Seldinger technique. This most likely results from the relatively inflexible guidewire causing extrasystoles as it contacts the endocardium. Ventricular fibrillation during guidewire insertion has been reported. The same investigators reported a 70% reduction in the incidence of arrhythmias when guidewire insertion was limited to 22 cm.

There are also reports of complete heart block due to guidewire insertion during central venous cannulation. These cases can be successfully managed using a temporary transvenous or external pacemaker. This complication has previously been reported with PA catheterization. The problem most likely resulted from excessive insertion of the guidewire, with impingement of the wire in the region of the right bundle branch. It is recommended that the length of guidewire insertion be limited to the length necessary to reach the SVC-RA junction to avoid these complications. It is also imperative to monitor the patient appropriately (e.g., ECG and pulse monitoring) and to have resuscitative drugs and equipment immediately available when performing central venous catheterization.

Strict aseptic technique is required to minimize catheter-related infections. Full barrier precautions during insertion of central venous catheters have been shown to decrease the incidence of catheter-related infections.[8] Subcutaneous tunneling of central venous catheters inserted into the internal jugular and femoral veins, antiseptic barrier-protected hub for central venous catheters, and antiseptic/antibiotic-impregnated short-term central venous catheters have been shown to reduce catheter-related infections. Hospital policies differ with respect to the permissible duration of catheterization at particular sites, but routine replacement of central venous catheters to prevent catheter-related infections is not recommended.

PULMONARY ARTERIAL PRESSURE MONITORING

The introduction of the flow-directed PA catheter was a quantum advance in the monitoring of patients in the perioperative period. Since the 1970s, its use has increased the amount of diagnostic information that can be obtained at the bedside in critically ill patients. It is impressive to observe large changes in the PAP and PCWP with almost no reflection in the CVP. Connors and coworkers prospectively analyzed 62 consecutive PA catheterizations. They found that fewer than one half of a group of clinicians correctly predicted the PCWP or CO and that more than 50% made at least one change in therapy based on data from the PA catheterization. Waller and Kaplan demonstrated that a group of experienced cardiac anesthesiologists and surgeons who were blinded to the information from PA catheterization during CABG surgery were unaware of any problem during 65% of severe hemodynamic abnormalities. Similarly, Iberti and Fisher showed that ICU physicians were unable to accurately predict hemodynamic data on clinical grounds and that 60% made at least one change in therapy and 33% changed their diagnosis based on PA catheter data*. The clinical significance of these changes has been questioned because the weight of evidence-based medicine on the subject does not support improvements in outcome related to PA catheter monitoring, and the overall use of the PA catheter has decreased 60–80% over the past decade. Nevertheless, with increasing numbers of patients with multisystem organ dysfunction undergoing cardiac surgical procedures, PA catheter monitoring is prevalent in cardiac surgical settings. An understanding of the potential benefits and pitfalls of PA catheterization is therefore essential for anesthesiologists.

Specific information that can be gathered with the PA catheter and the quantitative measurements of cardiovascular and pulmonary function that can be derived from this information are listed in Tables 9-1 and 9-2.

One of the main reasons that clinicians measure PCWP and PA diastolic pressure (PADP) is that these parameters are estimates of LAP, which is an estimate of left ventricular end-diastolic pressure (LVEDP). LVEDP is an index of left ventricular end-diastolic volume (LVEDV), which correlates well with left ventricular preload. The relationship between LVEDP and LVEDV is described by the left ventricular compliance curve. This nonlinear curve is affected by many factors, such as ventricular hypertrophy and myocardial ischemia. The PCWP and PADP do not directly measure LV preload. The relationship of these parameters is diagrammed in Figure 9-6.

The PCWP and PADP pressures will not accurately reflect LVEDP in the presence of incorrect position of the PA catheter tip, pulmonary vascular disease, high levels of PEEP, or mitral valvular disease. The patency of vascular channels between the distal port of the PA catheter and the LA is necessary to ensure a close relationship between the PCWP and LAP. This condition is met only in the dependent portions

*These and other references can be found in the chapter in the large reference textbook, Kaplan's Cardiac Anesthesia, 5th edition, Elsevier, NY, 2006.

Table 9-1   Normal Intracardiac Pressures

Location/Pressure	Mean (mm Hg)	Range (mm Hg)
Right atrial	5	1-10
Right ventricular	25/5	15-30/0-8
Pulmonary arterial systolic/ diastolic	23/9	15-30/5-15
Mean pulmonary arterial	15	10-20
Pulmonary capillary wedge	10	5-15
Left atrial	8	4-12
Left ventricular end-diastolic	8	4-12
Left ventricular systolic	130	90-140

Table 9-2   Derived Hemodynamic Parameters

Parameter/Formula	Normal Values
Cardiac index: $CI = CO/BSA$	2.8-4.2 L/min/m^2
Stroke volume: $SV = CO \times 1000/HR$	50-110 mL/beat
Stroke index: $SI = SV/BSA$	30-65 mL/beat/m^2
Left ventricular stroke work index: $LVSWI = 1.36 \times (MAP - PCWP) \times SI/100$	45-60 g•m/m^2
Right ventricular stroke work index: $RVSWI = 1.36 \times (MPAP - CVP) \times SI/100$	5-10 g•m/m^2
Systemic vascular resistance: $SVR = (MAP - CVP) \times 80/CO$	900-1400 dynes•s•cm^{-5}
Systemic vascular resistance index: $SVRI = (MAP - CVP) \times 80/CI$	1500-2400 dynes•s•cm^{-5}/m^2
Pulmonary vascular resistance: $PVR = (MPAP - PCWP) \times 80/CO$	150-250 dynes•s•cm^{-5}
Pulmonary vascular resistance index: $PVRI = (MPAP - PCWP) \times 80/CI$	250-400 dynes•s•cm^{-5}/m^2

BSA = body surface area; CI = cardiac index; CO = cardiac output; CVP = central venous pressure; HR = heart rate; LVSWI = left ventricular stroke work index; MAP = mean arterial pressure; PAP = pulmonary arterial pressure; PCWP = pulmonary capillary wedge pressure; PVR = pulmonary vascular resistance; PVRI = pulmonary vascular resistance index; RVSWI = right ventricular stroke work index; SI = stroke index; SV = stroke volume; SVR = systemic vascular resistance; SVRI = systemic vascular resistance index.

of the lung (West's zone III), in which the pulmonary venous pressure exceeds the alveolar pressure. Otherwise, the PCWP will reflect the alveolar pressure, not the LAP. Because PEEP decreases the size of West's zone III, it has been shown to adversely affect the correlation between the PCWP and LAP, especially in the hypovolemic patient. Nevertheless, the correlation of PCWP and LAP could be maintained in the presence of PEEP by placing the catheter tip below the left atrium. The acute respiratory distress syndrome (ARDS) seems to prevent the transmission of increased alveolar pressure to the pulmonary interstitium. This preserves the relationship between the PCWP and LAP during the application of PEEP. It is not considered prudent, however, to temporarily disconnect patients from PEEP to measure preload.

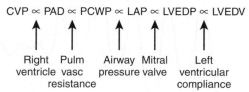

$$CVP \propto PAD \propto PCWP \propto LAP \propto LVEDP \propto LVEDV$$

Right ventricle · Pulm vasc resistance · Airway pressure · Mitral valve · Left ventricular compliance

Figure 9-6 The left ventricular end-diastolic volume (LVEDV) is related to left ventricular end-diastolic pressure (LVEDP) by the left ventricular compliance. The LVEDP is related to the left atrial pressure (LAP) by the diastolic pressure gradient across the mitral valve. The pulmonary capillary wedge pressure (PCWP) is related to the LAP by the pulmonary capillary resistance. The pulmonary artery diastolic pressure (PAD) is an estimate of the PCWP. The central venous pressure (CVP) reflects the PAD if right ventricular function is normal.

BOX 9-6 *Conditions Resulting in Discrepancies between Pulmonary Capillary Wedge Pressure and Left Ventricular End-Diastolic Pressure*

PCWP > LVEDP

- Positive-pressure ventilation
- Positive end-expiratory pressure
- Increased intrathoracic pressure
- Non–West lung zone III pulmonary artery catheter placement
- Chronic obstructive pulmonary disease
- Increased pulmonary vascular resistance
- Left atrial myxoma
- Mitral valve disease (e.g., stenosis, regurgitation)

PCWP < LVEDP

- Noncompliant left ventricle (e.g., ischemia, hypertrophy)
- Aortic regurgitation (premature closure of the mitral valve)

LVEDP > 25 mm Hg

LVEDP = left ventricular end-diastolic pressure; PCWP = pulmonary capillary wedge pressure.

Adapted from Tuman KJ, Carrol CC, Ivankovich AD: Pitfalls in interpretation of pulmonary artery catheter data. Cardiothorac Vasc Anesth Update 2:1, 1991.

The presence of large V waves in the PCWP tracing of patients with mitral regurgitation leads to an overestimation of the LVEDP. In patients with mitral stenosis, using the PCWP instead of the LAP to assess the transmitral gradient has been shown to overestimate the severity of mitral stenosis. However, when the PCWP was adjusted for the time delay through the pulmonary vasculature, the mean LAP and mean PCWP correlated well. It has been demonstrated that there is a significant positive gradient between the PCWP and the LAP in the initial hour after CPB. Box 9-6 is a summary of conditions that may alter the relationship between the PCWP and the LVEDP.

Placement of the Pulmonary Artery Catheter

The considerations for the insertion site of a PA catheter are the same as for CVP catheters. The right IJV approach remains the technique of choice because of the direct path between this vessel and the right atrium. The placement of PA catheters

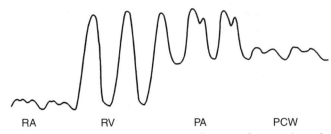

RA   RV   PA   PCW

Figure 9-7   The waveforms encountered during the flotation of a PA catheter from the venous circulation to the pulmonary capillary wedge (PCW) position. Notice the sudden increase in systolic pressure as the catheter enters the right ventricle (RV), the sudden increase in diastolic pressure as the catheter enters the pulmonary artery (PA), and the decrease in mean pressure as the catheter reaches the PCW position. RA = right atrium.

through subclavian vein introducers may be complicated by kinking of the catheter when the sternum is retracted during cardiothoracic surgery.

Passage of the PA catheter from the vessel introducer to the PA can be accomplished by monitoring the pressure waveform from the distal port of the catheter or under fluoroscopic guidance. Waveform monitoring is the more common technique for perioperative right-sided heart catheterization. First, the catheter must be advanced through the vessel introducer (15 to 20 cm) before inflating the balloon. The inflation of the balloon facilitates further advancement of the catheter through the right atrium and right ventricle into the PA. Normal intracardiac pressures are shown in Table 9-1. The pressure waveforms seen during advancement of the PA catheter are illustrated in Figure 9-7. The RA waveform is seen until the catheter tip crosses the tricuspid valve and enters the right ventricle. In the right ventricle, there is a sudden increase in SBP but little change in DBP compared with the RA tracing. Arrhythmias, particularly premature ventricular complexes, usually occur at this point but almost always resolve without treatment once the catheter tip has crossed the pulmonary valve. The catheter is rapidly advanced through the right ventricle toward the PA.

As the catheter crosses the pulmonary valve, a dicrotic notch appears in the pressure waveform and there is a sudden increase in diastolic pressure. The PCWP tracing is obtained by advancing the catheter 3 to 5 cm farther until there is a change in the waveform associated with a drop in the measured mean pressure. Deflation of the balloon results in reappearance of the PA waveform and an increase in the mean pressure value. Using the right IJV approach, the right atrium is entered at 25 to 35 cm, the right ventricle at 35 to 45 cm, the PA at 45 to 55 cm, and the PCWP at 50 to 60 cm in most patients.

If the catheter does not enter the PA by 60 cm, the balloon should be deflated. It should be withdrawn into the right atrium, and another attempt should be made to advance the catheter into proper position. Excessive coiling of the catheter in the right ventricle should be avoided to prevent catheter knotting. The balloon should be inflated only for short periods to measure the PCWP. The PA waveform should be continually monitored to be certain that the catheter does not float out into a constant wedge position because this may lead to PA rupture or pulmonary infarction. The PA catheter is covered by a sterile sheath that must be secured at both ends to prevent contamination of the external portion of the catheter. Not infrequently, the PA catheter must be withdrawn a short distance because the extra catheter in the right ventricle floats out more peripherally into the PA over time as the catheter softens.

The time for the entire PA catheter insertion procedure is 10 to 15 minutes in experienced hands. Many clinicians believe that the PA catheter should be inserted before the induction of anesthesia. Studies showed that PA catheter insertion in the awake patient did not result in myocardial ischemia or deleterious hemodynamic

III

BOX 9-7 *Indications for Pulmonary Artery Catheterization*

- Assessment of volume status
- Cardiac output measurements
- Hemodynamic measurements
- Respiratory or oxygen transport measurements

---

changes after preanesthetic medication and with continuation of all preoperative cardiac medications. A chest radiograph should be obtained postoperatively in all patients to check the position of the PA catheter. Most catheters pass into the right middle or lower lobes. The location of the PA catheter can also be checked by TEE imaging of the catheter in the RA, RV, and pulmonary artery.

Indications

The indications for PA catheterization are given in Box 9-7. The ability of PA catheters to positively influence patient outcome has never been conclusively proved in large-scale, prospective studies. There remains considerable controversy regarding the risk/benefit ratio of PA catheters. Many studies have reported no change or even worse outcome in patients who were monitored with PA catheters. Randomized trials on patients with myocardial infarction seemed to confirm these data, whereas earlier prospective studies on surgical patients showed improved outcome.[9-11]

Major problems with PA catheter outcome studies include flaws in study design and insufficient statistical power. The most common design flaws were a lack of therapeutic protocols or treatment algorithms and inadequate randomization, which introduce observer bias.[12] Physician knowledge is another confounding variable, as demonstrated in multicenter studies that indicated competency in interpreting PA catheter–derived data was lacking in many individuals and depended on such factors as the level of training and the frequency of use. As many as 47% of physicians could not correctly determine the PCWP to within 5 mm Hg.

Another problem with PA catheter outcome studies is the clinical setting, specifically operating room versus ICU. Patients in the ICU might have disease too far advanced to make invasive hemodynamic monitoring useful. Studies that have reported improved outcome used invasive hemodynamic monitoring to optimize oxygen delivery in the perioperative period.

The operative procedures and medical conditions that are cited as indications for PA catheterization in the perioperative period remain controversial and vary by institution. In a global sense, the indications for using a PA catheter are assessing volume status, measuring CO, measuring $S\bar{v}o_2$, and deriving hemodynamic parameters. In 2003, the American Society of Anesthesiologists (ASA) Task Force on Pulmonary Artery Catheterization published updated practice guidelines for PA catheterization (http://www.asahq.org/publicationsAndServices/pulm_artery.pdf).[13] These guidelines emphasized that patient, surgery, and practice setting had to be considered. Generally, the routine use of PA catheters is indicated in high-risk patients (e.g., ASA 4 or 5) and high-risk procedures (e.g., where large fluid changes or hemodynamic disturbances are expected). The practice setting is important, because there is evidence that inadequate training or experience may increase the risk for perioperative complications associated with the use of a PA catheter. It is recommended that the routine use of a PA catheter should be confined to centers with adequate training and experience in the perioperative management of patients with the PA catheter (Box 9-8). A summary of procedural indications that is relatively aggressive is shown in Box 9-9.

BOX 9-8 *American Society of Anesthesiologists' Practice Guidelines for Pulmonary Artery Catheter Use*

Opinions

- PA catheterization provides new information that may change therapy, with poor clinical evidence of its effect on clinical outcome or mortality.
- There is no evidence from large, controlled studies that preoperative PA catheterization improves outcome regarding hemodynamic optimization.
- Perioperative PA catheter monitoring of hemodynamic parameters leading to goal-directed therapy has produced inconsistent data in multiple studies and clinical scenarios.
- Having immediate access to PA catheter data allows important preemptive measures for selected subgroups of patients who encounter hemodynamic disturbances that require immediate and precise decisions about fluid management and drug treatment.
- Experience and understanding are the major determinants of PA catheter effectiveness.
- PA catheterization is inappropriate as routine practice in surgical patients and should be limited to cases in which the anticipated benefits of catheterization outweigh the potential risks.
- PA catheterization can be harmful.

Recommendations

- The appropriateness of routine PA catheterization depends on a combination of patient-related, surgery-related, and practice setting–related factors.
- Perioperative PA catheterization should be considered in patients who present with significant organ dysfunction or major comorbidity that poses an increased risk for hemodynamic disturbances or instability (e.g., ASA IV or V patients).
- Perioperative PA catheterization in surgical settings should be considered based on the hemodynamic risk of the individual case rather than generalized surgical setting–related recommendations. High-risk surgical procedures are those in which large fluid changes or hemodynamic disturbances can be anticipated and procedures that are associated with a high risk of morbidity and mortality.
- Because of the risk of complications from PA catheterization, the procedure should not be performed by clinicians or nursing staff or done in practice settings where competency in safe insertion, accurate interpretation of results, and appropriate catheter maintenance cannot be guaranteed.
- Routine PA catheterization is not recommended when the patient, procedure, or practice setting poses a low or moderate risk for hemodynamic changes.

III

BOX 9-9 *Clinical Indications for Pulmonary Artery Catheter Monitoring*

Major Procedures Involving Large Fluid Shifts or Blood Loss in Patients with

- Severe unstable coronary artery disease or poor left ventricular function (congestive heart failure)
- Cardiogenic or septic shock or with multiple organ failure
- Right-sided heart failure, pulmonary hypertension, or pulmonary embolism
- Hemodynamic instability requiring inotropes or intra-aortic balloon counterpulsation
- Surgery of the aorta requiring cross-clamping
- Hepatic transplantation
- Massive ascites requiring major surgery

The use of the PA catheter has significantly contributed to the understanding and care of patients with cardiac disease. Nevertheless, further large-scale randomized controlled trials are needed to clearly define which, if any, patient populations benefit from PA catheter monitoring. The body of evidence is inconclusive. The risks associated with perioperative PA catheter monitoring may outweigh the benefits in low-to-moderate risk patients, whereas high-risk patients undergoing major surgery probably benefit from right-sided heart catheterization. One major caveat is that the data derived from PA catheter monitoring must be interpreted correctly and treatment protocols should be followed to derive maximal benefit. In summary, using an evidence-based medicine approach, PA catheter monitoring does not improve patient outcome in most patient populations and may actually be harmful in certain circumstances.

Complications

The complications associated with PA catheter placement include almost all of those detailed in the section on CVP placement. The ASA Task Force on Pulmonary Artery Catheterization concluded that serious complications due to PA catheterization occur in 0.1% to 0.5% of patients monitored with a PA catheter. Higher estimates are found in the literature and probably represent different patient populations, hospital settings, level of experience with PA catheter management, and other factors.

Arrhythmias

The most common complications associated with PA catheter insertion are transient arrhythmias, especially premature ventricular contractions (PVCs). However, fatal arrhythmias have rarely been reported. Intravenous lidocaine has been used in attempts to suppress these arrhythmias, with mixed results. However, a positional maneuver entailing 5-degree head-up and right lateral tilt was associated with a statistically significant decrease in malignant arrhythmias (compared with the Trendelenburg position) during PA catheter insertion.

Complete Heart Block

Complete heart block may develop during PA catheterization in patients with preexisting left bundle-branch block (LBBB). This potentially fatal complication is most likely due to electrical irritability from the PA catheter tip causing transient right bundle-branch block (RBBB) as it passes through the RV outflow tract. The incidence of developing RBBB was 3% in a prospective series of patients undergoing PA catheterization. However, none of the patients with preexisting LBBB developed complete heart block in that series. In another study of 47 patients with LBBB, complete heart block occurred in 2 patients with recent-onset LBBB. It is imperative to have an external pacemaker immediately available or to use a pacing PA catheter when placing a PA catheter in patients with LBBB.

Endobronchial Hemorrhage

Iatrogenic rupture of the PA has become more common since the advent of PA catheter monitoring in the ICU and operating room.[14] Several risk factors have emerged: advanced age, female sex, pulmonary hypertension, mitral stenosis, coagulopathy, distal placement of the catheter, and balloon hyperinflation. Balloon inflation in distal pulmonary arteries is probably accountable for most episodes of PA rupture because of the high pressures generated by the balloon. Hypothermic CPB may also increase risk due to distal migration of the catheter tip with movement of the heart and hardening of the PA catheter. It is now common practice to pull the PA catheter back 3 to 5 cm when CPB is instituted.

9

It is important to consider the cause of the hemorrhage when forming a therapeutic plan. If the hemorrhage is minimal and a coagulopathy coexists, correction of the coagulopathy may be the only necessary therapy. Protection of the uninvolved lung is of prime importance. Tilting the patient toward the affected side, placement of a double-lumen endotracheal tube, and other lung-separation maneuvers should protect the contralateral lung. Strategies proposed to stop the hemorrhage include the application of PEEP, placement of bronchial blockers, and pulmonary resection. The clinician is obviously at a disadvantage unless the site of hemorrhage is known. A chest radiograph will usually indicate the general location of the lesion. Although the cause of endobronchial hemorrhage may be unclear, the bleeding site must be unequivocally located before surgical treatment is attempted. A small amount of radiographic contrast dye may help to pinpoint the lesion if active hemorrhage is present. In severe hemorrhage and with recurrent bleeding, transcatheter coil embolization has been used. This may emerge as the preferred treatment method.

Pulmonary Infarction

Pulmonary infarction is a rare complication of PA catheter monitoring. An early report suggested that there was a 7.2% incidence of pulmonary infarction with PA catheter use. However, continuously monitoring the PA waveform and keeping the balloon deflated when not determining the PCWP (to prevent inadvertent wedging of the catheter) were not standard practice at that time. Distal migration of PA catheters may also occur intraoperatively owing to the action of the right ventricle, uncoiling of the catheter, and softening of the catheter over time. Inadvertent catheter wedging occurs during CPB because of the diminished RV chamber size and retraction of the heart to perform the operation. Embolization of thrombus formed on a PA catheter could also result in pulmonary infarction.

Catheter Knotting and Entrapment

Knotting of a PA catheter usually occurs as a result of coiling of the catheter within the right ventricle. Insertion of an appropriately sized guidewire under fluoroscopic guidance may aid in unknotting the catheter. Alternatively, the knot may be tightened and withdrawn percutaneously along with the introducer if no intracardiac structures are entangled. If cardiac structures, such as the papillary muscles, are entangled in the knotted catheter, then surgical intervention may be required. Sutures placed in the heart may inadvertently entrap the PA catheter.

Valvular Damage

Withdrawal of the catheter with the balloon inflated may result in injury to the tricuspid or pulmonary valves. Placement of the PA catheter with the balloon deflated may increase the risk of passing the catheter between the chordae tendineae. Septic endocarditis has also resulted from an indwelling PA catheter.

Pacing Catheters

The possible indications for placement of a pacing PA catheter are shown in Box 9-10. The actual use in a group of 600 patients undergoing cardiac surgery is shown in Table 9-3.[15]

A multipurpose PA catheter contains five electrodes for bipolar atrial, ventricular, or atrioventricular (AV) sequential pacing. The intraoperative success rates for atrial, ventricular, and AV sequential capture have been reported as 80%, 93%, and 73%, respectively.

The Paceport and A-V Paceport catheters have lumina for the introduction of a ventricular wire (Paceport) or for atrial and ventricular wires (A-V Paceport) for temporary transvenous pacing. The success rate for ventricular pacing capture was

III

BOX 9-10 *Indications for Perioperative Placement of Pacing Pulmonary Artery Catheters*

- Sinus node dysfunction or bradycardia
- Second-degree (Mobitz II) atrioventricular block
- Complete (third-degree) atrioventricular block
- Digitalis toxicity
- Need for atrioventricular sequential pacing
- Aortic stenosis (need to maintain sinus rhythm)
- Severe left ventricular hypertrophy or noncompliant left ventricle
- Idiopathic hypertrophic subaortic stenosis/hypertrophic obstructive cardiomyopathy
- Need for an intracardiac electrogram

Table 9-3 **Use of Pacing Pulmonary Artery Catheters According to the Presence or Absence of Different Indications**

Indication	Indication Present*	Indication Present/ Pacing PAC Used[†] (%)	Indication Absent*	Indication Absent/ Pacing PAC Used[†] (%)	*P* Value
Sinus node dysfunction	24	6 (25.0)	576	32 (5.5)	0.002
First-degree AV block	52	1 (1.9)	548	37 (6.7)	0.24
Second-degree AV block	1	1 (100)			
Complete AV block	15	5 (33.3)	585	33 (5.6)	0.001
LBBB	41	5 (12.1)	559	33 (5.9)	0.17
RBBB	32	0 (0)	568	38 (6.6)	0.25
LAH	17	1 (5.8)	583	37 (6.3)	1.0
RBBB and LAH	5	0 (0)	595	38 (6.3)	1.0
Reoperation/ with other indications present	61	14 (23.0)	539	24 (4.4)	<0.001
Reoperation/ no other indications present	51	1 (1.9)	549	37 (6.7)	0.24
Aortic stenosis	88	11 (12.0)	512	27 (5.2)	0.02
Mitral stenosis	17	1 (5.8)	583	37 (6.3)	1.0
Aortic insufficiency	40	9 (22.5)	560	29 (5.1)	<0.001
Mitral regurgitation	65	7 (10.7)	535	31 (5.7)	0.17

*Total number of patients.
†Total number and percentage of patients with or without each indication.
AV = atrioventricular; LAH = left anterior block; LBBB = left bundle-branch block; PAC = pulmonary artery catheter; RBBB = right bundle-branch block.
From Risk SC, Brandon D, D'Ambra MN, et al: Indications for the use of pacing pulmonary artery catheters in cardiac surgery. J Cardiothorac Vasc Anesth 6:275, 1992.

9

96% for the Paceport. The success rates for atrial and ventricular pacing capture before CPB were 98% and 100%, respectively, in a study of the A-V Paceport.

Mixed Venous Oxygen Saturation Catheters

Monitoring the $S\bar{v}o_2$ is a means of providing a global estimation of the adequacy of oxygen delivery relative to the needs of the various tissues. The formula for $S\bar{v}o_2$ calculation can be derived by modifying the Fick equation and assuming that the effect of dissolved oxygen in the blood is negligible:

$$S\bar{v}o_2 = Sao_2 - \frac{Vo_2}{CO \cdot 1.34 \cdot Hb}$$

A decrease in the $S\bar{v}o_2$ can indicate one of the following situations: decreased CO; increased oxygen consumption; decreased arterial oxygen saturation; or decreased hemoglobin (Hb) concentration. To measure $S\bar{v}o_2$, blood is aspirated from the distal port of the PA catheter slowly, so as not to contaminate the sample with oxygenated alveolar blood.

The addition of fiberoptic bundles to PA catheters has enabled the continuous monitoring of $S\bar{v}o_2$ using reflectance spectrophotometry. The catheter is connected to a device that includes a light-emitting diode and a sensor to detect the light returning from the PA. $S\bar{v}o_2$ is calculated from the differential absorption of various wavelengths of light by the saturated and desaturated hemoglobin.

If it is assumed that there is constant oxygen consumption and arterial oxygen content, changes in $S\bar{v}o_2$ should reflect changes in CO. Several investigators have come to the conclusion that it provides a valuable measure of CO during surgery. The $S\bar{v}o_2$ has been shown to correlate with cardiac index during CABG surgery when oxygen consumption is constant, but not with the cardiac index when oxygen consumption is changing, such as during shivering after anesthesia. The usefulness of the catheter may primarily be its ability to continuously monitor the balance between oxygen delivery and consumption,[16] and $S\bar{v}o_2$ may also help predict survival after acute myocardial infarction.

III

CARDIAC OUTPUT MONITORING

The CO is the amount of blood pumped to the peripheral circulation by the heart each minute. It is a measurement that reflects the status of the entire circulatory system, not just the heart, because it is governed by autoregulation from the tissues. The CO is equal to the product of the SV and the heart rate. Preload, afterload, heart rate, and contractility are the major determinants of the CO. The measurement of CO is of particular interest in patients with cardiac disease.

Indicator Dilution

The indicator dilution method is based on the observation that, for a known amount of indicator introduced at one point in the circulation, the same amount of indicator should be detectable at a downstream point. The amount of indicator detected at the downstream point is equal to the product of CO and the change in indicator concentration over time. CO is calculated using the Stewart-Hamilton equation:

$$CO = I \times 60 \div \int C \, dt$$

in which CO is cardiac output, I is amount of indicator injected, and $\int C\ dt$ is the integral of indicator concentration over time (60 converts seconds to minutes).

Cold saline (i.e., thermodilution) or lithium ions are used as the indicator, whereas dye (e.g., indocyanine green) or radioisotopes are rarely used in current practice. Blood flow is directly proportional to the amount of the indicator delivered and inversely proportional to the amount of indicator that is present at a sampling site distal to the injection site.

Thermodilution

INTERMITTENT THERMODILUTION CARDIAC OUTPUT

The thermodilution method, using the PA catheter, is the most commonly used method at present for invasively measuring CO in the clinical setting. With this technique, multiple COs can be obtained at frequent intervals using an inert indicator, and without blood withdrawal. A bolus of cold fluid is injected into the right atrium, and the resulting temperature change is detected by the thermistor in the PA. When a thermal indicator is used, the modified Stewart-Hamilton equation is used to calculate CO:

$$CO = \frac{V(T_B - T_I) \times K_1 \times K_2}{\int_0^\infty \Delta T_B(t)dt}$$

in which CO is the cardiac output (L/min), V is the volume of injectate (mL), T_B is the initial blood temperature (°C), T_I is the initial injectate temperature (°C), K_1 is the density factor, K_2 is the computation constant, and $\int_0^\infty \Delta T_B(t)dt$ is the integral of blood temperature change over time.

Solution of this equation is performed by a computer that integrates the area under the temperature versus time curve. CO is inversely proportional to the area under the curve.

The temperature-versus-time curve is the crux of this technique, and any circumstances that affect it have consequences for the accuracy of the CO measurement. Specifically, anything that results in less "cold" reaching the thermistor, more "cold" reaching the thermistor, or an unstable temperature baseline will adversely affect the accuracy of the technique. Less "cold" reaching the thermistor would result in overestimation of the CO. This could be caused by a smaller amount of indicator, an indicator that is too warm, a thrombus on the thermistor, or partial "wedging" of the catheter. Conversely, underestimation of the CO will occur if excessive volume of injectate, or injectate that is too cold, is used to perform the measurement. Intracardiac shunts have unpredictable effects that depend on the anatomy and physiology of individual patients. Variations of up to 80% in measured CO occur when the rate of administration of intravenous crystalloid infusions caused fluctuations in baseline blood temperature. The rapid temperature decrease seen after hypothermic CPB has been shown to result in the underestimation of CO by 0.6 to 2.0 L/min. The normal changes in the PA that occur with each respiratory cycle appear to be exaggerated in the early phase after hypothermic CPB. This may cause peak-to-peak errors in estimation of intermittent CO of up to 50% if initiated at different times during the ventilatory cycle. This effect was significantly decreased with thermal equilibration, approximately 30 minutes after CPB. This problem is less prevalent currently, because hypothermic CPB is used less commonly.

The precision of the thermodilution CO technique is not very good but can be improved by ensuring that, for each determination, the rate and duration of the injection are kept as constant as possible. Whenever possible, 10-mL volumes of injectate should be used and the timing of the injection in the respiratory cycle should be the same.

CONTINUOUS THERMODILUTION CARDIAC OUTPUT

Pulmonary artery catheters with the ability to measure CO continuously were introduced into clinical practice in the 1990s. The method that has gained the most clinical use functions by mildly heating the blood in a pseudorandom stochastic fashion. In vitro as well as in vivo studies have shown that a good correlation exists between this method and other measures of CO.

There was a poor correlation between intermittent and continuous thermodilution CO ($r = 0.273$) in the first 45 minutes after CPB. In contrast, there was an excellent correlation between intermittent and continuous CO measurements obtained in more physiologically stable periods. Perhaps the reason for this observation lies in the unstable thermal baseline after hypothermic CPB.

The routine use of continuous CO catheters in cardiac surgery patients has not been shown to improve outcome, and they are more expensive than standard PA catheters. Bolus thermodilution CO still holds its place as the gold standard of CO measurements in the clinical setting.[17]

ARTERIAC PRESSURE-BASED CARDIAC OUTPUT

Recently, the FloTrac/Vigileo system has been introduced into clinical pratice. It is a unique system that measures CO from the radial artery catheter and does not require calibration. This device has been shown to be accurate in cardiac surgial patients. It measures beat-to-beat stroke volume, and calculate stroke volume variation as a predictor of fluid responsiveness or dynamic preload. Abnormal arterial pressure waveforms (eg: aortic regurgitation) will lead to incorrect CO measurements with this pulse contour technique.[18]

ANALYSIS AND INTERPRETATION OF HEMODYNAMIC DATA

The information provided by hemodynamic monitoring permits the calculation of various derived parameters that assist in evaluating patients clinically. The formulas, normal values, and units for the calculation of various hemodynamic parameters are presented in Table 9-2. These parameters include the SVR, pulmonary vascular resistance (PVR), SV, left ventricular stroke work (LVSW), and right ventricular stroke work (RVSW). As an example of information that may be obtained, graphs of PCWP versus SV can be constructed for individual patients; these "Starling curves" provide insight into the contractile state of the heart. Although these parameters are easily derived using the standard formulas, many modern monitors perform these calculations. To compare data among patients of different body weights and types, the various hemodynamic parameters may be normalized by indexing them to body surface area.

Systemic and Pulmonary Vascular Resistances

Systemic vascular resistance represents an estimation of the afterload of the left ventricle. Afterload is roughly defined as the force that impedes or opposes ventricular contraction. Higher SVR results in increased LV systolic wall stress. This has clinical significance because LV wall stress is one of the major determinants of myocardial oxygen consumption. Elevations in wall stress have been observed in patients with LV enlargement due to systemic hypertension, aortic stenosis, and aortic regurgitation.

Clinically, calculations of SVR are used to assess the response to inotropic, vasodilatory, and vasoconstrictive agents.[19] For example, a patient who is hypotensive despite a high normal CO has a low SVR. The SVR is calculated, and then therapy is instituted (e.g., a vasoconstrictor). A repeat calculation of the SVR enables the clinician to titrate the therapy to the appropriate endpoint. Despite this common use in the operating room and ICU setting, there is good evidence that SVR is not an accurate indicator of true afterload. Nevertheless, SVR remains the clinical technique for measuring afterload at the present time.

PVR remains the traditional measure of afterload of the right ventricle. Systolic PAP may provide a better estimation of RV afterload. PVR and PAP do provide some clinically useful information regarding the pulmonary vasculature and are readily available in patients with PA catheters. The PVR should be used in conjunction with other hemodynamic data to assess the response of the pulmonary vasculature to pharmacologic therapy and physiologic changes.

Frank-Starling Relationships

Myocardial function depends on the contractile state and the preload of the ventricle (sarcomere length at end-diastole). The relationship between the ventricular preload and myocardial work (ventricular stroke work) is the Frank-Starling relationship. The slope of the curve indicates the contractile state of the myocardium (Fig. 9-8). For clinical purposes, it is usually not feasible to measure actual end-diastolic volumes (can be estimated with TEE), and approximations of end-diastolic pressure, such as the PCWP or LAP, are often substituted. This introduces error, because the relationship between end-diastolic pressure and volume is usually nonlinear (as described by the diastolic ventricular compliance curve) and is dynamic. Unfortunately, the Frank-Starling relationship is extremely sensitive to changes in afterload. Patients with LV or RV dysfunction may have severe decrements in SV with increased SVR or PVR, respectively.

MONITORING CORONARY PERFUSION

The coronary perfusion pressure (CPP) is usually defined as the aortic diastolic blood pressure (DAP) minus the LVEDP:

$$CPP = DAP - LVEDP$$

Elevation of the LVEDP will decrease the gradient of blood flow to the vulnerable subendocardial tissue during diastole as will a decrease in the DBP. If coronary artery disease is present, significant stenosis will decrease the coronary artery DBP well below the aortic DBP, and elevation of LVEDP can seriously jeopardize the subendocardium. An increase in the LVEDP is detrimental in two ways: decreased coronary blood flow and increased myocardial oxygen demand ($M\bar{v}o_2$), which explain the severe ischemia seen with overdistention of the left ventricle. Tachycardia is also extremely detrimental because it decreases coronary filling time and increases oxygen demand. Subendocardial ischemia is commonly produced by a combination of tachycardia and elevated LVEDP.

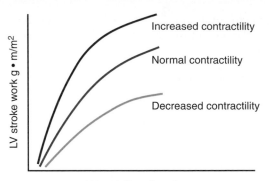

Figure 9-8 The graph of left ventricular (LV) stroke work versus LV preload (i.e., end-diastolic volume) is known as the Frank-Starling relationship. Shifting of the curve upward and to the left represents increased contractility. Shifting of the curve downward and to the right represents decreased contractility. Alterations in afterload significantly affect the curve.

ELECTROCARDIOGRAPHY

Interpretation of the ECG is often considered the domain of the cardiologist, but clinicians providing perioperative and critical care also derive important information from it by the standard 12-lead tracing or as a continuous "monitoring" modality.

The practicing anesthesiologist relies on the ECG to make critical decisions at many phases of the perioperative period in patients undergoing cardiac or noncardiac (particularly vascular) surgery.[20]

Lead Systems

Einthoven established electrocardiography using three extremities as references: the left arm, right arm, and left leg. He recorded the difference in potential between the left arm and right arm (lead I), between the left leg and right arm (lead II), and between the left leg and left arm (lead III). Because the signals recorded were differences between two electrodes, these leads were called *bipolar*. The positive or negative polarity of each of the limbs was chosen by Einthoven to result in positive deflections of most of the waveforms and has no innate physiologic significance. He postulated that the three limbs defined an imaginary equilateral triangle with the heart at its center.

Wilson refined and introduced the unipolar precordial leads into clinical practice. To implement these leads, he postulated a mechanism whereby the absolute level of electrical potential could be measured at the site of the exploring precordial electrode (the positive electrode). A negative pole with zero potential was formed by joining the three limb electrodes in a resistive network in which equally weighted signals cancel each other out. He called this the *central terminal*. He described three additional limb leads (VL, VR, and VF). These leads measured new vectors of activation, and in this way the hexaxial reference system for determination of electrical axis was established. He subsequently introduced the six unipolar precordial V leads in 1935 (Fig. 9-9).

Detection of Myocardial Ischemia

Pathophysiology of ST-Segment Responses

The ST segment is the most important portion of the QRS complex for evaluating ischemia (Box 9-11). The origin of this segment, at the J point, is easy to locate. Its end, which is generally accepted as the beginning of any change of slope of the

III

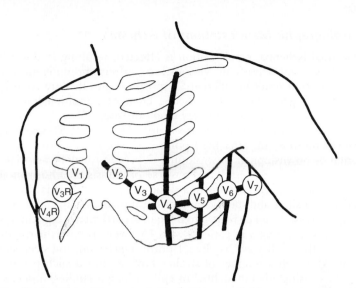

Figure 9-9 The locations of the precordial leads. *Heavy vertical lines* represent the midclavicular, anterior, axillary, and midaxillary lines (*from left to right*). V_1 and V_2 are referenced to the fourth intercostal space and V_4 to the fifth space. V_3 lies on a line between V_2 and V_4. V_5 and V_6 lie on a horizontal line from V_4. Additional precordial leads can be obtained on the right side (V_3R, V_4R), as well as extending farther left from V_6 (V_7). (From Friedman HH: Diagnostic Electrocardiography and Vectorcardiography. New York, McGraw-Hill, 1985, p 41; with permission of The McGraw-Hill Companies.)

BOX 9-11 *Monitoring for Myocardial Ischemia*

- (Preoperative) clinical symptoms
- Electrocardiogram (leads II, V_3, V_4, V_5)
- Transesophageal echocardiography
- Pulmonary artery catheterization

9

T wave, is more difficult to determine. In normal individuals there may be no discernible ST segment as the T wave starts with a steady slope from the J point, especially at rapid heart rates. The TP segment has been used as the isoelectric baseline from which changes in the ST segment are evaluated, but with tachycardia this segment is eliminated, and during exercise testing the PR segment is used. The PR segment is used in all ST-segment analyzers.

Repolarization of the ventricle proceeds from the epicardium to the endocardium, opposite to the vector of depolarization. The ST segment reflects the midportion, or phase 2, of repolarization during which there is little change in electrical potential. It is usually isoelectric. Ischemia causes a loss of intracellular potassium, resulting in a *current of injury*. The electrophysiologic mechanism accounting for ST-segment shifts (elevation or depression) remains controversial. The two major theories are based on a loss of resting potential as current flows from the uninjured to the injured area (i.e., diastolic current) and on a true change in phase 2 potential as current flows from the injured to the uninjured area (i.e., systolic current). With subendocardial injury, the ST segment is depressed in the surface leads. With epicardial or transmural injury, the ST segment is elevated.[21,22]

Electrocardiographic Manifestations of Ischemia

With myocardial ischemia, repolarization is affected, resulting in downsloping or horizontal ST-segment depression. Various local effects and differences in vectors during repolarization result in different ST morphologies that are recorded by the different leads. It is generally accepted that ST changes in multiple leads are associated with more severe degrees of coronary artery disease.

The classic criterion for ischemia is 0.1 mV (1 mm) of ST-segment depression measured 60 to 80 ms after the J point.[23-25] The slope of the segment must be horizontal or downsloping. Downsloping depression may be associated with a greater number of diseased vessels and a worse prognosis than horizontal depression. Slowly upsloping depression with a slope of 1 mV/s or less is also used but is considered less sensitive and specific (and difficult to assess clinically). Nonspecific ST-segment depression can be related to drug use, particularly digoxin. Interpretation of ST-segment changes in patients with LV hypertrophy is particularly controversial given the tall R-wave baseline, J-point depression, and steep slope of the ST segment. Although a number of studies have excluded such patients, others (including those using other modalities or epidemiologic studies) observed that LV hypertrophy is a highly significant predictor of adverse cardiac outcome.

The criteria for ischemia with ST-segment elevation ($\geq$0.1 mV in $\geq$2 contiguous leads) are used in conjunction with clinical symptoms or elevation of biochemical markers to diagnose acute coronary syndromes. It usually results from transmural ischemia, but it may potentially represent a *reciprocal change* in a lead oriented opposite to the primary vector with subendocardial ischemia. Perioperative ambulatory monitoring studies have also included more than 0.2 mV in any single lead as a criterion, but ST-segment elevation is rarely reported in the setting of noncardiac surgery. It is commonly observed, however, during weaning from CPB in cardiac surgery and during CABG surgery (on and off pump) with interruption of coronary flow in a native or graft vessel. ST-segment elevation in a Q-wave lead should not be analyzed for acute ischemia, although it may indicate the presence of a ventricular aneurysm.

Clinical Lead Systems for Detecting Ischemia

Early clinical reports of intraoperative monitoring using the V_5 lead in high-risk patients were based on observations during exercise testing, in which bipolar configurations of V_5 demonstrated high sensitivity for myocardial ischemia detection (up to 90%). Subsequent studies using 12-lead monitoring (torso mounted for stability during exercise) confirmed the sensitivity of the lateral precordial leads. Some studies, however, reported higher sensitivity for leads V_4 or V_6 compared with V_5, followed by the inferior leads (in which most false-positive responses were reported).

The factors responsible for precipitating ischemia during exercise testing and surgical settings may differ. For example, during exercise stress testing, most ischemia is demand related, whereas in the perioperative period a larger proportion may be related to reduced oxygen supply. The most sensitive leads during exercise testing, however, are useful in the perioperative setting.

Intraoperative Lead Systems

Detection of perioperative myocardial ischemia has received considerable attention over the past several decades and more recently with publication of several studies of clinical monitoring and therapy (e.g., perioperative β-blockade). Many of these studies demonstrated associations of perioperative ischemia with adverse cardiac outcomes in adults undergoing a variety of cardiac and noncardiac surgical procedures. The ease of use of new ST-segment trending software in operating room monitors has resulted in its routine use.

The recommended leads for intraoperative monitoring, based on several clinical studies, do not differ substantially from those used during exercise testing.[26] Clinical studies using continuous 12-lead ECG analysis reported that almost 90% of responses involved ST-segment depression alone (75% in V_5 and 61% in V_4). In approximately 70% of patients, significant changes were observed in multiple leads. The sensitivity of each of the 12 leads is shown in Figure 9-10. When considered in combination (as occurs clinically), the use of leads V_4 and V_5 increased sensitivity to 90%, whereas sensitivity for the standard clinical combination of leads II and V_5 was 80%. Use of leads V_2 through V_5 and lead II captured all episodes (Table 9-4).

A larger clinical study of patients undergoing vascular surgery using a longer period of monitoring (up to 72 hours) with more specific criteria for ischemia (>10 minute duration of episode) extended these observations. It was reported that V_3 was most sensitive for ischemia (87%) followed by V_4 (79%), whereas V_5 alone was only 66% sensitive. In the subgroup of patients in whom prolonged ischemic episodes ultimately culminated in infarction, V_4 was most sensitive (83%). In this study, all myocardial infarctions were non–Q-wave events detected by troponin elevation. Use of two precordial leads detected 97% to 100% of changes. Based on analysis of the resting isoelectric levels of each of the 12 leads (a unique component of this study), it was recommended that V_4 was the best single choice for monitoring of a single precordial lead, because it was most likely to be isoelectric relative to the resting 12-lead preoperative ECG. In contrast, the baseline ST segment was more likely above isoelectric in V_1 through V_3 and below isoelectric in V_5 and V_6. Surprisingly, no episodes of ST elevation occurred in this study.

A cohort of vascular patients monitored in the ICU for the first postoperative day with continuous 12-lead monitoring used a threshold of 20 minutes for an ischemic

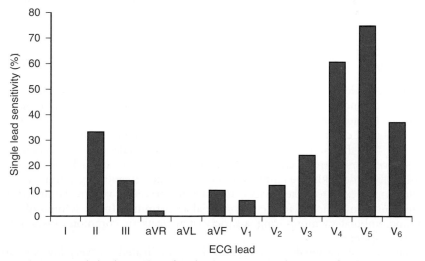

Figure 9-10 Single-lead sensitivity for the intraoperative detection of ischemia based on 51 episodes detected in 25 patients undergoing noncardiac surgery. Sensitivity was calculated by dividing the number of episodes detected in that lead by the total number of episodes. Sensitivity was greatest in lead V_5, and the lateral leads (I, aVL) were insensitive. (From London MJ, Hollenberg M, Wong MG, et al: Intraoperative myocardial ischemia: Localization by continuous 12-lead electrocardiography. Anesthesiology 69:232, 1988.)

Table 9-4	Sensitivity for Different Electrocardiographic Lead Combinations	
Number of Leads	Combination	Sensitivity (%)
1 lead	II	33
	V_4	61
	V_5	75
2 leads	II/V_5	80
	II/V_4	82
	V_4/V_5	90
3 leads	V_3/V_4/V_5	94
	II/V_4/V_5	96
4 leads	II/V_2-V_5	100

Data from London MJ, Hollenberg M, Wong MG, et al: Intraoperative myocardial ischemia: Localization by continuous 12-lead electrocardiography. Anesthesiology 69:232, 1988.

episode. Eleven percent of 149 patients met the criteria, with ST-segment depression in 71% and ST-segment elevation alone in 18% (12% had both). Most changes were detected in V_2 (53%) and V_3 (65%). Using the standard two-lead system (II and V_5), only 41% of episodes would have been detected.

The use of multiple precordial leads, although appealing, is not likely to become common clinical practice, owing to the limitations of existing monitors (and cables). Even if such equipment were available, it is likely that considerable resistance would occur from practitioners due to the extra effort associated with this approach. Perhaps, in the future, when lower cost wireless technologies are perfected, this approach may become a clinical reality; in the meantime, a combination of leads V_5 and II remains the clinical choice of most practitioners.

Arrhythmia and Pacemaker Detection

Use of inferior leads allows superior discrimination of P-wave morphology, facilitating visual diagnosis of arrhythmias and conduction disorders. Although esophageal (and even intracardiac) leads allow the greatest sensitivity in detecting P waves, these are rarely used clinically. Nevertheless, they should be kept in mind for difficult diagnoses. With the increasing use of implantable defibrillators and automatic external defibrillators to treat ventricular fibrillation and ventricular tachycardia, there is considerable interest in the refinement of arrhythmia detection algorithms and their validation. As expected, the devices' accuracy for detecting ventricular arrhythmias is high but is much lower for detecting atrial arrhythmias. In the settings of critical care and ambulatory monitoring, a variety of artifacts are common causes of false-positive responses.

Detection of pacemaker spikes may be complicated by very-low-amplitude signals related to bipolar pacing leads, amplitude varying with respiration, and total-body fluid accumulation. Most critical care and ambulatory monitors incorporate pacemaker spike enhancement for small high-frequency signals (typically 5 to 500 mV with 0.5- to 2-ms pulse duration) to facilitate recognition. However, this can lead to artifact if there is high-frequency noise within the lead system.

III

SUMMARY

- Patients with severe cardiovascular disease and those undergoing surgery associated with rapid hemodynamic changes should be adequately monitored at all times.
- Adequate monitoring is based on specific patient, surgical, and environmental factors.
- Standard monitoring for cardiac surgery patients includes invasive blood pressure, electrocardiography, central venous pressure, urine output, temperature, capnometry, pulse oximetry, and intermittent blood gas analysis.
- Electrocardiography remains the gold standard for myocardial ischemia monitoring. Thermodilution PA catheters and left atrial pressure catheters are invasive monitors. The risks and benefits should be considered for each patient.
- The Society of Cardiovascular Anesthesiologists and the American Society of Echocardiography have published recommendations for intraoperative PA catheter and TEE use in various clinical settings.
- Evidence-based data on clinical outcome and monitoring in cardiac anesthesia are difficult to obtain owing to difficulties in conducting large prospective trials.

REFERENCES

1. Dorje P, Tremper K: Systolic pressure variation: A dynamic measure of the adequacy of intravascular volume. Semin Anesth Periop Med Pain 24:147, 2005
2. Barbeau GR, Arsenault F, Dugas L, et al: Evaluation of the ulnopalmar arterial arches with pulse oximetry and plethysmography: Comparison with the Allen's test in 1010 patients. Am Heart J 147:489, 2004
3. Armstrong PJ, Han DC, Baxter JA, et al: Complication rates of percutaneous brachial artery access in peripheral vascular angiography. Ann Vasc Surg 17:107, 2003
4. Hind D, Calvert N, McWilliams R, et al: Ultrasonic locating devices for central venous cannulation: Meta-analysis. BMJ 327:361, 2003
5. Riopelle J, Ruiz D, Hunt J, et al: Circumferential adjustment of ultrasound probe position to determine the optimal approach to the internal jugular vein: A noninvasive geometric study in adults. Anesth Analg 100:512, 2005
6. Troianos CA, Kuwik R, Pasqual J, et al: Internal jugular vein and carotid artery anatomic relation as determined by ultrasonography. Anesthesiology 85:43, 1996
7. Parry G: Trendelenburg position, head elevation and a midline position optimize right internal jugular vein diameter. Can J Anaesth 51:379, 2004
8. Pawar M, Mehta Y, Kapoor P, et al: Central venous catheter-related bloodstream infections: Incidence, risk factors, outcome, and associated pathogens. J Cardiothorac Vasc Anesth 18:304, 2004
9. Sandham JD: Pulmonary artery catheter use—refining the question. Crit Care Med 32:1070, 2004
10. Chittock DR, Dhingra VK, Ronco JJ, et al: Severity of illness and risk of death associated with pulmonary artery catheter use. Crit Care Med 32:911, 2004
11. Sandham JD, Hull RD, Brant RF, et al: A randomized, controlled trial of the use of pulmonary artery catheters in high-risk surgical patients. N Engl J Med 348:5, 2003
12. Vender J: Pulmonary artery catheter utilization: The use, misuse, or abuse, J Cardiothorac Vasc Anesth 20:295-299, 2006
13. American Society of Anesthesiologists Task Force on Pulmonary Artery Catheterization: Practice guidelines for pulmonary artery catheterization: An updated report by the American Society of Anesthesiologists Task Force on Pulmonary Artery Catheterization. Anesthesiology 99:988, 2003
14. Abreu AR, Campos MA, Krieger BP: Pulmonary artery rupture induced by a pulmonary artery catheter: A case report and review of the literature. J Intensive Care Med 19:291, 2004
15. Risk SC, Brandon D, D'Ambra MN, et al: Indications for the use of pacing pulmonary artery catheters in cardiac surgery. J Cardiothorac Vasc Anesth 6:275, 1992
16. Reinhart K, Kuhn HJ, Hartog C, Bredle DL: Continuous central venous and pulmonary artery oxygen saturation monitoring in the critically ill. Intensive Care Med 30:1572, 2004
17. Zollner C, Goetz AE, Weis M, et al: Continuous cardiac output measurements do not agree with conventional bolus thermodilution cardiac output determination. Can J Anaesth 48:1143, 2001

9

18. Manecke GR: Cardiac output from the arterial catheter: Deceptively simple. J Cardiothorac Vasc Anesth 21:629, 2007
19. Bashore T: Afterload reduction in chronic aortic regurgitation: It sure seems like a good idea. J Am Coll Cardiol 45:1031, 2005
20. Weinfurt PT: Electrocardiographic monitoring: An overview. J Clin Monit 6:132, 1990
21. Tsuda H, Tobata H, Watanabe S, et al: QRS complex changes in the V_5 ECG lead during cardiac surgery. J Cardiothorac Vasc Anesth 6:658, 1992
22. Crescenzi G, Scandroglio AM, Pappalardo F, et al: ECG changes after CABG: The role of the surgical technique. J Cardiothorac Vasc Anesth 18:38, 2004
23. Horacek BM, Wagner GS: Electrocardiographic ST-segment changes during acute myocardial ischemia. Card Electrophysiol Rev 6:196, 2002
24. Carley SD: Beyond the 12 lead: Review of the use of additional leads for the early electrocardiographic diagnosis of acute myocardial infarction. Emerg Med (Fremantle) 15:143, 2003
25. Zimetbaum PJ, Josephson ME: Use of the electrocardiogram in acute myocardial infarction. N Engl J Med 348:933, 2003
26. London MJ: Multilead precordial ST-segment monitoring: "The next generation?" Anesthesiology 96:259, 2002

III

Chapter 10

Intraoperative Echocardiography

Ronald A. Kahn, MD • Stanton K. Shernan, MD •
Steven N. Konstadt, MD • Stuart J. Weiss, MD •
Joseph S. Savino, MD

Few areas in cardiac anesthesia have developed as rapidly as the field of intraoperative echocardiography. In the early 1980s, when transesophageal echocardiography (TEE) was first used in the operating room, its main application was the assessment of global and regional left ventricular (LV) function. Since that time there have been numerous technical advances: biplane and multiplane probes; multifrequency probes; enhanced scanning resolution; color flow, pulsed wave, and continuous wave Doppler; automatic edge detection; Doppler tissue imaging; three-dimensional (3D) reconstruction; and digital image processing. With these advances, the number of clinical applications of TEE has markedly increased. The common applications of TEE include (1) assessment of valvular anatomy and function, (2) evaluation of the thoracic aorta, (3) detection of intracardiac defects, (4) detection of intracardiac masses, (5) evaluation of pericardial effusions, (6) detection of intracardiac air and clots, and (7) assessment of biventricular systolic and diastolic function. In many of these evaluations, TEE is able to provide unique and critical information that was not previously available in the operating room (Box 10-1).

BOX 10-1 *Common Applications of Transesophageal Echocardiography*

- Assessment of valvular anatomy and function
- Evaluation of the thoracic aorta
- Detection of intracardiac defects
- Detection of intracardiac masses
- Evaluation of pericardial effusions
- Detection of intracardiac air and clots
- Assessment of biventricular systolic and diastolic function

BASIC CONCEPTS

Properties of Ultrasound

In echocardiography, the heart and great vessels are insonated with ultrasound, which is sound above the human audible range. The ultrasound is sent into the thoracic cavity and is partially reflected by the cardiac structures. From these reflections, distance, velocity, and density of objects within the chest are derived.

Wavelength, Frequency, and Velocity

An ultrasound beam is a continuous or intermittent train of sound waves emitted by a transducer or wave generator. It is composed of density or pressure waves and can exist in any medium with the exception of a vacuum. Ultrasound waves are characterized by their wavelength, frequency, and velocity. *Wavelength* is the distance between the two nearest points of equal pressure or density in an ultrasound beam, and *velocity* is the speed at which the waves propagate through a medium. As the waves travel past any fixed point in an ultrasound beam, the pressure cycles regularly and continuously between a high and a low value. The number of cycles per second (Hertz) is called the *frequency* of the wave. Ultrasound is sound with frequencies above 20,000 Hz, which is the upper limit of the human audible range. The relationship among the frequency (f), wavelength (λ), and velocity (v) of a sound wave is defined by the formula:

$$v = f \cdot \lambda$$

Piezoelectric crystals convert the energy between ultrasound and electrical signals. When presented with a high-frequency electrical signal, these crystals produce ultrasound energy, which is directed toward the areas to be imaged. Commonly, a short ultrasound signal is emitted from the piezoelectric crystal. After ultrasound wave formation, the crystal "listens" for the returning echoes for a given period of time and then pauses before repeating this cycle. This cycle length is known as the *pulse repetition frequency* (PRF). This cycle length must be long enough to provide enough time for a signal to travel to and return from a given object of interest. Typically, PRFs vary from 1 to 10 kHz, which results in 0.1- to 1.0-ms intervals between pulses. When reflected ultrasound waves return to these piezoelectric crystals they are converted into electrical signals, which may be appropriately processed and displayed. Electronic circuits measure the time delay between the emitted and received echo. Because the speed of ultrasound through tissue is a constant, this time delay can be converted into the precise distance between the transducer and tissue.

Imaging Techniques

M Mode

The most basic form of ultrasound imaging is M-mode echocardiography. In this mode, the density and position of all tissues in the path of a narrow ultrasound beam (i.e., *along a single line*) are displayed as a scroll on a video screen. The scrolling produces an updated, continuously changing time plot of the studied tissue section, several seconds in duration. Because this is a timed *motion display* (normal cardiac tissue is always in motion), it is called M mode. Because only a very limited part of the heart is being observed at any one time and because the image requires considerable interpretation, M mode is not currently used as a primary imaging technique. This mode is, however, useful for the precise timing of events within the cardiac cycle and is often used in combination with color flow Doppler imaging for the timing of abnormal flows.

Two-Dimensional Mode

By rapid, repetitive scanning along *many different radii* within an area in the shape of a fan (sector), echocardiography generates a 2D image of a section of the heart. This image, which resembles an anatomic section and, thus, can be more easily interpreted, is called a *two-dimensional scan.* Information on structures and motion in the plane of a 2D scan is updated 30 to 60 times per second. This repetitive update produces a "live" (real-time) image of the heart. Scanning 2D echo devices image the heart by using either a mechanically steered transducer or, as is common in many of the modern devices, an electronically steered ultrasound beam (phased-array transducer).

Doppler Techniques

Most modern echocardiographic scanners combine Doppler capabilities with their 2D imaging capabilities. After the desired view of the heart has been obtained by 2D echocardiography, the Doppler beam, represented by a cursor, is superimposed on the 2D image. The operator positions the cursor as parallel as possible to the assumed direction of blood flow and then empirically adjusts the direction of the beam to optimize the audio and visual representations of the reflected Doppler signal. At the present time, Doppler technology can be used in at least four different ways to measure blood velocities: pulsed wave, high repetition frequency, continuous wave, and color flow.

Color Flow Mapping

Advances in electronics and computer technology have allowed the development of color flow Doppler ultrasound scanners capable of displaying real-time blood flow within the heart as colors while also showing 2D images in black and white. In addition to showing the location, direction, and velocity of cardiac blood flow, the images produced by these devices allow estimation of flow acceleration and differentiation of laminar and turbulent blood flow.

A location in the heart where the scanner has detected flow toward the transducer (the top of the image sector) is assigned the color red. Flow away from the direction of the top is assigned the color blue. This color assignment is arbitrary and determined by the equipment manufacturer and the user's color mapping. In the most common color flow coding scheme, the faster the velocity (up to a limit), the more intense is the color. Flow velocities that change by more than a preset value within a brief time interval (flow variance) have the color green added to either the red or the blue. Both rapidly accelerating laminar flow (change in flow speed) and turbulent

10

BOX 10-2 *Diagnostic Applications for Contrast Echocardiography*

- Assessment of congenital heart disease
- Enhancement of endocardial borders for qualitative assessment of wall motion abnormalities
- Measurement of left ventricular function
- Quantification of valvular regurgitation
- Enhancement of color flow Doppler signals
- Assessment of myocardial perfusion
- Measurements of perfusion area after coronary artery bypass graft surgery
- Assessment of quality of coronary bypass grafts and cardioplegia distribution
- Correct assessment of the results of surgery for ventricular septal defect

flow (change in flow direction) satisfy the criteria for rapid changes in velocity. In summary, the brightness of the red or blue colors at any location and time is usually proportional to the corresponding flow velocity while the hue is proportional to the temporal rate of change of the velocity.

Contrast Echocardiography

Normally, red blood cells scatter ultrasound waves weakly, resulting in their black appearance on ultrasound examination. Contrast echocardiography is performed by injecting nontoxic solutions containing gaseous microbubbles. These microbubbles present additional gas-liquid interfaces, which substantially increase the strength of the returning signal. This augmentation in signal strength may be used to better define endocardial borders, optimize Doppler envelope signals, and estimate myocardial perfusion.

Contrast echocardiography has been used to image intracardiac shunts, valvular incompetence, and pericardial effusions. In addition, LV injections of hand-agitated microbubble solutions have been used to identify semiquantitative LV endocardial edges, cardiac output, and valvular regurgitation (Box 10-2).

Contrast agents are microbubbles, consisting of a shell surrounding a gas. Initial contrast agents were agitated free air in either a saline or blood/saline solution. These microbubbles were large and unstable, so they were unable to cross the pulmonary circulation; they were effective only for right-sided heart contrast. Because of their thin shell, the gas quickly leaked into the blood with resultant dissolution of the microbubble. Agents with a longer persistence were subsequently developed.[1]

EQUIPMENT

All of the currently available TEE probes employ a multifrequency transducer that is mounted on the tip of a gastroscope housing. The majority of the echocardiographic examination is performed using ultrasound between 3.5 and 7 MHz. The tip can be directed by the adjustment of knobs placed at the proximal handle. In most adult probes there are two knobs; one allows anterior and posterior movement, and the other permits side-to-side motion. Multiplane probes also include a control to rotate the echocardiographic array from 0 to 180 degrees. Thus, in combination with the ability to advance and withdraw the probe and to rotate it, many echocardiographic windows are possible. Another feature common to most probes is the inclusion of a temperature sensor to warn of possible heat injury from the transducer to the esophagus.

BOX 10-3 *Complications from Intraoperative Transesophageal Echocardiography*

- Injury from direct trauma to the airway and esophagus
  - Esophageal bleeding, burning, tearing
  - Dysphagia
  - Laryngeal discomfort
  - Bacteremia
  - Vocal cord paralysis
- Indirect effects
  - Hemodynamic and pulmonary effects of airway manipulation
  - Distraction from patient

Currently, most adult echocardiographic probes are multiplane (variable orientation of the scanning plane), whereas pediatric probes are either multiplane or biplane (transverse and longitudinal orientation, parallel to the shaft). The adult probes usually have a shaft length of 100 cm and are between 9 and 12 mm in diameter. The tips of the probes vary slightly in shape and size but are generally 1 to 2 mm wider than the shaft. The size of these probes requires the patient to weigh at least 20 kg. Depending on the manufacturer, the adult probes contain between 32 and 64 elements per scanning orientation. In general, the image quality is directly related to the number of elements used. The pediatric probes are mounted on a narrower, shorter shaft with smaller transducers. These probes may be used in patients as small as 1 kg.

An important feature that is often available is the ability to alter the scanning frequency. A lower frequency, such as 3.5 MHz, has greater penetration and is more suited for the transgastric view. It also increases the Doppler velocity limits. Conversely, the higher frequencies yield better resolution for detailed imaging. One of the limitations of TEE is that structures very close to the probe are seen only in a very narrow sector. Newer probes may also allow a broader near-field view. Finally, newer probes may possess the ability to scan simultaneously in more than one plane.

10

COMPLICATIONS

Complications resulting from intraoperative TEE can be separated into two groups: injury from direct trauma to the airway and esophagus and indirect effects of TEE (Box 10-3). In the first group, potential complications include esophageal bleeding, burning, tearing, dysphagia, and laryngeal discomfort. Many of these complications could result from pressure exerted by the tip of the probe on the esophagus and the airway. Although in most patients even maximal flexion of the probe will not result in pressure above 17 mm Hg, occasionally, even in the absence of esophageal disease, pressures greater than 60 mm Hg will result.

Further confirmation of the low incidence of esophageal injury from TEE is apparent in the few case reports of complications. In the world's literature, there are only a few reports of a fatal esophageal perforation and benign Mallory-Weiss tear after intraoperative TEE.

The second group of complications that result from TEE includes hemodynamic and pulmonary effects of airway manipulation and, particularly for new TEE operators, distraction from patient care. Fortunately, in the anesthetized patient there are rarely hemodynamic consequences to esophageal placement of the probe and there are no studies that specifically address this question. One potential hemodynamic effect of TEE, even in the well-anesthetized patient, is direct cardiac irritation from the probe with resultant atrial and ventricular arrhythmias. More important for the anesthesiologist are the problems of distraction from patient care. Although these reports are infrequent in the literature, the authors know of several endotracheal tube disconnections that went unnoticed to the point of desaturation during TEE. Additionally, there have been instances in which severe hemodynamic abnormalities have been missed because of fascination with the images or the controls of the echocardiograph machine. Clearly, new echocardiographers should enlist the assistance of an associate to watch the patient during the examination. This second anesthesiologist will become unnecessary after sufficient experience is gained. It is also important to be sure that all of the respiratory and hemodynamic alarms are activated during the echocardiographic examination.

SAFETY GUIDELINES AND CONTRAINDICATIONS

To ensure the continued safety of TEE, the following recommendations are made. The probe should be inspected before each insertion for cleanliness and structural integrity. If possible, the electrical isolation should also be checked. The probe should be inserted gently and, if resistance is met, the procedure aborted. Minimal transducer energy should be used and the image frozen when not in use. Finally, when not imaging, the probe should be left in the neutral, unlocked position to avoid prolonged pressure on the esophageal mucosa.

Absolute contraindications to TEE in intubated patients include esophageal stricture, diverticula, tumor, recent suture lines, and known esophageal interruption. Relative contraindications include symptomatic hiatal hernia, esophagitis, coagulopathy, esophageal varices, and unexplained upper gastrointestinal bleeding. Despite these relative contraindications, TEE has been used in patients undergoing hepatic transplantation without reported sequelae.

III

TECHNIQUE OF PROBE PASSAGE

The passage of a TEE probe through the oral and pharyngeal cavities in anesthetized patients may be challenging at times. The usual technique is to place the well-lubricated probe in the posterior portion of the oropharynx with the transducer element pointing inferiorly and anteriorly. The remainder of the probe may be stabilized by looping the controls and the proximal portion of the probe over the operator's neck and shoulder. The operator's left hand then elevates the mandible by inserting the thumb behind the teeth, grasping the submandibular region with the fingers, and then gently lifting. The probe is then advanced against a slight but even resistance, until a loss of resistance is detected as the tip of the probe passes the inferior constrictor muscle of the pharynx. This usually occurs 10 cm past the lips in neonates to 20 cm past the lips in adults. Further manipulation of the probe is performed under echocardiographic guidance.

Difficult TEE probe insertion may be caused by the probe tip abutting the pyriform sinuses, vallecula, posterior tongue, or an esophageal diverticulum. Overinflation of the endotracheal tube cuff could also obstruct passage of the probe. Maneuvers that might aid the passage of the probe include changing the neck position, realigning the

TEE probe, and applying additional jaw thrust by elevating the angles of the mandible. The probe may also be passed with the assistance of laryngoscopy. The probe should never be forced past an obstruction. This could result in airway trauma or esophageal perforation.

ANATOMY AND TRANSESOPHAGEAL ECHOCARDIOGRAPHY VIEWS

Multiplane Transesophageal Echocardiography Probe Manipulation: Descriptive Terms and Technique

The process of obtaining a comprehensive intraoperative multiplane TEE examination begins with a fundamental understanding of the terminology and technique for probe manipulation (Fig. 10-1).[2] Efficient probe manipulation minimizes esophageal injury and facilitates the process of acquiring and sweeping through 2D image planes. Horizontal imaging planes are obtained by moving the TEE probe up and down (proximal and distal) in the esophagus at various depths relative to the incisors (upper esophageal: 20 to 25 cm; midesophageal: 30 to 40 cm; transgastric: 40 to 45 cm; deep transgastric: 45 to 50 cm) (Table 10-1). Vertical planes

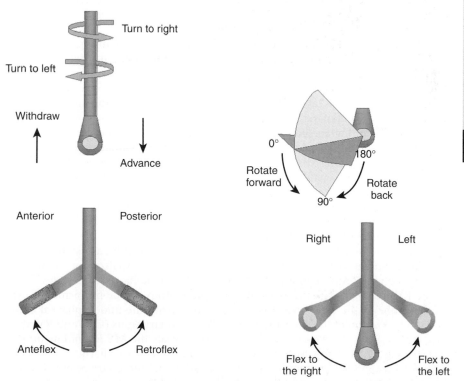

Figure 10-1 Ways to adjust the probe. *Top left,* Probe movement in the esophagus. *Top right,* Scanning angles obtained by crystal rotation. *Bottom left,* Movement of the tip forward and back. *Bottom right,* Movement of the tip from side to side.

are obtained by manually turning the probe to the patient's left or right. Further alignment of the imaging plane can be obtained by manually rotating one of the two control wheels on the probe handle, which flexes the probe tip to the left or right direction or in the anterior or posterior plane. Multiplane probes may further facilitate interrogation of complex anatomic structures, such as the mitral valve (MV), by allowing up to 180 degrees of axial rotation of the imaging plane without manual probe manipulation.

The Comprehensive Intraoperative Transesophageal Echocardiography Examination: Imaging Planes and Structural Analysis

Left and Right Ventricles

The LV should be carefully examined for global and regional function using multiple transducer planes, depths, and rotational and angular orientations (Fig. 10-2). Analysis of segmental function is based on a qualitative visual assessment that includes the following grading system of both LV wall thickness and motion (endocardial border excursion) during systole: 1 = normal (>30% thickening); 2 = mild hypokinesis (10% to 30% thickening); 3 = severe hypokinesis (<10% thickening); 4 = akinesis (no thickening); 5 = dyskinesis (paradoxical motion). The *midesophageal (ME) four-chamber view* at 0 to 20 degrees (see Fig. 10-2A) and *two-chamber view* at approximately 80 to 100 degrees (see Fig. 10-2B) enable visualization of the septal and lateral as well as the inferior and anterior segments at the basal, mid, and apical level segments, respectively. The *ME long-axis (LAX) view* at 120 to 160 degrees (see Fig. 10-2C) allows evaluation of the remaining anteroseptal and posterior LV segments. Because the LV is usually oriented inferiorly to the true horizontal plane, slight retroflexion of the probe tip may be required to minimize LV foreshortening. The *transgastric (TG) mid short-axis (SAX) view* at 0 to 20 degrees (see Fig. 10-2D) is the most commonly used view for monitoring LV function because it allows a midpapillary assessment of the LV segments supplied by the corresponding coronary arteries (right [RCA], left circumflex [CX], and left anterior descending [LAD]). This view also enables qualitative and quantitative evaluation of pericardial effusions. Advancing or withdrawing the probe at the transgastric depth enables LV evaluation at the respective apical and basal levels (*TG basal short-axis view;* see Fig. 10-2F). Further evaluation of the LV can be obtained at the midpapillary transgastric depth by rotating the probe forward to the *TG two-chamber view* (80 to 100 degrees) (see Fig. 10-2E) and *TG long-axis view* (90 to 120 degrees) (see Fig. 10-2J).

Right ventricular (RV) regional and global function can be assessed from the ME four-chamber view (see Fig. 10-2A), which allows visualization of the septal and free walls. Although a formal segmental scheme has not been developed for the RV free wall, regional assessment of the septum can be performed. Turning the probe to the right and advancing slightly from the midesophageal depth allows visualization of the tricuspid valve (TV), coronary sinus (CS), and RV apex. Rotating the probe between 60 and 90 degrees reveals the *ME RV inflow-outflow view* (see Fig. 10-2M), in which the RA, TV, inferior RV free wall, right ventricular outflow tract (RVOT), pulmonic valve (PV), and main pulmonary artery (PA) can be viewed "wrapping around" the centrally oriented AV. This view often allows optimal Doppler beam alignment to evaluate the TV and can also be helpful for directing PA catheter floating and positioning. The *TG mid short-axis view*

Table 10-1 The Comprehensive Intraoperative Multiplane Transesophageal Echocardiographic Examination

Probe Tip Depth (from lips): Upper Esophageal (20 to 25 cm)

View	*Aortic arch: long axis*
Multiplane angle range	0°
Anatomy imaged	Aortic arch; left brachiocephalic vein; left subclavian and carotid arteries; right brachiocephalic artery
Clinical utility	Ascending aorta and arch pathology: atherosclerosis, aneurysms, and dissections
	Aortic CPB cannulation site evaluation
View	*Aortic arch: short axis*
Multiplane angle range	90°
Anatomy imaged	Aortic arch; left brachiocephalic vein; left subclavian and carotid arteries; right brachiocephalic artery; main pulmonary artery and pulmonic valve
Clinical utility	Ascending aorta and arch pathology: atherosclerosis, aneurysms and dissections; pulmonary embolus; pulmonary valve evaluation (insufficiency, stenosis, Ross procedure)
	Pulmonary artery catheter placement

Probe Tip Depth: Midesophageal (30 to 40 cm)

View	*Four chamber*
Multiplane angle range	0° to 20°
Anatomy imaged	Left ventricle and atrium
	Right ventricle and atrium
	Mitral and tricuspid valves
	Interatrial and interventricular septa
	Left pulmonary veins: slight probe withdrawal and turning to left
	Right pulmonary veins: slight probe withdrawal and turning to right
	Coronary sinus: slight probe advancement and turning to right
Clinical utility	Ventricular function: global and regional
	Intracardiac chamber masses: thrombus, tumor, air; foreign bodies
	Mitral and tricuspid valve evaluation: pathology, pathophysiology
	Congenital or acquired interatrial and ventricular septal defects evaluation
	Hypertrophic obstructive cardiomyopathy evaluation
	Ventricular diastolic evaluation via transmitral and pulmonary vein Doppler flow profile analysis
	Pericardial evaluation: pericarditis; pericardial effusion
	Coronary sinus evaluation: coronary sinus catheter placement; dilation secondary to persistent left superior vena cava
View	*Mitral commissural*
Multiplane angle range	60° to 70°
Anatomy imaged	Left ventricle and atrium
	Mitral valve

10

Table continued on following page

Table 10-1 The Comprehensive Intraoperative Multiplane Transesophageal Echocardiographic Examination (Continued)

Probe Tip Depth: Midesophageal (30 to 40 cm)

Clinical utility	Left ventricular function: global and regional Left ventricular and atrial masses: thrombus, tumor, air; foreign bodies Mitral valve evaluation: pathology, pathophysiology Ventricular diastolic evaluation via transmitral Doppler flow profile analysis
View	*Two chamber*
Multiplane angle range	80° to 100°
Anatomy imaged	Left ventricle, atrium and atrial appendage Mitral valve Left pulmonary veins: turning probe to left Coronary sinus (short axis or long axis by turning probe tip to left)
Clinical utility	Left ventricular function: global and regional Left ventricular and atrial masses: thrombus, tumor, air; foreign bodies Mitral valve evaluation: pathology, pathophysiology Ventricular diastolic evaluation via transmitral and pulmonary vein Doppler flow profile analysis Coronary sinus evaluation: coronary sinus catheter placement; dilation secondary to persistent left superior vena cava
View	*Long axis*
Multiplane angle range	120° to 160°
Anatomy imaged	Left ventricle and atrium Left ventricular outflow tract Aortic valve Mitral valve Ascending aorta
Clinical utility	Left ventricular function: global and regional Left ventricular and atrial masses: thrombus, tumor, air; foreign bodies Mitral valve evaluation: pathology, pathophysiology Ventricular diastolic evaluation via transmitral Doppler flow profile analysis Aortic valve evaluation: pathology, pathophysiology Ascending aorta pathology: atherosclerosis, aneurysms, dissections Hypertrophic obstructive cardiomyopathy evaluation
View	*Right ventricular inflow-outflow ("wrap-around")*
Multiplane angle range	60° to 90°
Anatomy imaged	Right ventricle and atrium Left atrium Tricuspid valve Aortic valve Right ventricular outflow tract Pulmonic valve and main pulmonary artery
Clinical utility	Right ventricular and right and left atrial masses: thrombus, embolus, tumor, foreign bodies Pulmonic valve and subpulmonic valve: pathology; pathophysiology Pulmonary artery catheter placement Tricuspid valve: pathology; pathophysiology Aortic valve: pathology; pathophysiology

III

Probe Tip Depth: Midesophageal (30 to 40 cm)

View	*Aortic valve: short axis*
Multiplane angle range	30° to 60°
Anatomy imaged	Aortic valve
	Interatrial septum
	Coronary ostia and arteries
	Right ventricular outflow tract
	Pulmonary valve
Clinical utility	Aortic valve: pathology; pathophysiology
	Ascending aorta pathology: atherosclerosis, aneurysms and dissections
	Left and right atrial masses: thrombus, embolus, air, tumor,
	Foreign bodies
	Congenital or acquired interatrial septal defects evaluation
View	*Aortic valve: long axis*
Multiplane angle range	120° to 160°
Anatomy imaged	Aortic valve
	Proximal ascending aorta
	Left ventricular outflow tract
	Mitral valve
	Right pulmonary artery
Clinical utility	Aortic valve: pathology; pathophysiology
	Ascending aorta pathology: atherosclerosis, aneurysms and dissections
	Mitral valve evaluation: pathology, pathophysiology
View	*Bicaval*
Multiplane angle range	80° to 110°
Anatomy imaged	Right and left atrium
	Superior vena cava (long axis)
	Inferior vena cava orifice: advance probe and turn to right to visualize inferior vena cava in the long axis, liver, hepatic and portal veins
	Interatrial septum
	Right pulmonary veins: turn probe to right
	Coronary sinus and thebesian valve
	Eustachian valve
Clinical utility	Right and left atrial masses: thrombus, embolus, air, tumor, foreign bodies
	Superior vena cava pathology: thrombus, sinus venosus atrial septal defect
	Inferior vena cava pathology (thrombus, tumor)
	Femoral venous catheter placement
	Coronary sinus catheter placement
	Right pulmonary vein evaluation: anomalous return, Doppler evaluation for left ventricular diastolic function
	Congenital or acquired interatrial septal defects evaluation
	Pericardial effusion evaluation
View	*Ascending aortic: short axis*
Multiplane angle range	0° to 60°
Anatomy imaged	Ascending aorta
	Superior vena cava (short axis)
	Main pulmonary artery
	Right pulmonary artery
	Left pulmonary artery (turn probe tip to left)
	Pulmonic valve

Table continued on following page

Table 10-1   The Comprehensive Intraoperative Multiplane Transesophageal Echocardiographic Examination (Continued)

Probe Tip Depth: Midesophageal (30 to 40 cm)

Clinical utility	Ascending aorta pathology: atherosclerosis, aneurysms and dissections
	Pulmonic valve: pathology; pathophysiology
	Pulmonary embolus/thrombus evaluation
	Superior vena cava pathology: thrombus, sinus venosus atrial septal defect
	Pulmonary artery catheter placement
View	*Ascending aorta: long axis*
Multiplane angle range	100° to 150°
Anatomy imaged	Ascending aorta
	Right pulmonary artery
Clinical utility	Ascending aorta pathology: atherosclerosis, aneurysms and dissections
	Anterograde cardioplegia delivery evaluation
	Pulmonary embolus/thrombus
View	*Descending aorta: short axis*
Multiplane angle range	0°
Anatomy imaged	Descending thoracic aorta
	Left pleural space
Clinical utility	Descending aorta pathology: atherosclerosis, aneurysms and dissections
	Intra-aortic balloon placement evaluation
	Left pleural effusion
View	*Descending aorta: long axis*
Multiplane angle range	90° to 110°
Anatomy imaged	Descending thoracic aorta
	Left pleural space
Clinical utility	Descending aorta pathology: atherosclerosis, aneurysms and dissections
	Intra-aortic balloon placement evaluation
	Left pleural effusion

Probe Tip Depth: Transgastric (40 to 45 cm)

View	*Basal short axis*
Multiplane angle range	0° to 20°
Anatomy imaged	Left and right ventricle
	Mitral valve
	Tricuspid valve
Clinical utility	Mitral valve evaluation ("fish-mouth view"): pathology, pathophysiology
	Tricuspid valve evaluation: pathology, pathophysiology
	Basal left ventricular regional function
	Basal right ventricular regional function
View	*Mid short axis*
Multiplane angle range	0° to 20°
Anatomy imaged	Left and right ventricle
	Papillary muscles
Clinical utility	Mid left and right ventricular regional and global function
	Intracardiac volume status
View	*Two chamber*
Multiplane angle range	80° to 100°

III

Probe Tip Depth: Transgastric (40 to 45 cm)

Anatomy imaged	Left ventricle and atrium
	Mitral valve: chordae and papillary muscles
	Coronary sinus
Clinical utility	Left ventricular regional and global function (including apex)
	Left ventricular and atrium masses: thrombus, embolus, air, tumor, foreign bodies
	Mitral valve: pathology and pathophysiology
View	*Long axis*
Multiplane angle range	90° to 120°
Anatomy imaged	Left ventricle and outflow tract
	Aortic valve
	Mitral valve
Clinical utility	Left ventricular regional and global function
	Mitral valve: pathology and pathophysiology
	Aortic valve: pathology and pathophysiology
View	*Right ventricular inflow*
Multiplane angle range	100° to 120°
Anatomy imaged	Right ventricle and atrium
	Tricuspid valve: chordae and papillary muscles
Clinical utility	Right ventricular regional and global function
	Right ventricular and atrium masses: thrombus, embolus, tumor, foreign bodies
	Tricuspid valve: pathology and pathophysiology

Probe Tip Depth: Deep Transgastric (45 to 50 cm)

View	*Long axis*
Multiplane angle range	0° to 20° (anteflexion)
Anatomy imaged	Left ventricle and outflow tract
	Interventricular septum
	Aortic valve and ascending aorta
	Left atrium
	Mitral valve
	Right ventricle
	Pulmonic valve
Clinical utility	Aortic valve and subaortic pathology and pathophysiology
	Mitral valve pathology and pathophysiology
	Left and right ventricular global function
	Left and right ventricular masses: thrombus, embolus, tumor,
	Foreign bodies
	Congenital or acquired interventricular septal defect evaluation

10

(see Fig. 10-2D) displays the crescent-shaped, thinner-walled RV to the left of the LV (i.e., to the right side of the LV).

Mitral Valve

The echocardiographic evaluation of the MV requires a thorough assessment of its leaflets (anterior and posterior), annulus, and the subvalvular apparatus (chordae tendineae, papillary muscles, and adjacent LV walls) to locate lesions and define the etiology and severity of the pathophysiology. The mitral leaflets can be further divided into posterior leaflet scallops—lateral (P1), middle (P2), and medial (P3)—that correspond with respective anterior leaflet sections—lateral third (A1), middle third (A2), and medial third (A3). The leaflets are united at the anterolateral and

III

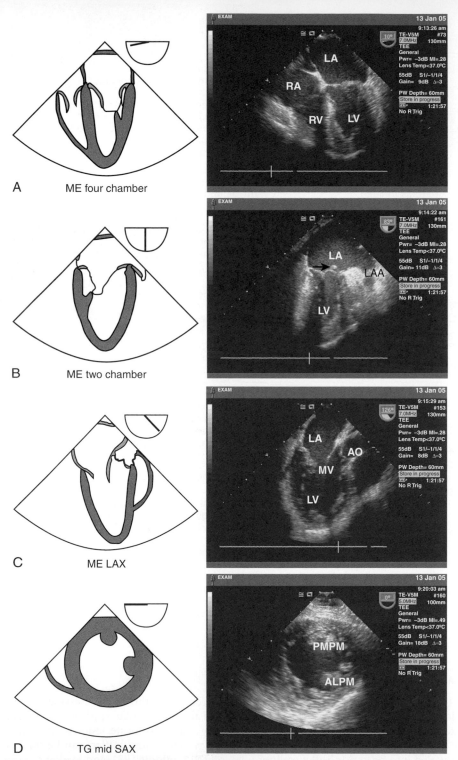

A ME four chamber

B ME two chamber

C ME LAX

D TG mid SAX

Figure 10-2 Schematic drawings and corresponding echo images of the comprehensive TEE examination. **A,** ME four-chamber view. **B,** ME two-chamber view; the *arrow* points to a prolapsing posterior mitral leaflet. **C,** ME LAX view. **D,** TG mid SAX view.

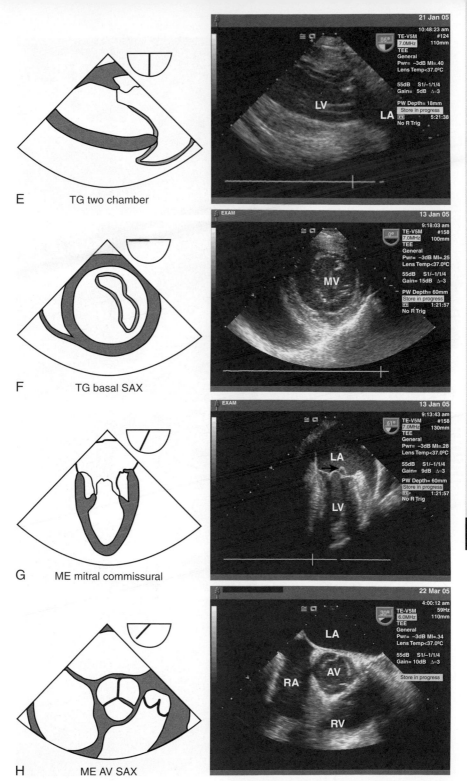

E, TG two-chamber view. **F,** TG basal SAX view. **G,** ME mitral commissural view; the *arrow* points to a prolapsing posterior mitral leaflet. **H,** ME AV SAX view. *Continued*

III

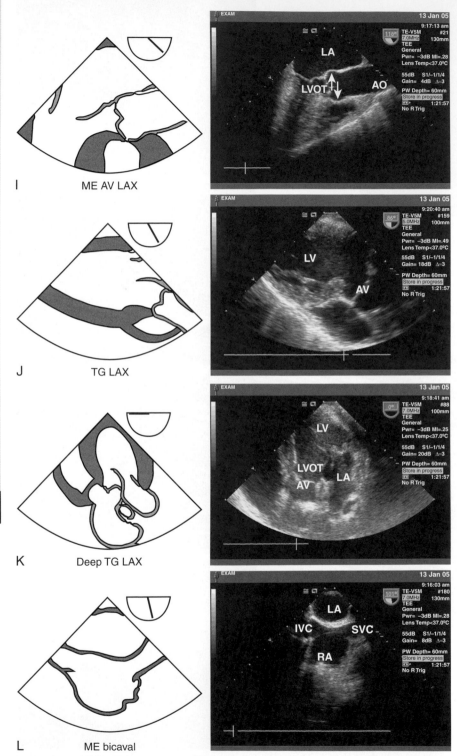

I ME AV LAX

J TG LAX

K Deep TG LAX

L ME bicaval

Fig. 10-2, cont'd I, ME AV LAX view; the *arrows* point to the aortic sinuses. **J,** TG LAX view. **K,** Deep TG LAX view. **L,** ME bicaval view.

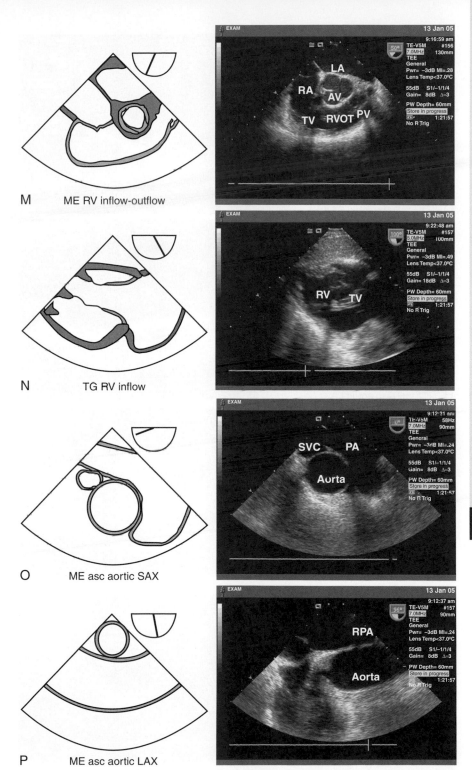

M

ME RV inflow-outflow

N

TG RV inflow

O

ME asc aortic SAX

P

ME asc aortic LAX

M, ME RV inflow-outflow view. **N,** TG RV inflow view. **O,** ME asc aortic SAX view. **P,** ME asc aortic LAX view.

Continued

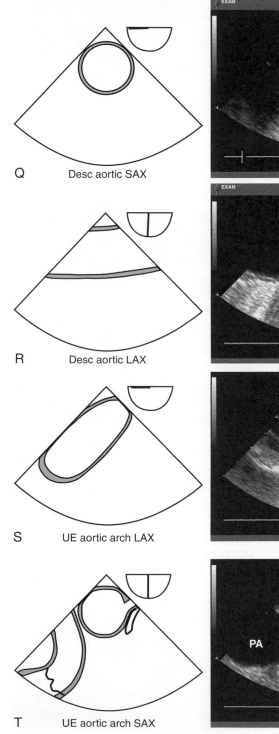

Q   Desc aortic SAX

R   Desc aortic LAX

S   UE aortic arch LAX

T   UE aortic arch SAX

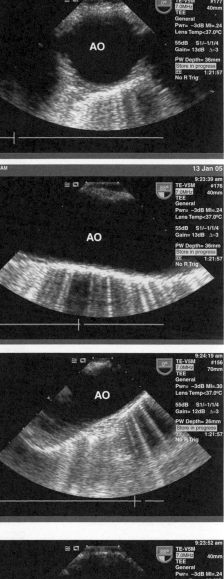

Fig. 10-2, cont'd Q, Desc aortic SAX view. **R,** Desc aortic LAX view. **S,** UE aortic arch LAX view. **T,** UE aortic arch SAX view. ME=mid-esophageal; SAX=short axis; LAX=long axis; AV=aortic valve; RV=right ventricle; TG=transgastric; UE=upper esophageal; asc=ascending aorta; desc=descending aorta; LA=left atrium; MV=mitral valve; LVOT=left ventricular outflow tract; RA=right atrium; LV=left ventricle; TV=tricuspid valve; PV=pulmonic valve; RVOT=right ventricular outflow tract; ALPM=anterior lateral papillary muscle; PMPM=posterior medial papillary muscle; IVC=inferior vena cava; SVC=superior vena cava.

posteromedial commissures. The ME four-chamber view (see Fig. 10-2A) displays the larger appearing anterior leaflet (A3) to the left of the posterior leaflet (P1). Anteflexing the probe provides imaging of the anterior aspect of the MV, while gradual advancement of the probe and retroflexion shifts the image plane to the posterior aspect of MV. Maintaining the probe at the ME depth and rotating the multiplane angle forward to 60 to 70 degrees develops the *ME mitral commissural view* (see Fig. 10-2G) in which A2 is flanked by P1 on the right and P3 on the left, giving A2 the appearance of a "trap door" as it moves in and out of the imaging plane throughout the cardiac cycle.

Aortic Valve, Aortic Root, and Left Ventricular Outflow

The three cusps of the semilunar AV are best visualized simultaneously in the *ME AV short-axis view* (see Fig. 10-2H), which is obtained by rotating the probe forward to 30 to 60 degrees. The noncoronary cusp is superior, lying adjacent to the atrial septum, the right cusp is inferiorly imaged, and the left cusp lies to the right pointing in the direction of the LA appendage (LAA). This view permits planimetry of the AV orifice, evaluation of congenital anomalies of the AV (e.g., bicuspid AV), and qualitative assessment of aortic regurgitation (AR) when color flow Doppler imaging is used. The *ME AV long-axis view* (see Fig. 10-2I) can be obtained at the same depth while rotating the probe to 120 to 160 degrees, allowing for visualization of the left ventricular outflow tract (LVOT), AV annulus and leaflets (right and either noncoronary or left), sinuses of Valsalva, sinotubular junction, and proximal ascending aorta. This view is particularly useful for evaluating AR with color flow Doppler imaging, systolic anterior motion of the MV, and proximal aortic pathology (dissections, aneurysms). Rotating the probe back to 90 to 120 degrees and advancing into the stomach to the transgastric level develops the *TG long-axis view* (see Fig. 10-2J). In this view, the LVOT and AV are oriented to the right and inferiorly in the displayed image, thereby providing an optimal window for parallel Doppler beam alignment for the assessment of flows and pressure gradients (aortic stenosis, hypertrophic obstructive cardiomyopathy). Rotating the probe back further to 0 to 20 degrees, advancing deep into the stomach and anteflexing the tip so that it lies adjacent to the LV apex allows for the development of the *deep TG long-axis view* (see Fig. 10-2K), which also provides optimal Doppler beam alignment for measuring transaortic valve and LVOT flow velocities and may also provide an additional window for assessing flows through muscular VSDs and LV apical pathology (thrombus, aneurysms).

Tricuspid Valve

The echocardiographic evaluation of the TV requires a thorough assessment of its three leaflets (anterior, posterior, and septal), annulus, chordae tendineae, papillary muscles, and corresponding RV walls. In the ME four-chamber view (see Fig. 10-2A), the septal TV leaflet is displayed on the right side and the posterior TV leaflet on the left side of the annulus. Rotating the multiplane angle to 60 to 90 degrees develops the ME RV inflow-outflow view (see Fig. 10-2M), which displays the posterior TV leaflet

10

on the left side of the image and the anterior TV leaflet on the right side of the image adjacent to the AV. The *TG RV inflow view* (see Fig. 10-2N) is obtained by advancing the probe into the stomach and rotating to 100 to 120 degrees. This view is ideal for visualizing the chordae tendineae and papillary muscles in the RV. Rotating back to the TG mid short-axis view at 0 to 20 degrees and slightly withdrawing the probe provides a cross-sectional view of the TV, displaying the anterior leaflet in the far field, the posterior leaflet to the left in the near field, and the septal leaflet on the right side of the image.

Pulmonic Valve and Pulmonary Artery

The pulmonic valve (PV) is a trileaflet, semilunar valve. The ME AV short-axis view (see Fig. 10-2H) displays the transition between the RVOT and PV. Rotating the probe back toward 0 degrees and withdrawing slightly develops the *ME ascending aortic short-axis view* (see Fig. 10-2O), displaying the transition between the RV and main PA and its bifurcation. Although the right PA is usually easy to visualize by turning the probe to the right, the left PA is often obscured by the interposing, air-filled, left main-stem bronchus. This view can be used in the Doppler echocardiographic assessment of PV pathophysiology because of the parallel alignment of the beam relative to the flow and can also be used to locate pulmonary emboli. The ME RV inflow-outflow (see Fig. 10-2M) view can also be used to assess RV, PV, and main PA.

Left Atrium, Left Atrial Appendage, Pulmonary Veins, and Atrial Septum

The LA is the closest cardiac structure to the TEE probe when positioned in the esophagus. Consequently, the LA is usually easily displayed in the superior aspect of the 2D image sector. The ME four-chamber view (see Fig. 10-2A) displays the LA almost in its entirety with the LAA oriented to its superior and lateral aspect when the probe is slightly withdrawn. The muscular ridges of the pectinate muscles within the LAA should not be confused with thrombi. Slight further withdrawal of the probe and turning it to the left allows the left upper pulmonary vein (LUPV) to be imaged as it enters the LA from the anterior to posterior direction separated from the lateral border of the LAA by the "warfarin ridge." In contrast to the LUPV, which is usually optimally aligned for parallel Doppler beam alignment, the left lower pulmonary vein (LLPV) enters the LA just below the LUPV in a lateral-to-medial direction and is more perpendicularly aligned. Pulmonary venous Doppler flow-velocity profiles are useful for the qualitative and quantitative assessment of LV diastolic function. Turning the probe to the right at this depth reveals the right upper pulmonary vein (RUPV) entering the LA in an anterior-to-posterior direction. The right lower pulmonary vein (RLPV) can sometimes be visualized as it enters perpendicular to the long axis of the LA, by slightly advancing the probe.

The interatrial septum (IAS), consisting of thicker limbus regions flanking the thin fossa ovalis, can also be imaged in the ME four-chamber view. Benign lipomatous hypertrophy of the IAS must be distinguished from pathologic lesions such as atrial myxomas. The patency of the IAS and presence of PFO or congenital atrial septal defects (ASDs) should be assessed with Doppler echocardiography and intravenous injections of agitated saline or other contrast agents. Advancing and rotating the probe to 80 to 100 degrees develop the ME two-chamber view (see Fig. 10-2B), which allows for further imaging of the LA from left to right. The LAA and LUPV can be seen by turning the probe slightly to the left. Rotating the probe to the right at this level and adjusting the multiplane angle to 80 to 110 degrees develop the *ME bicaval view* (see Fig. 10-2L), which delineates the superior vena cava (SVC) entering the RA

III

to the right of the image and the inferior vena cava (IVC) entering from the left. The IAS can be seen in the middle of the image separating the LA and RA.

Right Atrium and Coronary Sinus

The RA can be most easily visualized in the ME four-chamber view (see Fig. 10-2A) by turning the probe to the patient's right side. In this view, the entire RA can be visualized for size, overall function, and the presence of masses (thrombi, tumors). Rotating the multiplane angle to 80 to 110 degrees develops the *ME bicaval view* (see Fig. 10-2L), which displays the RA and its internal structures (eustachian valve, Chiari network, crista terminalis). The SVC can be imaged entering the RA on the right, superior to the right atrial appendage (RAA), and the IVC enters the RA on the left of the display. Advancing and turning the probe to the right allow for a qualitative evaluation of the intrahepatic segment of the IVC and hepatic veins. Pacemaker electrodes and central venous catheters for hemodynamic monitoring or cardiopulmonary bypass (CPB) can be easily imaged in this view.

The coronary sinus (CS) lies posteriorly in the atrioventricular groove, emptying into the RA at the inferior extent of the atrial septum. The CS can be viewed in long axis entering the RA just superior to the tricuspid annulus by advancing and slightly retroflexing the probe from ME four-chamber view (see Fig. 10-2A). The CS can be imaged cross-sectionally in short axis in the ME two-chamber (see Fig. 10-2B) view in the upper left of the display. Turning the probe to the left in this view often allows visualization of the CS in long axis as it traverses the atrioventricular groove. The CS and thebesian valve can also be visualized in the *ME bicaval* view (see Fig. 10-2L) on the upper right of the image as the CS enters the RA at an obtuse angle, by turning the probe to leftward simultaneously with retro- and leftward flexion. Echocardiographic visualization of the CS can be useful for directing the placement of CS catheters used for CPB with retrograde cardioplegia.

Thoracic Aorta

The proximal and mid-ascending thoracic aorta can be visualized in short axis in the *ME ascending aortic short-axis view* (see Fig. 10-2O). Advancing and withdrawing the probe should enable visualization of the thoracic aorta from the sinotubular junction to a point 4 to 6 cm superior to the AV and allow inspection for aneurysms and dissections. Rotating the multiplane angle to 100 to 150 degrees develops the *ME ascending aortic long-axis view* (see Fig. 10-2P), which optimally displays the parallel anterior and posterior walls for measuring proximal and mid-ascending aortic diameters. This view can also be obtained from the ME AV long-axis view (see Fig. 10-2I) by slightly withdrawing and turning the probe to the left.

TEE imaging of the aortic arch is often obscured by the interposing, air-filled trachea. The most optimal views of the aortic arch are obtained by withdrawing the probe from the ME ascending aortic short-axis view at 0 degrees (see Fig. 10-2O) and rotating to the left to obtain the *upper esophageal aortic arch long-axis view* (see Fig. 10-2S), which displays the proximal arch followed by the mid arch, the great vessels (brachiocephalic, left carotid and left subclavian artery), and distal arch before it joins the proximal descending thoracic aorta imaged in cross section. Alternatively, rotating the probe to 90 degrees develops the *upper esophageal aortic arch short-axis view* view (see Fig. 10-2T). Turning the probe to the left, this view delineates the transition of the distal arch with the proximal descending thoracic aorta. Turning the probe to the right and slightly withdrawing it allows for the mid arch and great vessels to be imaged on the right side of the screen, followed by the distal ascending aorta when the probe is subsequently advanced

10

and rotated forward to 120 degrees (ME ascending aortic long-axis view [see Fig. 10-2P]). Epiaortic scanning may be particularly useful for assessing the extent of ascending aortic and arch pathology (e.g., aneurysms, dissection, atherosclerosis) to determine cross-clamping and cannulation sites for CPB.

A short-axis image of the descending thoracic aorta is obtained by turning the probe leftward from the ME four-chamber view (see Fig. 10-2A) to produce the *descending aortic short-axis* view (see Fig. 10-2Q). Rotating the multiplane angle of the probe from 0 degrees to 90 to 110 degrees produces a long-axis image, the *descending aortic long-axis* view (see Fig. 10-2R). The descending thoracic aorta should be interrogated in its entirety, beginning at the distal aortic arch by continually advancing the probe and turning slightly to the left until the celiac and superior mesenteric arteries are visualized branching tangentially from the anterior surface of the abdominal aorta when the probe is in the stomach. Thorough examination of the descending thoracic aorta may be necessary to evaluate the distal extent of an aneurysm or dissection. In addition, the descending aortic short- and long-axis views can be useful for confirming appropriate intra-aortic balloon positioning.

CLINICAL APPLICATIONS

Ventricular Function

Cardiovascular function, such as the global indices of muscle contraction or regional indices described by segmental wall motion, is assessed by analyzing moving echocardiographic images. Assessment of global and regional ventricular function has become the cornerstone for evaluating patients with ischemic heart disease (IHD). The dynamic assessment of ventricular function with echocardiography is based on derived indices of muscle contraction and relaxation. Echocardiographic indices of LV function that incorporate endocardial border outlines and Doppler techniques can be used to estimate CO, stroke volume (SV), ejection fraction (EF), and parameters of ventricular relaxation and filling.

Global LV performance is directly related to preload, contractility, and afterload. Cardiac output reflects systolic function and is an important factor in oxygen delivery. Alteration in LV diastolic function may result from systolic dysfunction or, in as many as 40% of patients, may be the primary and main etiology of cardiac failure.

Visual Estimation of Function

In routine clinical work, the anesthesiologist-echocardiographer must make visual estimates of ventricular wall motion and overall function. These depend on the ability of the individual to interpret the images and correctly "quantify" subjective assessments of ventricular function. The clinician may be aided by video recordings of prior function or video images stored on split screens. These estimations of global ventricular function are usually performed in the short-axis view of the LV, but additional information can also be gained by assessing the long-axis views of the LV. In this assessment, the observer examines the end-diastolic image and compares it with the end-systolic frame to determine the degree of ejection. The rate of ejection is also estimated.

Regional wall motion abnormalities (RWMAs) may be identified on visual inspection of echocardiographic images by anesthesiologists. Several studies have documented that an educated visual analysis of echocardiographic images provides a better estimation of LVEF than more sophisticated and time-consuming computer techniques.

III

Preload/Diastolic Function

End-Diastolic Dimensions

Whereas in conventional hemodynamics preload is often estimated by measuring left-sided heart filling pressures (pulmonary capillary wedge pressure [PCWP], left atrial pressure [LAP], or LV end-diastolic pressure [LVEDP]), in echocardiography it can be determined by measuring LV end-diastolic dimensions. End-diastolic dimensions provide a better index of preload than the PCWP. When PCWP and end-diastolic volume (EDV), derived from short-axis areas at the level of the papillary muscles, were compared as predictors of cardiac index (CI) in patients undergoing coronary artery bypass grafting (CABG), a strong correlation was observed between end-diastolic area (EDA), or EDV, and CI, whereas no significant correlation was found between PCWP and CI.

TEE is often, for practical reasons, limited to a single short-axis view at the level of the papillary muscles. Some evidence suggests that short-axis EDAs measured at this level correlate reasonably well with measurements obtained by on-heart echocardiography and with EDVs measured simultaneously using radionuclides. There are two main echocardiographic signs of decreased preload: (1) decrease in EDA ($<5.5 \text{ cm}^2/\text{m}^2$) invariably reflects hypovolemia; and (2) obliteration of the end-systolic area (ESA) ("the kissing ventricle sign") accompanies the decrease in EDA in severe hypovolemia.

Myocardial Ischemia Monitoring

Regional Wall Motion and Systolic Wall Thickness

The relationship of echocardiographic indices of regional myocardial function to ischemia has been compared with changes that occur with the surface ECG, PCWP, and the onset of chest pain. As early as 1935 it was recognized that acute myocardial ischemia results in abnormal inward motion and thickening of the affected myocardial region. Since then, RWMAs have been shown to occur within seconds of inadequate blood flow or oxygen supply. These abnormal contraction patterns typically occur at the same time as regional lactate production.

Diagnosis of Ischemia

The precise sequence of functional changes that occur in the myocardium after interruption of flow has been studied in models of acute ischemia, including percutaneous transluminal coronary angioplasty (PTCA). Abnormalities in diastolic function usually precede abnormal changes in systolic function. Normal function is critical for LV filling and is dependent on ventricular relaxation, compliance, and atrial contraction. Diastolic ventricular function can be assessed by monitoring the rate of filling associated with changes in the chamber dimensions. Regional systolic function can be estimated by echocardiographic determination of wall thickening and wall motion during systole in both long- and short-axis views of the ventricle. The short-axis view of the LV at the papillary muscle level displays myocardium perfused by the three main coronary arteries and is, therefore, very useful. However, because the short-axis view does not image the ventricular apex and this is a very common location of ischemia, the long-axis and longitudinal ventricle views are also clinically important.[3]

As the myocardial oxygen supply/demand balance worsens, graded RWMAs progress from mild hypokinesia to severe hypokinesia, akinesia, and finally dyskinesia. *Normal contraction* is defined as greater than 30% thickening of the ventricular wall. *Mild hypokinesia* refers to inward contraction that is slower and less vigorous than normal during systole, with ventricular wall thickening of 10% to 30%.

10

BOX 10-4 *Limitations of Transesophageal Echocardiography*

Incompatibility: induction, laryngoscopy, intubation, emergence, extubation
Artifact interference: electronic, septum, bundle-branch block
Lack of specificity: tethering effect, scar, afterload changes, stunned myocardium

Severe hypokinesia is defined as less than 10% wall thickening. The precise distinction between varying degrees of hypokinesia can be difficult. *Akinesia* refers to the absence of wall motion or no inward movement of the endocardium during systole. *Dyskinesia* refers to paradoxical wall motion or movement outward during ventricular systole.

Limitations

Although TEE appears to have many advantages over traditional intraoperative monitors of myocardial ischemia, there remain potential limitations as well (Box 10-4). The most obvious limitation of TEE monitoring is the fact that ischemia cannot be detected during critical periods, such as induction, laryngoscopy, intubation, emergence, and extubation. In addition, the adequacy of RWMA analysis may be influenced by artifact.

The septum in particular must be given special consideration with respect to wall motion and wall thickness assessment. The septum is composed of two parts: the lower muscular portion and the basal membranous portion. The basal septum does not exhibit the same degree of contraction as the lower muscular part. At the most superior basal portion, the septum is attached to the aortic outflow track. Its movement at this level is normally paradoxical during ventricular systole. The septum is also a unique region of the LV, because it is a region of the RV as well and is therefore influenced by forces from both ventricles. In addition, sternotomy, pericardiotomy, and CPB have been found to alter the translational and rotational motion of the heart within the chest, which may cause changes in ventricular septal motion.

Another potential problem of RWMA assessment is evaluation of the dyssynchronous contraction that occurs as a result of a bundle-branch block or ventricular pacing. In these situations, the system used to assess RWMAs must compensate for global motion of the heart and evaluate not only regional endocardial wall motion but also myocardial thickening.

Not all RWMAs are indicative of myocardial ischemia or infarction. Clearly, under normal conditions, all hearts do not contract in a homogeneous and consistent manner. It is reasonable to assume, however, that most of the time an acute change in the regional contraction pattern of the heart during surgery is likely attributable to myocardial ischemia. An important exception to this rule may apply in models of acute coronary artery occlusion. In these models, it has been established that myocardial function becomes abnormal in the center of an ischemic zone, but it is also true that the myocardial regions adjacent to the ischemic zones become dysfunctional as well. Several studies have reported that the total area of dysfunctional myocardium commonly exceeds the area of ischemic or infarcted myocardium. The impairment of function in nonischemic tissue has been thought to be caused by a "tethering effect." Tethering, or the attachment of noncontracting tissue that is normally perfused, probably accounts for the consistent overestimation of infarct size by echocardiography when compared with postmortem studies.

Another limitation of RWMA analysis during surgery is that it does not differentiate stunned or hibernating myocardium from acute ischemia, nor does it differentiate the cause of ischemia between increased oxygen demand and decreased oxygen supply. Finally, it should be noted that areas of previous ischemia or scarring may become unmasked by changes in afterload and appear as new RWMAs. This is particularly important in vascular surgery, in which major abrupt changes in afterload occur.

Outcome Significance

Data regarding the significance of intraoperative detection of RWMAs suggest that transient abnormalities unaccompanied by hemodynamic or ECG evidence of ischemia may not represent significant myocardial ischemia and are usually not associated with postoperative morbidity. Hypokinetic myocardial segments appear to be associated with minimal perfusion defects compared with the significant perfusion defects that accompany akinetic or dyskinetic segments. Hence, hypokinesia may be a less predictive marker for postoperative morbidity.[4]

Intraoperative TEE has helped predict the results of CABG. Following CABG of previously dysfunctional segments, immediate improvement of regional myocardial function (which is sustained) has been demonstrated. In addition, prebypass compensatory hypercontracting segments have been reported to revert toward normal immediately after successful CABG. Persistent RWMAs after CABG appear to be related to adverse clinical outcomes, and lack of evidence of RWMAs after CABG has been shown to be associated with a postoperative course without cardiac morbidity.

A formalized approach to the acquisition of data and decision-making (Fig. 10-3) enhances the quality of the intraoperative echocardiogram, its interpretation, and the confidence with which the findings are communicated to other members of the operative and nonoperative teams. The broad database that is required to formulate an intelligent decision includes provider- and patient-specific data. Patient-specific data include history and demographics, preoperative diagnostic examinations, admitting diagnosis and comorbidities, the patient's wishes, recommendations of referring physicians, and intraoperative data. Intraoperative data include hemodynamic data, visual inspection, surgical input, and the TEE examination. A systematic TEE examination of the heart and great vessels permits the acquisition and interpretation of qualitative and quantitative echocardiographic data applied to intraoperative decision-making. The provider-specific data are composed of an accumulated database of knowledge acquired from training, experience, and continuous medical education.

10

INTRAOPERATIVE TRANSESOPHAGEAL ECHOCARDIOGRAPHY: INDICATIONS

The first decision by the echocardiographer is whether TEE is indicated. Application of intraoperative TEE in the care of the patient with mitral disease is widely accepted. Even in this area, however, there is a paucity of data supporting an improved outcome for intraoperative patients cared for with TEE compared with no TEE. The decision to perform TEE during cardiac surgery is substantiated by practice expectations and consensus opinion.[5] In an attempt to develop an evidence-based approach to this expanding technology, the American Society of Anesthesiologists (ASA) and the Society of Cardiovascular Anesthesiologists (SCA) co-sponsored a task force to develop guidelines for defining the indications for perioperative TEE.[2,6] Despite the scarcity of outcome data to support the application of TEE in the perioperative period, TEE had rapidly been adopted by cardiac surgeons and cardiac anesthesiologists as a routine monitoring

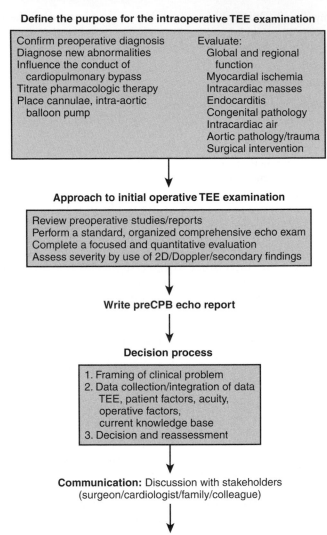

Define the purpose for the intraoperative TEE examination

Confirm preoperative diagnosis
Diagnose new abnormalities
Influence the conduct of
   cardiopulmonary bypass
Titrate pharmacologic therapy
Place cannulae, intra-aortic
   balloon pump

Evaluate:
   Global and regional
     function
   Myocardial ischemia
   Intracardiac masses
   Endocarditis
   Congenital pathology
   Intracardiac air
   Aortic pathology/trauma
   Surgical intervention

Approach to initial operative TEE examination

Review preoperative studies/reports
Perform a standard, organized comprehensive echo exam
Complete a focused and quantitative evaluation
Assess severity by use of 2D/Doppler/secondary findings

Write preCPB echo report

Decision process

1. Framing of clinical problem
2. Data collection/integration of data
   TEE, patient factors, acuity,
   operative factors,
   current knowledge base
3. Decision and reassessment

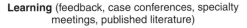

Communication: Discussion with stakeholders
(surgeon/cardiologist/family/colleague)

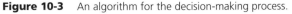

Learning (feedback, case conferences, specialty
meetings, published literature)

Figure 10-3   An algorithm for the decision-making process.

and diagnostic modality during cardiac surgery. In 1996, the task force published their guidelines designed to establish the scientific merit of TEE and justification of its use in defined patient cohorts. The indications were grouped into three categories based on the strength of the supporting evidence/expert opinion that TEE improves outcome (Box 10-5). Category I indications suggested strong evidence/expert opinion that TEE was useful in improving clinical outcome. Category II indications suggested there was weak evidence/expert opinion that TEE improves outcome in these settings. Category III indications suggested there was little or no scientific merit or expert support for the application of TEE in these settings.

BOX 10-5 Indications for the Use of Transesophageal Echocardiography

Category I

- Heart valve repair
- Congenital heart surgery
- Hypertrophic obstructive cardiomyopathy
- Endocarditis
- Acute aortic dissection
- Acute, unstable aortic aneurysm
- Aortic valve function in the setting of aortic dissection
- Traumatic thoracic aortic disruption
- Pericardial tamponade

Category II

- Myocardial ischemia and coronary artery disease
- Increased risk of hemodynamic disturbances
- Heart valve replacement
- Aneurysms of the heart
- Intracardiac masses
- Intracardiac foreign bodies
- Air emboli
- Intracardiac thrombi
- Massive pulmonary emboli
- Traumatic cardiac injury
- Chronic aortic dissection
- Chronic aortic aneurysm
- Detection of aortic atheromatous disease as a source of emboli
- Evaluating the effectiveness of pericardiectomies
- Heart-lung transplantation
- Mechanical circulatory support

Category III

- Other cardiomyopathy
- Emboli during orthopedic procedures
- Uncomplicated pericarditis
- Pleuropulmonary disease
- Placement of intra-aortic balloon pump, pulmonary artery catheter
- Monitoring the administration of cardioplegia

Modified from published guidelines of the American Society of Anesthesiologists and the Society of Cardiovascular Anesthesiologists.

10

CASE STUDIES OF INTRAOPERATIVE TEE

Case Study 1   CARDIAC FUNCTION AND REGIONAL WALL MOTION ABNORMALITIES

FRAMING

Ventricular function is a predictor of outcome after heart surgery and a predictor of long-term outcome in patients with cardiovascular disease. Patients with compensated congestive heart failure may have severely decreased EF with minimal

Continued on following page

symptoms. Regional ventricular dysfunction is most commonly caused by myocardial ischemia or infarction. Hence, there is an imperative to detect ventricular dysfunction and institute treatment in an attempt to prevent acute or long-term consequences.

Is ventricular function normal or abnormal? Is the abnormal function global or regional? What is the coronary distribution that relates to an RWMA? Is the ventricle big or small? Is the myocardium thinned or hypertrophied? Is the abnormal function new or old? Does the medical or surgical intervention improve or deteriorate ventricular function?

DATA COLLECTION

LV systolic function is assessed echocardiographically based on regional and global wall motion. Methods of assessment include changes in regional wall thickness, radial shortening with endocardial excursion, fractional area change (FAC), and systolic displacement of the mitral annulus. Off-line measurements of EF can be calculated using Simpson's rule. FAC is the most common metric used to assess global LV function. Other measures include end-diastolic area (EDA), end-systolic area (ESA), and meridional wall stress.

Regional assessment provides an index of myocardial well-being that can be linked to coronary anatomy and blood flow. Although the measurement of coronary blood flow is not achieved by TEE, the perfusion beds and corresponding myocardium for the left anterior descending (LAD), left circumflex (LCX), and right coronary (RCA) arteries are relatively distinct and can be scrutinized by TEE using multiplane imaging. The transgastric and long-axis imaging views of the LV are the most widely used for evaluating wall motion abnormalities. Digital archival systems have gained popularity for their ability to capture a single cardiac cycle that can then be examined more closely as a continuous cine loop. Cine loops can also permit side-by-side display of images obtained under varying conditions (e.g., prebypass and postbypass). Regional myocardial ischemia produces focal changes in the corresponding ventricular walls before changes occur on the ECG. Changes progress from normal wall motion to hypokinesis or akinesis. Dyskinesis, thinning, and calcification of the myocardium suggest a nonacute process, likely a prior infarction.

DISCUSSION

Preexisting ventricular dysfunction suggests increased risk for surgery and poorer long-term outcome. The presence of such ventricular dysfunction may deteriorate intraoperatively, requiring the need for marked pharmacologic or mechanical support. A patient with a preoperative EF of 10% scheduled for coronary artery bypass grafting (CABG) and MV repair is at increased risk of intraoperative ischemia, acute heart failure, and difficulty maintaining hemodynamic stability during the immediate postbypass period. Anticipating such problems, placement of an intra-aortic balloon pump or femoral arterial catheter is considered during the prebypass period (Fig. 10-4). The same patient is likely to benefit from the administration of inotropic agents.

A marked decrement or unexpected decrease in global cardiac function after release of the aortic cross-clamp can be caused by poor myocardial preservation during cross-clamping or distention of the heart during bypass. The risk of such incidents can be reduced by the monitoring of the electrical activity of the heart and pulmonary artery pressures and for distention of the RV and LV. Effective venting of the heart is often difficult to discern by visual inspection alone, especially with the use of minimally invasive surgery through small incisions. TEE imaging can diagnose ventricular distention produced by AV insufficiency.

Not all preexisting regional wall motion abnormalities benefit from coronary revascularization. Regions of akinesia and dyskinesia are usually the result of a myocardial infarction and may reflect nonviable myocardium, although "hibernating" myocardium is possible. Hypokinetic segments are generally viable and may represent active ischemia. Preoperative positron emission tomography (PET) scanning can detect hibernating myocardium and may be cost-effective to guide CABG.[7] The detection of hibernating myocardium in an area of chronic ischemia and regional hypokinesis will direct the surgeon to revascularize the corresponding stenosed coronary artery. In contrast, an occluded coronary artery with downstream infarction may not benefit from revascularization, as contractile function may be irreversibly lost. However, in this latter scenario, revascularization postinfarction may provide some benefit in decreasing the risk of ventricular aneurysm formation.

III

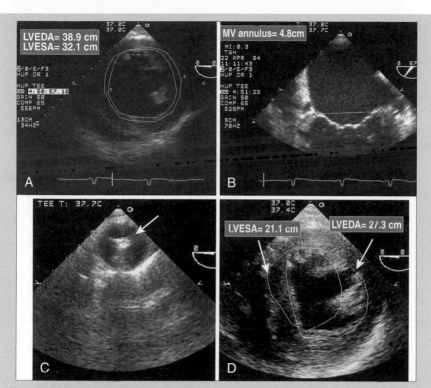

Figure 10-4 The prebypass transesophageal echocardiography (TEE) examination may have predictive value for postbypass circulatory management. A 63-year-old woman with a past medical history of hypertension, congestive heart failure, pulmonary edema, dilated cardiomyopathy, diabetes, and obesity was scheduled for coronary artery bypass grafting (CABG) and mitral valve (MV) repair. The preoperative evaluation documented moderate to severe mitral regurgitation (MR) with reversal of systolic pulmonary vein blood flow velocity. The prebypass TEE mid-esophageal four-chamber view showed a markedly dilated left ventricle (LV) and mildly dilated right ventricle (RV) with mildly decreased global dysfunction. **A)** The transgastric view was characterized by severe global dysfunction and a LV end-diastolic diameter of 6.6 cm. The fractional area change (FAC) was 17% [FAC = (LV end-diastolic area − LV end-systolic area)/LV end-diastolic area × 100]. Revascularization alone was unlikely to significantly improve MV function. **B)** The mid-esophageal bicommissural view of the MV demonstrated marked dilation of the MV annulus (major axis = 4.8 cm) and tethering of the leaflets below the valve plane that was caused by LV chamber dilation. A femoral arterial catheter was inserted for monitoring of central aortic pressure and/or possibly placing an intra-aortic balloon pump. The patient underwent a CABG × 3 and MV annuloplasty for moderate MR. The separation from bypass was difficult, requiring milrinone, epinephrine, vasopressin, and placement of an intra-aortic balloon pump. **C)** TEE, which was used to initially confirm the location of the femoral guidewire, was later used to position the balloon pump just downstream to the left subclavian artery. **D)** Worsening of RV function that was characterized by increased central venous pressure, new-onset tricuspid regurgitation, and a hypokinetic RV can be appreciated by ventricular septal flattening and dilation of the RV. The LV ejection fraction did not decrease as might be expected; after correcting MR, the FAC improved slightly from 17% to 22% post-bypass. Cardiac function continued to improve, and the counterpulsation device was removed without complication on the first day after surgery. The infusions of milrinone and epinephrine were continued for several days.

10

If the intraoperative examination reveals new ventricular dysfunction, the intraoperative team must determine the etiology and severity and plan a treatment. Other causes of RWMAs such as conduction abnormalities (left bundle-branch block or ventricular pacing) can be difficult to distinguish. Treatment of myocardial ischemia may include optimizing hemodynamics; administering anticoagulants, nitrates, calcium channel blockers, or β-blockers; inserting an intra-aortic balloon pump; or instituting CPB and coronary revascularization. The presence of a new-onset RWMA after separation from bypass is worrisome for myocardial ischemia. Even the patient without coronary artery disease remains at risk because of hypotension, shower of air or debris into the coronary circulation, or coronary spasm. The patient with coronary artery disease undergoing coronary revascularization may have all the above risks, technical difficulties at the anastomotic site, injury to the native coronary (e.g., stitch caught the back wall), or occlusion of the coronary graft by thrombosis or aortic dissection. The coronary arteries, grafts, and anastomoses should be carefully inspected for patency and flow. Graft patency in the operating room is difficult to determine. Techniques include manual stripping and refill, measuring coronary flow by hand-held Doppler, or administration of echocardiographic contrast agents. A new RWMA in the distribution of a new coronary graft can prompt the decision-making strategies listed in Table 10-2.

Table 10-2 Management Strategies for New-Onset Myocardial Ischemia Post Bypass

Diagnosis	Plausible Treatment
Coronary graft occlusion	Revise coronary graft
Coronary air emboli	Increase coronary perfusion pressure, administer coronary dilators
Coronary calcium/atheroma emboli	Support circulation
Dissection of the aortic root	Repair dissection
Coronary spasm	Administer coronary dilators

Case Study 2   MANAGEMENT OF ISCHEMIC MITRAL REGURGITATION

FRAMING

Ischemic heart disease is the most common cause of mitral insufficiency in the United States. Mechanisms of valve incompetence are varied and include annular dilatation, papillary muscle dysfunction from active ischemia or infarction, papillary muscle rupture, or ventricular remodeling from scar, often leading to a tethering effect of the subvalvular apparatus. Mitral regurgitation leads to pulmonary hypertension, pulmonary vascular congestion, and pulmonary edema with functional disability. Ventricular function deteriorates as the LV becomes volume overloaded with corresponding chamber dilatation. Left untreated, severe MR from ischemic heart disease has a poor prognosis, hence the imperative for diagnosis and treatment.[8] Patients presenting for surgical coronary revascularization often have concomitant MR of a mild or moderate degree. The intraoperative team is confronted with the decision of whether to surgically address the MV during the coronary operation.

Does MR warrant mitral surgery? What is the mechanism of the regurgitation? What is the grade of the MR? Is the MR likely to improve by coronary revascularization alone?

DATA COLLECTION

Pertinent data, including preoperative functional status and evaluation, need to be considered to appropriately interpret and place the intraoperative data in context. The preoperative echocardiogram and ventriculogram need to be reviewed. The intraoperative hemodynamic data are coupled with TEE information to complete the dataset needed to move forward with the decision-making process. The severity of MR on TEE is measured by the vena contracta, maximum area of the regurgitant jet, regurgitant orifice area, and pulmonary vein blood flow velocities. Wall motion assessment and the ECG are used for detecting reversible myocardial dysfunction that may benefit from revascularization. The hemodynamic and TEE data are coupled with provocative testing of the MV in an attempt to emulate the working conditions of the MV in an awake, unanesthetized state. It is not uncommon that preoperative mild to moderate MR with a structurally normal valve totally resolves under the unloading conditions of general anesthesia.[9]

DISCUSSION

Most cases of ischemic MR are categorized as "functional" rather than structural. In a study of 482 patients with ischemic MR, 76% had functional ischemic MR, compared with 24% having significant papillary muscle dysfunction. The mechanism of ischemic MR is attributed to annular dilatation, secondary to LV enlargement and regional LV remodeling with papillary muscle displacement, causing apical tethering and restricted systolic leaflet motion. The importance of local LV remodeling with papillary muscle displacement as a mechanism for ischemic MR has been reproduced in an animal model.

The MR is prioritized in accordance with principal diagnosis (e.g., coronary artery disease), comorbidities, functional disability, and short- and long-term outcome. Ischemic MR is quantitated and the mechanism of valve dysfunction is defined. Intraoperative MR is compared with preoperative findings. Discrepancies between the preoperative and intraoperative assessment of the valve may reflect the pressure and volume unloading effects of general anesthesia. In patients with functional ischemic MR who have 1 to 2+ MR, the MV is often not repaired or replaced. However, the need for surgical intervention in patients with 2+ MR under anesthesia remains a point of debate and has not been definitively answered by prospective studies. MV surgery is typically recommended to improve functional status and long-term outcome for patients with 3+ ischemic MR or greater. Ignoring significant ischemic MR at the time of CABG can limit the functional benefit derived from surgery.

The risks to the patient of not surgically altering the MV and anticipated residual regurgitation is weighed against the risk of atriotomy, mitral surgery, extending cardiopulmonary and aortic cross-clamp times, and the likelihood that the coronary surgery will be successful at decreasing the severity of MR. Added risk includes commitment to a mechanical prosthesis should a reparative procedure prove unsuccessful. MR due to acute ischemia may resolve after restoration of coronary blood flow (Fig. 10-5). The reversibility of the regurgitation is difficult to predict: factors supporting reversibility (and hence no immediate need to surgically address the valve) include a structurally normal MV, normal LA and LV dimension, including the mitral annulus, and RWMAs associated with transient regurgitation and pulmonary edema. Revascularization of the culprit myocardium with improvement in regional function may be all that is necessary to restore normal mitral coaptation.[10] Myocardial infarction with a fixed wall motion defect or aneurysm, chronically dilated left-sided heart, dilated annulus, or other structural abnormalities that are not reversible (ruptured papillary muscle or chordae, leaflet prolapse, leaflet perforation) suggest myocardial revascularization is unlikely to correct the valvular incompetence.

The decision to proceed or not to proceed with mitral surgery in the setting of ischemic heart disease is institution and surgeon dependent. Centers may elect to surgically address any degree of MR detected during the preoperative or intraoperative workup of a patient scheduled for coronary surgery. Less aggressive sites elect to proceed with coronary revascularization, followed by repeat scrutiny of the ventricular wall motion and MV. If revascularization has not corrected the MR, the surgeon proceeds with CPB and mitral surgery. With the advent of off-pump coronary artery bypass surgery, this process has gained another level of complexity, because decisions to proceed with mitral repair will commit the patient to CPB. Off-pump mitral surgical procedures may be possible in the near future.

Continued on following page

10

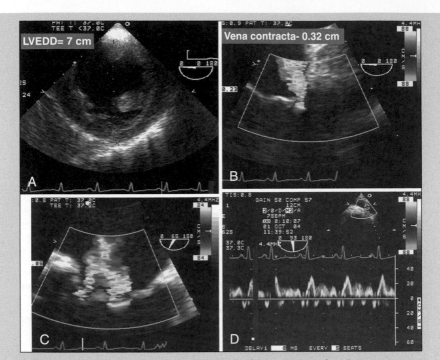

Figure 10-5 Evaluation of mitral regurgitation (MR) in a patient undergoing coronary artery bypass grafting. A 63-year-old man was scheduled to undergo off-pump coronary artery revascularization. The patient had a history of progressive congestive heart failure without evidence of acute pulmonary edema. The physical examination was significant for diffuse laterally displaced point of maximum impulse (PMI) and a systolic murmur at the apex that radiated to the axilla. The patient received an intraoperative transesophageal echocardiography (TEE) examination to evaluate the severity of MR. **A)** The left ventricle (LV) was significantly dilated with an LV end-diastolic dimension of 7 cm and had depressed systolic function with an estimated ejection fraction of 40%. The MR was characterized by color-flow Doppler imaging to be a central jet of mild to moderate severity. **B)** The grading of MR was based on the area of the regurgitant jet and the vena contracta viewed in a bicommissural view. The pathogenesis of MR was believed to be functional and resulted from restricted leaflet mobility caused by the dilated LV. **C)** The coaptation of the anterior and posterior leaflets was below the valve plane. **D)** The absence of reversal of pulmonary vein blood flow measured in the left lower pulmonary vein supported the assessment of moderate MR. Because the annulus was not significantly dilated (the minor axis measured 2.97 cm) and the MR graded as only mild to moderate, the surgeon proceeded with his initial plan of off-pump coronary artery bypass grafting. The MR decreased immediately after revascularization, and the patient's symptoms were expected to further improve with afterload reduction.

Case Study 3	**MANAGEMENT OF PREVIOUSLY UNDIAGNOSED AORTIC VALVE DISEASE**

FRAMING

A relatively common clinical scenario for the echocardiographer is to assess the significance of previously unrecognized AV pathology. This discussion has pertinence for the echocardiographer faced with the new diagnosis of a bicuspid valve, AS, or insufficiency.

What are the symptoms that brought the patient to medical attention? What is the patient's baseline function? What is the anatomy of the AV? What is the severity of AR or of AS? How do the intraoperative findings of AV disease differ from the preoperative assessment? Would surgical repair or replacement of the AV benefit the patient's short- or long-term outcome? What is the planned procedure, and how would the risks be changed if the procedure was altered to address the new finding? Does another health care provider need to be involved in the decision of whether to surgically address the valve? Is the pathology of the AV significant enough to require surgical intervention at this time?

DATA COLLECTION AND CHARACTERIZATION OF THE AORTIC VALVE

Multiplane TEE permits an accurate assessment of AV area, valvular pathology, severity of regurgitation and stenosis, and detection of secondary cardiac changes. In the case of AS, the severity of valvular dysfunction is determined by measuring the transvalvular pressure gradient, by calculating the AV area using the continuity equation, and by planimetry of the AV systolic orifice. Planimetry of the AV orifice with TEE is more closely correlated with the catheterization-determined valve area (using the Gorlin formula) than the value derived from TTE ($r=0.91$ vs. 0.84). The severity of AR by TEE is generally graded with color flow Doppler imaging with measurement of the width of the regurgitant jet relative to the width of the LV outflow tract. TEE is sensitive to even the most trivial amount of AR. Jet areas measured by TEE tend to be larger, and their severity is graded as greater compared with AR assessed by TTE. Determining the clinical significance of AR typically requires assessment of more than just regurgitant grade, although severe 4+ AR is never left unaddressed.

The etiology and extent of AV disease can be best delineated by TEE, as shown in Figure 10-6. The relatively high resolution of the AV and associated structures in the near field of the midesophageal short- and long-axis views permits an accurate assessment of the severity and mechanism of valvular disease. The aortic leaflets should be inspected in the midesophageal long-axis view for the presence of vegetations, perforation, restriction, thickening/calcification, malcoaptation, and leaflet prolapse. The presence of subvalvular disease, such as a discrete fibrous subaortic membrane, can also be reliably excluded. The ascending aorta from the valve to the right pulmonary artery also should be viewed in long axis. This view is usually optimal for examining associated pathology of the aortic root and ascending aorta (e.g., aortoannular ectasia, bicuspid valve, type A aortic dissection).

AS is caused by calcification of the AV and rheumatic heart disease. Bicuspid AVs are at greater risk compared with the general population. AS produces a systolic pressure gradient between the LV and aorta. Secondary findings are dependent on where the patient's condition is along the natural course of the disease. Secondary findings often contribute to the decision-making process, because they infer the

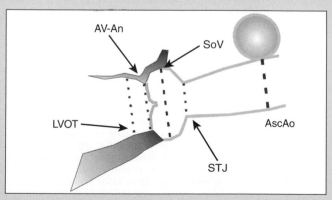

Figure 10-6 Anatomy of the aortic root. This schematic figure of the aortic valve in long axis shows the components of the aortic root, which include sinotubular junction (STJ), sinus of Valsalva (SoV), and the annulus of the aortic valve (AV-An). LVOT = left ventricular outflow tract; AscAo = ascending aorta.

Continued on following page

effects or consequences of the disease. AS is commonly associated with LV hypertrophy and abnormal filling of the LV. The diastolic function is often impaired owing to a thickened, noncompliant LV. Hence, MV and pulmonary vein blood flow velocities would demonstrate a blunted passive filling phase of the ventricle. Systolic function is often normal or hyperdynamic. The LV chamber size is normal or small. However, longstanding AS results in progressive ventricular systolic dysfunction and heart failure. The LV becomes dilated with compromised contractile function. As the ventricle fails, CO decreases with a resultant decrease in trans-AV pressure gradient. Hence, the pressure gradient across an AV may be misleading as a measure for severity of AS.

NATURAL COURSE OF AORTIC STENOSIS

The natural course of AS in the adult begins with a prolonged asymptomatic period associated with minimal mortality. Progression of the disease is manifested by a reduction in the valve area and an increase in the transvalvular systolic pressure gradient. The progression is quite variable, exhibiting a decrease in effective valve area ranging from 0.1 to 0.3 cm^2/yr. AV calcification, as depicted by echocardiography, has been suggested to be an independent predictor of outcome. Patients with no or mild valvular calcification, compared with those with moderate or severe calcification, had significantly increased rates of event-free survival at 1 and 4 years (92% vs. 60% and 75% vs. 20%, respectively). Decisions regarding valve replacement for mild or moderate AV disease in the setting of cardiac surgery for another cause are complicated by the variability in the natural progression of the disease. The pathogenesis of AS is an active process having many similarities to the progression of atherosclerosis. AV calcification is not a random degenerative process but an actively regulated disease associated with hypercholesterolemia, inflammation, and osteoblast activity. More aggressive medical control of these processes might be expected to have a positive impact on outcome by retarding the degenerative process.

ASSESSMENT OF MILD AND MODERATE AORTIC STENOSIS

The intraoperative management of mild to moderate AS at the time of cardiac surgery remains controversial. A patient arrives in the operating room scheduled for a CABG but is discovered to also have mild or moderate AS that was unappreciated preoperatively. The operative team must decide whether to surgically address the AV. The ACC/AHA task force recommends valve replacement at the time of coronary surgery if the asymptomatic patient has severe AS but acknowledges there are very limited data to support intervention in the case of mild or moderate AS. It is in this exact scenario that the rate of progression of AS is of value but it is rarely obtainable. A rapidly calcifying valve in a young patient that is becoming rapidly stenotic would sway the operative team to perform an aortic valve replacement (AVR). A combined double cardiac procedure (CABG/AVR) increases the initial perioperative risk, as well as those risks associated with long-term prosthetic valve implantation. A delay in AVR and commitment to a second heart operation in the future subjects the patient to the risk of a repeated sternotomy in the setting of patent coronary grafts and its associated morbidities. If the AV is not operated on during the initial presentation for CABG, the development of symptomatic AS may be quite delayed or may not happen.

A review of 1,344,100 patients in the national database of the Society of Thoracic Surgeons having CABG, CABG/AVR, or AVR alone culminated in a decision paradigm recommendation. The study assumed rates of AV disease progression (pressure gradient of 5 mm Hg/yr), valve-related morbidity, and age-adjusted mortality rates that were obtained from published reports.[11] The authors proposed three factors in the consideration of CABG or AVR/CABG: age (life expectancy), peak pressure gradient, and rate of progression of the AS (if known). Since the latter is difficult to discern, the analysis assumed an average rate of disease progression and recommended patients should undergo AVR/CABG when the pressure gradient exceeds 30 mm Hg. The threshold (AS pressure gradient) to perform both procedures is increased for patients older than 70 years of age because the reduced life expectancy diminishes the likelihood that they will become symptomatic from the AV disease. Whether to perform a concomitant AVR at the time of revascularization was also addressed by Rahimtoola, who advocated a less aggressive approach.[12] One problem with both studies is that they analyzed the transvalvular pressure gradient, which may be a misleading measure of the degree of stenosis of the AV, as its value is dependent on CO. A low CO and flow rate will produce a low transvalvular pressure gradient, even in the setting of a severely stenotic AV. However, in the setting of preserved ventricular systolic function and mild or moderate AS, a pressure gradient is a useful metric. The variable rate of disease progression and the controversy regarding the indications for "prophylactic" AVR preclude a simple algorithm for dealing with this patient cohort. Increased age, lack of symptoms, minimal LV hypertrophy, with a valve area suggesting milder disease, and a pressure gradient less than 30 mm Hg would sway the decision to not replace the AV. In an asymptomatic young patient, a severely calcified valve, bicuspid valve, and LV hypertrophy in the setting of moderate stenosis, and a pressure gradient greater than 30 mm Hg would suggest that an AVR might be beneficial in the long term. It is often useful to include the patient's primary cardiologist and family in the decision-making process.

ASSESSMENT OF LOW PRESSURE GRADIENT AORTIC STENOSIS

Patients with LV dysfunction and decreased CO in the setting of AS often present with only modest transvalvular pressure gradients (<30 mm Hg). Distinguishing patients with a low CO and severe AS from patients with mild to moderate AS can be challenging (Fig. 10-7). The standard for assessing severity of AS is AV area, typically calculated using either a continuity method or by planimetry. Patients with low-gradient AS with severe LV dysfunction who received an AVR had improved survival and functional status compared with patients who did not have a valve replacement.[13]

A low pressure gradient related to LV dysfunction may not open the AV to its maximum capacity. Dobutamine challenge in a patient with low pressure gradient AS can be useful in establishing true AV area. The ability to distinguish between true AV stenosis and a state of "pseudostenosis" relies on characteristic changes in hemodynamic and structural measurements in response to the augmented CO. The test is not typically performed in the operative setting but rather as a preoperative evaluation. The increase in calculated AV area is related to the increase in the CO and is attributed to partial reversal of primary cardiac dysfunction. If dobutamine improves CO and increases AV area, it is likely the baseline calculations overestimated the severity of the AS. The dobutamine challenge is conducted as follows: patients with low-gradient AS receive intravenous dobutamine at 5 μg/kg/min with stepwise increases in dose. Patients may exhibit a significant increase in AV area (0.8 cm² to 1.1 cm²) and a decline in valve resistance after dobutamine challenge. Patients with fixed, high-grade AS would demonstrate no change in valve area and an increase in valve resistance. The 2003 ACC/AHA/ASE Task Force gave a class IIb recommendation (usefulness/efficacy is less well established by evidence/opinion) for the use of dobutamine echocardiography in the evaluation of patients with low-gradient AS and ventricular dysfunction.[14] In addition to its role in distinguishing between true stenosis and pseudostenosis, low-dose dobutamine echocardiography is helpful in risk stratifying of patients with severe true AS. Patients with augmented contractile function after dobutamine administration have an improved outcome after surgery.[15]

Continued on following page

10

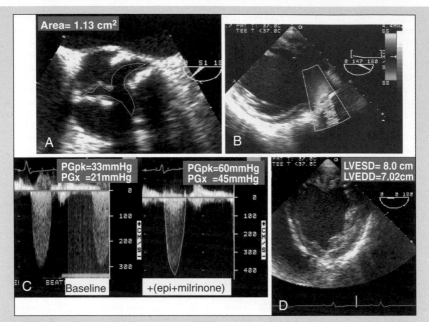

Figure 10-7 Low pressure gradient severe aortic stenosis. A 76-year-old cachetic man was scheduled to undergo corrective surgery for severe mitral regurgitation (MR) and possibly clinically significant aortic stenosis (AS). **A)** The midesophageal short-axis view of the aortic valve (AV) showed a highly calcified trileaflet valve with restricted mobility. The measurement of AV area, 1.13 cm², which was obtained by planimetry, was believed to underestimate the severity of AS because of the shadowing artifacts related to the severity of calcification. **B)** The transgastric long axis view of the left ventricle (LV) was obtained, and the velocity profiles of blood flow within the LV outflow tract and the AV were measured. **C)** Although the patient had a diagnosis of severe AS, the maximal and mean pressure gradients were 33 mm Hg and 21 mm Hg, respectively. The area of the AV was calculated to be 0.83 cm² using the continuity equation. **D)** The LV function was characterized by a severe dilated cardiomyopathy with an ejection fraction of 8%, LVESD of 7 cm, and LVEDD of 8 cm. The diagnosis of low pressure gradient AS was considered, and infusions of epinephrine and milrinone were started. Cardiac performance improved from 2.4 L/min to 4.5 L/min, and the pressured gradients increased to 60 mm Hg, peak, and 45 mm Hg, mean. Although the calculated valve area that was recorded under conditions of inotrope support slightly increased to 0.9 cm², transesophageal echocardiography (TEE) clarified that the marked increase in the pressure gradient was consistent with a diagnosis of low-gradient AS and confirmed the presence of cardiac reserve.

Case Study 4   ACUTE AORTIC SYNDROMES

FRAMING

The unstable patient with suspected acute aortic disease or injury is often the most challenging of TEE cases. There are few more crucially important decisions that are posed to the intraoperative echocardiographer than to quickly and accurately diagnose the nature and extent of acute aortic injury. Hypotension and respiratory distress may prevent a complete and comprehensive evaluation before surgery. Patient history is often unobtainable. The echocardiographer becomes a detective. Clues are quickly gathered from the available clinical presentation, past history, and associated physical findings. The TEE is often the only modality used to establish the diagnosis and define the surgical plan.

It is midnight on a gloomy rainy night. The hospital helicopter pilot calls in "young woman, unrestrained driver, deceleration injury, steering wheel impact, chest contusion, unconscious, hypotensive. She is intubated with bilateral breath sounds. Her blood pressure is 70/40 mm Hg with an HR = 125 sinus tachycardia. She is being fluid resuscitated and being transported directly to the cardiac operating room." The patient is too unstable for magnetic resonance imaging (MRI) or computed tomography (CT). The patient arrives with a portable chest radiograph obtained as she traveled through the emergency department, showing a widened mediastinum. The vital signs have not changed except that she is receiving dopamine at 10 μg/kg/min. Pulses are palpable in the groins and the neck (Fig. 10-8). The attending surgeon turns to the echocardiographer-anesthesiologist and asks, "I need to know whether this is an anterior injury with heart contusion, injury to the ascending aorta, tamponade with blood in the pericardium, or a transected aorta or does the patient have a nonoperable injury? The former will require a sternotomy. The transections will require a left thoracotomy. If we make the incorrect decision, the patient will surely die." The patient is stabilized in the operating room and the TEE probe is inserted. After the diagnosis is made, the patient is positioned and prepped accordingly for the definitive surgery.

The sensitivity and specificity of TEE to detect and diagnose injury or disease of the thoracic aorta are significantly better than the sensitivity and specificity of TTE and are comparable to findings on CT and MRI.[16] TEE provides information regarding cardiac performance and the presence of other critically important sequelae that may be important in determining the approach and timing for surgical intervention. Hence, TEE is indicated even if MRI or CT has confirmed the diagnosis.

Can consent be obtained from the patient or family members? In these emergency circumstances, it may be more prudent to proceed with the TEE examination rather than delaying diagnosis and treatment in an attempt to find family members. What is the differential diagnosis of a widened mediastinum? How does TEE discriminate the different causes of a widened mediastinum? Is the TEE performed in the awake distressed patient, or is the TEE done under more controlled conditions of an anesthetized, intubated patient? Is there a risk of cervical spine injury? Is there a risk of esophageal injury? Can insertion of the TEE probe further compromise the patency of mediastinal structures? Is there fluid in the pericardium? What is the biventricular function? Is there myocardial rupture? Is there aortic rupture? Is the thoracic aorta intact? Is there an intimal flap and a dissection? Is there a transection? Is there a pleural or periaortic effusion/hematoma? What factors determine the urgency of intervention and strategies for management?

DATA COLLECTION

Because the diagnosis and cause for instability are not established, the entire mediastinum, including the left pleural space, is interrogated before definitive therapy is initiated. Rarely is there not enough time to do a complete TEE examination. The operative team can often proceed with confidence in the management of these critically ill patients with only TEE to guide the treatment. The primary event in aortic dissection is a tear and separation of the aortic intima. It is uncertain whether the inciting event is a primary rupture of the intima with secondary dissection of the media or hemorrhage within the media and subsequent rupture of the overlying intima. Systolic ejection forces blood into the aortic media through a tear that leads to the separation of the intima from the surrounding media, creating a false lumen. Blood flow may exist in both the false and true lumens through communicating fenestrations. Aortic dissections are classified by one of two anatomic schemes (the DeBakey and Stanford classifications). Transection is diagnosed through the detection of paraaortic hematoma near the isthmus and a "step-up" in the internal media wall.

DISCUSSION

Acute dissections (Stanford type A or DeBakey type I or type II) involving the ascending aorta or arch are considered acute surgical emergencies. In contrast, dissections confined to the descending aorta (distal to the left subclavian artery; Stanford type B or DeBakey type III) are treated medically unless the patient demonstrates proximal extension, hemorrhage, or malperfusion. From the International Registry of Acute Aortic Dissection (IRAD), 73% of the 384 patients with type B dissections were managed medically; in-hospital mortality was 10%.[17] The long-term survival rate after applying medical therapy is 60% to 80% at 4 to 5 years and 40% to 45% at 10 years.

Continued on following page

10

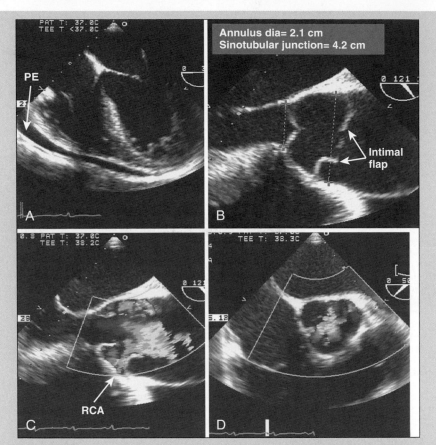

Annulus dia= 2.1 cm
Sinotubular junction= 4.2 cm

PE

Intimal flap

RCA

A   B   C   D

Figure 10-8 Acute aortic syndrome as the etiology of hemodynamic compromise. A 62-year-old previously healthy, unrestrained driver had a motor vehicle accident. On arrival to the emergency department, the patient was hypotensive (BP=90/45) and tachycardic (HR=120). He described an episode of loss of consciousness that was associated with severe chest pain but could not recall if the syncopal episode preceded the accident. The chest radiograph was significant for several fractured ribs, widened mediastinum, and a pleural effusion. The patient became progressively more unstable and was transferred to the operating room to perform diagnostic transesophageal echocardiography (TEE) and definitive surgical procedure if necessary. The echocardiographer performed a quick transthoracic echocardiographic examination that confirmed the presence of pericardial effusion with findings that were consistent for tamponade. After fluid resuscitation and induction of anesthesia, a TEE examination was performed. **A)** The midesophageal four-chamber view showed presence of a pericardial effusion (PE) that compromised right atrial filling. **B)** The mid-esophageal long-axis view of the aortic valve revealed a type A dissection that was characterized by intimal flaps within the aortic root and that extended distally into the descending thoracic aorta. The annulus of the aortic valve was of normal size, but the sinus and root were markedly enlarged (diameter of sinotubular junction=4.22 cm). **C)** The dissection extended into the noncoronary and right coronary sinus segments, narrowing blood flow at the coronary ostia (*arrow*). Although the ECG did not show acute ischemia, the right ventricular function and inferior wall of the left ventricle were mildly hypokinetic. **D)** Although an effaced aortic root, ascending aortic aneurysm, and acute dissection in this age group are suggestive of congenital bicuspid valve, the short-axis view of the aortic valve showed a trileaflet valve with a coaptation defect with aortic insufficiency at the noncoronary cusp. The surgeon resuspended the aortic valve and replaced the ascending aorta and hemiarch with a tube graft. The valve repair was successful with only +1 aortic insufficiency and cardiac return to normal after surgery.

Survival is best in patients with noncommunicating and retrograde dissections. From the IRAD registry, in-hospital mortality for surgical patients was significantly higher (32%). The increased rate of mortality for surgically treated patients is likely influenced by selecting a cohort of patients with more advanced disease and complicated course (malperfusion, leakage, extension). The overall reported short- and long-term outcomes are similar for medically treated patients with type B dissections. Of 142 patients with type aortic dissections, there was a trend toward lower mortality with medical therapy compared with surgical treatment at 1 year (15% vs. 33%). Both groups had similar survival at 5 and 10 years (60% and 35%).

Ascending aortic dissections (involving the aortic root, ascending aorta, or arch) are acute surgical emergencies, because of the high risk for a life-threatening complication such as AR, cardiac tamponade, myocardial infarction, rupture, and stroke. The mortality rate is as high as 1% to 2% per hour early after symptom onset. Neither acute myocardial ischemia nor cerebral infarction should contraindicate urgent intervention. Although patients with stroke in progress may be at increased risk for hemorrhagic cerebral infarction due to intraoperative anticoagulation, leading to hemorrhagic stroke, the authors have seen several patients who experienced dramatic neurologic recovery. Operative mortality for ascending aortic dissections at experienced centers varies from 7% to 36%, well below the greater than 50% mortality with medical therapy.[18]

Traumatic aortic rupture is a life-threatening vascular injury that often results in lethal hemorrhage. In a multicenter trial of 274 patients, the overall mortality rate reached 31%, with 63% of deaths attributable to aortic rupture. Aortic transection and rupture usually occur at the aortic isthmus (between the left subclavian and the first intercostal arteries) and result from shear forces generated by unrestrained frontal collisions. Although aortography had been considered the gold standard for the diagnosis of transection, TEE and contrast-enhanced spiral CT and MRI are currently favored, especially for patients with renal insufficiency.[19] Intravascular ultrasonography has been proposed as a potential diagnostic tool for the identification of limited aortic injuries. Traumatic aortic rupture needs to be distinguished from an aortic dissection. Imaging of a dissected aorta typically reveals true and false lumens at multiple levels. The focal aortic injury of aortic transection is quite localized and may be overlooked when performing a cursory examination. A second potential diagnostic problem is that protuberant atherosclerotic changes of the aorta may be difficult to differentiate from partial aortic tears. The thick and irregular intraluminal flap, which corresponds to disruption of both intimal and medial aortic layers, can be imaged in both the short- and long-axis planes in the vicinity of the isthmus. In the longitudinal view, the medial flap is nearly perpendicular to the aortic wall because traumatic lesions are usually confined within a few centimeters distal to the left subclavian. The formation of a localized contained rupture of the false aneurysm is common. Color flow Doppler imaging and spectral Doppler imaging can be used to detect turbulence associated with nonlaminar flow at the aortic defect and the presence of a pressure gradient. Traditional treatment includes immediate surgical intervention using a right lateral decubitus approach and resection of the aorta with insertion of a tube graft. Deployment of endovascular stent grafts has been successful. Two series that included a total of 16 patients having aortic transection reported successful repair with no mortality or serious morbidity.[20] However, the application of this device under such conditions poses a high risk for left subclavian malperfusion and paraplegia. The decision regarding appropriate management and time course of therapy will depend on the technical availability and expertise within the institution and the forthcoming results of clinical trials that use newer, less invasive technologies.

10

SUMMARY

- An ultrasound beam is a continuous or intermittent train of sound waves emitted by a transducer or wave generator that is composed of density or pressure. Ultrasound waves are characterized by their wavelength, frequency, and velocity.
- Waves interact with the medium in which they travel and with one another, and the manner in which waves interact with a medium is determined by its density and homogeneity. When a wave is propagated through an inhomogeneous medium, it is partly absorbed, partly reflected, and partly scattered.
- Doppler frequency shift analysis can be used to obtain blood flow velocity, direction, and acceleration of red blood cells, where the magnitude and direction of the frequency shift are related to the velocity and direction of the moving target.
- Doppler shifts above the Nyquist limit will create artifacts described as "aliasing" or "wraparound," and blood flow velocities will appear in a direction opposite to the conventional one. To optimize Nyquist limits, the ultrasound frequency should be low and the sampling frequency should be high.
- Normally, red blood cells scatter ultrasound waves weakly, resulting in a black appearance on ultrasonic examination. Contrast echocardiography uses gas microbubbles to present additional gas-liquid interfaces, which substantially increase the strength of the returning signal. This augmentation in signal strength may be used to better define endocardial borders, optimize Doppler envelope signals, and estimate myocardial perfusion.
- *Axial resolution* is the minimum separation between two interfaces located in a direction parallel to the ultrasound beam so that they can be imaged as two different interfaces. *Lateral resolution* is the minimum separation of two interfaces aligned along a direction perpendicular to the beam. *Elevational resolution* refers to the ability to determine differences in the thickness of the imaging plane.
- Absolute contraindications to transesophageal echocardiography in intubated patients include esophageal stricture, diverticula, tumor, recent suture lines, and known esophageal interruption. Relative contraindications include symptomatic hiatal hernia, esophagitis, coagulopathy, esophageal varices, and unexplained upper gastrointestinal bleeding.
- Horizontal imaging planes are obtained by moving the transesophageal echocardiography probe up and down (upper esophageal: 20 to 25 cm; midesophageal: 30 to 40 cm; transgastric: 40 to 45 cm; deep transgastric: 45 to 50 cm). Multiplane probes may further facilitate interrogation of complex anatomic structures by allowing up to 180 degrees of axial rotation of the imaging plane without manual probe manipulation.
- The dynamic assessment of ventricular function with echocardiography is based on derived indices of muscle contraction and relaxation. Echocardiography indices of left ventricular function that incorporate endocardial border outlines and Doppler techniques can be used to estimate cardiac output, stroke volume, ejection fraction, and parameters of ventricular relaxation and filling.
- Decision making by TEE requires "Framing" the problem, "Data collection", and a comprehensive TEE examination.

REFERENCES

1. Miller AP, Nanda NC: Contrast echocardiography: New agents. Ultrasound Med Biol 30:425, 2004
2. Shanewise J, Cheung A, Aronson S, et al: ASE/SCA guidelines for performing a comprehensive intraoperative multiplane transesophageal echocardiography examination: Recommendations of the American Society of Echocardiography Council for Intraoperative Echocardiography and the Society of Cardiovascular Anesthesiologists Task Force for Certification in Perioperative Transesophageal Echocardiography. Anesth Analg 89:870, 1999
3. Weyman AF: The year in echocardiography. J Am Coll Cardiol 45:48, 2005
4. Fleisher L, Welskopf R: Real-time intraoperative monitoring of myocardial ischemia in noncardiac surgery. Anesthesiology 92:1183, 2000
5. Kallmeyer IJ, Collard CD, Fox JA, et al: The safety of intraoperative transesophageal echocardiography: A case series of 7200 cardiac surgical patients. Anesth Analg 92:1126, 2001
6. Practice guidelines for perioperative transesophageal echocardiography. A report by the American Society of Anesthesiologists and the Society of Cardiovascular Anesthesiologists Task Force on Transesophageal Echocardiography. Anesthesiology 84:986, 1996
7. Kozman H, Cook JR, Wiseman AH, et al: Presence of angiographic coronary collaterals predicts myocardial recovery after coronary bypass surgery in patients with severe left ventricular dysfunction. Circulation 98:II-57, 1998
8. Grigioni F, Enriquez-Sarano M, Zehr KJ, et al: Ischemic mitral regurgitation: Long-term outcome and prognostic implications with quantitative Doppler assessment. Circulation 103:1759, 2001
9. Grewal KS, Malkowski MJ, Piracha AR, et al: Effect of general anesthesia on the severity of mitral regurgitation by transesophageal echocardiography. Am J Cardiol 85:199, 2000
10. Guy TS, Moainie SL, Gorman JH, III et al: Prevention of ischemic mitral regurgitation does not influence the outcome of remodeling after posterolateral myocardial infarction. J Am Coll Cardiol 43:377, 2004
11. Smith WT, Ferguson TB Jr., Ryan T, et al: Should coronary artery bypass graft surgery patients with mild or moderate aortic stenosis undergo concomitant aortic valve replacement? A decision analysis approach to the surgical dilemma. J Am Coll Cardiol 44:1241, 2004
12. Rahimtoola SH: "Prophylactic" valve replacement for mild aortic valve disease at time of surgery for other cardiovascular disease? No. J Am Coll Cardiol 33:2009, 1999
13. Pereira JJ, Lauer MS, Bashir M, et al: Survival after aortic valve replacement for severe aortic stenosis with low transvalvular gradients and severe left ventricular dysfunction. J Am Coll Cardiol 39:1356, 2002
14. Cheitlin MD, Armstrong WF, Aurigemma GP, et al: ACC/AHA/ASE 2003 guideline update for the clinical application of echocardiography—summary article: A report of the American College of Cardiology/American Heart Association Task Force on Practice Guidelines (ACC/AHA/ASE Committee to Update the 1997 Guidelines for the Clinical Application of Echocardiography). J Am Coll Cardiol 42:954, 2003
15. Monin JL, Quere JP, Monchi M, et al: Low-gradient aortic stenosis: Operative risk stratification and predictors for long-term outcome: A multicenter study using dobutamine stress hemodynamics. Circulation 108:319, 2003
16. Feindel CM, David TE: Aortic valve sparing operations: Basic concepts. Int J Cardiol 97:61, 2004
17. Suzuki T, Mehta RH, Ince H, et al: Clinical profiles and outcomes of acute type B aortic dissection in the current era: Lessons from the International Registry of Aortic Dissection (IRAD). Circulation 108(Suppl II):II-312, 2003
18. Nienaber CA, Eagle KA: Aortic dissection: New frontiers in diagnosis and management: I. From etiology to diagnostic strategies. Circulation 108:628, 2003
19. Goarin JP, Cluzel P, Gosgnach M, et al: Evaluation of transesophageal echocardiography for diagnosis of traumatic aortic injury. Anesthesiology 93:1373, 2000
20. Ott MC, Stewart TC, Lawlor DK, et al: Management of blunt thoracic aortic injuries: Endovascular stents versus open repair. J Trauma 56:565, 2004

10

Chapter 11

Central Nervous System Monitoring

Harvey L. Edmonds, Jr., PhD

Nearly half of the 1 million patients undergoing cardiac surgery each year worldwide will likely experience persistent cognitive decline.[1] The direct annual cost to U.S. insurers for brain injury from just one type of cardiac surgery, myocardial revascularization, is estimated at $4 billion. Furthermore, the same processes that injure the central nervous system (CNS) also appear to cause dysfunction of other vital organs. Thus, there are enormous clinical and economic incentives to improve CNS protection during cardiac surgery.

Historically, there has been little enthusiasm for neurophysiologic monitoring during cardiac surgery because of the presumed key role of macroembolization. It is widely assumed that most brain injuries during adult cardiac surgery result from cerebral embolization of atheromatous or calcified material dislodged from sclerotic blood vessels during their manipulation. Until the introduction of myocardial revascularization without cardiopulmonary bypass (CPB) or aortic clamp application, these injuries often have been viewed as unavoidable and untreatable.

Technical developments have begun to alter this perception. First, CNS injuries still occur despite reductions in aortic manipulation with the new approaches to coronary artery bypass and aortic surgery.[2] Second, neurophysiologic studies have implicated hypoperfusion and dysoxygenation as major causative factors in CNS injury (Box 11-1). Because these functional disturbances are often detectable and correctable there is an impetus to examine the role of neurophysiologic monitoring in CNS protection.

ELECTROENCEPHALOGRAPHY

Electroencephalographic (EEG) monitoring for ischemia detection has been performed since the first CPB procedures, but this long experience is not broad. Limited use appears to have several causes.

> **BOX 11-1** *Factors Contributing to Brain Injury during Cardiac Surgery*
>
> • Atheromatous emboli from aorta manipulation
> • Lipid microemboli from recirculation of unwashed cardiotomy suction
> • Gaseous microemboli from air leakage and cavitation
> • Cerebral hypoperfusion from dysautoregulation
> • Cerebral hyperperfusion
> • Cerebral hyperthermia

First, small, practical, and affordable EEG monitors have only recently become available.

Second, the traditional diagnostic approach to EEG analysis depended on complex pattern recognition of 16-channel analog waveforms to identify focal ischemic changes. Because this analytic format necessitated extensive training and constant vigilance, cardiac surgery EEG monitoring directly by anesthesia providers has often been viewed as impractical. However, it has been shown that a four-channel recording, which included bilateral activity from both the anterior and posterior circulation, was effective in identifying focal ischemia. In addition, computerized processing of EEG signals provides simplified trend displays that have helped to overcome many of the earlier complexities.

Third, EEG analysis during cardiac surgery was often confounded by anesthetics, hypothermia, and roller-pump artifacts. Fortunately, the troublesome roller pumps have been replaced with centrifugal pumps or eliminated entirely; moderate to deep hypothermia is now usually applied only in aortic arch reconstruction; and fast-track anesthesia protocols avoid marked EEG suppression.

Physiologic Basis of Electroencephalography

EEG-directed interventions designed to correct cerebral hypoperfusion during cardiac surgery require an appreciation of the underlying neurophysiologic substrate. Scalp-recorded EEG signals reflect the temporal and spatial summation of long-lasting (10 to 100 ms) postsynaptic potentials, which arise from columnar cortical pyramidal neurons (Fig. 11-1).

EEG rhythms represent regularly recurring waveforms of similar shape and duration. These signal oscillations depend on the synchronous excitation of a neuronal population. The descriptive nature of conventional EEG characterizes the oscillations (measured in cycles per second [cps] or Hertz [Hz]) as sinusoids that were classified according to their amplitude and frequency. The terminology used to describe the frequency bands of the most common oscillatory patterns is illustrated in Figure 11-2 and listed in Box 11-2.

Practical Considerations of Electroencephalographic Recording and Signal Processing

Standardized electrode placement is based on the International 10-20 System (Fig. 11-3). It permits uniform spacing of electrodes, independent of head circumference, in scalp regions known to correlate with specific areas of cerebral cortex. Four anatomic landmarks are used: the nasion, inion, and preauricular points.

11

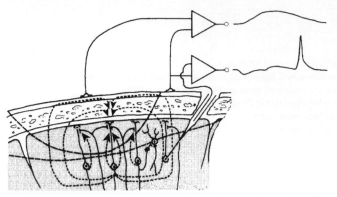

Figure 11-1 The production of EEG waves. Scalp electrodes record potential differences that are caused by postsynaptic potentials in the cell membrane of cortical neurons. The closed loops of the *lighter dashed lines* represent the summation of extracellular currents produced by the postsynaptic potentials. Open segments of the *heavier dashed lines* connect all points having the same voltage level. The two scalp electrodes record changes in the voltage difference over time (*top trace at upper right*). The *lower trace* from a microelectrode inserted in a single cortical neuron has little direct relationship to the summated EEG wave. (Modified from Fisch BJ: EEG Primer, 3rd ed. New York, Elsevier, 1999.)

The frequency range involved in production of the EEG waveform is termed its *bandwidth*. The upper and lower bandwidth boundaries are controlled by filters that reject frequencies above and below the EEG bandwidth. Both the appearance of the unprocessed EEG waveform and the value of univariate numeric EEG descriptors such as the mean frequency may be heavily influenced by signal bandwidth. The same cerebral biopotential recorded by different EEG devices may result in dissimilar waveforms and numeric values.

Display of Electroencephalographic Information

Time-Domain Analysis

Traditional display of the EEG is a graph of biopotential voltage (*y*-axis) as a function of time and, consequently, is described as a time-domain process. The objective of a diagnostic EEG is to identify the most likely cause of a detected abnormality at one moment in time. Typically, a diagnostic EEG is obtained under controlled conditions, using precisely defined protocols. Recorded EEG appearance is visually compared with reference patterns. Interpretation is based on recognition of unique waveform patterns that are pathognomonic for specific clinical conditions. In contrast, the goal of EEG monitoring is to identify clinically important change from an individualized baseline. Unlike diagnostic EEG interpretation, monitoring requires immediate assessment of continuously fluctuating signals in an electronically hostile, complex, and poorly controlled recording environment. Therefore, of necessity, interpretation relies less on pattern recognition and more on statistical characterization of change. Simple numerical descriptors thus may appropriately form an integral part of EEG monitoring.

Both EEG diagnostic and monitoring interpretations are based, in part, on the "Law of the EEG" (Box 11-3). It states that amplitude and dominant frequency are inversely related. Simultaneous decreases in both amplitude and frequency may indicate ischemia or anoxia (Fig. 11-4).

Awake—low voltage—random, fast

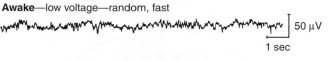

50 μV

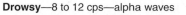

1 sec

Drowsy—8 to 12 cps—alpha waves

Stage 1—3 to 7 cps—theta waves

Theta waves

Stage 2—12 to 14 cps—sleep spindles and K complexes

Sleep spindle   K complex —

Delta sleep—½ to 2 cps—delta waves >75 μV

REM sleep—low voltage—random, fast with sawtooth waves

Sawtooth waves Sawtooth waves

Figure 11-2 The specific EEG characteristics of the different stages of the human sleep-wake cycle are shown. Note the appearance of the four most common frequency bands from the lowest frequency delta, through theta and alpha to high-frequency beta. An even higher gamma frequency band (25 to 55 cps) is also described. (Modified from Yli-Hankala A [ed]: Handbook of Four-Channel EEG in Anesthesia and Critical Care. Helsinki, GE Medical, Datex-Ohmeda Division, 2004.)

11

BOX 11-2	*EEG Frequency Bands*
Delta	0.5 to 2 Hz
Theta	3 to 7 Hz
Alpha	8 to 12 Hz
Beta	13 to 24 Hz
Gamma	25 to 55 Hz

Time domain analysis of traditional electroencephalography uses linear amplitude voltage and time scales. The amplitude range of EEG signals is quite large (several hundred microvolts) and univariate statistical measures of its central tendency and dispersion may contain clinically useful information. Furthermore, amplitude variation may present clinically significant changes in reactivity that can be

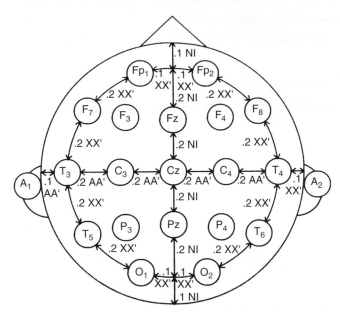

Figure 11-3 The position of the electrodes in the International 10-20 system according to scalp measurements. The sagittal hemicircumference (labeled AA') is measured from the root of one zygoma (just anterior to the ear) to the other, across the vertex. The third measurement is the ipsilateral hemicircumference (XX') measured from a point 10% of the coronal hemicircumference above the zygoma. Through these intersecting lines all of the scalp electrodes may be located, except frontal (F3, F4) and parietal (P3, P4). The frontal and parietal electrodes are placed along the frontal or parietal coronal line midway between the middle electrode and the electrode marked in the circumferential ring.

BOX 11-3   *Law of the EEG*

- In the absence of a pathologic process, EEG amplitude and frequency are inversely related.
- Simultaneous decrease may indicate ischemia, anoxia, or excessive hypnosis.
- Simultaneous increase may indicate seizure or artifact.

---

obscured by frequency-domain analysis. Advances in the technology of EEG amplitude integration have prompted a resurgent interest in this attractively simple approach, particularly in pediatrics.

Frequency Domain Analysis

An alternative method, frequency domain analysis, is exemplified by the prismatic decomposition of white light into its component frequencies (i.e., color spectrum). As the basis of spectral analysis, the Fourier theorem states that a periodic function can be represented, in part, by a sinusoid at the fundamental frequency and an infinite series of integer multiples (i.e., harmonics). The Fourier function at a specific frequency equals the amplitude and phase angle of the associated sinusoid. Graphs of amplitude and phase angle as functions of frequency are called Fourier spectra (i.e., spectral analysis). The EEG amplitude spectral scale (Fig. 11-5) squares voltage values to eliminate troublesome negative values. Squaring changes the unit of amplitude measure from microvolts to either picowatts (pW) or nanowatts (nW). However, a power amplitude scale tends to overemphasize large-amplitude changes.

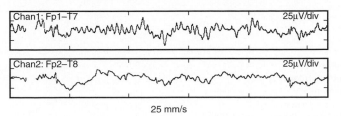

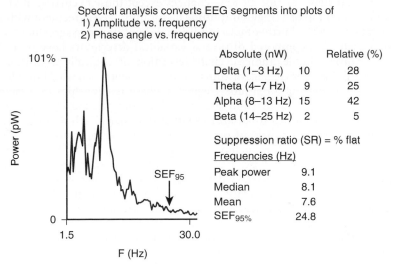

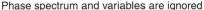

25 mm/s

Figure 11-4 This two-channel EEG recording was made immediately after induction of anesthesia, prior to head repositioning for insertion of a central venous catheter. Anesthetic induction apparently uncovered a preexisting asymmetry that was not evident in the waking EEG. Although the patient had a history of an earlier mild cerebrovascular accident and transient ischemic attacks, he appeared neurologically normal at preoperative assessment. (Modified from Yli-Hankala A [ed]: Handbook of Four-Channel EEG in Anesthesia and Critical Care. Helsinki, GE Medical, Datex-Ohmeda Division, 2004.)

Spectral analysis converts EEG segments into plots of
1) Amplitude vs. frequency
2) Phase angle vs. frequency

	Absolute (nW)	Relative (%)
Delta (1–3 Hz)	10	28
Theta (4–7 Hz)	9	25
Alpha (8–13 Hz)	15	42
Beta (14–25 Hz)	2	5

Suppression ratio (SR) = % flat

Frequencies (Hz)

Peak power	9.1
Median	8.1
Mean	7.6
$SEF_{95\%}$	24.8

Phase spectrum and variables are ignored

Figure 11-5 EEG frequency spectral pattern obtained from a patient anesthetized with 1 MAC isoflurane. It illustrates some of the many univariate numeric EEG descriptors.

11

Clinically important changes in lower amplitude components that are readily discernible in the linearly scaled unprocessed EEG waveform may become invisible in power spectral displays.

Simplification of the large amount of spectral information generally has been achieved through the use of univariate numeric descriptors. Most commonly, the power contained in a specified traditional EEG frequency band (delta, theta, alpha, or beta) is calculated in absolute, relative, or normalized terms.

The most widely used univariate frequency descriptors are (1) peak power frequency (the single frequency of the spectrum that contains the highest amplitude) (Box 11-4), (2) median power frequency (frequency below which 50% of the spectral power occurs), (3) mean spectral frequency (sum of power contained at each frequency of the spectrum times its frequency divided by the total power), (4) spectral edge frequency (SEF; frequency below which a predetermined fraction, usually 95%, of the spectral power occurs), and (5) suppression ratio (SR; percent of flat-line EEG contained within sampled epochs).

BOX 11-4 *Common Univariate EEG Descriptors Detecting Ischemia*

- Total power
- Peak power frequency
- Mean frequency
- Median frequency
- 95% Spectral edge frequency (SEF)
- Suppression ratio (SR)

Pronk evaluated computer-processed univariate descriptors of EEG changes occurring before, during, and after CPB.[3] Mean spectral frequency alone was sufficient to adequately describe all EEG changes except those occurring at very low amplitudes. Addition of a single-amplitude factor improved agreement with visual interpretation to 90%. Further factor addition did not improve agreement.

Multivariate (i.e., composed of several variables) descriptors have been developed to improve simple numeric characterization of clinically important EEG changes. With this approach, algorithms are used to generate a single number that represents the pattern of amplitude-frequency-phase relationships occurring in a single epoch. Several commercially available monitors provide unitless numbers that have been transformed to an arbitrary 0-to-100 scale. Each monitor provides a different probability estimate of patient response to verbal instruction. Current examples of these descriptors include the bispectral index (BIS), the patient state index (PSI), and spectral entropy.[4,5] BIS and PSI are empirically derived proprietary indices developed from proprietary patient databases. In contrast, spectral entropy is neither empirical nor proprietary but rather represents the novel application of long-established physical sciences entropy equations to the analysis of cranial biopotentials. Each product is designed to require the use of proprietary self-adhesive forehead sensors. Collectively, these products are now in widespread use as objective measures of hypnotic effect (Box 11-5).

Most hypnotics decrease EEG complexity (i.e., variability) in a dose-related fashion. This long-established observation provides the rationale for the use of nonproprietary spectral entropy analysis as an objective measure of hypnotic effect.[6] The absence of an empiric rule-based approach avoids the need for arbitrary weighting coefficients and minimizes the potentially distorting influences of very low- and very high-amplitude EEG signals.

The use of pseudo-three-dimensional plots to display successive power spectra as a function of time was popularized by Bickford, who coined the term *compressed spectral array* (CSA). This technique now represents one of the most common displays of computer-processed EEG in the frequency domain. Popularity stems from enormous data compression. For example, the essential information contained in a 4-hour EEG recording consuming more than 1000 pages of unprocessed waveforms can be displayed in CSA format on a single page.

With CSA (Fig. 11-6), successive power spectra of brief (2- to 60-second) EEG epochs are displayed as smoothed histograms of amplitude as a function of frequency. Spectral compression is achieved by partially overlaying successive spectra, with time represented on the z-axis. Hidden-line suppression improves clarity by avoiding overlap of successive traces. Although the display is aesthetically attractive, it has limitations. The extent of data loss due to spectral overlapping depends on the nonstandard axial rotation that varies among EEG monitors.

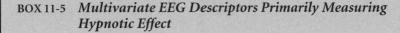

BOX 11-5 *Multivariate EEG Descriptors Primarily Measuring Hypnotic Effect*

- Bispectral index (BIS)
- Patient state index (PSI)
- Spectral entropy

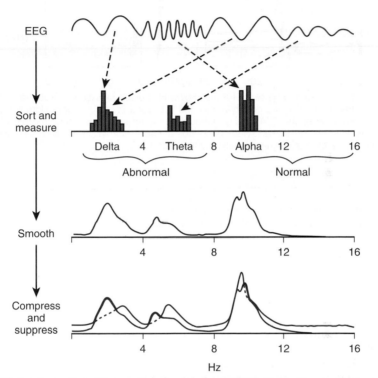

Figure 11-6 Generation of a compressed spectral array (CSA) display. *Top panel* represents the unprocessed EEG time domain waveform. The *second panel* depicts Fourier transformation of the signal into the frequency domain. Smoothing of spectral data contained in individual frequency bins occurs in the *third panel*, whereas compressed sequencing of successive spectra with hidden-line suppression occurs in the *bottom panel*. (Modified from Myers RR, Stockard JJ, Fleming NI, et al: Br J Anaesth 45:664, 1973.)

An alternative to the CSA display to reduce data loss is the density-modulated spectral array (DSA) that uses a two-dimensional dot matrix plot of time as a function of frequency (Fig. 11-7). The density of dots indicates the amplitude at a particular time-frequency intersection (e.g., an intense large spot indicates high amplitude). Clinically significant shifts in frequency may be detected earlier and more easily than with CSA.

In summary, a quick assessment of EEG change in either the time or frequency domain focuses on (1) maximal peak-to-peak amplitude, (2) relation of maximal amplitude to dominant frequency, (3) amplitude and frequency variability, and (4) new or growing asymmetry between homotopic (i.e., same position on each cerebral hemisphere) EEG derivations. These objectives are generally best achieved through the viewing of both unprocessed and processed displays with a clear understanding of the characteristics and limitations of each (Box 11-6).

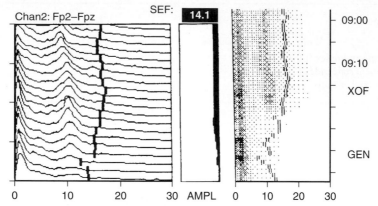

Figure 11-7 The same EEG segments are shown in the compressed spectral array (CSA, *left*), total power trend (*middle*), and density-modulated spectral array (DSA, *right*). Note the improved amplitude resolution of the CSA display, although some information is obscured by foreground peaks. (Modified from Yli-Hankala A [ed]: Handbook of Four-Channel EEG in Anesthesia and Critical Care. Helsinki, GE Medical, Datex-Ohmeda Division, 2004.)

BOX 11-6 *Measures That Define EEG Changes*

- Maximum peak-to-peak amplitude (or total power)
- Relation of maximum amplitude to dominant frequency
- Amplitude and frequency variability
- Right-left symmetry

Electroencephalography for Injury Prevention during Cardiac Surgery

There is normally a tight coupling among cerebral cortical synaptic activity, metabolism, and blood flow. Such coupling is necessary because of the large energy requirements of interneuronal communication. Indeed, at least 60% of neuronal oxygen and glucose is consumed in the processes of synaptic and axonal transmission, whereas the remainder is used to maintain cellular integrity. Neurons rapidly adjust their signaling capabilities to conserve vital energy stores. Even a slight new imbalance between supply and consumption of energy substrates is manifested by altered synaptic activity. The EEG provides a sensitive measure of this synaptic change and represents an early warning of developing injury. Identification and correction of the physiologic imbalance may then avert serious injury (Box 11-7).

Although the EEG is a very sensitive indicator of cerebrocortical synaptic depression, possibly signifying cerebral ischemia or hypoxia, it is not specific. EEG suppression may also be the result of cooling or hypnotic agents. Fortunately, the time course of EEG suppression and information available from other monitors usually permit distinction between potentially harmful (e.g., ischemia) and harmless (e.g., hypothermia) causes.

Documentation of Preexisting Electroencephalographic Abnormalities

Because there is a high likelihood of latent cerebrovascular disease in many older cardiac surgery patients, it is essential to examine the waking EEG for signs of marked asymmetry before the induction of anesthesia. This serves both to alert the anesthesia

BOX 11-7   *Important Considerations during EEG Interpretation*

- EEG change signifies imbalance, not necessarily injury.
- The EEG is sensitive to imbalance but not specific for its cause.
- EEG prediction of neurologic outcome is good but not perfect.

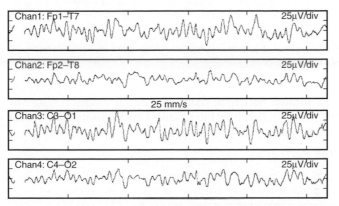

Figure 11-8   This four-channel unprocessed EEG display indicates developing cerebrocortical suppression in the right hemisphere (channel 2: Fp2–T8; channel 4: C4–O2) associated with head turning for pulmonary artery catheter placement. Symmetrical traces were restored with return of the head to a neutral position (not shown). This transient EEG change before surgical incision emphasizes the importance of obtaining a baseline EEG record before anesthetic induction to document any preexisting asymmetry or other abnormalities. (Modified from Yli-Hankala A [ed]: Handbook of Four-Channel EEG in Anesthesia and Critical Care. Helsinki, GE Medical, Datex-Ohmeda Division, 2004.)

provider to the patient's increased vulnerability and to document the previously unappreciated risk.

Objective Measurement of Hypnotic Effect

Recording the transition from wakefulness to unresponsiveness permits detection of unusual sensitivity or resistance to general anesthetics. Such information is vital during fast-track anesthesia protocols to avoid excessive or inadequate anesthesia.

Head Position

Because of the diffuse nature of atherosclerotic vascular disease, many elderly patients are at increased risk for positional focal or regional cerebral ischemia that may occur before incision. Head rotation for surgical positioning or insertion of a pulmonary artery catheter may compress a vital carotid or vertebral artery. Such ischemia is generally identified by marked depression in the affected frontotemporal EEG derivation (Fig. 11-8).

Vascular Obstruction and Flow Misdirection

Manipulation or torsion of the aorta or vena cava may result in regional or global cerebral ischemia. During CPB, the aortic cannula can misdirect either cardiac or pump flow away from one or more head vessels while leaving the radial artery pressure unaltered. Alternatively, a malpositioned venous cannula may impair return

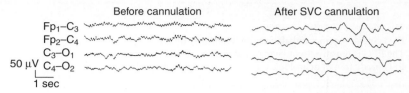

Figure 11-9 Insertion of a 14-Fr venous cannula in this pediatric patient during repair of an atrial septal defect caused a sudden diffuse EEG slowing. The heart rate and blood pressure remained unchanged, although the central venous pressure rose from 6 to 45 mm Hg. Cannula repositioning restored both the former EEG pattern and central venous pressure. (Modified from Rodriguez RA, Cornel G, Semelhago L, et al: Ann Thorac Surg 64:1820, 1997. Copyright 1997, with permission of the Society of Thoracic Surgeons.)

from the head without noticeable change in central venous pressure or return flow to the venous reservoir. Resulting intracranial hypertension leads to ischemic depression of the EEG (Fig. 11-9).

Nonpulsatile Perfusion

Nonpulsatile perfusion used with CPB and some new left ventricular assist devices may result in microcirculatory collapse in susceptible regions of the cerebral cortex, despite "acceptable" radial artery pressures. EEG-guided increases in arterial pressure, circulating volume, or both may be needed to restore perfusion in the microvasculature.

Hemodilution

Hemodilution is used to improve vital organ perfusion by reducing viscosity. However, it may cause inadequate delivery of oxygenated hemoglobin to a high-demand brain, even though hematocrit and systemic venous oxygen saturation are within normal limits. EEG deterioration may thus serve as an objective indicator for transfusion.

Hypocarbia and Hypercarbia

Cerebral arteries normally constrict in response to decreased carbon dioxide tension or hydrogen ion concentration. With reactive arteries, hypocarbia may lead to cerebral ischemia, because flow is reduced 4%/mm Hg (CO_2). In this circumstance, return to normocarbia can markedly improve cerebral perfusion. Conversely, hypercarbia may steal blood from the dilated vessels of an already underperfused region, resulting in focal EEG slowing. This circumstance may be exacerbated by the use of volatile anesthetics causing cerebral vasodilation.

Cooling

During cardiac surgery requiring deep hypothermic circulatory arrest, the EEG provides an effective method for assessing the effects of cooling. Optimal brain temperature may be viewed as a balance between decreased cerebral oxygen consumption and increased risk of coagulopathy. Actual brain temperature cannot be measured directly and appears to be influenced by many variables, including the rate of cooling as well as acid-base and anesthetic management. The EEG is often used to assess the functional consequences of brain cooling, because a flat-line pattern signifies cortical synaptic quiescence. The wide interpatient variation in flat-line temperature is the rationale for EEG guidance of the cooling process. Alternative use of a fixed temperature criterion increases the risks of both excessive and inadequate brain cooling.

III

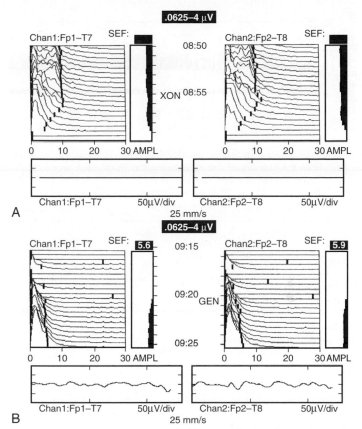

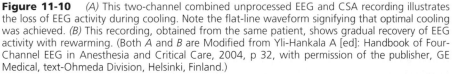

Figure 11-10 *(A)* This two-channel combined unprocessed EEG and CSA recording illustrates the loss of EEG activity during cooling. Note the flat-line waveform signifying that optimal cooling was achieved. *(B)* This recording, obtained from the same patient, shows gradual recovery of EEG activity with rewarming. (Both *A* and *B* are Modified from Yli-Hankala A [ed]: Handbook of Four-Channel EEG in Anesthesia and Critical Care, 2004, p 32, with permission of the publisher, GE Medical, text-Ohmeda Division, Helsinki, Finland.)

11

As nasopharyngeal or tympanic temperature decreases to 28°C (Fig. 11-10), there is a gradual loss of absolute spectral power across all frequency bands. Although the reversible decreases in absolute spectral band power are quite large, computing these changes as relative spectral band power minimizes these changes, suggesting that initial brain cooling exerts a similar decrease in spectral power across all frequency bands and cortical regions.[7] Cooling below 28°C leads to progressive slowing of the residual EEG until the EEG waveform becomes a flat line.

Rewarming

After circulatory arrest, the EEG documents the recovery of synaptic function during rewarming. However, rapid rewarming may result in cerebral ischemia due to cold-triggered vasoparesis, which uncouples cerebral blood flow and metabolism.

Myocardial Revascularization without Extracorporeal Support

The most recent significant advance in cardiac surgery has been myocardial revascularization on a beating heart. Avoidance of CPB may protect patients from the many potential hazards of this nonphysiologic insult. In addition, its potential economic

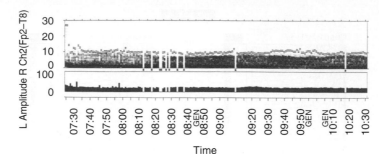

Figure 11-11 Note the stability of the EEG during this myocardial revascularization without cardiopulmonary bypass. (Modified from Yli-Hankala A [ed]: Handbook of Four-Channel EEG in Anesthesia and Critical Care. Helsinki, GE Medical, Datex-Ohmeda Division, 2004.)

BOX 11-8 *Important Imbalances Identified with EEG*

- Preexisting EEG abnormality
- Hypnotic effect
- Head malposition
- Hypocarbia-induced cerebral ischemia
- Malperfusion syndrome
- Need for blood replacement
- Optimal cooling and rewarming technique
- Seizures

---

advantages promise widespread application. Figure 11-11 illustrates the typical remarkable stability of the EEG during a beating heart coronary revascularization despite transient hypotension and bradycardia.

Seizure Detection

Certain anesthetics and adjuvants such as etomidate, enflurane, sevoflurane, and the opioid analgesics may produce seizure-like EEG activity, although the clinical manifestations may be obscured by neuromuscular blockade. Perioperative EEG seizure activity in infant cardiac surgery patients was associated with a 10-point decline in expected intelligence quotient when subsequently measured in the patients' fifth year after surgery (Box 11-8).

AUDITORY EVOKED POTENTIALS

Auditory evoked potentials (AEPs) assess specific areas of the brainstem, midbrain, and auditory cortices. Because of their simplicity, objectivity, and reproducibility, AEPs are suitable for monitoring patients during cardiovascular surgery. Specific applications of AEP monitoring in this environment are the assessment of temperature effects on brainstem function and evaluation of hypnotic effect.

Acoustic stimuli trigger a neural response integrated by a synchronized neuronal depolarization that travels from the auditory nerve to the cerebral cortex. Scalp-recorded signals, obtained from electrodes located at the vertex and ear lobe, contain both the AEPs and other unrelated EEG and EMG activity. Extraction of the relatively low-amplitude AEPs from the larger amplitude background activity requires signal-averaging techniques. Because the AEP character remains constant for each stimulus repetition, averaging of many repetitions suppresses the inconstant background. For the AEP sensory stimulus, acoustic clicks are the most commonly used. These broadband signals are generated by unidirectional rectangular short pulses (40 to 500 µs) with frequency spectra below 10 kHz.

The specific benefit of AEPs to cardiac surgery derives from their temperature sensitivity, because cooling slows both axonal conduction and synaptic transmission. A decrease of tympanic or nasopharyngeal temperature from 35° to 25°C doubles wave V latency. Further cooling will eventually suppress waves III to V completely, signifying the virtual elimination of synaptic transmission within the brainstem auditory circuits. Brainstem AEPs (BAEPs) document complete deep hypothermic electrocerebral silence before temporary circulatory arrest.[8]

The critical protective action of hypothermia on the brain cannot be accurately assessed by thermometry because of marked individual differences in thermal compartmentation throughout the body. Even within the brain, cooling technique (e.g., rapid vs. slow, alpha-stat vs. pH-stat acid-base balance, α-adrenergic blockade vs. none) may result in substantial thermal inhomogeneity within the cerebrum. Therefore, hypothermia-induced electrocortical silence (i.e., flat EEG) does not necessarily indicate cessation of synaptic activity within deep brain structures. The high metabolic rates of some of these structures (e.g., basal ganglia and inferior colliculus) render them particularly vulnerable to ischemic injury. EEG quiescence plus a loss of BAEP waves III to V ensures thorough cooling of the brain core. This approach appears to offer an optimal neuroprotective environment during temporary cessation of cerebral perfusion (Box 11-9).

TRANSCRANIAL DOPPLER ULTRASONOGRAPHY

Ultrasound Technology

Ultrasonic probes of a clinical transcranial Doppler (TCD) sonogram contain an electrically activated piezoelectric crystal that transmits low power 1- to 2-mHz acoustic vibrations (i.e., insonation) through the thinnest portion of temporal bone (i.e., acoustic window) into brain tissue. Blood constituents (predominantly erythrocytes), contained in large arteries and veins, reflect these ultrasonic waves back to the probe, which also serves as a receiver. Because of laminar blood flow, erythrocytes traveling in the central region of a large blood vessel move with higher velocity than those near the vessel wall. Thus, within each vascular segment (i.e., sample volume), a series of echoes associated with varying velocities is created. The frequency differences between the insonation signal and each echo in the series are proportional to the associated velocity, and this velocity is determined from the Doppler equation. Although several large intracranial arteries may be insonated through the temporal window, the middle cerebral artery (MCA) is generally monitored during cardiac surgery because it carries approximately 40% of the hemispheric blood flow.

The cerebral oximeter has detected potentially catastrophic cerebral desaturation due to great vessel torsion during cardiac manipulation. Desaturation often appears to be the result of compromised venous return. Particularly in pediatric cardiac operations and in myocardial revascularization without CPB, cardiac manipulation may produce sudden large rSo_2 decreases without any appreciable change in mean arterial pressure or arterial oxygen saturation.

Fukada and coworkers reported cerebral oximetric detection and successful correction of a malperfusion syndrome during acute type A aortic dissection repair.[16] Although parallel recording of radial and femoral arterial pressures is widely used to detect malperfusion, no pressure difference was seen in this case owing to maintenance of perfusion in the leftmost arch branch. Malperfusion-related cerebral ischemia may often be identified by EEG or somatosensory evoked potentials, but these signals are susceptible to compromise by electrocautery, deep anesthesia, and hypothermia. Cerebral oximetry is also used during extracorporeal membrane oxygenation to detect regional deficiencies in brain perfusion associated with carotid cannulation.

rSo_2 Responsiveness to CO_2

Acid-base management during CPB remains controversial, particularly during deep cooling. Some propose that the higher CO_2 tension afforded by pH-stat acid-base management results in fewer neurologic complications. Vijay and colleagues observed that during adult near-normothermic myocardial revascularization, vasopressor-induced perfusion pressure increases alone were sometimes inadequate to correct decreased rSo_2 occurring during CPB. In this situation, judiciously applied permissive hypercapnia often was effective in restoring rSo_2 to baseline.[17]

Despite these seeming benefits, hypercapnia has potentially deleterious effects. Hypercapnia-induced cardiac output and heart rate also increase myocardial oxygen demand, whereas cerebral vasodilation may exacerbate preexisting intracranial hypertension. Cerebral oximetry provides a convenient method to document appropriate bihemispheric CO_2 reactivity (Box 11-13). In addition, continuous measurement of brain oxygen saturation permits CO_2 titration to achieve optimal tissue perfusion at the lowest risk. Individualized management of CO_2 tension facilitated by cerebral oximetry enhances the opportunity for anesthesia providers and perfusionists to positively affect the outcome of cardiovascular surgery.

BOX 11-13 *Important Imbalances Identified by Cerebral Oximetry*

- Preexisting cerebral oxygen imbalance
- Position-related asymmetry
- Cerebral arterial CO_2 reactivity and autoregulation
- Need for blood replacement
- Volume status
- Perfusion cannula malposition
- Malperfusion syndrome
- Optimal brain cooling and rewarming
- Successful supplementary cerebral perfusion during circulatory arrest

---

NEUROMONITORING AND OUTCOME

Outcome studies of EEG monitoring primarily have concentrated on process variables, describing occurrences of ischemic EEG changes and their possible association with neurologic complications. To date, the results of only one adequately powered prospective randomized study on EEG clinical and economic benefit have been published. Myles and associates demonstrated a significant 82% decrease in awareness with BIS monitoring. This finding replicated the results of a large nonrandomized study, which showed that BIS monitoring was associated with a 78% decrease in awareness. Both these results are consistent with a number of smaller, nonrandomized studies.[18,19]

There are two outcome studies that have examined the impact of multimodality neuromonitoring using a combination of EEG, TCD, and cerebral oximetry[20,21] (Fig. 11-18). Both found a 2.7-day reduction in length of stay associated with multimodality neuromonitoring. The study of Edmonds also noted an 11% reduction in hospital expenses.[20] In addition to the substantial reductions in hospital stay, charges, and neurologic complications, the results suggested possible benefit to other vital organ systems. This finding is not unexpected because the same processes that injure the brain may also injure other organs. Future studies of neuromonitoring efficacy should not overlook these important accessory benefits. In addition, Lozano and Mossad reviewed studies of neuromonitoring during pediatric cardiac surgery and showed that the monitoring was associated with enhanced outcomes (Table 11-1).[22]

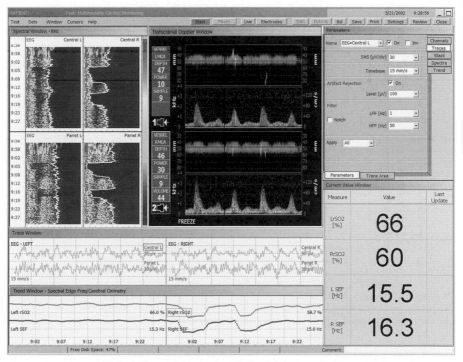

Figure 11-18 Multimodality neuromonitoring (EEG, TCD, and cerebral oximetry) viewed on a single computer screen. Note the loss in right hemisphere EEG high-frequency activity with associated declines in both SEF and rSo$_2$ and the presence of emboliform HITS in the power M-mode and spectral TCD displays. (Courtesy of Howard Bailin, Axon Instruments, Hauppauge, NY.)

Table 11-1   Multimodality Neuromonitoring for Cardiac Surgery

Modality	Function
Electroencephalography	Cortical synaptic activity
Middle latency auditory evoked potentials	Subcortical-cortical activity
Brainstem auditory evoked potentials	Brainstem synaptic activity
Transcranial Doppler	Blood flow change and emboli
Cerebral oximetry	Cortical oxygen balance

SUMMARY

- Cardiac surgery–associated brain injury is common, multifactorial, and often preventable.
- Electroencephalography can detect cerebral ischemia/hypoxia and seizures and measure hypnotic effect.
- Middle-latency auditory evoked potentials objectively document inadequate hypnosis.
- Brainstem auditory evoked potentials measure the effects of cooling and rewarming on deep brain structures.
- Transcranial Doppler ultrasonography assesses the direction and character of blood flow through large intracranial arteries and identifies microemboli.
- Cerebral oximetry, using spatially resolved transcranial near-infrared spectroscopy, provides a continuous measure of change in the balance of cerebral oxygen supply and demand.
- Used in concert, these technologies can reduce the incidence of brain injury and ensure the adequacy of hypnosis.

REFERENCES

1. Newman MF, Kirchner JL, Phillips-Bute B, et al: Longitudinal assessment of neurocognitive function after coronary artery bypass surgery. N Engl J Med 344:395, 2001
2. Kilo J, Dzerny M, Gorlitzer M, et al: Cardiopulmonary bypass affects cognitive brain function after coronary artery bypass grafting. Ann Thorac Surg 72:1926, 2001
3. Pronk RAF: EEG Processing in Cardiac Surgery. Utrecht, Inst Med Physics TNO, 1982
4. Gugino LD, Chabot RJ, Prichep LSD, et al: Quantitative EEG changes associated with loss and return of consciousness in healthy adult volunteers anaesthetized with propofol or sevoflurane. Br J Anaesth 87:421, 2001
5. Vakkuri A, Yli-Hankala A, Talja P, et al: Time-frequency balanced spectral entropy as a measure of anesthetic effect in central nervous system during sevoflurane, propofol, and thiopental anesthesia, Acta Anaesthesiol Scand 48:145, 2004
6. Viertiö-Oja H, Maja V, Särkelä M, et al: Description of the Entropy™ algorithm as applied in the Datex-Omeda S/5™ Entropy Module. Acta Anaesthesiol Scand 48:154, 2004
7. Gugino LD, Chabot RJ, Aglio LS, et al: QEEG changes during cardiopulmonary bypass: Relationship to postoperative neuropsychological function. Clin Electroencephalogr 30:53, 1999
8. Kumar A, Bhattacharya A: Evoked potential monitoring in anaesthesia and analgesia. Anaesthesia 55:225, 2000
9. Gugino LD, Aglio LS, Edmonds HL Jr: Neurophysiological monitoring in vascular surgery. Bailliere's Clin Anaesth 14:17, 2000
10. Edmonds HL Jr: Emboli and renal dysfunction in CABG patients [editorial]. J Cardiothorac Vasc Anesth 18:545, 2004
11. Watzman HM, Kurth CD, Montenegro LM, et al: Arterial and venous contributions to near-infrared cerebral oximetry. Anesthesiology 93:947, 2000

12. Pigula FA, Siewers RD, Nemoto E: Hypothermic cardiopulmonary bypass alters oxygen/glucose uptake in the pediatric brain. J Thorac Cardiovasc Surg 121:366, 2001
13. Monk TG, Reno KA, Olsen BS, et al: Postoperative cognitive dysfunction is associated with cerebral oxygen desaturations. Anesthesiology 93:A167, 2000
14. Madsen PL, Nielsen HB, Christiansen P: Well-being and cerebral oxygen saturation during acute heart failure in humans. Clin Physiol 20:158, 2000
15. Bar-Yosef S, Sanders EG, Grocott HP: Asymmetric cerebral near-infrared oximetric measurements during cardiac surgery. J Cardiothorac Vasc Anesth 17:773, 2003
16. Fukada J, Morishita K, Kawaharada N: Isolated cerebral perfusion for intraoperative cerebral malperfusion in type A aortic dissection. Ann Thorac Surg 75:266, 2003
17. Vijay V, McCusker K, Stasko A, et al: Cerebral oximetry-directed permissive hypercapnia enhances cerebral perfusion during CPB for heart failure surgery. Heart Surg Forum 6:205, 2003
18. Myles PS, Leslie K, McNeil J, et al: Bispectral index monitoring to prevent awareness during anesthesia: The B-Aware randomized controlled trial. Lancet 363:1757, 2004
19. Ekman A, Lindholm M-L, Lenmarken C, et al: Reduction in the incidence of awareness using BIS monitoring, Acta Anaesthesiol Scand 48:20, 2004
20. Edmonds HL Jr: Multi-modality neurophysiologic monitoring for cardiac surgery. Heart Surg Forum 5:225, 2002
21. Laschinger J, Razumovsky AY, Stierer KA, et al: Cardiac surgery: Value of neuromonitoring. Heart Surg Forum 6:204, 2003
22. Lozano S, Mossad E: Cerebral function monitors during pediatric cardiac surgery: Can they make a difference? J Cardiothorac Vasc Anesth 18:645, 2004

11

Chapter 12

Coagulation Monitoring

Linda Shore-Lesserson, MD

<table>
<tr><td>

Monitoring Heparin Effect

Activated Coagulation Time
Heparin Resistance
Heparin-Induced Thrombocytopenia
Measurement of Heparin Sensitivity
Heparin Concentration
High-Dose Thrombin Time

Heparin Neutralization

Protamine Effects on Coagulation Monitoring
Monitoring for Heparin Rebound

Heparin Neutralization Monitors

Thrombin Time
Bedside Tests of Heparin Neutralization
Heparinase

Tests of Coagulation

Bedside Tests of Coagulation
Fibrinogen Level

</td><td>

Monitoring Fibrinolysis

Viscoelastic Tests
End Products of Fibrin Degradation
Monitoring the Thrombin Inhibitors
Hirudin
Bivalirudin

Monitoring Platelet Function

Platelet Count
Bleeding Time
Aggregometry
Platelet-Mediated Force Transduction

Bedside Platelet Function Testing

Thromboelastography
Thromboelastography Modifications
Tests of Platelet Response to Agonist

Summary

References

</td></tr>
</table>

The need to monitor anticoagulation during and after surgery is the reason that the cardiac surgical arena has evolved into a major site for the evaluation and use of hemostasis monitors. The rapid and accurate identification of abnormal hemostasis has been the major impetus toward the development of point-of-care tests that can be performed at the bedside or in the operating room. The detection and treatment of specific coagulation disorders in a timely and cost-efficient manner are major goals in hemostasis monitoring for the cardiac surgical patient.

MONITORING HEPARIN EFFECT

Cardiac surgery had been performed for decades using empirical heparin dosing in the form of a bolus and subsequent interval dosing. Empirical dosing continued because of the lack of an easily applicable bedside test to monitor the anticoagulant effects of heparin.

The first clotting time to be used to measure heparin's effect was the whole-blood clotting time (WBCT), or the Lee-White WBCT. This simply requires whole blood to be placed in a glass tube, maintained at 37°C, and manually tilted until blood fluidity is no longer detected. This test fell out of favor for monitoring the cardiac surgical patient because it was so labor intensive and required the undivided attention of the person performing the test for periods up to 30 minutes. Although the glass surface of the test tube acts as an activator of factor XII, the heparin doses used for cardiac surgery prolong the WBCT to such a profound degree that the test is impractical as a monitor of the effect of heparin during cardiac surgery. To speed the clotting time so that the test was appropriate for clinical use, activators were added to the test tubes and the activated coagulation time (ACT) was introduced into practice.

Activated Coagulation Time

The ACT was first introduced by Hattersley in 1966 and is still the most widely used monitor of heparin effect during cardiac surgery. Whole blood is added to a test tube containing an activator—diatomaceous earth (celite) or kaolin. The presence of activator augments the contact activation phase of coagulation, which stimulates the intrinsic coagulation pathway. ACT can be performed manually, whereby the operator measures the time interval from when blood is injected into the test tube to when clot is seen along the sides of the tube. More commonly, the ACT is automated as it is in the Hemochron and Hemotec systems. In the automated system, the test tube is placed in a device that warms the sample to 37°C. The Hemochron device (International Technidyne Corp., Edison, NJ) rotates the test tube, which contains celite activator and a small iron cylinder, to which 2 mL of whole blood is added. Before clot forms, the cylinder rolls along the bottom of the rotating test tube. When clot forms, the cylinder is pulled away from a magnetic detector, interrupts a magnetic field, and signals the end of the clotting time. Normal ACT values range from 80 to 120 seconds. The Hemochron ACT can also be performed using kaolin as the activator in a similar manner (Fig. 12-1).

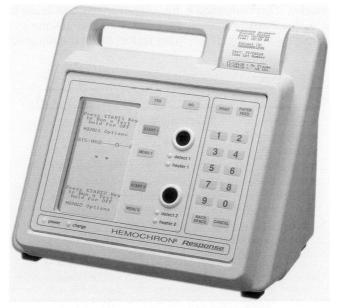

Figure 12-1 The Hemochron Response is a dual-chamber point-of-care coagulation monitor that is capable of measuring clotting times that are compatible with Hemochron technology. This system has software capability for calculation, data management, and storage of results. (Courtesy of International Technidyne Corp., Edison, NJ, http://www.itcmed.com)

The Hemotec ACT device (Medtronic Hemotec, Parker, CO) is a cartridge with two chambers that contain kaolin activator and is housed in a heat block. Blood (0.4 mL) is placed into each chamber and a daisy-shaped plunger is raised and passively falls into the chamber. The formation of clot will slow the rate of descent of the plunger, and this decrease in velocity of the plunger is detected by a photo-optical system that signals the end of the ACT test. The Hemochron and Hemotec ACTs have been compared in a number of investigations and have been found to differ significantly at low heparin concentrations.[1] However, differences in heparin concentration, activator concentration, and the measurement technique make comparison of these tests difficult and have led to the realization that the Hemochron ACT result and the Hemotec ACT result are not interchangeable. In adult patients given 300 U/kg of heparin for cardiopulmonary bypass (CPB), the Hemochron and Hemotec (Hepcon) ACTs were both therapeutic at all time points; however, at two points, the Hemochron ACT was statistically longer. This difference was even more pronounced in pediatric patients, who have higher heparin consumption rates. The apparent "overestimation" of ACT by the Hemochron device during hypothermic CPB may be due to the different volumes of blood that each assay warms to 37°C.

The ACT test can be modified by the addition of heparinase. Using this modification, the coagulation status of the patient can be monitored during CPB while the anticoagulant effects of heparin are eliminated. Because this test is a side-by-side comparison of the untreated ACT to the heparinase ACT, it also has the advantage of being a rapid test for the assessment of a circulating heparin-like substance or for residual heparinization after CPB.

With the introduction of ACT monitoring into the cardiac surgical arena, clinicians have been able to more accurately titrate heparin and protamine dosages. As a result, many investigators report reductions in blood loss and transfusion requirements, although many of these studies used retrospective analyses. The improvements in postoperative hemostasis documented with ACT monitoring are potentially attributed to better intraoperative suppression of microvascular coagulation and improved monitoring of heparin reversal with protamine.

ACT monitoring of heparinization is not without pitfalls, and its use has been criticized because of the extreme variability of the ACT and the absence of a correlation with plasma heparin levels (Fig. 12-2). Many factors have been suggested to alter the

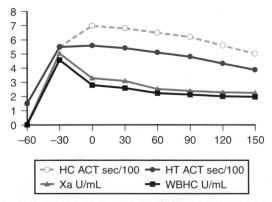

Figure 12-2 Anticoagulation measured at baseline (−60 minutes), heparinization (−30 minutes), and six time points after institution of cardiopulmonary bypass (CPB). Note the close correlation between the anti–factor Xa (Xa) activity and whole blood heparin concentration (WBHC), which does not parallel the change in Hemochron (HC ACT) or Hemotec activated coagulation time (HT ACT). (Modified from Despotis GJ, Summerfield AL, Joist JH: Comparison of activated coagulation time and whole blood heparin measurements with laboratory plasma anti-Xa heparin concentration in patients having cardiac operations. J Thorac Cardiovasc Surg 108:1076-1082, 1994.)

ACT, and these factors are prevalent during cardiac surgical procedures. When the extracorporeal circuit prime is added to the patient's blood volume, hemodilution occurs and may theoretically increase ACT. Evidence suggests that this degree of hemodilution alone is not enough to actually alter ACT. Hypothermia increases ACT in a "dose-related" fashion. It has been shown that although hemodilution and hypothermia significantly increase the ACT of a heparinized blood sample, similar increases do not occur in the absence of added heparin. The effects of platelet alterations are a bit more problematic. At mild to moderate degrees of thrombocytopenia, the baseline and heparinized ACT are not affected. It is not until platelet counts are reduced to below 30,000 to 50,000/μL that ACT may be prolonged. Patients treated with platelet inhibitors such as prostacyclin, aspirin, or platelet membrane receptor antagonists have a prolonged heparinized ACT compared with patients not treated with platelet inhibitors. This ACT prolongation is not exclusively related to decreased levels of platelet factor 4 (PF4) (PF4 is a heparin-neutralizing substance), because it also occurs when blood is anticoagulated with substances that are not neutralized by PF4. Platelet lysis, however, significantly shortens the ACT due to the release of PF4, and other platelet membrane components, which may have heparin-neutralizing activities. Anesthesia and surgery also decrease the ACT and create a hypercoagulable state, possibly by creating a thromboplastic response or through activation of platelets.

During CPB, heparin decay varies substantially and its measurement is problematic because hemodilution and hypothermia alter the metabolism of heparin. In a CPB study, the consumption of heparin varied from 0.01 to 3.86 U/kg/min and there was no correlation between the initial sensitivity to heparin and the rate of heparin decay. In the pediatric population, the consumption of heparin is increased above that of adult levels. The heparin administration protocol for pediatric patients undergoing CPB should account for a large volume of distribution, increased consumption, and a shorter elimination half-life. In monitoring the effects of heparin in pediatric patients, the minimum acceptable ACT value should be increased or an additional monitor should be used.

Heparin Resistance

Heparin resistance is documented by an inability to raise the ACT of blood to expected levels despite an adequate dose and plasma concentration of heparin. In many clinical situations, especially when heparin desensitization or a heparin inhibitor is suspected, heparin resistance can be treated by administering increased doses of heparin in a competitive fashion. If an adequately prolonged clotting time is ultimately achieved using higher-than-expected doses of heparin, a better term than *heparin resistance* would be *heparin tachyphylaxis* or "altered heparin responsiveness." During cardiac surgical procedures, the belief that a safe minimum ACT value of 300 to 400 seconds is required for CPB is based on a few clinical studies and a relative paucity of scientific data. However, inability to attain this degree of anticoagulation in the heparin-resistant patient engenders the fear among cardiac surgical providers that the patient will experience a microvascular consumptive coagulopathy or that clots will form in the extracorporeal circuit.

Many clinical conditions are associated with heparin resistance. Sepsis, liver disease, and pharmacologic agents represent just a few (Table 12-1). Many investigators have documented decreased levels of antithrombin III (ATIII) secondary to heparin pretreatment, whereas others have not found decreased ATIII levels.[2] In patients receiving preoperative heparin infusions, lower baseline ACT was the only risk factor found for predicting heparin resistance compared with patients not receiving preoperative heparin.

12

Table 12-1   Disease States Associated with Heparin Resistance

Disease State	Comment
Newborn	Decreased ATIII levels until 6 months of age
Venous thromboembolism	May have increased factor VIII level
	Accelerated clearance of heparin
Pulmonary embolism	Accelerated clearance of heparin
Congenital ATIII deficiency	40% to 60% of normal ATIII concentration
Type I	Reduced synthesis of normal/ abnormal ATIII
Type II	Molecular defect within the ATIII molecule
Acquired ATIII deficiency	<25% of normal ATIII concentration
Preeclampsia	Levels unchanged in normal pregnancy
Cirrhosis	Decreased protein synthesis
Nephrotic syndrome	Increased urinary excretion of ATIII
DIC	Increased consumption of ATIII
Heparin pretreatment	85% of normal ATIII concentration due to accelerated clearance
Estrogen therapy	Decreased protein synthesis
Cytotoxic drug therapy (L-asparaginase)	Decreased protein synthesis

ATIII = antithrombin III; DIC = disseminated intravascular coagulation.

Patients receiving preoperative heparin therapy traditionally require larger heparin doses to achieve a given level of anticoagulation when that anticoagulation is measured by the ACT. Presumably, this "heparin resistance" is due to deficiencies in the level or activity of ATIII. Other possible causes include enhanced factor VIII activity and platelet dysfunction causing a decrease in ACT response to heparin. In vitro addition of ATIII enhances the ACT response to heparin. ATIII concentrate is now available and represents a reasonable method of treating patients with documented ATIII deficiency.[3]

Heparin-Induced Thrombocytopenia

The syndrome known as heparin-induced thrombocytopenia (HIT) develops in anywhere from 5% to 28% of patients receiving heparin. HIT is commonly categorized into two subtypes. HIT type I is characterized by a mild decrease in platelet count and is the result of the proaggregatory effects of heparin on platelets. HIT type II is considerably more severe, most often occurs after more than 5 days of heparin administration (average onset time, 9 days), and is mediated by antibody binding to the complex formed between heparin and PF4. Associated immune-mediated endothelial injury and complement activation cause platelets to adhere, aggregate, and form platelet clots, or "white clots." Among patients developing HIT II, the incidence of thrombotic complications approximates 20%, which in turn may carry a mortality rate as high as 40%. Demonstration of heparin-induced proaggregation of platelets confirms the diagnosis of HIT type II. This can be accomplished with a heparin-induced serotonin release assay or a specific heparin-induced platelet activation assay. A highly specific enzyme-linked immunosorbent assay for the heparin/PF4 complex has been developed and has been used to delineate the course of IgG and IgM antibody responses in patients exposed to unfractionated heparin during cardiac surgery. Bedside antibody tests are being developed that may speed the diagnosis of this condition.

The options for treating these patients are few. If the clinician has the luxury of being able to discontinue the heparin for a few weeks, often the antibody disappears and allows a brief period of heparinization for CPB without complication.[4] Changing the tissue source of heparin was an option when bovine heparin was predominantly in use. Some types of low-molecular-weight heparin (LMWH) have been administered to patients with HIT, but reactivity of the particular LMWH with the patient's platelets should be confirmed in vitro. Supplementing heparin administration with pharmacologic platelet inhibition using prostacyclin, iloprost, aspirin, or aspirin and dipyridamole has been reported, all with favorable outcomes. Tirofiban with unfractionated heparin has been used in this clinical circumstance. Plasmapheresis may be used to reduce antibody levels. The use of heparin could be avoided altogether through anticoagulation with direct thrombin inhibitors such as argatroban, hirudin, or bivalirudin. These thrombin inhibitors have become standard of care in the management of the patient with HIT II. Monitoring their effects during CPB is more complex.

Measurement of Heparin Sensitivity

Even in the absence of heparin resistance, patient response to an intravenous bolus of heparin is extremely variable. The variability stems from different concentrations of various endogenous heparin-binding proteins such as vitronectin and PF4. This variability exists whether measuring heparin concentration or the ACT; however, variability seems to be greater when measuring the ACT. Because of the large interpatient variation in heparin responsiveness and the potential for heparin resistance, it is critical that a functional monitor of heparin anticoagulation (with or without a measure of heparin concentration) be used in the cardiac surgical patient. A threefold range of ACT response to a 200-U/kg heparin dose and similar discrepancy in heparin decay rates was documented, and therefore, the use of individual patient dose-response curves is needed to determine the optimal heparin dose. This is the concept on which point-of-care individual heparin dose-response (HDR) tests are based.

An HDR curve can be generated manually using the baseline ACT and the ACT response to an in vivo or in vitro dose of heparin. Extrapolation to the desired ACT provides the additional heparin dose required for that ACT. Once the actual ACT response to the heparin dose is plotted, further dose-response calculations are made based on the average of the target ACT and the actual ACT (Fig. 12-3). This methodology was first described by Bull and associates and forms the scientific basis for the automated dose-response systems manufactured by Hemochron and Hemotec. The Hemochron RxDx system uses the heparin-response test (HRT), which is an ACT with a known quantity of in vitro heparin (3 IU/mL). Using an algorithm that incorporates the patient's baseline ACT, estimated blood volume, and HRT, a dose-response curve is generated that enables calculation of the heparin dose required to attain the target ACT. The patient's heparin sensitivity can be calculated in seconds/IU/mL by dividing the HRT by 3 IU/mL.

The RxDx system also provides an individualized protamine dose using the protamine response test (PRT). This is an ACT with one of two specific quantities of protamine, depending on the amount of circulating heparin suspected (2 IU/mL or 3 IU/mL). Using the patient's heparinized ACT, the PRT, and an estimate of the patient's blood volume, the protamine dose needed to return the ACT to baseline can be calculated based on a protamine-response curve. Jobes and coworkers reported that the heparin dose directed by the RxDx system resulted in ACT values well above the target ACT. In their patients, in vivo heparin sensitivity was higher than in vitro sensitivity. RxDx also resulted in lower protamine doses, lower

12

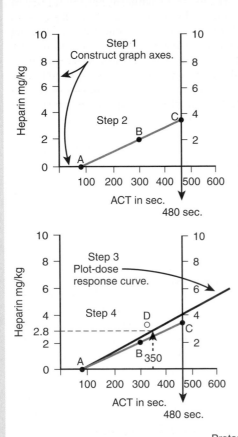

Step 1
Construct graph axes.

Step 2

Step 3
Plot-dose response curve.

Step 4

ACT in sec.

480 sec.

Heparin mg/kg

Step 2

Determine initial ACT (A) and administer 2 mg/kg heparin, then measure ACT (B) and plot both values.

Extrapolate an imaginary line through "A" and "B" to intersect with 480 second line to find point "C."

Example: 3.5 mg/kg heparin is needed to produce 480 sec. ACT or 1.5 mg/kg in addition to the 2 mg/kg heparin already given.

Step 3

After required heparin has been given, measure ACT. Plot point "D."

If point "D" does not superimpose on point "C," then a dose-response curve is drawn from "A" to a point midway between "C" and "D."

Step 4

After 60 minutes, measure the ACT. Determine amount of heparin in patient's circulation from the dose-response curve.

Example: Assume an ACT of 350 sec.; the heparin level would be 2.8 mg/kg. To return to 480 sec., 1.2 mg/kg of heparin is needed.

Step 5

To reverse anticoagulation, circulating heparin level is determined as in step 4. The neutralizing dose of protamine is heparin level mg/kg × 1.3.
Example: ACT of 325 seconds is measured. Heparin level is 2.6 mg/kg, and 3.4 mg/kg protamine is required.

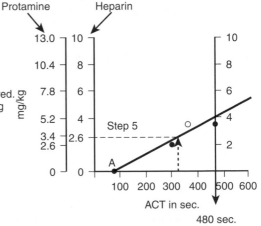

Protamine   Heparin

mg/kg

Step 5

ACT in sec.

480 sec.

Figure 12-3 Construction of a dose-response curve for heparin. ACT = activated coagulation time. (From Bull BS, Huse WM, Brauer FS, et al: Heparin therapy during extracorporeal circulation: II. The use of a dose-response curve to individualize heparin and protamine dosage. J Thorac Cardiovasc Surg 69:685-689, 1975.)

postoperative mediastinal tube losses, and reduced transfusion requirements compared with a ratio-based system of heparin/protamine administration.[5] In a larger study that standardized the treatment of heparin rebound, the reduced protamine dose was confirmed; however, the reductions in bleeding were not substantiated. The use of a protamine dose-response curve has been shown to successfully reduce the protamine dose in vascular surgery compared with standard weight-based protamine dosing.[6]

The Hepcon HMS system uses the HDR cartridge in the Hepcon instrument (Fig. 12-4). Each cartridge houses six chambers. Chambers 1 and 2 contain heparin at a concentration of 2.5 U/mL, chambers 3 and 4 contain heparin at a concentration of 1.5 U/mL, and chambers 5 and 6 do not contain heparin. Once information regarding patient weight, height, and CPB prime volume is entered, the information that can be obtained from this test includes the baseline ACT (chambers 5 and 6) and an HDR slope. The dose-response slope, which is the increase in ACT from 1.5 U/mL to 2.5 U/mL heparin, is extrapolated to the desired target ACT or target heparin concentration and the heparin dose is calculated.

Heparin Concentration

Proponents of ACT measurement to guide anticoagulation for CPB argue that a functional assessment of the anticoagulant effect of heparin is mandatory and that the variability in ACT represents a true variability in the coagulation status of the patient. Opponents argue that during CPB the sensitivity of the ACT to heparin is altered and ACT does not correlate with heparin concentration or with anti–factor Xa activity measurement. Heparin concentration can be measured using the Hepcon HMS system (Medtronic Hemotec), which uses an automated protamine titration technique. With a cartridge with four or six chambers containing tissue thromboplastin

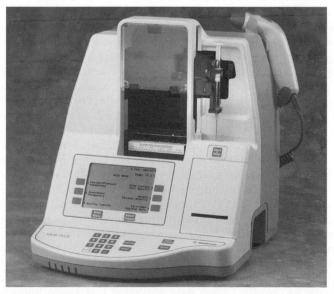

Figure 12-4 The HMS heparin management system has an automated dispenser that places the appropriate volume of whole blood into each chamber of the test cartridge. A variety of assays can be performed in this instrument, depending on the cartridge used. (Courtesy of Medtronic Inc., Parker, CO, http://www.medtronic.com/cardsurgery/bloodmgmt/hmsplus.html)

12

and a series of known protamine concentrations, 0.2 mL of whole blood is automatically dispensed into the chambers. The first channel to clot is the channel whose protamine concentration most accurately neutralizes the heparin without a heparin or a protamine excess. Because protamine neutralizes heparin in the ratio of 1 mg of protamine per 100 U of heparin, the concentration of heparin in the blood sample can be calculated. A cartridge that monitors heparin concentration over a wide range can be used first, followed by another cartridge that can measure heparin concentrations within a narrower range. The maintenance of a stable heparin concentration rather than a specific ACT level usually results in higher doses of heparin being administered because the hemodilution and hypothermia on CPB increase the sensitivity of the ACT to heparin. The measure of heparin concentration has been shown to more closely correlate with anti–factor Xa activity measurements than the ACT during CPB, although the precision and bias of the test may not prove to be acceptable for exclusive use clinically.

In a prospective randomized trial, Despotis and colleagues demonstrated that by using a transfusion algorithm in association with Hepcon-based heparin management, chest tube drainage was minimally reduced and transfusion of non–red blood cell products could be significantly reduced relative to a group of patients who had ACT-based heparin management.[7] They attributed their results to better preservation of the coagulation system by high heparin doses because the doses of heparin administered in the Hepcon group were nearly twice the doses used in the ACT management group. The Hepcon, remains one of the more sensitive tests for detecting residual heparinization after protamine reversal because the heparin concentration can be measured by protamine titration to levels as low as 0.4 IU/mL.

High-Dose Thrombin Time

A functional test of heparin-induced anticoagulation that correlates well with heparin levels is the high-dose thrombin time (HiTT; International Technidyne Inc., Edison, NJ). The TT is a clotting time that measures the conversion of fibrinogen to fibrin by thrombin. The TT is prolonged by the presence of heparin and by hypofibrinogenemias or dysfibrinogenemias. Because the TT is sensitive to very low levels of heparin, a high dose of thrombin is necessary in the TT to accurately assay the high doses of heparin used for CPB. The HiTT is performed by adding whole blood to a prewarmed, prehydrated test tube that contains a lyophilized thrombin preparation. After the addition of 1.5 mL of blood, the tube is inserted into a Hemochron well and the time to clot formation is measured. In vitro assays indicate that HiTT is equivalent to the ACT in evaluation of the anticoagulant effects of heparin at heparin concentrations in the range of 0 to 4.8 IU/mL. Unlike ACT, HiTT is not altered by hemodilution and hypothermia and has been shown to correlate better with heparin concentration than the ACT during CPB. While on CPB, heparin concentration and HiTT decrease while the Hemochron and the Hepcon ACT increase. Another potential advantage of HiTT monitoring occurs for patients receiving aprotinin therapy. In the presence of heparin, aprotinin augments the celite ACT, possibly because its kallikrein-inhibiting capacity prolongs activation of the intrinsic coagulation pathway by XIIa. This should not be interpreted to represent enhanced anticoagulation. The kaolin ACT is less affected by aprotinin therapy than the celite ACT, perhaps because kaolin, unlike celite, *activates* the intrinsic pathway by stimulation of factor XI directly. Others have suggested that kaolin binds to aprotinin and reduces the anticoagulant effect of aprotinin in vitro. However, the heparinized kaolin ACT is still somewhat prolonged in the presence of aprotinin. HiTT is not affected by aprotinin therapy and can be used as a measure of heparinization for CPB patients receiving aprotinin therapy. The high-dose thromboplastin time is another measure of anticoagulation that is not affected by aprotinin therapy. The high-dose thromboplastin time is a whole blood clotting time in which celite is replaced by 0.3 mL of rabbit brain thromboplastin to which 1.2 mL of blood is added. This test measures the time to coagulation via activation of the extrinsic pathway. This pathway of coagulation is also stimulated during pericardiotomy due to the rich thromboplastin environment of the pericardial cavity.

HEPARIN NEUTRALIZATION

Protamine Effects on Coagulation Monitoring

Reversal of heparin-induced anticoagulation is most frequently performed with protamine. Biologically, protamine binds to positively charged groups such as phosphate groups and may have important properties in angiogenesis and immune function. Different successful dosing plans have been proposed. The recommended dose of protamine for heparin reversal is 1 to 1.3 mg protamine per 100 U heparin; however, this dose often results in a protamine excess.

In addition to hemodynamic sequelae, protamine has adverse effects on coagulation.[8] Large doses prolong the WBCT and the ACT, possibly via thrombin inhibition. In animals and in humans, protamine has been associated with thrombocytopenia, likely due to activation of the complement cascade. The anticoagulant effect of protamine may also be due to inhibition of platelet aggregation, alteration in the platelet surface membrane, or depression of the platelet response to various agonists. These alterations in platelet function result from the presence of the heparin-protamine complex, not protamine alone. Protamine-heparin complexes activate ATIII in vitro and result in complement activation. The anticoagulant effects of free protamine occur when protamine is given in doses in excess of those used clinically; however, the risk of free protamine being the cause of a hemostatic defect is small, given the rapid clearance of protamine relative to heparin.

Monitoring for Heparin Rebound

The phenomenon referred to as heparin rebound describes the reestablishment of a heparinized state after heparin has been neutralized with protamine. Various explanations for heparin rebound have been proposed. The most commonly postulated is that rapid distribution and clearance of protamine occur shortly after protamine administration, leaving unbound heparin remaining after protamine clearance. Furthermore, endogenous heparin antagonists have an even shorter life span than protamine and are eliminated rapidly, resulting in free heparin concentrations. Also possible is the release of heparin from tissues considered heparin storage sites (endothelium, connective tissues). Endothelial cells bind and depolymerize heparin via PF4. Uptake into the cells of the reticuloendothelial system, vascular smooth muscle, and extracellular fluid may account for the storage of heparin that contributes to reactivation of heparin anticoagulation, referred to as *heparin rebound*.

Residual low levels of heparin can be detected by sensitive heparin concentration monitoring in the first hour after protamine reversal and can be present for up to 6 hours postoperatively. Increased bleeding as a result of heparin rebound may

12

273

occur, specifically when higher doses of heparin have been administered. Monitoring for heparin rebound can be accomplished using tests that are sensitive to low levels of circulating heparin. These tests are also useful monitors for confirmation of heparin neutralization at the conclusion of CPB.

HEPARIN NEUTRALIZATION MONITORS

To administer the appropriate dose of protamine at the conclusion of CPB, it would be ideal to measure the concentration of heparin present and give the dose of protamine necessary to neutralize only the circulating heparin. As a result of heparin metabolism and elimination, which vary considerably among individuals, the dose of protamine required to reverse a given dose of heparin decreases over time. Furthermore, protamine antagonizes the anti-IIa effects of heparin more effectively than the anti-Xa effects and thus varies in its potency depending on the source of heparin and its anti-IIa properties. Administration of a large fixed dose of protamine or a dose based on the total heparin dose given is no longer the standard of care and may result in an increased incidence of protamine-related adverse effects. An optimal dose of protamine is desired because unneutralized heparin results in clinical bleeding and an excess of protamine may produce an undesired coagulopathy. The use of individualized protamine dose-response curves uniformly results in a reduced protamine dose and has been shown to reduce postoperative bleeding.[9] One such dose-response test, the Hemochron PRT test, is an ACT performed on a heparinized blood sample that contains a known quantity of protamine. With knowledge of the ACT, PRT, and the estimated blood volume of the patient, the protamine dose needed to neutralize the existing heparin level can be extrapolated. The Hepcon instrument also has a protamine dose-response test, which is the protamine titration assay. The chamber that clots first contains the dose of protamine that most closely approximates the circulating dose of heparin. By measuring the circulating heparin level, the protamine dose required for its neutralization is calculated based on a specified heparin/protamine dose ratio.

At the levels of heparinization needed for cardiac surgery, tests that are sensitive to heparin become not clottable. ACT is relatively insensitive to heparin and is ideal for monitoring anticoagulation at high heparin levels but is too insensitive to accurately diagnose incomplete heparin neutralization. ACT had a high predictive value for adequate anticoagulation (confirmed by laboratory activated partial thromboplastin time [aPTT]) when greater than 225 seconds but was poorly predictive for inadequate anticoagulation when less than 225 seconds. The low levels of heparin present when heparin is incompletely neutralized are best measured by other more sensitive tests of heparin-induced anticoagulation, such as heparin concentration, aPTT, and TT. Thus, after CPB, confirmation of return to the unanticoagulated state should be performed with a sensitive test for heparin anticoagulation[10] (Box 12-1).

Thrombin Time

Thrombin time is the time it takes for the conversion of fibrinogen to fibrin clot when blood or plasma is exposed to thrombin. Fibrin strands form in seconds. Detection of fibrin formation using standard laboratory equipment involves incubation of the blood or plasma sample within the chamber in which an optical or electrical probe sits. A detector senses either movement of the probe or the creation of an electrical field (electrical detection) due to fibrin formation and hence signals the end of the test. Hemochron manufactures a point-of-care TT test that uses a lyophilized

---

BOX 12-1 *Heparin Neutralization*

- The most benign form of bleeding after cardiac surgery is due to residual heparinization.
- Treatment is with either protamine or another heparin-neutralizing product.
- Transfusion of allogeneic blood products is rarely indicated.
- Residual heparin can be measured by using:
  - A protamine titration assay
  - A heparin neutralized thrombin time assay
  - A heparinase ACT compared with ACT or
  - Any other heparinase test that compares itself with the test without heparinase added.

---

preparation of thrombin in a Hemochron test tube to which 1 mL of blood is added. Identification of fibrin formation in a Hemochron machine uses the standard Hemochron technology described previously with the ACT. The manufacturer suggests that the normal TT is 39 to 53 seconds for whole blood and 43 to 68 seconds for citrated blood. Because the TT specifically measures the activity of thrombin, it is very sensitive to heparin-induced enhancement of ATIII activity. It is a useful test in the post-CPB period for differentiating the cause of bleeding when both prothrombin time (PT) and aPTT are prolonged, because it excludes the intrinsic and extrinsic coagulation pathway limbs and evaluates the conversion of factor I to Ia. The TT is elevated in the presence of heparin, hypofibrinogenemia, dysfibrinogenemia, amyloidosis, or antibodies to thrombin. The TT is also elevated in the presence of fibrin degradation products if the systemic fibrinogen concentration is low.

The TT is an appropriate laboratory test for monitoring the degree of fibrinolytic activity in patients receiving thrombolytic therapy. Measurements of the quantity of fibrinogen, plasminogen, or plasma proteins generated during fibrinolysis are difficult to interpret and yield no prognostic information for dose adjustments. Thrombolytic agents activate the fibrinolytic system to generate plasmin, which then causes clot dissolution and decreases the quantities of fibrinogen and fibrin. This effect can be monitored using the TT. The TT should be measured at baseline (before institution of fibrinolytic therapy) and 3 to 4 hours after therapy is initiated. If it is prolonged by 1.5 to 5 times the baseline value, therapy should be considered effective. If the TT is prolonged by greater than 7 times the baseline value, an increased risk of bleeding is incurred; if the TT is not prolonged at all, therapy has failed to activate fibrinolysis.

Bedside Tests of Heparin Neutralization

Hepcon measures heparin concentration via a protamine titration assay. Cartridges with varying ranges of protamine concentration are available for use. The cartridge with the lower concentration of protamine in the titration is useful for the detection of residual circulating heparin and is sensitive to levels of heparin as low as 0.2 U/mL. Whole blood PT and aPTT assays are sensitive to deficiencies in coagulation factors and overly sensitive to low levels of heparin (aPTT); they lack specificity in assessing residual heparinization. The heparin-neutralized thrombin time (HNTT) is a TT assay with a small dose of protamine sufficient to neutralize 1.5 U/mL of heparin. Because the TT is elevated in the presence of heparin, hypofibrinogenemia, or dysfibrinogenemia, to discriminate among these three causes, HNTT and TT should be performed together. A normal HNTT in the presence of an elevated TT virtually confirms residual heparin effect and would indicate the need for protamine administration. If HNTT is prolonged as well as the TT, the cause of bleeding may be attributed either to a fibrinogen problem or to a concentration of heparin higher than that which could be neutralized by the HNTT. In one study comparing bedside monitors of anticoagulation, the TT-HNTT difference bore a significant correlation with the aPTT elevation. Using the line of best fit, aPTT elevation of 1.5 times the control corresponded to a 31-second difference in the TT and HNTT, indicating a convenient threshold value of TT-HNTT for the administration of protamine.

Heparinase

Heparinase (Neutralase I) is an enzyme that specifically degrades heparin by catalyzing cleavage of the saccharide bonds found in the heparin molecule. As demonstrated by the ACT, heparinase in a dose of 5 µg/kg has been shown to successfully neutralize heparin effects in healthy volunteers and in patients who have undergone CPB. A dose of 7 µg/kg has been demonstrated to be even more efficacious in returning ACT to baseline values. Doses sufficient to neutralize a dose of 300 U/kg had no significant hemodynamic effects in a canine model.[11] Investigators have not found any platelet-depressive effects of heparinase in contrast to the well-documented platelet dysfunction associated with protamine therapy. Return to the unanticoagulated state after the use of heparinase has been confirmed using ACT monitoring or heparin concentration monitoring.

TESTS OF COAGULATION

Standard tests of coagulation, the PT and the aPTT, are performed on plasma to which the anticoagulant citrate has been added. Because these tests are performed on plasma, they require centrifugation of blood and are generally not feasible for use at the bedside. The aPTT tests the integrity of the intrinsic and the final coagulation pathways and is more sensitive to low levels of heparin than the ACT. Factors IX and X are most sensitive to heparin effects, and thus the aPTT will be prolonged even at very low heparin levels. The test uses a phospholipid substance to simulate the interaction of the platelet membrane in activating factor XII. (Thromboplastin is a tissue extract containing tissue factor and phospholipid. The term *partial thromboplastin* refers to the use of the phospholipid portion only.) The aPTT is prolonged in the presence of deficiencies of factors XII, XI, IX, and VIII, HMWK, and kallikrein. The aPTT reaction is considerably slower than the PT; and in order to speed activation of factor XII, an activator such as celite or kaolin is added to the assay. After incubation of citrated plasma with phospholipid and activator, calcium is added and the time to clot formation is measured. Normal aPTT is 28 to 32 seconds, which is often expressed as a ratio with a control plasma sample from the same laboratory. This is important because partial thromboplastin reagents have different sensitivities to heparin and many have nonlinear responses to heparin in various concentration ranges.

PT measures the integrity of the extrinsic and common coagulation pathways. PT will be prolonged in the presence of factor VII deficiency, warfarin sodium (Coumadin) therapy, or vitamin K deficiency. Large doses of heparin also prolong the PT because of inactivation of factor II. The addition of thromboplastin to citrated plasma results in activation of extrinsic coagulation. After a 3-minute incubation and recalcification, the time to clot formation is measured and is recorded as the

PT. Normal PT is 12 to 14 seconds; however, due to differences in the quality and lot of the thromboplastin used, absolute PT values are not standardized and are difficult to compare across different testing centers. The international normalized ratio (INR) has been adopted as the standard for coagulation monitoring. The INR is an internationally standardized laboratory value that is the ratio of the patient's PT to the result that would have been obtained if the International Reference Preparation (IRP) had been used instead of the laboratory reagents. Each laboratory uses reagents with a specific sensitivity (International Sensitivity Index [ISI]) relative to the IRP. The ISI of a particular set of reagents is provided by each manufacturer so that the INR can be reported.

Bedside Tests of Coagulation

PT and aPTT tests performed on whole blood are available for use in the operating room or at the bedside. The Hemochron PT test tube contains acetone-dried rabbit brain thromboplastin to which 2 mL of whole blood is added and the tube is inserted into a standard Hemochron machine. Normal values range from 50 to 72 seconds and are automatically converted by a computer to the plasma equivalent PT and INR. Hemochron aPTT contains kaolin activator and a platelet factor substitute and is performed similarly to the PT. The aPTT is sensitive to heparin concentrations as low as 0.2 U/mL and displays a linear relationship with heparin concentration up to 1.5 U/mL.

The Ciba Corning Biotrack 512 coagulation monitor for evaluating bedside PT and aPTT uses 0.1 mL of whole blood placed into a disposable plastic cartridge for either PT or aPTT. The sample is drawn by capillary action into a heated chamber where exposure to reagents occurs. The PT uses rabbit brain thromboplastin. The aPTT uses soybean phosphatide as the platelet substitute and bovine brain sulfatide as the activator. From the reaction chamber, blood traverses a reaction path where clot formation is detected by a laser optical system. The resulting time to clot formation is converted to a ratio of the control value by a microprocessor that has control values encoded.

Many investigators have studied the Ciba Corning Biotrack system for monitoring anticoagulation in different clinical scenarios. For patients receiving oral anticoagulant therapy, the Biotrack 512 monitor has been found to be suitable for monitoring PT and INR. The bedside Biotrack aPTT with the laboratory aPTT and heparin level in patients receiving therapeutic heparinization after interventional cardiac catheterization have been compared. The authors found a strong correlation ($r = 0.89$) between the Biotrack aPTT and the aPTT from the hospital laboratory. The correlation between Biotrack aPTT and heparin level was not strong, probably because of the many other factors such as heparin neutralization and clearance that affect the heparin concentration in vivo. Another study in patients receiving heparin compared the Ciba Corning Biotrack aPTT assay with standard laboratory aPTT and documented that Biotrack was less sensitive to heparin than the laboratory aPTT; however, the correlation coefficient of these two tests was $r = 0.82$. In patients on warfarin therapy, the Biotrack aPTT was more sensitive than the laboratory aPTT and yielded consistently higher results for the aPTT value. In another study in patients being anticoagulated for nonsurgical applications, the bedside aPTT was similar to the standard aPTT in its prediction of treatment in simple therapeutic algorithms. However, in more complex clinical situations, there was less agreement between the bedside aPTT and laboratory aPTT.[12]

In a comparison of bedside coagulation monitors after cardiac surgical procedures, acceptable accuracy and precision levels for Hemochron and Ciba Corning Biotrack

12

PT in comparison with standard laboratory plasma PT, were documented, making them potentially valuable for use in the perioperative period. Neither Hemochron nor Ciba Corning aPTT reached this level of clinical competence compared with standard laboratory tests. Others have documented that this monitor seems to be more precise for PT than for aPTT. Because of rapid turn-around times, these point-of-care coagulation monitors may be useful in predicting patients who will bleed after cardiac surgery and have also been successfully used in transfusion algorithms to decrease the number of allogeneic blood products given to cardiac surgical patients.[13]

Fibrinogen Level

Fibrinogen concentration is traditionally measured using either clottable protein methods, endpoint detection techniques, or immunochemical tests. Of the former, the most commonly used fibrinogen assay relies on the method of Clauss. This method involves a 10-fold dilution of plasma, which ensures that fibrinogen is the rate-limiting step in clot formation. Subsequently, an excess of thrombin is added to the sample and the time to clot formation is measured. The clotting time is inversely related to the fibrinogen concentration. Because this assay relies on detection of actual clot, it can be affected by fibrin degradation products, polymerization inhibitors, or other inhibitors of fibrin formation. Because of the thrombin excess, small clinical concentrations of heparin do not affect fibrinogen determination according to the Clauss technique.

A whole blood point-of-care fibrinogen assay is available using the Hemochron system. The specific test tube contains a lyophilized preparation of human thrombin, snake venom extract, protamine, buffers, and calcium stabilizers. The test tube is incubated with 1.5 mL of distilled water and heated in the Hemochron instrument for 3 minutes. Whole blood is placed into a diluent vial, where it is 50% diluted, and from this vial, 0.5 mL of diluted whole blood is placed into the specific fibrinogen test tube. The clotting time is measured using standard Hemochron technology as described previously. The fibrinogen concentration is determined by comparison with a standard curve for this test. Normal fibrinogen concentration of 180 to 220 mg/dL correlates with a clotting time of 54 ± 2.5 seconds. Fibrinogen deficiency of 50 to 75 mg/dL correlates with a clotting time of 150 ± 9.0 seconds.

Unlike the method of Clauss, the endpoint detection assays rely on the detection of changes in turbidity of plasma when clot is formed. This technique does not require the maintenance of a stable cross-linked fibrin product and therefore does not report underestimated fibrinogen measurements due to the presence of inhibitors. Immunochemical measures of fibrinogen concentration are a direct and accurate measurement technique; however, they are expensive and time consuming and require specialized laboratory facilities.

MONITORING FIBRINOLYSIS

Fibrinolysis, the dissolution of fibrin, is the normal modifier of hemostasis that ensures that coagulation does not proceed unchecked. It occurs in the vicinity of a clot and dissolves clot when local endothelial healing occurs. Fibrinolysis is mediated by the serine protease plasmin, which is the product of the cleavage of plasminogen by tissue plasminogen activator. Fibrinolysis is a normal phenomenon in response to clot formation; when it occurs systemically, it represents a pathologic condition.

III

Fibrinolysis can be primary or secondary. Primary fibrinolysis occurs when fibrinolytic activators are released or produced in excess and do not represent a response to the coagulation process. Examples of primary fibrinolysis include the release of plasminogen activators during liver transplantation surgery and the exogenous administration of fibrinolytic agents such as streptokinase. During primary fibrinolysis, plasmin cleaves fibrinogen, yielding fibrinogen degradation products. These end products can be measured using immunologic techniques.

When fibrinolysis is a result of enhanced activation of the coagulation system, secondary fibrinolysis ensues. A well-known extreme form of secondary fibrinolysis is seen during disseminated intravascular coagulation, when both systemic coagulation and fibrinolysis are occurring in excess. During CPB, fibrinolysis is most likely secondary to the microvascular coagulation that is occurring despite attempts at suppression using high doses of heparin.

The identification of fibrinolysis can be accomplished through either direct measurement of the clot lysis time (manual or viscoelastic tests) or measurement of the end products of fibrin degradation. The manual clot lysis time simply involves the placement of whole blood into a test tube. This blood clots in a matter of minutes. Visual inspection determines the endpoint for observation of clot lysis, and this time period is the clot lysis time. This technique is considerably time consuming and requires constant observation by the person performing the test.

Viscoelastic Tests

Viscoelastic tests measure the unique properties of the clot as it is forming, organizing, strengthening, and lysing. As a result, fibrinolysis determination by this methodology requires that time elapse during which clot formation is occurring. It is subsequent to clot formation and platelet-fibrin linkages that clot lysis parameters can be measured. For this reason, viscoelastic tests often require longer than 1 hour to detect the initiation of fibrinolysis; however, if fibrinolysis is enhanced, results can often be obtained in 30 minutes.

End Products of Fibrin Degradation

Other methods for quantifying fibrinolysis include measurement of the end products of fibrin degradation. Fibrin degradation products are the result of the cleavage of fibrin monomers and polymers and can be measured using a latex agglutination assay. When plasmin cleaves cross-linked fibrin, dimeric units are formed that comprise one D-domain from each of two adjacent fibrin units. These "D-dimers" are frequently measured by researchers in clinical and laboratory investigations. They are measured by either enzyme-linked immunosorbent assays or latex agglutination techniques and thus are not available for on-site use. Controversy still exists regarding whether D-dimer level or fibrin degradation products are the most sensitive test for detecting fibrinolysis, but most agree that the presence of D-dimers is the most specific for cross-linked fibrin degradation.[14]

Monitoring the Thrombin Inhibitors

A new class of drugs, the selective thrombin inhibitors, is a viable alternative to heparin anticoagulation for CPB. These agents include hirudin, argatroban, and other experimental agents. A major advantage of these agents over heparin is that they are able to effectively inhibit clot-bound thrombin in an ATIII-independent fashion. The platelet thrombin receptor is believed to be the focus of thrombin's procoagulant effects in states of thrombosis such as after coronary artery angioplasty. Because

12

surface-bound thrombin is more effectively suppressed, thrombin generation can be reduced at lower levels of systemic anticoagulation than are achieved during anti-coagulation by the heparin-ATIII complex. This translates into less bleeding despite the lack of a clinically useful antidote for the thrombin antagonists.[15] Thrombin antagonists are also not susceptible to neutralization by PF4 and thus are not neutralized at endothelial sites where activated platelets reside. They are also useful in patients with HIT in whom the administration of heparin and subsequent antibody-induced platelet aggregation would be dangerous.

Hirudin

Hirudin, a coagulation inhibitor isolated from the salivary glands of the medicinal leech (*Hirudo medicinalis*), is a potent inhibitor of thrombin that, unlike heparin, acts independently of ATIII and inhibits clot-bound thrombin as well as fluid-phase thrombin. Hirudin does not require a cofactor and is not susceptible to neutralization by PF4. This would seem to be beneficial in patients in whom platelet activation and thrombosis are potential problems. Recombinant hirudin (r-hirudin) was administered as a 0.25-mg/kg bolus and an infusion to maintain the hirudin concentration at 2.5 µg/mL as determined by the ecarin clotting time in studies by Koster and coworkers.[16] The ecarin clotting time, modified for use in the TAS analyzer, has been used in large series of patients with HIT. Compared with standard treatment with heparin or LMWHs, r-hirudin–treated patients maintained platelet counts and hemoglobin levels and had few bleeding complications if renal function was normal. Hirudin is a small molecule (molecular weight 7 kDa) that is eliminated by the kidney and is easily hemofiltered at the end of CPB.

Bivalirudin

Bivalirudin is a small 20–amino acid molecule with a plasma half-life of 24 minutes. It is a synthetic derivative of hirudin and thus acts as a direct thrombin inhibitor. Bivalirudin binds to both the catalytic binding site and the anion-binding exosite on fluid phase and clot-bound thrombin. The part of the molecule that binds to thrombin is actually cleaved by thrombin itself, so the elimination of bivalirudin activity is independent of specific organ metabolism. Bivalirudin has been used successfully as an anticoagulant in interventional cardiology procedures as a replacement for heparin therapy. In fact, in interventional cardiology, bivalirudin has been associated with less bleeding and equivalent ischemic outcomes compared with heparin plus a platelet inhibitor. This may be the result of bivalirudin being both an antithrombin anticoagulant and an antithrombin at the level of the platelet. Merry and colleagues showed equivalence with regard to bleeding outcomes and an improvement in graft flow after off-pump cardiac surgery when bivalirudin was used (0.75-mg/kg bolus, 1.75-mg/kg/hr infusion).[17] Case reports confirm the safety of bivalirudin use during CPB, although current trials are under way. Monitoring of anticoagulant activity is performed using the ecarin clotting time with similar prolongation to that seen with hirudin anticoagulation.[18] The ecarin clotting time has a closer correlation with anti-IIa activity and plasma drug levels than does the ACT. For this reason, standard ACT monitoring during antithrombin therapy is not preferred if ecarin clotting time can be measured.

The anticoagulant effects of the thrombin antagonists can be monitored using the ACT, aPTT, or the TT. The bleeding time may also be prolonged.

Bivalirudin has been favorably compared with heparin in patients undergoing coronary angioplasty for unstable angina. The half-life of aPTT prolongation is approximately 40 minutes, and reductions in formation of fibrinopeptide A are evidence of thrombin inhibition and fibrinogen preservation. Careful monitoring should be used because there may be a rebound prothrombotic state after cessation of therapy, which could lead to recurrence of anginal symptoms (Box 12-2).

MONITORING PLATELET FUNCTION

Circulating platelets adhere to the endothelium via platelet surface receptors that bind exposed collagen and become activated. This initiates platelet activation, because collagen is a potent platelet activator. The unstimulated platelet, which is discoid in shape, undergoes a conformational change when activated. The activated platelet is spherical, extrudes pseudopodia, and expresses an increased number of activated surface receptors that can be measured to quantify the degree of platelet reactivity. The intensity of this platelet activation occurs in proportion to the quantity and nature of the platelet stimulus and increases in a graded fashion with increasing concentrations of agonists. The glycoprotein (GP) IIb/IIIa receptor is the primary receptor responsible for fibrinogen binding and the formation of the platelet plug.

Platelet Count

Numerous events occur during cardiac surgical procedures that predispose patients to platelet-related hemostasis defects. The two major categories are thrombocytopenia and qualitative platelet defects. Thrombocytopenia commonly occurs during cardiac surgery as a result of hemodilution, sequestration, and destruction by nonendothelial surfaces. Platelet counts commonly fall to 100,000/μL or slightly below; however, the final platelet count is greatly dependent on the starting value and the duration of platelet destructive interventions (i.e., CPB). Between 10,000/μL and 100,000/μL, bleeding time decreases directly; however, at platelet counts greater than 50,000/μL, neither the bleeding time nor platelet count has any correlation with postoperative bleeding in cardiac surgical patients. On the other hand, platelet size or mean platelet volume does have some correlation with hemostatic function. Larger, younger platelets are more hemostatically active than smaller ones. Mean platelet volume multiplied by the platelet count gives an estimation of overall platelet mass and is referred to as the *plateletcrit*. It is important to appreciate the inverse relationship between platelet volume and platelet count when using a measure such as the plateletcrit to assess the viability of the existing platelet population. Because the mean platelet volume is dependent on the method of specimen collection, the anticoagulant used, and temperature of the storage conditions, its reproducibility is dependent on standardized laboratory procedures.

Qualitative platelet defects occur more commonly than thrombocytopenia during CPB procedures. The range of possible causes of platelet dysfunction includes

12

traumatic extracorporeal techniques, pharmacologic therapy, hypothermia, and fibrinolysis; the hemostatic insult increases with the duration of time spent on CPB. The use of bubble oxygenators, noncoated extracorporeal circulation, and cardiotomy suctioning may cause platelets to become activated, initiate the release reaction, and partly deplete platelets of the contents of their alpha granules. Many of these changes are only transiently associated with CPB. The hematologic changes associated with CPB have been characterized. While the platelet count falls and reaches a plateau at 2 hours after CPB, mean platelet volume reaches its nadir at 2 hours after CPB and then begins to rise during the ensuing 72 hours. The relative thrombocytopenia seen up to 72 hours after cardiac surgery is not consistently associated with a bleeding diathesis. Similarly, the clotting proteins fibrinogen, factor VIII/von Willebrand factor (vWF), and factor VIII-C also rise to levels above baseline in the 2 to 72 hours after CPB.

Large doses of heparin have been shown to reduce the ability of the platelets to aggregate and to reduce clot strength. This effect is not reversed when protamine is administered; however, it may be mitigated by the prophylactic administration of aprotinin. The adverse effects of heparin on platelet function may be due to its ability to inhibit the formation of thrombin, the most potent invivo platelet activator. However, heparin also activates the fibrinolytic system, a system that, through plasmin and other activators, has the ability to depress platelet function through other mechanisms. Additionally, various degrees of fibrinolysis occur after CPB. Circulating plasmin causes dissolution of the GPIb platelet receptor and decreases the adhesiveness of platelets. Because fibrinolysis is partly responsible for the platelet dysfunction seen after heparin administration and CPB, the efficacy of antifibrinolytic agents as hemostatic drugs can be better appreciated. In addition to reducing platelet adhesiveness to vWF, the fibrin degradation products formed depress platelet responsiveness to agonists.

Protamine-heparin complexes and protamine alone also contribute to platelet depression after CPB. Mild to moderate degrees of hypothermia are associated with reversible degrees of platelet activation and platelet dysfunction, which may be partly mitigated by the use of aprotinin therapy. Overall, the potential coagulation benefits of normothermic CPB compared with hypothermic CPB require further study in well-conducted randomized trials (Box 12-3).

Bleeding Time

The bleeding time is performed by creating a skin incision and measuring the time to clot formation via the platelet plug. The Ivy bleeding time is performed on the volar surface of the forearm above which a cuff is inflated to 40 mm Hg (above venous pressure). Using a template, two parallel incisions are made and the incisions blotted with filter paper every 30 seconds until no further bleeding occurs. The time from incision to cessation of blood seepage is the template bleeding time. The Duke bleeding time is performed on the earlobe and has advantages for cardiac surgery because the earlobe is more accessible and less likely to be subjected to the peripheral vasoconstriction seen after hypothermia. However, because neither the width/depth of the incision nor the venous pressure can be controlled in the Duke bleeding time, the Ivy bleeding time is considered the superior test. Normal bleeding time is 4 to 10 minutes.

Numerous prospective blinded investigations have confirmed that bleeding time has little or no value in predicting excessive hemorrhage after cardiac surgery. Even in patients receiving therapeutic doses of aspirin, an increase in bleeding time does not necessarily translate into an increase in mediastinal tube drainage or transfusions

> ### BOX 12-3 *Platelet Function*
>
> - The measure of platelet count does not correlate with bleeding after cardiac surgery.
> - Patients frequently have extreme degrees of thrombocytopenia but do not bleed because they have adequate platelet function.
> - It is the measure of platelet function that correlates temporally with the bleeding course seen after cardiac surgery.
> - The thromboelastogram maximal amplitude, mean platelet volume, and other functional platelet tests are very useful in transfusion algorithms.

if reinfusion and blood conservation techniques are used aggressively. There is substantial evidence that platelet-directed therapy in the form of platelet transfusions or desmopressin acetate shortens a prolonged bleeding time in patients with clinical hemorrhage. Because the bleeding time does not follow the temporal course of postoperative coagulopathy, the bleeding time may be a nonspecific and impractical test for detecting an existing platelet defect but may be suitable for following patient response to platelet-directed therapies.

Aggregometry

Activated platelets undergo aggregation, which is initially a reversible process. Activation also induces the release of substances from alpha and dense platelet granules and platelet lysosomes. Because platelet granules contain many platelet agonists, the release of granular contents further stimulates platelet activation and is responsible for the secondary phase of platelet aggregation. This secondary phase of platelet aggregation is dependent on the release of thromboxane and other substances from the platelet granules, is an energy-consuming process, and is irreversible.

Aggregometry is a useful research tool for measuring platelet responsiveness to a variety of different agonists. The end result, platelet aggregation, is an objective measure of platelet activation. Platelet aggregometry uses a photo-optical instrument to measure light transmittance through a sample of whole blood or platelet-rich plasma. Platelet-rich plasma undergoes a decrease in light transmittance on the early phase of platelet activation due to the change in platelet shape from discoid to spherical. When exposed to a platelet agonist such as thrombin, adenosine diphosphate (ADP), epinephrine, collagen, or ristocetin, the initial reversible aggregation phase results in increased light transmittance due to the platelet aggregates that decrease the turbidity of the sample. The larger the platelet aggregates, the greater is the transmittance of light. In the absence of further activation, disaggregation occurs and the plasma sample becomes turbid. However, when the platelet release reaction occurs, thromboxane and other activators are released from the platelet alpha granules and the phase of secondary, or irreversible, aggregation occurs. This results in a further increase in light transmittance.

Platelet-Mediated Force Transduction

An instrument that measures the force developed by platelets during clot retraction has been shown to be directly related to platelet concentration and function[19] (Hemodyne). The apparatus consists of a cup and a parallel upper plate. The cup is filled with blood or the platelet-containing solution, and the upper plate is lowered onto the clotting solution. Clot forms and adheres to the outer edges of the cup and

12

to the plate above. A thin layer of oil is deposited onto the surfaces that are exposed to air. The upper plate is coupled to a displacement transducer that translates displacement due to platelet retraction into a force. Normal values for platelet force development have been suggested by the investigators. The antiplatelet effects of heparin have been evaluated using this force retractometer. Using this instrument, investigators have shown that high heparin concentrations completely abolish platelet force generation. Furthermore, the concentration of protamine required to reverse the anticoagulant effects of heparin is not sufficient to reverse these antiplatelet effects. The antiplatelet effects of protamine alone have also been evaluated using this monitor.

BEDSIDE PLATELET FUNCTION TESTING

Thromboelastography

The coaguloviscometers that were developed in the 1920s formed the basis of viscoelastic coagulation testing that is now known as thromboelastography. Thromboelastography in its current form was developed by Hartert in 1948 and has been used in many different clinical scenarios to diagnose coagulation abnormalities.[20] Although not yet truly portable, the thromboelastograph (TEG; Haemoscope, Skokie, IL) can be performed "on site" either in the operating room or in a laboratory and provides a rapid whole blood analysis that yields information about clot formation and clot dissolution. Within minutes, information is obtained regarding the integrity of the coagulation cascade, platelet function, platelet-fibrin interactions, and fibrinolysis. The principle is as follows: whole blood (0.36 mL) is placed into a plastic cuvette into which a plastic pin is suspended; this plastic pin is attached to a torsion wire that is coupled to an amplifier and recorded; a thin layer of oil is added to the surface of the blood to prevent drying of the specimen; and the cuvette oscillates through an arc of 4 degrees, 45 minutes at 37°C. When the blood is liquid, movement of the cuvette does not affect the pin. However, as clot begins to form, the pin becomes coupled to the motion of the cuvette and the torsion wire generates a signal that is recorded. The recorded tracing can be stored by computer, and the parameters of interest are calculated using a simple software package. Alternatively, the tracing can be generated on line with a recording speed of 2 mm/min. The tracing generated has a characteristic conformation that is the signature of the TEG (Fig. 12-5).

The specific parameters measured by the TEG include the reaction time (R value), coagulation time (K value), a angle, maximal amplitude (MA), amplitude 60 minutes after the MA (A60), and clot lysis indices at 30 and 60 minutes after MA (LY30 and LY60, respectively). The reaction time, R, represents the time for initial fibrin formation and is a measure of the intrinsic coagulation pathway, the extrinsic coagulation pathway, and the final common pathway. R is measured from the start of the bioassay until fibrin begins to form and the amplitude of the tracing is 2 mm. Normal values vary depending on the types of activator used and range from 7 to 14 minutes using celite activator and are as short as 1 to 3 minutes using tissue factor activator. The K value is a measure of the speed of clot formation and is measured from the end of the R time to the time that the amplitude reaches 20 mm. Normal values (3 to 6 minutes) also vary with the type of activators used. The a angle, another index of speed of clot formation, is the angle formed between the horizontal axis of the tracing and the tangent to the tracing at 20-mm amplitude. Alpha values normally range from 45 to 55 degrees. Because both the K value and the a angle are measures of the speed of clot strengthening, each is improved by high levels of functional fibrinogen. MA (normal is 50 to 60 mm) is an index of clot strength as determined

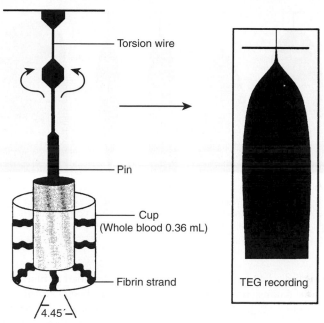

Torsion wire

Pin

Cup
(Whole blood 0.36 mL)

Fibrin strand

TEG recording

4.45°

Figure 12-5 Schematic diagram of the thromboelastograph instrumentation (*left*) and a sample tracing (*right*). A whole blood sample is placed into the cup into which a plastic pin is suspended. This plastic pin is attached to a torsion wire that is coupled to an amplifier and recorder. See text for details. (From Mallett SV, Cox DJA: Thromboelastography. Br J Anaesth 69:307-313, 1992.)

by platelet function, the cross-linkage of fibrin, and the interactions of platelets with polymerizing fibrin. The peak strength of the clot, or the shear elastic modulus "G," has a curvilinear relation with MA and is defined as G = (5000 · MA)/ (96 – MA). The percent reduction in MA after 30 minutes reflects the fibrinolytic activity present and is normally not more than 7.5%.

Characteristic TEG tracings can be recognized to be indicative of particular coagulation defects. A prolonged R value indicates a deficiency in coagulation factor activity or level and is seen typically in patients with liver disease and in patients on anticoagulants such as warfarin or heparin. MA and a angle are reduced in states associated with platelet dysfunction or thrombocytopenia and are even further reduced in the presence of a fibrinogen defect. LY 30, or the lysis index at 30 minutes after MA, is increased in conjunction with fibrinolysis. These particular signature tracings are depicted in Figure 12-6.

TEG is a useful tool for diagnosing and treating perioperative coagulopathy in patients undergoing cardiac surgical procedures due to a variety of potential coagulation defects that may exist. Within 15 to 30 minutes, on-site information is available regarding the integrity of the coagulation system, the platelet function, fibrinogen function, and fibrinolysis. With the addition of heparinase, TEG can be performed during CPB and can provide valuable and timely information regarding coagulation status.[21] Because TEG is a viscoelastic test and evaluates whole blood hemostasis interactions, it is suggested that TEG is a more accurate predictor of postoperative hemorrhage than routine coagulation tests that analyze individual components of the hemostasis system. A number of clinical trials have confirmed that in cardiac surgical patients TEG has a greater predictive value and greater specificity than routine coagulation tests for diagnosing patients known as "bleeders." Tuman

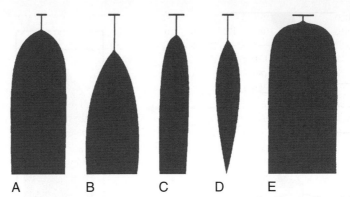

Figure 12-6 Signature thromboelastograph tracings. Tracing identification from left to right. A = normal; B = coagulation factor deficiency; C = platelet dysfunction or deficiency; D = fibrinolysis; E = hypercoagulability. (From Mallett SV, Cox DJA: Thromboelastography. Br J Anaesth 69:307-313, 1992.)

and associates studied 42 patients, of whom 9 were classified as bleeders.[21] A routine coagulation screen consisting of ACT, PT, aPTT, and platelet count had only a 33% accuracy for predicting bleeding, whereas TEG and Sonoclot (Sienco Inc., Morrison, CO) (another viscoelastic test) had 88% and 74% accuracy, respectively. Other investigators have also found that TEG abnormalities predict postoperative bleeding and, using TEG parameters, they were also able to identify a population of patients who respond to therapy with desmopressin acetate.

In a large retrospective evaluation in more than 1000 patients, Spiess and associates found that the institution of a transfusion algorithm using TEG resulted in a significant reduction in the incidence of mediastinal exploration and in the rate of transfusion of allogeneic blood products.[22] Because of its ease of use and application at the bedside, TEG has been used in many research settings to assess drug effects on platelet function and clot strength.

Thromboelastography Modifications

Thromboelastography was originally performed using recalcified citrated whole blood or celite activator. The addition of recombinant human tissue factor as an activator can accelerate the rate of thrombin formation and thus the formation of fibrin. This serves to shorten the time required for development of the MA. Because the MA is primarily reflective of clot strength and platelet function, this information can be obtained more quickly with tissue factor enhancement. The recombinant tissue factor is a thromboplastin agent and is available from a number of manufacturers.[23]

An application of TEG in the clinical arena is its use in monitoring GPIIb/IIIa receptor blockade and ADP receptor blockade in patients treated with specific antiplatelet agents. TEG with tissue factor acceleration speeds the appearance of MA and is accurate for monitoring the platelet inhibition by large concentrations of GPIIb/IIIa receptor blockers. Using this technique with platelet-rich plasma, the reduction of the MA has been used as an index of platelet inhibition by GPIIb/IIIa receptor blockers in the catheterization laboratory. Comparison with the baseline MA yields a relative measure of the degree of platelet inhibition.

Because the MA is a function of the platelet-fibrinogen interaction, a reduction in the MA can be accomplished by the addition of potent GPIIb/IIIa receptor blockade to the assay. The resultant MA, in the presence of excessively high GPIIb/IIIa

III

receptor blockade, is primarily due to the fibrinogen concentration and the strength of fibrin alone. This value (called MA_f) correlates strongly with plasma fibrinogen concentration.

The thienopyridine ADP-receptor blockers clopidogrel and ticlopidine are widely used in cardiovascular medicine. The ability to measure the platelet defect induced by these drugs is very difficult unless sophisticated laboratory techniques such as ADP-aggregometry are used. Aggregometry yields accurate results; however, it is not readily available in the perioperative period as a point-of-care test. Native TEG analysis does not measure the thienopyridine-induced platelet defect because the formation of thrombin in the assay has an overwhelming effect on the development of the TEG MA. A modification of the TEG removes thrombin from the assay and studies a nonthrombin clot, strengthened by the addition of ADP. Figure 12-7 depicts the different signature TEG tracings that are used to calculate the platelet contribution to MA when a platelet inhibitor is present. This assay was specifically created to measure the platelet inhibition by ADP antagonists such as clopidogrel and is referred to as the platelet mapping assay. The MA_{kh} is the maximal activation of platelets and fibrin and is the largest amplitude that can be achieved. The MA_f is the MA that is obtained when a thrombin-depleted fibrin clot is formed without a platelet contribution. The MA_{pi} is the MA_f contribution plus the platelet contribution. MA_{pi} is created by adding an activator such as ADP to the MA_f assay (for clopidogrel testing). Only platelets that can be activated by ADP contribute to the MA_{pi}. The following formula calculates the percent reduction in platelet activity using this assay.

$$100 - \left[\left(MA_{pi} - MA_f \right) / \left(MA_{kh} - MA_f \right) \right] \times 100$$

Clopidogrel, ticlopidine, and even aspirin inhibition can now be studied at the point-of-care using this modification.[24]

Tests of Platelet Response to Agonist

HemoSTATUS

Despite the introduction of numerous point-of-care coagulation analyzers that allow for rapid determination of a patient's coagulation status, the qualitative measure of platelet function, at the bedside, remains an elusive challenge. HemoSTATUS (Medtronic Inc., Parker, CO) is a point-of-care platelet function assay that uses the Hepcon monitoring system to measure platelet reactivity. A six-channel cartridge measures the heparinized kaolin-activated ACT without platelet activator (channels 1 and 2) and with incrementally increasing doses of platelet-activating factor [PAF] (channels 3 to 6). The ACT of the PAF-activated channels will be shortened due to the ability of activated platelets to speed coagulation.

The potential ability to measure the qualitative function of platelets using a point-of-care assay provides innumerable advantages for clinicians caring for cardiac surgical patients. Platelet dysfunction is one of the more common hemostasis defects incurred during CPB, yet it is difficult to specifically measure platelet function rapidly and at the bedside. Viscoelastic tests conveniently measure platelet function, but their use in transfusion algorithms is limited by a lack of specificity to the measure of platelet dysfunction. Transfusion algorithms have been suggested to result in reduced transfusions in cardiac surgical patients and have incorporated only the measure of platelet number, because the on-site ability to measure platelet function has been so elusive. Inclusion of a measure of platelet function into a transfusion algorithm would potentially reduce allogeneic transfusions even further.

An initial investigation of HemoSTATUS in cardiac surgical patients was performed by Despotis and colleagues.[25] The authors studied 150 patients and

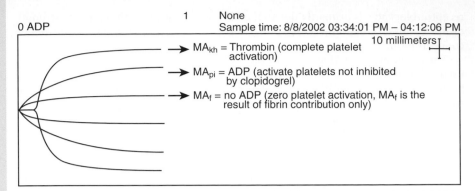

Figure 12-7 Thromboelastograph tracings using the modification to measure platelet inhibition by the thienopyridine drugs clopidogrel or ticlopidine. The measurements made are the maximal amplitude allowing thrombin activation of platelets (MA_{kh}). This is the standard kaolin-activated MA. Also measured is the maximal amplitude measuring only the fibrinogen component of MA (MA_f) using a fibrinogen activator, and the maximal amplitude measuring the platelet contribution to MA by platelets able to be activated by ADP (MA_{pi}). This is using a fibrinogen activator plus ADP. Only platelets that are responsive to ADP will contribute to the MA_{pi}.

conducted multivariate analyses to evaluate the relationship between postoperative blood loss and multiple demographic, operative, and hemostatic measurements. They demonstrated a significant correlation between HemoSTATUS measurements on arrival in the intensive care unit (ICU) and 4-hour postoperative mediastinal tube drainage ($r = -0.85$, channel 5; $r = -0.82$, channel 6). Using receiver operating characteristic (ROC) curves for the detection of excessive mediastinal tube drainage, the accuracy of a number of hemostasis assays was measured. The highest predictability for bleeding was found in both the channel 5 clot ratio and the bleeding time. The PT, aPTT, and platelet count had much lower predictive value. HemoSTATUS-derived clot ratios also had the capability to detect enhanced platelet function after the administration of pharmacologic platelet therapy (desmopressin acetate) and after the transfusion of platelet concentrates. Subsequent investigations in cardiac surgical patients have confirmed a significant yet weak correlation of HemoSTATUS with postoperative bleeding but have not found this test to be superior to TEG or routine coagulation tests in its predictive value.

Other Platelet Function Tests

Ultegra (Accumetrics, San Diego, CA), or "rapid platelet function assay," is a point-of-care monitor designed specifically to measure the platelet response to a thrombin-receptor-agonist peptide (TRAP). This technology was approved by the U.S. Food and Drug administration for use as a platelet function assay.

The Platelet Function Analyzer (PFA-100) (Dade Behring, Miami, FL) is a monitor of platelet adhesive capacity that is valuable in its diagnostic abilities to identify drug-induced platelet abnormalities, platelet dysfunction of von Willebrand's disease, and other acquired and congenital platelet defects.

"Platelet Works" Ichor (Array Medical, Somerville, NJ) is a test that uses the principle of the platelet count ratio to assess platelet reactivity. The instrument is a Coulter counter that measures the platelet count in a standard EDTA-containing tube. Platelet count is also measured in tubes containing the platelet agonist ristocetin, ADP, epinephrine, collagen, or thrombin. Addition of blood to these agonist tubes causes platelets to activate, adhere to the tube, and be effectively eliminated from the platelet count. The ratio of the activated platelet count to the nonactivated platelet count is a function of the reactivity of the platelets. Early investigation in cardiac surgical patients indicates that this assay is useful in providing a platelet count and that it is capable of measuring the platelet dysfunction that accompanies CPB.

SUMMARY

- Monitoring the effect of heparin is done using an activated coagulation time (ACT), a functional test of heparin anticoagulation. The ACT is susceptible to elevation due to hypothermia, hemodilution, and the use of aprotinin (celite ACT).
- Heparin resistance can be congenital or acquired. Pretreatment heparin exposure predisposes a patient to altered heparin responsiveness due to either antithrombin III (ATIII) depletion, platelet activation, or activation of extrinsic coagulation.
- Heparin-induced thrombocytopenia type I is benign and is a normal aggregation response of platelets to heparin. Heparin-induced thrombocytopenia type II is an abnormal immunologic response to the heparin/platelet factor 4 complex and is sometimes associated with overt thrombosis.
- Protamine neutralization of heparin can be associated with "protamine reactions," which include vasodilatory hypotension, anaphylactoid reactions, and pulmonary hypertensive crises (types 1, 2, and 3).
- Before considering a transfusion of plasma, it is important to document that the effect of heparin has been neutralized. This can be done using a heparinase-neutralized test or a protamine-neutralized test.
- Point-of-care tests are available for use in transfusion algorithms that can measure coagulation factor activity (international normalized ratio, activated partial thromboplastin time) and platelet function.
- Fibrinolysis is common after cardiopulmonary bypass when antifibrinolytic therapy is not used.
- New thrombin inhibitor drugs are available for anticoagulation in patients who cannot receive heparin. These can be monitored using the ecarin clotting time or a modified ACT. Bivalirudin and hirudin are the two new drugs that have been used most often in cardiac surgery.
- Platelet dysfunction is the most common reason for bleeding after cardiopulmonary bypass. There are point-of-care tests that can be used to measure specific aspects of platelet function.
- The degree of platelet inhibition as measured by standard or point-of-care instruments has been shown to correlate with decreased ischemic outcomes after coronary intervention. However, cardiac surgical patients who are receiving antiplatelet medication are at increased risk for postoperative bleeding.

12

REFERENCES

1. Reich DL, Zahl K, Perucho MH, Thys DM: An evaluation of two activated clotting time monitors during cardiac surgery. J Clin Monit 8:33, 1992
2. Linden MD, Schneider M, Baker S, et al: Decreased concentration of antithrombin after preoperative therapeutic heparin does not cause heparin resistance during cardiopulmonary bypass. J Cardiothorac Vasc Anesth 18:131, 2004
3. Levy JH, Montes F, Szlam F, Hillyer CD: The in vitro effects of antithrombin III on the activated coagulation time in patients on heparin therapy. Anesth Analg 90:1076, 2000
4. Warkentin TE, Greinacher A: Heparin-induced thrombocytopenia and cardiac surgery. Ann Thorac Surg 76:638, 2003

5. Jobes DR, Aitken GL, Shaffer GW: Increased accuracy and precision of heparin and protamine dosing reduces blood loss and transfusion in patients undergoing primary cardiac operations. J Thorac Cardiovasc Surg 110:36, 1995

6. Szalados JE, Ouriel K, Shapiro JR: Use of the activated coagulation time and heparin dose-response curve for the determination of protamine dosage in vascular surgery. J Cardiothorac Vasc Anesth 8:515, 1994

7. Despotis GJ, Joist JH, Hogue Jr CW, et al: The impact of heparin concentration and activated clotting time monitoring on blood conservation: A prospective, randomized evaluation in patients undergoing cardiac operation. J Thorac Cardiovasc Surg 110:46, 1995

8. Warkentin TE, Crowther MA: Reversing anticoagulants both old and new. Can J Anaesth 49:S11, 2002

9. LaDuca FM, Zucker ML, Walker CE: Assessing heparin neutralization following cardiac surgery: Sensitivity of thrombin time-based assays versus protamine titration methods. Perfusion 14:181, 1999

10. Shigeta O, Kojima H, Hiramatsu Y, et al: Low-dose protamine based on heparin-protamine titration method reduces platelet dysfunction after cardiopulmonary bypass. J Thorac Cardiovasc Surg 118:354, 1999

11. Levy JH, Cormack JG, Morales A: Heparin neutralization by recombinant platelet factor 4 and protamine. Anesth Analg 81:35, 1995

12. Werner M, Gallagher JV, Ballo MS, Karcher DS: Effect of analytic uncertainty of conventional and point-of-care assays of activated partial thromboplastin time on clinical decisions in heparin therapy. Am J Clin Pathol 102:237, 1994

13. Nuttall GA, Oliver WC, Beynen FM, et al: Determination of normal versus abnormal activated partial thromboplastin time and prothrombin time after cardiopulmonary bypass. J Cardiothorac Vasc Anesth 9:355, 1995

14. Whitten CW, Greilich PE, Ivy R, et al: D-dimer formation during cardiac and noncardiac thoracic surgery. Anesth Analg 88:1226, 1999

15. Lincoff AM, Bittl JA, Kleiman NS, et al: Comparison of bivalirudin versus heparin during percutaneous coronary intervention (the Randomized Evaluation of PCI Linking Angiomax to Reduced Clinical Events [REPLACE] trial). Am J Cardiol 93:1092, 2004

16. Koster A, Hansen R, Grauhan O, et al: Hirudin monitoring using the TAS ecarin clotting time in patients with heparin-induced thrombocytopenia type II. J Cardiothorac Vasc Anesth 14:249, 2000

17. Merry AF, Raudkivi PJ, Middleton NG, et al: Bivalirudin versus heparin and protamine in off-pump coronary artery bypass surgery. Ann Thorac Surg 77:925, 2004

18. Koster A, Spiess B, Chew DP, et al: Effectiveness of bivalirudin as a replacement for heparin during cardiopulmonary bypass in patients undergoing coronary artery bypass grafting. Am J Cardiol 93:356, 2004

19. Carr ME Jr : In vitro assessment of platelet function. Transfus Med Rev 11:106, 1997

20. Spiess BD: Thromboelastography and cardiopulmonary bypass. Semin Thromb Hemost 21:27, 1995

21. Tuman KJ, McCarthy RJ, Djuric M, et al: Evaluation of coagulation during cardiopulmonary bypass with a heparinase-modified thromboelastographic assay. J Cardiothorac Vasc Anesth 8:144, 1994

22. Spiess BD, Gillies BS, Chandler W, Verrier E: Changes in transfusion therapy and reexploration rate after institution of a blood management program in cardiac surgical patients. J Cardiothorac Vasc Anesth 9:168, 1995

23. Shore-Lesserson L, Manspeizer HE, DePerio M, et al: Thromboelastography-guided transfusion algorithm reduces transfusions in complex cardiac surgery. Anesth Analg 88:312, 1999

24. Bliden KP, Dichiara J, Tantry U, et al: Increased risk in patients with high platelet aggregation receiving chronic clopidogrel therapy. J Amer Coll Cardiol 49:657, 2007

25. Despotis GJ, Levine V, Saleem R, et al: Use of point-of-care test in identification of patients who can benefit from desmopressin during cardiac surgery: A randomised controlled trial. Lancet 354:106, 1999

III

Section IV
Anesthesia Techniques for Cardiac Surgical Procedures

Chapter 13

Anesthesia for Myocardial Revascularization

Martin J. London, MD • Alexander Mittnacht, MD • Joel A. Kaplan, MD

Providing anesthesia care for patients undergoing coronary artery bypass grafting (CABG) continues to be a challenging yet rewarding endeavor. Surgical, anesthetic, and technologic advances continue to drive changes in clinical routines at a rapid pace, even at a time when the numbers of cases have declined because of the growth of percutaneous coronary interventions (PCIs).

Cardiac anesthesiologists who have been in practice for the past several decades have seen a variety of anesthetic and surgical practices come into vogue and fall out of favor based on new research and economic pressures. Perhaps the most striking example is the rise and fall of high-dose opioid anesthesia, which was initially driven by concern about excessive cardiovascular depression by volatile anesthetics in the 1970s and further accelerated in the mid-1980s by concerns about potential coronary steal with isoflurane. The prolonged postoperative mechanical ventilation resulting from the shift to high-dose opioids was also thought important to reduce stress on the recently revascularized myocardium. However, during the following decade, this approach was completely reversed by new basic and clinical research, such as lack of evidence for adverse effects of volatile agents, particularly as related to potential effects of coronary vasodilation on coronary steal, and by strong evidence of their benefits via rapid preconditioning; by social and economic factors (i.e., safety and efficacy of fast-tracking for most patients and recognition that time on the ventilator for many patients is an uncomfortable experience); and by the rapid rise in off-pump coronary artery bypass grafting (OPCAB), which by avoiding adverse physiologic effects of cardiopulmonary bypass (CPB) facilitates more rapid emergence and recovery in many patients.[1,2] Given the increasing emphasis on pain control in all surgical patients and its reported association with enhanced postoperative outcome in a variety of surgical subgroups, there has been a resurgence in the use of neuraxial techniques in cardiac surgery, particularly in European and Asian countries.[3] Although not commonly used in the United States because of logistical issues and liability concerns, the rapidly growing literature base mandates that clinicians familiarize themselves with their potential benefits and risks.

EPIDEMIOLOGY AND RISK ASSESSMENT

In 2001, coronary artery disease (CAD) was estimated to occur in 13.2 million individuals in the United States (6.4%), resulting in approximately 500,000 deaths, 2 million hospital discharges, and a societal cost of $133 billion. CABG surgery is clearly the established cornerstone of treatment of advanced degrees of CAD. Although its absolute frequency has recently declined, there is no doubt that it will remain a common procedure and that its complexity will continue to increase for many decades to come. An understanding of the basic epidemiology of CABG surgery and of risk assessment for patients undergoing it is important for the anesthesiologist for a variety of reasons, including interactions with surgeons and cardiologists; enhancing clinical management of patients by recognizing high-risk characteristics and situations where preoperative management may not be adequate (such that delay of a planned elective procedure or additional perioperative interventions are required); developing a better sense of long-term trends in surgical practice that may impact on future practice volume (e.g., growth or decline of CABG techniques); and changes in complexity of such procedures that may influence reimbursement or additional training requirements.

Preoperative risk assessment for patients undergoing CABG has evolved dramatically over the past 2 decades. The Department of Veterans Affairs in the 1970s established the first large-scale, multicenter surgical outcomes database applying rigorous statistical methodology for comparing outcomes between centers. This group and others have pioneered methodology for adjusting for different severity of illness between patients (i.e., risk adjustment) using multiple preoperative and perioperative variables thought to be of intrinsic value (usually by expert consensus) that could be easily captured and have high consistency of definition.

The Society of Thoracic Surgeons (STS) instituted a voluntary clinical database system with this approach in the early 1990s that has continued to grow rapidly as cardiac surgical groups are increasingly interested in benchmarking their practices against others.[4] Many tertiary centers (e.g., Cleveland Clinic) and regional consortiums of hospitals (e.g., Northern New England Cardiovascular Disease Study Group) maintain databases, and some publish statistical models. Many states have established and maintain risk-adjusted mandatory reporting systems for hospital and individual surgeon performance (with New York State being an early and influential pioneer). A new scoring system (EuroSCORE) based on outcomes in 128 centers in eight European countries has received increasing attention. It appears to compare favorably with the STS model in North American patients.[5] It is freely accessible by means of an interactive web-based calculator (www.euroscore.org) and is decidedly simpler and faster to use than the STS's scoring system, which is now also freely accessible to the public at http://www.sts.org/sections/stsnationaldatabase/riskcalculator/index.html.

PATHOPHYSIOLOGY OF CORONARY ARTERY DISEASE

Anatomy

The anesthesiologist should be familiar with coronary anatomy if only to interpret the significance of angiographic findings. The coronary circulation and common sites for placement of distal anastomoses during CABG are shown in Figures 13-1 to 13-3.

The right coronary artery (RCA) arises from the right sinus of Valsalva and is best seen in the left anterior oblique view on coronary cineangiography. It passes anteriorly for the first few millimeters; it then follows the right atrioventricular (AV) groove and curves posteriorly within the groove to reach the crux of the heart, the area where the interventricular septum (IVS) meets the AV groove. In 84% of cases, it terminates as the posterior descending artery (PDA), which is its most important branch, being the sole supply to the posterior-superior IVS. Other important branches are those to the sinus node in 60% of patients and the AV node in approximately 85% of patients. Anatomists consider the RCA to be dominant when it crosses the crux of the heart and continues in the AV groove regardless of the origin of the PDA. Angiographers, however, ascribe dominance to the artery, right coronary or left coronary (circumflex), that gives rise to the PDA.

The vertical and superior orientation of the RCA ostium allows easy passage of air bubbles during aortic cannulation, CPB, or open valve surgery. In sufficient concentration (e.g., coronary air embolus), myocardial ischemia involving the inferior LV wall segments and the right ventricle may occur (Fig. 13-4). In contrast, the near

13

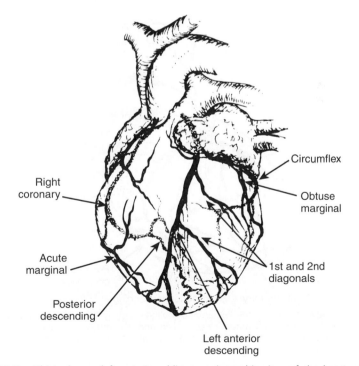

Figure 13-1   Thirty-degree left anterior oblique angiographic view of the heart, which best shows the right coronary artery. *Arrows* indicate common sites of distal vein graft anastomoses. (From Stiles QR, Tucker BL, Lindesmith GG, et al: Myocardial Revascularization: A Surgical Atlas. Boston, Little, Brown, 1976.)

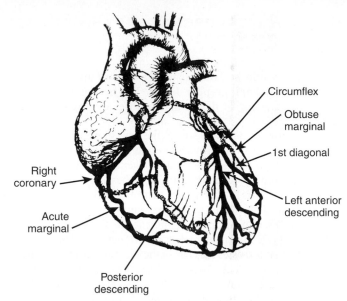

Figure 13-2 Ten-degree right anterior oblique angiographic view of the heart, which best shows the left main coronary artery dividing into the circumflex and left anterior descending arteries. *Arrows* indicate common sites of distal vein graft anastomoses. (Adapted from Stiles QR, Tucker BL, Lindesmith GG, et al: Myocardial Revascularization: A Surgical Atlas. Boston, Little, Brown, 1976.)

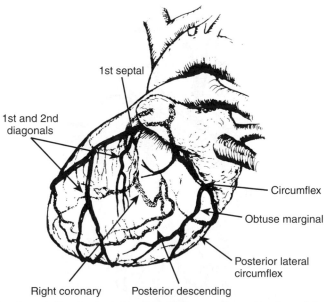

Figure 13-3 Seventy-five-degree left anterior oblique angiographic view of the heart, which best shows branches of the left anterior descending and circumflex coronary arteries. (Adapted from Stiles QR, Tucker BL, Lindesmith GG, et al: Myocardial Revascularization: A Surgical Atlas. Boston, Little, Brown, 1976.)

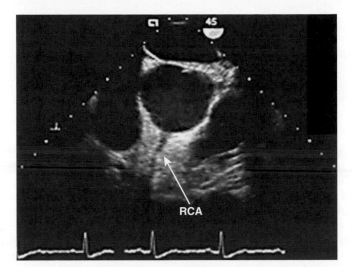

Figure 13-4   The vertical and superior orientation of the right coronary artery arising from the aortic root is identified by transesophageal echocardiography (TEE). The TEE transducer in the esophagus is on the top of the screen, and the patient's chest wall is on the bottom. Retained air preferentially enters the right coronary artery (RCA), which may cause inferior ischemia, depending on the amount of air and the coronary perfusion pressure. Elevation of perfusion pressure using phenylephrine is often used to treat coronary air embolus. The left main artery (not visible) arises at approximately 3 o'clock on this image. (Image courtesy of Martin J. London, MD, University of California, San Francisco, CA [www.ucsf.edu/teeecho].)

perpendicular orientation of the left main coronary ostium makes air embolization much less common.

The left coronary artery arises from the left sinus of Valsalva as the left main coronary artery. This is best seen in a shallow right anterior oblique projection. The left main coronary artery courses anteriorly and to the left, where it divides in a space between the aorta and pulmonary artery (PA). Its branches are the left anterior descending (LAD) and circumflex arteries. The LAD passes along the anterior intraventricular groove. It may reach only two thirds of the distance to the apex or extend around the apex to the diaphragmatic portion of the left ventricle. Major branches of the LAD are the diagonal branches, which supply the free wall of the left ventricle, and septal branches, which course posteriorly to supply the major portion of the IVS. Although there may be many diagonal and septal branches, the first diagonal and first septal branches serve as important landmarks in the descriptions of lesions of the LAD.

The circumflex arises at a sharp angle from the left main coronary artery and courses toward the crux of the heart in the AV groove. When the circumflex gives rise to the PDA, the circulation is said to be left dominant and the left coronary circulation supplies the entire IVS and the AV node. In approximately 40% of patients, the circumflex supplies the branch to the SA node. Up to four obtuse marginal (OM) arteries arise from the circumflex and supply the lateral wall of the left ventricle. All of the previously described epicardial branches give rise to small vessels that supply the outer third of the myocardium and penetrating vessels that anastomose with the subendocardial plexus. This capillary plexus is unique in that it functions as an end-arterial system. Each epicardial arteriole supplies a capillary plexus that forms an end loop rather than anastomosing with an adjacent capillary from another epicardial artery. Significant collateral circulation does not exist at the microcirculatory level. This capillary anatomy explains the very distinct areas of myocardial ischemia or infarction that can be related to disease in a discrete epicardial artery.

13

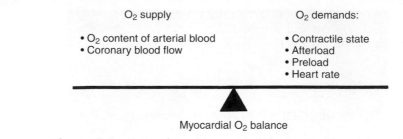

Figure 13-5 Factors determining myocardial oxygen supply and demand.

CAD most commonly affects the epicardial muscular arteries with rare intra-myocardial lesions. However, severe disorders of the microcirculation and primary impairment of coronary vascular reserve in normal coronary arteries have been described, especially in diabetics, female patients, and those with variant angina. Atherosclerosis in all organs is most common at the outer edges of vessel bifurcations, because in these regions blood flow is slower and changes direction during the cardiac cycle resulting in less net shear stress than in other regions with more steady blood flow and higher shear stress. Low shear stress has been shown to stimulate an atherogenic phenotype in the endothelium. Epicardial lesions can be single but are more often multiple. A combined lesion of the RCA and both branches of the left coronary artery is referred to as triple-vessel disease. The left coronary artery supplies the thickest portions of the left ventricle, at least the exterior two thirds of the IVS, and the greater part of the atria. Most bypass grafts are done on the left coronary system.

Venous drainage of the myocardium is primarily to the coronary sinus, which drains 96% of the LV free wall and septum, and the remainder of the venous return goes directly into the right atrium.[6] A small fraction may enter other cardiac chambers directly through the anterior-sinusoidal, anterior-luminal, and thebesian veins.

Myocardial Ischemia and Infarction

In patients with CAD, myocardial ischemia usually results from increases in myocardial oxygen demand (Fig. 13-5) that exceed the capacity of the stenosed coronary arteries to increase their oxygen supply. However, the determinants of myocardial oxygen balance are complex, and alterations may have several effects. For example, an increase in blood pressure (i.e., increased afterload) increases wall tension and oxygen demand while also increasing coronary blood flow (CBF). It is now appreciated that myocardial ischemia may occur without changes in systemic hemodynamics and in awake patients may occur in the absence of chest pain (i.e., silent ischemia), particularly in diabetic patients.

In atherosclerotic heart disease, the fundamental lesion is an intimal lipid plaque that causes chronic stenosis and episodic thrombosis, occurring most often in an epicardial coronary artery, thereby reducing myocardial blood supply. Characteristics of the vulnerable plaque include high lipid content, a thin fibrous cap, a reduced number of smooth muscle cells, and increased macrophage activity. The lipid core is the most thrombogenic component of the plaque. Fuster described five phases in the progression of CAD by plaque morphology. Phase 1 is a small plaque present in many people younger than 30 years and usually progresses very slowly depending on the presence of risk factors associated with CAD (i.e., elevated low-density lipoprotein cholesterol). Phase 2 is a plaque with a high lipid content that has the potential to rupture. If it ruptures, it will lead to thrombosis and increased stenosis (phase 5), possibly producing unstable angina or an acute coronary syndrome.

IV

The phase 2 plaque usually does not rupture; it instead progresses onto phases 3 and 4, with enlargement and fibrous tissue organization, which may ultimately produce an occlusive plaque at phase 5.[7]

ANESTHESIA FOR CORONARY ARTERY BYPASS GRAFTING

Conventional CABG with CPB is still the most commonly performed cardiac surgical procedure (Box 13-1). Fast-track management with early extubation (4 to 8 hours postoperatively) has become the standard of care in nearly all centers. OPCAB is increasing steadily, although its use tends to be very frequent in some centers or infrequent in others as various surgeons have become "early adopters" or are waiting for firm evidence-based recommendations from future randomized, controlled trials. However, anesthetic management of the sickest patients undergoing multivessel operations combined with valve repair or replacement, repeat operations, and other complex procedures (e.g., ventricular septal defect repairs along with CABG after acute myocardial infarction) has changed relatively little over the past decade as the long duration of surgery usually mandates greater cumulative doses of fixed anesthetic agents with overnight or even prolonged postoperative mechanical ventilation. However, many clinicians have adopted use of infusions of shorter-acting agents (e.g., sufentanil, propofol, remifentanil), avoided large cumulative dosing of fixed agents with potentially long half-lives (e.g., midazolam), and now rely on a volatile anesthesia "base," taking a "wait and see" attitude toward early extubation if surgery is "smooth" and physiologic parameters remain within acceptable limits (e.g., good urine output, normothermic, adequate hematocrit).

Premedication

The concept of "premedication" has been evolving with new knowledge and the increasing role of the cardiac anesthesiologist as a "perioperative physician." The cardiac anesthesiologist must be familiar with the potential benefits of administering (or hazards of not administering) a variety of cardiovascular medications, particularly anti-anginal medications, and ensure that appropriate medications are ordered for morning administration with sips of water.

Anxiolysis, Amnesia, and Analgesia

The purposes of premedication are to pharmacologically reduce apprehension and fear, to provide analgesia for potentially painful events before induction (e.g., vascular cannulation), and to produce some degree of amnesia. In patients with CAD, premedication may help prevent preoperative anginal episodes that are relatively commonly observed on continuous ambulatory ECG monitoring but are often silent clinically. Regardless of the drugs used, the clinician should be prepared to give intravenous drugs (e.g., benzodiazepines, opiates) when the patient arrives in the preoperative area to supplement inadequate sedation. All patients receive supplemental oxygen after premedication and are monitored with at least pulse oximetry during vascular cannulation (if performed before entry into the operating room suite).

A variety of drugs and regimens are used for sedation depending on the practice setting (e.g., same-day admission), the patient's condition, and the clinician's preferences. Use of oral, intramuscular, or intravenous benzodiazepines is very common and provides effective anxiolysis and some degree of amnesia. Diazepam remains popular as an oral premedicant (0.1 to 0.15 mg/kg), and midazolam is most popular intravenously (1 to 2 mg). Opioids, most commonly morphine

13

BOX 13-1   *Management Strategies for Anesthesia for Myocardial Revascularization*

Preoperative Evaluation and Management

Assessment of Cardiac Characteristics

1. Cardiac history and presenting symptoms
   - Acute unstable angina, acute myocardial infarction, congestive heart failure, cardiogenic shock highest risk (possible intra-aortic balloon pump, left ventricular assist device)
2. Coronary artery anatomy
   - Left main high-grade lesion, triple-vessel disease, proximal left anterior descending artery lesions: highest risk
   - Status of collateral circulation and microcirculation, diffuse distal disease
3. Ventricular function
   - Ejection fraction: >50%, low risk; <50%, intermediate risk; <25% to 30%, high risk
4. Valvular and structural anatomy and function
   - Best assessed by echocardiogram and/or cardiac catheterization
   - Concurrent aortic stenosis (potential for subendocardial ischemia), mitral regurgitation (may be related to acute or chronic ischemia, papillary rupture), aortic insufficiency (dilated ventricle, increased wall tension, problems with administration of anterograde cardioplegia, ventricular dilation during surgery), ventricular septal defect (acute), ventricular aneurysm or pseudoaneurysm
5. Electrocardiogram
   - Q waves (ischemic potential, reduced function), ST-T depression or elevation (ischemic potential)
   - Left bundle-branch block (advanced coronary artery disease, depressed function, potential complete heart block with passage of pulmonary artery catheter)
   - PR interval (prolongation with β-blockers and calcium channel blockers, progression to more advanced block)
   - Rhythm: atrial fibrillation, flutter, supraventricular tachycardia (instability during case, increased risk of perioperative cerebrovascular accident)
6. Chest radiograph
   - Cardiomegaly (depressed function, pericardial effusion or tamponade)
   - Aortic calcification (inability to cross-clamp aorta, "porcelain aorta")
   - Lung fields (acute or chronic heart failure, pleural effusions)

Assessment of Major Comorbidities

1. Carotid and cerebrovascular disease
   - Assess for presence of high-grade occlusive disease (unusual in absence of symptoms or previous cerebrovascular accident); carotid duplex ultrasound examination of all high-risk patients
2. Peripheral vascular disease
   - Usually obvious, aortic disease associated with inability to pass an intra-aortic balloon pump (IABP) in normal manner, difficult radial artery catheterization possible
3. Diabetes
   - Hyperglycemia associated with impaired endothelial function and attenuation of preconditioning
   - Serum potassium abnormalities with glucose or acid-base management
4. Renal disease
   - For dialysis patients, ensure recent dialysis and verify serum potassium level
   - Careful fluid and medication management
   - Systemic acidosis and hyperkalemia more likely
   - More frequent blood gas and electrolyte sampling required

IV

5. Pulmonary disease
  - Bronchospasm, air trapping, high dead space with slower inhalation agent uptake, atelectasis, segmental and lobar collapse possible

Preoperative Medication Management

1. β-Adrenergic blockers
  - Recommended for all patients unless contraindicated to reduce risk of ischemia
2. Calcium channel blockers
  - Higher incidence of heart block or need for pacing with concurrent β-blocker therapy
  - Efficacy in ischemia prevention controversial
3. Angiotensin-converting enzyme inhibitor
  - Clinical studies; increased propensity for hypotension during induction
4. Diuretics
  - Ensure adequate serum potassium levels
5. Statins
  - Beneficial anti-inflammatory effects and improved outcome independent of lipid lowering effects
6. Aspirin
  - Strong data to suggest it should be continued despite increased bleeding, especially for early and late graft patency and mortality
7. Other antiplatelet agents or glycoprotein IIb/IIIa inhibitors
  - Associated with increased bleeding; hold as appropriate, and treat with platelets, or recombinant factor VII as necessary
8. Heparin
  - Usually discontinued 4 hours preoperatively for stable patients, continued up to and through pre-CPB period for critical left main disease or acutely unstable angina patients
9. Insulin
  - Continuous infusion for poorly controlled hyperglycemia; insulin resistance may be encountered during hypothermic CPB
10. Oral hypoglycemic agents
  - Metformin is associated with lactic acidosis in patients developing perioperative low cardiac output; it is optimal to hold administration several half-lives preoperatively.
  - Glyburide experimentally blocks preconditioning by closure of ATP-mediated potassium channels.
11. Antibiotic prophylaxis
  - Cephazolin (1 g IV) or cefuroxime (1.5 g IV) less than 60 minutes before incision; vancomycin (1 g by slow infusion to avoid hypotension and flushing) or clindamycin (600 to 900 mg IV) for penicillin or cephalosporin allergy; adjust as appropriate for renal failure.
  - Repeat: cefazolin every 2 to 5 hours, cefuroxime every 3 to 4 hours, vancomycin every 6 to 12 hours, clindamycin every 3 to 6 hours; adjust as appropriate for renal failure.
12. Anxiolytic or analgesic premedication
  - Oral diazepam (5 to 10 mg) at least 1 hour before induction; supplement with intravenous fentanyl or midazolam as needed.
  - Intramuscular lorazepam (1 to 2 mg) or morphine (approximately 0.15 mg/kg) at least 1 hour before induction, depending on age, comorbidities, and anxiety level
  - Supplemental oxygen to avoid desaturation and ischemia
13. Preoperative epidural insertion
  - Uncommonly used in the United States, but it may reduce stress response, preserve adrenoreceptor function, and decrease time to extubation, pulmonary complications and pain scores.
  - Use for conscious off-pump coronary artery bypass has been reported.
  - Optimal to place at least 6 to 8 hours preoperatively to ensure adequate hemostasis

Box continued on following page

13

Intraoperative Management

1. Intravenous access
   - One or two large-bore peripheral intravenous catheters; fluid warmer for blood administration
2. ECG monitoring
   - V_3 to V_5 precordial lead monitoring most sensitive for ischemia; recommended for all patients with the exception of those with left bundle-branch block
   - Inferior lead for rhythm monitoring
3. Blood pressure monitoring
   - Radial artery catheter: right arm may be preferable because of potential effects of retraction for left internal mammary artery dissection (with newer surgical retractors, this is likely less problematic).
   - Backup cuff for arterial monitoring failure and correlation of pressures
4. Intrathecal medication
   - Low-dose intrathecal morphine (0.005 to 0.01 mg/kg) may reduce postoperative pain; use 25-gauge needle to minimize vascular trauma.
5. Anesthetic induction
   - Ensure surgeon and perfusionist are available in the rare event of cardiac arrest during induction, which may require emergency femoral-femoral CPB if the patient is unresponsive to conventional therapy.
   - Fast-tracking routines using reduced doses of opioids and or benzodiazepines are standard in most centers. Various combinations of opioid boluses with or without continuous infusion (fentanyl, 10 to 20 μg/kg; sufentanil, 2.5 to 5 μg/kg; remifentanil infusion) and volatile agents (isoflurane, sevoflurane, or desflurane) with or without supplemental intravenous drugs (midazolam, propofol or dexmedetomidine infusions) are used. Given the increasing evidence for preconditioning effects, liberal volatile agent use is encouraged. Avoid nitrous oxide because of the adverse impact of possible hypoxemia on myocardial oxygen delivery and the possible expanding effects on cerebral or coronary gaseous emboli.
   - Muscle relaxation with nondepolarizing neuromuscular blockers is almost always used.
   - Maintain heart rate as low as allowed based on adequate blood pressure and cardiac output to maximize coronary blood flow, which in the left ventricle occurs exclusively during diastole. The heart rate can be influenced by β-blocker or calcium channel blocker use, valvular disease, ejection fraction, or opioid dosing.
   - Maintain adequate perfusion pressure based on coronary, cerebrovascular, renal, and other involved organ systems, based on examination of preoperative values and reduction in demand during stable anesthetic.
   - Baseline arterial blood gas determination is recommended after intubation, along with routine clinical examination for proper endotracheal tube placement.
   - Baseline activated coagulation time is required before heparin administration; heparin dose-response system is used in many centers.
   - Foley placement for all patients
   - Temperature monitoring: bladder or esophageal (core temperature) and nasopharyngeal or tympanic (brain temperature) are recommended for all CPB cases to minimize temperature gradients during rewarming and to minimize risk of cerebral hyperthermia with potential cerebral venous desaturation (implicated in neurocognitive dysfunction).
   - Cerebral monitoring: bispectral or similar monitors (e.g., entropy, PSArray) are increasingly used in cardiac patients because of the increased risk of recall and for better titration of anesthetics, particularly with fast-track techniques. Efficacy remains controversial. Regardless of their use, care should be taken at all times to monitor for evidence of lightness, especially during periods of hemodynamic instability in which the anesthetic level is reduced.

6. Pulmonary artery catheter or central venous pressure catheter placement
   - Central venous pressure catheter is considered standard of care; pulmonary artery catheter use is very center specific.
   - Need for placement of pulmonary artery catheter before induction is controversial, but severe concurrent valve disease and a low ejection fraction are strong indications.
   - When using pulmonary artery catheter, ensure the catheter does not wedge inadvertently during surgical manipulation of the heart (closes the loop, advancing it outward). Transesophageal echocardiography (TEE) can easily verify positioning; otherwise, withdrawing the catheter several centimeters before institution of CPB is usually effective.
   - Avoid pulmonary artery catheter balloon inflation, particularly when the patient is heparinized or hypothermic.
7. Pharmacologic adjuncts
   - Antifibrinolytic therapy – Used primarily for CPB cases.
   - ε-Aminocaproic acid (Amicar): continuous infusion from skin incision and bolus dosing (5 g) after heparin administration and after CPB weaning are used with variable efficacy.
   - Tranexamic acid: strong evidence in the literature for efficacy
   - Corticosteroid administration – High dose before CPB; methylprednisolone (2 to 3 g) is used in some centers to block some components of inflammatory response.
8. Insertion of TEE
   - Use influenced by surgeon's preference, center's resources, anesthesia or cardiology expertise, and availability; routine use common in many centers for all patients.
   - Can be of particular value in guiding anesthetic (fluid administration, detection of new ischemia, verification of pulmonary artery catheter in proximal pulmonary artery) and surgery (verification of retrograde cardioplegia cannula, IABP tip relative to arch vessels, presence of aortic root and arch calcification, ulceration, or mobile components, placement of left ventricular vent, ischemic changes).
   - Stomach decompression before and after placement of probe is recommended to decrease risk of postoperative passive aspiration.
   - Esophageal perforation is rare but increasingly recognized as a complication that must be considered, especially with development of septic changes with new bilateral pleural effusions postoperatively.
9. Sternotomy
   - It is a very stimulating stress; ensure adequate anesthesia, especially if preparation and drape period is prolonged.
   - "Let down the lungs" to avoid potential pleural tear from sternal saw.
   - Repeat sternotomy
     - Uses different technique: oscillating saw on outer sternal table, wires removed manually, and blunt dissection with scissor used on the inner table of the sternum.
     - Risks include right ventricular perforation, damage to existing vein grafts, and ventricular fibrillation from electrocautery energy transmitted by a sternal wire
     - Use external defibrillation pads on all repeat sternotomy cases.
     - Ensure that blood (preferably 2 units checked) is close at hand during opening.
     - Usual presenting sign of right ventricular perforation is ventricular fibrillation, often with little obvious bleeding; emergent femoral-femoral CPB is usually required.

Management before Revascularization

1. Maintain "favorable hemodynamics," with low heart rate and maintenance of systemic blood pressure depending on the preoperative baseline, age, coronary anatomy, and presence of other compromised organs (e.g., brain, kidney). Hypotension with surgical manipulation of the heart and aorta is unavoidable but is usually treated with phenylephrine, volume supplementation, and Trendelenburg position. Close communication with the surgeon is essential.

Box continued on following page

13

2. Left internal mammary artery dissection: elevate table, rotate to left, and reduce tidal volumes (increase rate) to facilitate surgeon's exposure. Similar maneuvers are done for the less commonly performed right internal mammary artery dissection. Heparin is usually administered before clamping of the left internal mammary artery pedicle to avoid thrombosis. Papaverine is often injected retrograde by the surgeon, which occasionally causes hypotension.

3. Conventional coronary artery bypass grafting (CABG)
   - Passive hypothermia is likely protective, given the reduction in myocardial oxygen demands and cerebral protective effects.
   - Pre-bypass phlebotomy is popular in certain centers, although evidence of its efficacy is controversial. Blood may be sequestered before heparinization into storage bags, usually by central venous pressure catheter access, which may require additional fluid administration or by the right atrial cannula just before institution of bypass, usually with the assistance of phenylephrine.
   - Retrograde cardioplegia may be used alone or, more commonly, in combination with anterograde techniques. Perfusion of the right ventricle is limited by this technique. TEE can assist in placement and confirmation of the catheter in the coronary sinus.

4. Repeat cases
   - Atheroma in prior vein grafts is sandy and often loose. Sudden, profound ischemia may occur with surgical manipulation of grafts due to distal embolization. This may require emergent institution of CPB.
   - Adequate conduits are essential for performing anastomoses. This can be problematic in repeat cases.
   - Exposure for cannulation and of the left ventricle is often more complex because of adhesions and accounts for increased blood loss.

5. Off-pump CABG
   - Maintenance of normothermia is desirable to reduce bleeding and propensity toward ventricular fibrillation, and for facilitating intraoperative extubation if planned. Forced air and water blankets can be helpful.

6. Heparin administration
   - Administer 300 to 400 IU/kg. Higher dose required with heparin resistance (most commonly associated with prolonged preoperative administration). Resistance is usually easily treated with 1 unit of fresh frozen plasma or recombinant antithrombin III. Activated coagulation time between 450 and 500 seconds is required for institution of CPB.
   - Dosing of heparin for off-pump CABG cases is controversial, with centers using full- or low-dose regimens.
   - Only use kaolin-activated coagulation time tubes with concurrent aprotinin administration.
   - Mild hypotension due to vasodilation can occur with heparin administration.
   - For patients with heparin-induced thrombocytopenia, direct thrombin inhibitors have been used with success.

7. Cannulation
   - Aortic cannula
     - Examination of cannulation site by epicardial imaging may be used particularly if surgical palpation is suspicious for calcium or TEE examination reveals prominent distal arch or proximal aortic root disease. Surgical response to severe disease ranges from no change to "no touch" techniques to potential circulatory arrest.
     - Ensure that systemic pressure is lowered to lowest safe level (90 to 110 mm Hg systolic) during cannulation to minimize risk of dissection.
     - Adequate eye protection is required at all times and particularly during this period due to splash hazard.
     - Surgeon inspects lines for air bubbles before hooking up circuit.
     - Hypotension can be effectively treated by perfusionist infusing fluid.

IV

- Retrograde cannula: Inserted in the coronary sinus with insertion site near the right atrial appendage. TEE can guide approximately but is limited by its two-dimensional imaging. Proper placement can be verified by TEE, surgical palpation in great cardiac vein, and dark color of the coronary sinus blood. Pressure monitoring is used to ensure adequate infusion (if low, it is likely in the right ventricle; if excessively high, rupture could occur). Insertion can be difficult and cause major hemodynamic compromise and arrhythmias. For sick repeat or low ejection fraction, insertion after institution of CPB or preparation for rapid institution of CPB may occasionally be required because arrest may occur.
- Venous cannula: For isolated CABG, a single large-bore venous cannula is inserted through the right atrium into the inferior vena cava. It can be partially imaged by TEE in the bicaval view.
- Left ventricular vent: Inserted after institution of CPB via the left superior pulmonary vein in many but not all cases. Can be visualized on TEE short-axis view. Verification of absence of thrombus in the LV is essential in patient with a recent anterior wall MI or aneurysm.

Revascularization Management

1. Conventional CABG
   - On institution of CPB with full flow, discontinue mechanical ventilation. Passive insufflation of oxygen (200 mL/min) is usually continued. Discontinue all maintenance intravenous fluid. Turn off power to the TEE transducer if present. Verify pulmonary artery catheter tip position to avoid inadvertent wedging. Drain urine bag or mark value before CPB.
   - Myocardial preservation by surgeon and perfusionist involves anterograde or retrograde cardioplegia (or both), arrest with high-potassium cardioplegia, and in most centers, hypothermia (systemic, topical, and by cardioplegia).
2. Off-pump CABG
   - Left anterior descending and diagonal vessels
     - Only mild left ventricular displacement is required (packs under left ventricle with mild rotation of the left ventricle upward and to the left); hemodynamic effects are usually minimal in the absence of ischemia or a very low ejection fraction. Diagonal visualization requires additional rotation. Stabilizer placement is usually well tolerated. Hemodynamic changes (hypotension) are usually easily treated with fluids, Trendelenburg position, or phenylephrine.
   - Posterior descending and circumflex vessels
     - Moderate to severe left ventricular displacement (verticalization), most pronounced for circumflex anastomoses, is required. Application of an apical suction device is common, although other, simpler methods are used. With proper placement, hypotension is usually mild but more common than with left anterior descending or diagonal grafts. With improper placement or a large left ventricle or right ventricle, compressive effects on the right ventricle can be severe, leading to a major reduction in cardiac output. Opening of the right pleural space may accommodate the right ventricle, relieving the compression with hemodynamic improvement. Trendelenburg positioning is helpful for maintaining hemodynamics and for the surgeon's visualization.
   - Mechanical ischemic preconditioning (5-minute occlusion followed by 5-minute reperfusion) is used by some surgeons. However, evidence for efficacy, especially with concurrent volatile agent use, is weak.
   - Some clinicians use "reperfusion prophylaxis," similar to the cardiac catheterization lab setting during acute MI with lidocaine, thrombolytics, and magnesium sulfate. With routine off-pump CABG there is little evidence for this because most patients have native and collateral flow.
   - Ischemia during anastomosis can be treated with insertion of an intracoronary shunt. Some surgeons use these routinely, although there is concern regarding endothelial damage with their use; and many surgeons avoid them unless absolutely necessary.

13

Box continued on following page

• TEE can be helpful. However, with verticalization and application of a stabilizer, visualization of all walls and interpretation of wall motion can be difficult. ECG amplitude is often markedly diminished with verticalization for posterior descending artery and circumflex anastomoses. Detection of new mitral regurgitation strongly suggests new ischemia.

Management after Revascularization

1. CPB weaning
   • Plan ahead for potential inotrope and other vasoactive drug use based on presence of known predictors of difficult weaning, particularly low ejection fraction before CPB.
   • Epicardial leads (atrial and ventricular) should be placed. Atrioventricular block and bradycardia are common in patients with severe ischemia and those on β-blockers and calcium channel antagonists. Impaired diastolic relaxation is common, reducing the effectiveness of the Frank-Starling mechanism for augmentation of cardiac output. Heart rate plays a larger role, and maintaining heart rate at 80 to 90 beats per minute for several hours avoids ventricular distention. Frequent evaluation for return of the patient's underlying sinus rhythm is optimal because it may be associated with the best cardiac output.
   • Augmentation of cardiac index with catecholamines (epinephrine, dopamine, dobutamine) and/or phosphodiesterase inhibitors (amrinone, milrinone) may be required for low cardiac index (generally <2.0 L/min/m²) or elevation of pulmonary artery occlusion pressure (generally >18 to 20 mmHg).
   • Intra-aortic balloon counterpulsation is used when inotrope therapy alone is insufficient. IABP augments diastolic coronary perfusion and forward flow ("suction effect"). Aortic insufficiency is a relative contraindication to IABP. Evaluate with TEE to avoid ventricular distention, and check placement below the level of the left subclavian and carotid vessels.
2. Off-pump CABG
   • Assuming adequate anastomoses have been performed, cardiac index returns to normal levels immediately. Function may deteriorate if significant ischemia has occurred, although this is unusual.
3. Reversal of heparin and hemostasis
   • Protamine is usually administered empirically in a 1:1 ratio in the absence of use of automated systems such as the Heparin Dose Response System (Medtronic, Inc., Minneapolis, MN).
   • Avoid a rapid bolus. Exact infusion rates remain controversial.
4. Chest closure and transport
   • Remove TEE, and decompress stomach with orogastric tube.
   • Monitor blood pressure, ECG, and SaO₂ for transport.
   • Ensure chest tubes (if present) are on water seal because tension pneumothorax is a known hazard during transport.
   • Ensure patency of mediastinal drainage because tamponade is a known hazard.

(0.1 to 0.15 mg/kg) given by the intramuscular route, and fentanyl (50 to 75 μg), administered intravenously, are recommended to provide analgesia, particularly during radial artery cannulation. Scopolamine, usually given intramuscularly (0.2 to 0.4 mg) but occasionally intravenously, has been commonly used for its potent amnestic effects. Given its potential to induce delirium and disorientation, particularly in the elderly, it is less frequently used today. Acute toxicity associated with overdosage can be effectively reversed with physostigmine.

Management of Antianginal and Antihypertensive Medications

β-ADRENERGIC RECEPTOR ANTAGONISTS

For the newly trained anesthesiologist who is told to provide "perioperative β-blockade" to all patients with known CAD, or those with multiple risk factors undergoing major noncardiac (particularly vascular) surgery, it may come as a surprise that in 1972, a case series from the prestigious Cleveland Clinic admonished clinicians to withdraw such medication at least 2 weeks before CABG surgery reporting that 5 such patients died within 24 hours of surgery. Several years later, Kaplan and co-workers found that it was safe to continue β-blockade and that operative mortality was similar in patients in whom propranolol had been continued within 24 to 48 hours of surgery. Randomized trials evaluating the safety of administration of propranolol within 12 hours of surgery showed a significantly greater increase in the incidence of pre-CPB ischemia in patients withdrawn from propranolol (within 24 to 72 hours); they also recommended continuation of therapy up until the time of surgery. Further work in the 1980s documented the efficacy of continuation of β-blockers through surgery with regard to reducing pre-CPB ischemia. These studies were instrumental in laying the groundwork for the subsequent noncardiac surgery studies in the late 1980s. These led to the contemporary randomized perioperative β-blocker trials, which despite ongoing controversy regarding the exact efficacy of this therapy resulted in its becoming a clinical routine.[8] Several contemporary observational studies have documented associations of β-blocker therapy with reduction in perioperative mortality in CABG patients. The largest of these by Ferguson and colleagues[9] considered 629,877 patients in the STS database (1996 to 1999) in which a modest but statistically significant reduction in 30-day risk-adjusted mortality was reported (OR = 0.94, 95% CI = 0.91 to 0.97). This treatment effect was observed in many high-risk subgroups, although a trend toward increased mortality was seen in patients with an ejection fraction (EF) less than 30% (OR = 1.13; 95% CI, 0.96 to 1.33). Considerable efforts are being expended by major organizations (STS, ACC) in increasing compliance with existing guidelines for use of β-blockers at the time of hospital discharge (along with use of aspirin, statins, and angiotensin-converting enzyme [ACE] inhibitors).

OTHER MEDICATIONS

Aspirin (and other platelet inhibitors such as dipyridamole) have long been recognized to have strong efficacy in the prevention of early graft thrombosis after CABG, and are a well-recognized component of primary and secondary prevention strategies for all patients with ischemic heart disease. A large observational analysis reported substantial reduction in overall mortality (1.3% vs. 4.0%) and ischemic complications of the heart, brain, kidneys, and gastrointestinal tract when aspirin was administered within 48 hours after surgery. However, patients receiving aspirin immediately before surgery have more mediastinal bleeding and may receive more blood products. A consensus conference of the American College of Chest Physicians on antithrombotic and thrombolytic therapies recommended institution of aspirin within 6 hours after CABG surgery over continuation of preoperative therapy (level of evidence Ia).[10]

ACE inhibitors and statins are receiving attention as agents given a variety of important "pleiotropic" effects (e.g., effects independent of their primary actions of antihypertensive effects or lipid-lowering effects, respectively).[11] Potent anti-inflammatory effects and beneficial effects on endothelial function have been reported for both agents, as well as less clear effects on angiogenesis. Both agents are commonly administered acutely during PCI for their purported benefits. ACE inhibitors are widely

13

considered to be vasculoprotective, particularly with regard to ventricular remodeling after acute myocardial infarction, and they appear to reduce damage after ischemic reperfusion (likely related to reduction in ischemic-induced vasoconstriction and reduction in leukocyte adhesion). Statins have been reported to reduce circulating levels of adhesion molecules, which have been implicated in endothelial dysfunction after CPB. Both agents appear to have direct effects on platelet aggregation and plasminogen activator inhibitors. Of the two classes of drugs, the greatest interest appears to be on the statins because of the greater number of publications and intense concurrent interest with regard to cardioprotection for noncardiac (particularly vascular) surgery. Several investigators have published similar reports of efficacy in observational cohorts of CABG patients.

Monitoring

Electrocardiogram

On arrival in the operating room, the patient undergoing CABG should have routine monitors placed, including pulse oximetry, noninvasive BP, and the ECG. A multilead ECG system and recorder is extremely useful in managing patients with ischemic heart disease. Observing the oscilloscope screen alone results in failure to detect 50% to 80% of episodes of myocardial ischemia detected by continuous recording techniques. Although a continuous paper writeout is useful, online ST-segment trending systems may be more beneficial in the early diagnosis of myocardial ischemia. Recording capability is necessary to provide visual analysis and is invaluable in diagnosing arrhythmias. Transmural myocardial ischemia is a regional disorder; therefore, placement of leads in areas known angiographically to be at risk may increase ECG sensitivity for ischemia detection, whereas subendocardial ischemia is localized nearly exclusively to ST-segment depression in the lateral precordial leads.

Arterial Pressure Monitoring

The radial artery is usually cannulated for BP monitoring during CABG. Dissection of the internal mammary artery with forceful retraction of the sternum may result in tenting of the subclavian artery, with a resultant reduction in flow and inaccuracies in the displayed pressure. Some centers routinely monitor the side opposite the proposed internal mammary artery dissection to avoid this problem, whereas others use this side to detect the problem. The use of newer retractors makes this substantially less problematic. Others prefer to use the nondominant hand to avoid serious quality of life issues should the rare ischemic complication occur. The noninvasive blood pressure should be used as an accuracy check when there is any doubt. Radial arterial pressures are quite distal to the central circulation and have been shown to be inaccurate immediately after hypothermic CPB. Substantial reductions in radial arterial versus aortic pressure have been reported in several clinical investigations (10 to 30 mm Hg), often requiring 20 to 60 minutes after CPB to resolve. Alterations in forearm vascular resistance (decrease) are believed to be responsible for this common phenomenon. This problem can be overcome by temporarily transducing pressure directly from the aorta (by a needle or a cardioplegia cannula) or by insertion of a femoral arterial catheter.

Central Venous Cannulation

The placement of a central venous pressure (CVP) catheter is a standard of practice in cardiac anesthesia both for pressure measurement and for infusing vasoactive drugs. Some centers routinely place two catheters (a large introducer and a smaller

CVP catheter) in the central circulation to facilitate volume infusion and vasoactive or inotropic drug administration.

Pulmonary Artery Catheterization

The efficacy of PA catheterization in medical and surgical settings has evolved over the past 20 years from steadily increasing use in the 1980s and 1990s to distinctly lower use now. Increasing literature evidence from a variety of experimental designs has strongly suggested that despite the substantial amount of physiologic information obtained, major clinical outcomes are little influenced. Earlier studies suggested that clinicians were unable to accurately judge filling pressures based on clinical signs and that therapy could be influenced by these data in the surgical and medical settings. Intraoperatively, PA catheterization was also shown to detect decreased left ventricular (LV) compliance associated with myocardial ischemia. It also appeared better suited for monitoring high-risk patients.

Based on the existing literature it is not possible to give precise criteria for use of a PA catheter in CABG.[12] The higher the patient risk (based primarily on established preoperative clinical predictors), the more favorable is the risk-benefit ratio. Risk factors include the following:

1. Significant impairment of ventricular function (EF<40%, evidence of acute or chronic congestive heart failure, known elevation of left ventricular end-diastolic pressure (LVEDP) on preoperative catheterization, need for preoperative intra-aortic balloon pump (IABP), acute or chronic severe mitral regurgitation due to ischemia, ventricular septal defect after myocardial infarction, or other mechanical complications).
2. High risk for intraoperative ischemia or difficult revascularization (i.e., recent, large myocardial infarction or severe unstable angina, known poor revascularization targets or severe microcirculatory disease, reoperation, catheterization laboratory PCI "crash").
3. Severe comorbidities (e.g., renal failure, on or approaching need for dialysis; severe chronic obstructive pulmonary disease).
4. Combined procedures that significantly lengthen duration of surgery or add significant blood loss (e.g., CABG-carotid, other vascular procedures).

Although most of the recent clinical reports of patients undergoing OPCAB have used, and many recommend use of PA catheterization, it is not possible to give firm recommendations on this because of the lack of evidence-based data.

Transesophageal Echocardiography

It is appreciated that the earliest signs of myocardial ischemia include diastolic dysfunction followed by systolic segmental wall motion abnormalities that occur within seconds of acute coronary occlusion. Comparison of TEE with continuous (Holter) ECGs have shown a greater incidence of segmental wall motion abnormalities than ECG changes in patients with CAD. However, it is thought that new segmental wall motion abnormalities detected in the intraoperative period may frequently occur due to nonischemic causes, particularly changes in loading conditions, and alteration in electrical conduction in the heart. The use of inotropic agents or elevations of catecholamine levels can aggravate (by increased oxygen demand) or improve wall motion. Changes in preload and afterload are likely the most important factors in the CABG setting; transient reversible segmental wall motion abnormalities are commonly related to acute myocardial stunning due to ischemia before or during weaning from CPB. TEE is highly sensitive but not specific for myocardial ischemia. The short-axis midpapillary muscle view, commonly used because of its inclusion of myocardium supplied by the three major coronary arteries,

13

may entirely miss segmental wall motion abnormalities occurring in the basal or apical portions of the heart. These changes necessitate interrogation of additional components of the comprehensive TEE examination recommended by the ASE/SCA Task Force before and after CPB or after completion of revascularization in OPCAB. The ASA Practice Guidelines for TEE (which have not been revised since their initial publication in 1996) list the perioperative uses in patients with increased risk of myocardial ischemia or infarction as a category II indication (supported by weaker evidence and expert consensus). The indication is strengthened when ECG monitoring cannot be used to diagnose ischemia (e.g., in patients with left bundle-branch block, extensive Q waves, or ST-T abnormalities on the baseline ECG), and it is weakened when baseline segmental wall motion abnormalities are present (particularly akinesis or dyskinesis due to fibrotic, calcified, or aneurysmal myocardium). Use of perioperative TEE to evaluate myocardial perfusion, coronary anatomy, or graft patency is listed as a category III indication, but newer technology will upgrade this indication. Evaluation of ischemic mitral regurgitation by TEE may even influence the surgical management during CABG.[13]

Induction and Maintenance

Induction of anesthesia should take place in a calm and relaxed manner, preferably in a quiet operating room. Attention should be paid to the ambient room temperature because entry into an excessively cold operating room can elicit a sympathetic response increasing blood pressure and sometimes heart rate, particularly in the elderly and thin patients. Allaying the patient's anxiety with premedication and calm, reassuring verbal interaction is also critical. Preoxygenation should be used and monitoring should be in place, including PA catheterization in patients at very high risk, whose condition may be unstable during or after induction.

There are two main considerations in choosing an induction technique for patients undergoing CABG. The first is LV function. Patients with good LV function often have a strong sympathetic response to surgical stimulation and may require supranormal doses of anesthetics, plus the addition of β-blockers with or without vasodilators, to control these responses. Patients with poor LV function often do not tolerate normal doses of anesthetics and are unable to produce a significant hemodynamic response to sympathetic stimulation or the response may precipitate major reductions in cardiac output.

The second consideration is the desirability of early extubation. Time spent in the intensive care unit (ICU) is one of the most expensive aspects of hospital care for CABG and is heavily influenced by postoperative ventilator management. The patient with normal preoperative LV function, assuming an uneventful intraoperative course, will have recovered 90% of baseline LV function by 4 hours postoperatively and can usually be extubated within 4 to 6 hours postoperatively if attention is paid to adequate rewarming and postoperative analgesia and if high doses of respiratory depressant anesthetics (particularly opioids and benzodiazepines) have been avoided. With the routine application of fast-track techniques, some centers have adopted immediate extubation in the operating room. However, this remains relatively uncommon and requires the close cooperation of a highly coordinated team. Because this is not always the case (particularly in teaching institutions in which residents and fellows rotate for short intervals or in some private institutions in which staffing at night is relatively low), many centers take a more measured, less aggressive approach.

After the induction of anesthesia, the pre-bypass period (for conventional CABG) may last less than an hour (e.g., only one or two saphenous vein grafts harvested) or several hours (e.g., for dissection of the left internal mammary artery, right internal mammary artery, or radial or gastroepiploic arteries after a repeat sternotomy). Surgical stimulus may be severe, such as during sternotomy or dissection around

IV

the ascending aorta. Between 50% and 70% of patients in most series presenting for CABG have normal LV function (when not ischemic) and are capable of mounting significant blood pressure and heart rate responses to noxious stimuli, whereas others with poor LV function may require pharmacologic support of the blood pressure for such stimuli. It is evident that no single approach to anesthesia for CABG procedures is suitable for all patients. Most hypnotics, opioids, and volatile agents have been used in different combinations for the induction and maintenance of anesthesia with good results in the hands of experienced clinicians.

Primary Induction Agents

Considerations for choice of induction agent in the patient undergoing CABG are based on theoretical and practical clinical considerations. Desirable goals include avoidance of hypertension and tachycardia, which is most likely to occur in the patient with normal ventricular function, hypertension, and LV hypertrophy; avoidance of hypotension and excessive myocardial depression in a patient with depressed ventricular function or with severe flow-dependent stenoses; and provision of smooth intubating conditions with a lack of effect on airway resistance.

Thiopental has been used for decades for induction in this setting. Its predominant hemodynamic effects include reduction in mean arterial pressure and cardiac output accompanied by a modest increase in heart rate. These are believed to result from a combination of direct myocardial depression, venodilation, and a decrease in central sympathetic outflow. The use of thiopental in most centers has declined substantially in favor of propofol. Adverse effects on airway resistance, a greater propensity to elicit bronchospasm, and a greater association with postoperative nausea and vomiting are other potential factors.

The clinical effects of propofol are in general similar to those of thiopental. However, it has numerous advantages over thiopental based on its predictable pharmacokinetics and dynamics. Based on these, it has been widely adopted in the operating room for anesthesia delivery by computer-controlled devices and for postoperative ICU sedation. It is often used for sedation after CABG surgery.[14]

Benzodiazepines

Benzodiazepines are commonly used in combination with a narcotic to induce anesthesia for CABG. In most settings, midazolam has replaced diazepam given its numerous advantages (particularly water solubility, a shorter half-life, and absence of metabolites capable of accumulation prolonging sedative effects). Numerous clinical series of widely different sizes and designs, reporting on the efficacy of diazepam or, more commonly, midazolam used with high-dose opioids, were subsequently published. Moderate degrees of hypotension were reported in most studies primarily attributed to a reduction in systemic vascular resistance.

Opioids

These drugs are pure opioid agonists and none provides complete anesthesia as defined by predictable dose-response relations for suppression of the stress response and release of endogenous catecholamines even with high serum concentrations. Hypertension and tachycardia have been commonly reported in response to induction/intubation and surgical stimuli (particularly with sternotomy) in older studies of high-dose opioid anesthesia with fentanyl or sufentanil. Figure 13-6 demonstrates this lack of association of serum levels with hemodynamic responses.

To provide complete anesthesia if high-dose opioids are used, the usual practice is to supplement with inhaled or other intravenous agents (e.g., midazolam). This permits a reduction in the total dose of opioid and, particularly with volatile agents, more rapid return of respiratory drive facilitating early extubation.

13

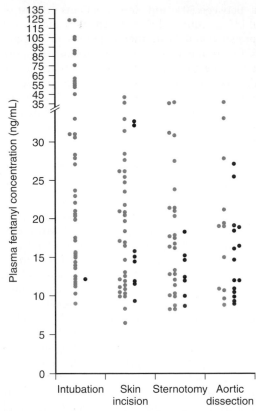

Figure 13-6　The plasma fentanyl concentration and number of patients with a hypertensive response at each event studied. *Filled circles* indicate hypertensive status; *open circles* indicate normotensive status. (From Wynands JE, Townsend GE, Wong P, et al: Blood pressure response and plasma fentanyl concentrations during high and very high-dose fentanyl anesthesia for coronary artery surgery. Anesth Analg 62:661, 1983.)

IV

Inhalation Anesthetics and Myocardial Protection

There is steadily increasing evidence that inhalation anesthetic agents have favorable properties in patients undergoing CABG surgery, particularly in comparison to total intravenous anesthesia approaches. Along with the now routine use of fast-track anesthesia techniques, there has been a major resurgence in their use as the primary anesthetic for cardioprotection, with opioids and benzodiazepines increasingly relegated to a "supplemental" status.

MYOCARDIAL PROTECTION AND PRECONDITIONING

Inhalation anesthetics are thought to protect the myocardium against ischemia by their ability to mimic ischemic preconditioning. They have been shown to reduce myocardial infarction size after periods of ischemia, protect the heart against postischemic LV dysfunction, and reduce the incidence of arrhythmias after cardiac surgery. Intravenous anesthetics such as propofol do not appear to have the same cardioprotective properties. There is increasing evidence from prospective randomized clinical studies in patients undergoing CABG surgery that volatile anesthetic agents should be part of the anesthetic regimen, particularly in patients at high risk for ischemic events.[15]

The exact mechanisms of preconditioning are still actively under investigation. After the administration of a preconditioning signal such as ischemia, inhalation anesthetics, opioids, bradykinin, or nitroglycerin, membrane-bound receptors (adenosine A_1, adrenergic, bradykinin, muscarinic, delta-1 opioid) coupled to inhibitory G-proteins are activated. Consequently, products of intracellular transduction pathways (e.g., protein kinase C, tyrosine kinases, mitogen-activated protein kinases) mediate the opening and stabilization of adenosine triphosphate (ATP)-sensitive mitochondrial K_{ATP} channels, the effectors thought to be mainly responsible for the preconditioning phenomenon. Increased formation of nitric oxide, free oxygen radicals, and enzymes such as cyclooxygenase-2 are also involved in the preconditioning process.

There is increasing evidence that the choice of anesthetic in patients at risk for cardiac events may have a significant effect on myocardial protection. Inhalation anesthetics have multiple cardioprotective effects, including triggering the preconditioning cascade and blunting of reperfusion injury. The mode of administration, dose, timing, differences between various inhalation agents, patient selection, and the impact on cardiac morbidity and mortality remain to be more precisely elucidated by larger randomized clinical trials.

SEVOFLURANE

Sevoflurane has been increasingly used during cardiac surgery owing to its favorable hemodynamic effects and cardioprotective properties. It is a potent trigger of the preconditioning cascade.[16] It has beneficial effects on intraoperative myocardial function after CPB, and it may also favorably influence long-term morbidity and mortality after CABG.

DESFLURANE

Desflurane has unique hemodynamic effects particularly in relation to sevoflurane. These have resulted in controversy regarding its use in patients with coronary artery disease. Desflurane decreases systemic vascular resistance, blood pressure, and LV systolic and diastolic function in a dose-dependent fashion. However, desflurane causes a significant increase in heart rate, PA pressure, and pulmonary capillary wedge pressure. This increased sympathetic activity is most pronounced when desflurane concentrations are increased rapidly and with higher absolute concentrations. The resulting increase in heart rate could possibly lead to myocardial ischemia in patients presenting with ischemic heart disease.

Desflurane has been shown to have preconditioning-like cardioprotective effects in vitro and in vivo.[17] It preconditions human myocardium by activation of K_{ATP} channels, stimulation of adenosine A_1 receptors, and nitric oxide release.

Desflurane has been used safely and effectively in CABG surgery worldwide. However, the clinician must remain aware of its sympathetic stimulating properties, particularly with rapid increases in concentration.

ISOFLURANE

Preconditioning with isoflurane has been documented in multiple studies. Its hemodynamic properties and its effect on the preconditioning cascade are similar to those of sevoflurane. When isoflurane was compared with sevoflurane in patients with cardiac disease undergoing noncardiac surgery, there was no significant difference in perioperative ischemic events, adverse cardiac outcomes, intraoperative hemodynamic stability, and inotropic support between the two groups. Isoflurane mimics ischemic preconditioning through activation of mitochondrial K_{ATP} channels and the generation of free radicals. Its preconditioning effect appears to be potentiated by concurrent opioid administration.

13

Neuromuscular Blocking Agents

All of the available neuromuscular blocking agents have been used to produce adequate intubation conditions and relaxation during CABG surgery. Traditionally, pancuronium had been advocated for use with high-dose narcotic techniques, because it offsets opioid-induced bradycardia. However, it has long been recognized that clinically significant tachycardia resulting in myocardial ischemia could occur during induction of anesthesia with high-dose fentanyl and pancuronium. With the increasing popularity of fast-track cardiac surgery, early extubation is now most desirable and the longer duration of action of pancuronium is a potential disadvantage. Several studies have compared the duration of action of pancuronium and rocuronium in patients undergoing cardiac surgery. Irrespective of a single intubating dose or a continuous infusion, patients receiving rocuronium had significantly less residual neuromuscular blockade and shorter time to extubation. Especially in fast-track cardiac surgery, shorter-acting neuromuscular blocking agents such as rocuronium are recommended to avoid residual paralysis and to allow for early extubation and ICU discharge. Neuromuscular transmission monitoring to assess for residual blockade and use of pharmacologic reversal is advisable especially if a fast-track anesthesia technique is used.

Intraoperative Awareness and Recall

Patients undergoing cardiac surgery have always been considered to be at increased risk due to anesthetic regimens intentionally devoid of cardiodepressant inhalation anesthetics and due to frequent periods of light anesthesia in the presence of hemodynamic instability resulting from surgical manipulation of the heart and great vessels, depressed contractility after CPB, or bleeding. The published incidence of awareness in patients undergoing cardiac surgery is significantly higher than that reported for general surgery with older reports of up to 23%. However, the introduction of fast-track anesthesia techniques and the recognition that inhalation agents are useful in intraoperative preconditioning before CPB have changed anesthetic regimens for cardiac surgery. It is now recognized that use of inhalation agents during cardiac surgery (including during CPB) reduces the risk of awareness.[18]

Choice of Technique

A wide variety of techniques have been used for anesthetic induction and maintenance for CABG. Hemodynamic alterations such as hypotension after induction, or hypertension and tachycardia at intubation, are not infrequent. They can be readily treated with small doses of vasopressors, such as phenylephrine or ephedrine for hypotension, or deepening anesthesia or adding β-blockade to treat hyperdynamic responses. No single technique was demonstrated to be superior in terms of reduced intraoperative ischemia, postoperative myocardial infarction, or death.

Interest in the use of thoracic epidural anesthesia (TEA) for cardiac surgery has steadily increased over the past 15 years. It has been long appreciated that thoracic sympathectomy has favorable effects on the heart and coronary circulation. Its coronary vasodilating effects have been well documented and it has been used to treat unstable angina for many years. There has been a resurgence in interest, and it is frequently used as a supplement to general anesthesia for cardiac surgery, particularly in Europe and Asia (Fig. 13-7). However, in the United States, medicolegal concerns about the rare but present danger of a devastating neurologic injury and the substantial logistical issues regarding placement the night before surgery, increased time to place relative to inducing general anesthesia, and the potential for cancellation of a case in event of bloody return are major limiting factors. The advent of fast-tracking could be considered a potential

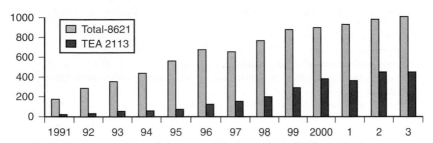

Figure 13-7 Frequency of use of thoracic epidural anesthesia (TEA) at a single center over the past 31 years (total of 2013 patients). All catheters were placed the day before surgery between C7 and T3. Dural puncture occurred in 0.9%, and temporary neurologic deficits occurred in 0.2%. No permanent deficits occurred. (From Chakravarthy M, Thimmangowda P, Krishnamurthy J, et al: Thoracic epidural anesthesia in cardiac surgical patients: A prospective audit of 2,113 cases. J Cardiothorac Vasc Anesth 19:44, 2005.)

driving force (e.g., ability to extubate faster and have a more comfortable patient with TEA), although most evidence suggests that a wide variety of techniques can be effectively used to facilitate early extubation and that the cardioprotective effects of volatile agents may be as effective as the beneficial effects of thoracic sympathectomy.

TEA in conscious patients (with supplemental intravenous sedation) appears to be increasingly used for off-pump CABG (OPCAB or minimally invasive direct CABG [MIDCAB] approaches) with reports from diverse settings (e.g., Germany, Turkey, India) and has been designated conscious off-pump coronary artery bypass grafting (COPCAB). In most series, 2% to 3% of catheters are unable to be placed in potential candidates and 2% to 3% of patients are converted to general anesthesia because of a large pneumothorax or incomplete analgesia. Patients were fast-tracked, an ICU stay was not used, and some were discharged from the hospital the day of surgery. Patient acceptance appeared to be quite high. No complications related to TEA were observed. This is clearly an area of growing interest and one that has potential advantages, particularly for countries with different health care systems, resource constraints, and sociocultural differences.

Safety concerns are a major consideration in use of TEA in this setting given chronic use of antiplatelet agents, use of systemic anticoagulation and platelet inhibition for acute therapy of unstable angina, and systemic anticoagulation and potential coagulopathy induced by CPB. The true incidence of serious complications (particularly epidural hematoma) is unknown. A widely quoted estimate is 1 in 1528 for TEA with 95% confidence. Intrathecal risks are quoted as 1 in 3610. These estimates were based on consideration of more than 4000 reported cases (cardiac surgery) in which no complications were reported. Chakravarthy and coworkers presented an audit of 2113 cardiac surgery TEA cases over a 13-year period with no permanent neurologic deficits, a 0.9% dural puncture rate, and 0.2% transient neurologic deficits.[19]

FAST-TRACK MANAGEMENT FOR CORONARY ARTERY BYPASS GRAFTING

The fast-track clinical pathway encompasses a variety of perioperative (and after hospital discharge) management strategies, but early extubation is the one that has received the greatest attention (Box 13-2). Because it is a simple, continuous variable

---

BOX 13-2 *Perioperative Goals of Fast-Track Management*

- Preoperative education
- Same-day admission whenever possible
- Anesthetic technique tailored to early extubation and effective early postoperative analgesia
- Flexibility in the use of recovery areas (e.g., use of postanesthesia care unit instead of an ICU)
- Early extubation incorporating nurse- or respiratory therapist–driven protocols for stable patients
- Early mobilization and removal of catheters, tubes, and similar devices
- Early ICU and hospital discharge for patients meeting criteria
- Early follow-up (e.g., telephone, office visits) after hospital discharge
- Formalized clinical pathway and interdisciplinary continuous quality improvement strategies

---

(e.g., hours to extubation), it is one that many observational reports and a smaller number of randomized, controlled trials have reported. It also appears to be the only one that has resulted in meta-analyses showing the practice is safe and effective.[20] Early extubation is acknowledged as a key component of the fast-track clinical pathway and one that was considered perhaps the most radical change in practice during the peak of scrutiny of the fast-track pathway (Box 13-3).

CORONARY ARTERY BYPASS GRAFTING WITHOUT CARDIOPULMONARY BYPASS

Off-pump coronary artery bypass grafting is the single greatest change in CABG techniques in the past 2 decades.[21,22] Although this term encompasses a range of surgical approaches (based on the degree of invasiveness encompassing full, limited, or no sternotomy), the technique that is most commonly performed is OPCAB with a full sternotomy. The precise number of such procedures performed remains largely speculative; however, it is likely in the 20–30% range at the present time. Surgeons appear to adopt it enthusiastically or not at all, an unsurprising finding given the unsettled state of the literature. Although the literature base is increasing rapidly, the final word is still years away (given several large ongoing randomized, controlled trials). However, it appears that OPCAB is as effective as routine CABG, is safer for certain patient subsets, and may be associated with improvement in several outcomes at slightly lower resource use. Its use is likely to increase, especially for high-risk patients with serious comorbidities associated with higher morbidity/mortality from CPB (e.g., severe cerebrovascular and renal disease). The clinician will immediately notice that the pace and tempo of anesthetic management differs substantially from that of conventional CABG. The focused involvement of the anesthesiologist is perhaps more important in OPCAB than during on-pump CABG (including use of TEE and PA catheterization).

Although OPCAB is perceived as a contemporary development, surgery on the beating heart was first performed in the 1950s and early 1960s, preceding the widespread use of CPB-based CABG because of the slower development and application of CPB techniques in the late 1960s. In the late 1980s and early 1990s, introduction of

IV

BOX 13-3 *Suggested Criteria for Early Extubation*

Systemic

- Body temperature stable and >36°C (96.8°F) or <38°C (100.4°F)
- Arterial pH > 7.30

Cardiovascular

- Stable hemodynamics on minimal or decreasing doses of inotrope or vasodilator therapy; cardiac index > 2.0 L/min/m², stable $S\bar{v}o_2$, minimal base deficit
- Stable cardiac rhythm or good response to pacing

Respiratory

- Spontaneous respiratory rate > 10 to 12 and < 25 to 30 breaths per minute, vital capacity > 10 mL/kg, maximal negative inspiratory force > −20 cm H_2O with minimal respiratory support (e.g., low levels of continuous positive airway pressure, pressure support)
- Adequate arterial blood gases: PaO_2 > 70 to 80 mm Hg (Fio_2 = 0.4 to 0.5), $PaCO_2$ < 40 to 45 mm Hg
- Chest radiograph without major abnormalities (e.g., minimal atelectasis)

Renal

- Adequate urine output (non–dialysis-dependent patients), stable electrolytes, and input/output values for patients on preoperative dialysis

Neurologic

- Awake, alert, cooperative, moving all extremities
- Adequate motor strength (e.g., hand grip); if not, consider relaxant reversal, especially for patients receiving pancuronium

Surgical

- Adequate hemostasis with decreasing or stable mediastinal drainage

---

the short-acting β-blocker esmolol led some surgeons to "experiment" with OPCAB (on the LAD) by lowering of the heart rate. However, it was not until the mid- to late 1990s when surgical researchers developed efficient mechanical stabilizer devices that minimized motion around the anastomosis site (independent of heart rate) that this technique became widespread. The ability to expose the posterior surface of the heart to access the posterior descending and the circumflex vessels using suction devices usually placed on the apex of the heart, pericardial retraction sutures, slings, or other techniques, without producing major hemodynamic compromise, was critical for multivessel application of this technique. This is commonly referred to as *verticalization*, in contrast to *displacement* for the LAD and diagonal anastomoses.

OPCAB extends the range of surgeon-induced hemodynamic changes the anesthesiologist encounters relative to routine CABG. The skilled cardiac anesthesiologist must be able to anticipate and communicate with the surgeon to minimize the adverse impact of these changes on the heart and other important organs. The surgical manipulations involve a variety of geometric distortions of cardiac anatomy (most notably compression of the right ventricle and, to a lesser degree, some distortion of the mitral valve annulus). The magnitude of distortion varies with the patient's individual anatomy (most notably the size and shape of the right and left ventricles), the skill of the surgeon in placement of stabilizer devices, use of "deep" pericardial stay sutures (which facilitate forward superior apical displacement for

13

LAD anastomosis), and manipulation of the pleural space (e.g., right pleural incision to create space for the compressed right ventricle). With a skilled surgeon, the changes are usually modest or easily treated with the Trendelenburg position, use of vasoconstrictors or inotropes, and judicious volume expansion. However, severe changes due to acute ischemia, mitral regurgitation, or unrecognized right ventricular compression may occur, necessitating emergent conversion to CPB.

Monitoring for Off-Pump Coronary Artery Bypass Grafting

Hemodynamic changes with OPCAB vary with location of the anastomosis and type of stabilizer or verticalizer system used, although most of the available hemodynamic data was obtained from low-risk patients. At present, there is no clear consensus or guidelines with regard to the type of monitoring recommended for OPCAB. Most observational studies have used fairly extensive monitoring with PA catheterization. TEE appears to be widely used, despite problems with imaging during the anastomotic period, particularly when the heart is verticalized. As with on-pump CABG, it is likely that as this procedure is more widely adopted and clinicians gain increasing familiarity, that monitoring recommendations, particularly for low-risk patients, will become less sophisticated.

Outcomes in Off-Pump Coronary Artery Bypass Grafting

Several investigators and working groups have comprehensively reviewed outcomes in patients undergoing OPCAB. Investigators have analyzed 37 randomized trials of 3369 patients with comparable treatment groups with the exception of a marginal difference in number of grafts performed (2.6 OPCAB versus 2.8 CABG).[21] All but one of the studies specifically excluded "high-risk" patients. Although various definitions were used, most excluded patients with low ejection fractions, repeat procedures, and renal failure, and several studies excluded patients with diseased circumflex vessels. As expected, not all studies reported on all outcomes. The investigators found no significant differences in 30-day or 1- to 2-year mortality, myocardial infarction, stroke (30 day and 1 to 2 years), renal dysfunction, need for IABP, wound infection, or reoperation for bleeding or reintervention (for ischemia). OPCAB was associated with a significant reduction in atrial fibrillation (OR = 0.58), numbers of patients transfused (OR = 0.43), respiratory infections (OR = 0.41), need for inotropes (OR = 0.48), duration of ventilation (weighted mean difference [WMD] of 3.4 hours), ICU length of stay (WMD of 0.3 day), and hospital length of stay (WMD of 1.0 days). Changes in neurocognitive dysfunction were not different in the immediate postoperative period; they were significantly improved at 2 to 6 months (OR = 0.57), but there were no differences seen at 12 months. The critical issue of graft patency was addressed in only four studies, and these varied substantially with regard to when this was assessed (3 months in two and 12 months in two). Only one study reported a difference (reduction in circumflex patency with OPCAB). Because of the small numbers of patients, the overall data for this category were considered inadequate for meta-analysis. A large-scale, randomized, controlled trial is being conducted by the Department of Veterans Affairs with evaluation of graft patency at 1 year postoperatively. Four randomized, controlled trials have analyzed quality of life. Various methods precluded inclusion in the meta-analysis, but it generally appears there is little difference between operations. Of the 20 trials reporting conversion rates, 8% of OPCAB patients required conversion to CABG, whereas only 1.7% were converted from CABG to OPCAB. The conversion rate for OPCAB in these low- to medium-risk patients is substantial and would be expected to be even higher in higher-risk patients with greater disease burdens, more complex lesions, or impaired ventricular function in whom tolerance of stabilization and verticalization may be less. The anesthesiologist must be prepared for rapid institution of CPB at all times.

The ultimate adoption of OPCAB resides in demonstration of similar rates of long-term graft patency. Given the longevity of most grafts, particularly the internal mammary artery (>15 years), this will take some time to be conclusively established. With ongoing technologic advances, it is likely this approach will continue to expand in numbers of patients and surgical complexity.

MYOCARDIAL ISCHEMIA DURING REVASCULARIZATION

Incidence of Myocardial Ischemia in Patients Undergoing Revascularization Surgery

In addition to providing anesthesia, a major concern of the anesthesiologist is the prevention and treatment of myocardial ischemia. Numerous laboratory and clinical studies have examined the incidence of myocardial ischemia in the perioperative period, as it relates to the administration of anesthetic drugs. Although the incidence of pre-bypass ischemia in patients appears to be between 10% and 50%, it is not at all clear that the anesthetic drug combination per se is a determinant of this incidence. Several studies have addressed whether the anesthetic technique (e.g., fast-track or early extubation, high thoracic epidural) is related to perioperative morbidity and myocardial ischemic events. An extensive meta-analysis of more than 30 randomized, controlled trials of patients undergoing cardiac surgery showed no difference in the relative risk of postoperative myocardial ischemia when early extubation protocols were compared with conventional extubation management.[22]

Hemodynamic Changes Related to Myocardial Ischemia

Besides ECG abnormalities, some hemodynamic changes should alert the anesthesiologist to the possibility of intraoperative myocardial ischemia. The association of tachycardia with hypotension or increased LV filling pressure (both of which reduce coronary perfusion pressure [CPP] is a particularly undesirable combination jeopardizing the oxygen supply-demand relationship. Figure 13-8 demonstrates how hypertension in the absence of tachycardia, in response to surgical stress (skin incision), can be associated with pulmonary hypertension, elevated pulmonary capillary wedge pressure, and prominent A and V waves on the PCWP waveform. Although ECG changes occurred later, the early hemodynamic abnormalities almost certainly were the result of ischemic LV dysfunction. Treatment included deepening anesthesia and administering a nitroglycerin infusion.

LV diastolic dysfunction detected with TEE is the earliest change identified after coronary artery occlusion, and it often precedes the development of abnormal systolic function. Regional wall motion abnormalities also have been described as early signs of ischemia. They occur within seconds of inadequate blood flow or oxygen supply. Regional wall motion abnormalities detected by TEE have been shown to be a more sensitive method of detecting myocardial ischemia in patients undergoing CABG compared with ST-segment changes. Myocardial ischemia on repositioning

13

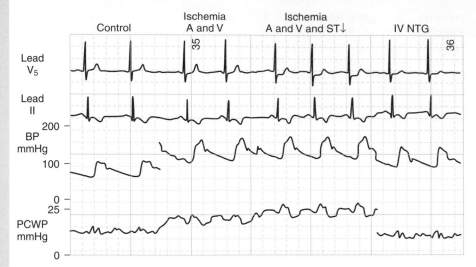

Figure 13-8   Nitroglycerin (NTG) relieved postintubation intraoperative myocardial ischemia, as evidenced by large A and V waves in the pulmonary capillary wedge pressure (PCWP) tracing and then by ST-segment depression. BP = blood pressure. (From Kaplan JA, Wells PH: Early diagnosis of myocardial ischemia using the pulmonary arterial catheter. Anesth Analg 60:789, 1981.)

the heart during OPCAB can be the cause of a sudden onset of mitral regurgitation or worsening of preexisting mitral regurgitation, both of which can be detected with TEE monitoring.

Intraoperative Treatment of Myocardial Ischemia

Close attention to hemodynamic control and rapid treatment of abnormalities are fundamental principles of the intraoperative management of the patient with CAD. If there is a hemodynamic abnormality that is temporally related to the onset of ischemia, it should be treated accordingly. Hemodynamic treatment to ensure an adequate CPP (diastolic BP – LVEDP) should be a priority, as should control of heart rate, the single most important treatable determinant of myocardial oxygen consumption. Table 13-1 summarizes the treatment of acute perioperative myocardial ischemia.[23,24]

Intravenous Nitroglycerin

Since the introduction in 1976 by Kaplan and colleagues of the V_5 lead to diagnose myocardial ischemia and intravenous nitroglycerin to treat it, nitroglycerin has been one of the mainstays in the treatment for perioperative myocardial ischemia. Intravenous nitroglycerin acts immediately to reduce LV preload and wall tension, primarily by decreasing venous tone in lower doses, whereas in larger doses it may also decrease arterial resistance and epicardial coronary arterial resistance. Nitroglycerin has been shown to consistently decrease LV filling pressure, systemic blood pressure, and myocardial oxygen consumption and to improve LV performance in patients with severe dysfunction. It is most effective in treating acute myocardial ischemia with induced ventricular dysfunction accompanied by sudden elevations in LVEDV, LVEDP, and PA pressure. These elevations in LV preload and wall tension further exacerbate perfusion deficits to the ischemic subendocardium and usually respond immediately to nitroglycerin.

Table 13-1   **Acute Treatments for Suspected Intraoperative Myocardial Ischemia***

Associated Hemodynamic Finding	Therapy	Dosage
Hypertension, tachycardia[†]	Deepen anesthesia	
	Intravenous (IV) β-blockade	Esmolol, 20-100 mg, +50-200 μg/kg/min PRN
		Metoprolol, 0.5-2.5 mg
		Labetalol, 2.5-10 mg
	IV nitroglycerin	Nitroglycerin, 33-330 μg/min[‡]
Normotension, tachycardia[†]	Ensure adequate anesthesia, change anesthetic regimen	
	IV β-blockade	β-blockade, as above
Hypertension, normal heart rate	Deepen anesthesia	
	IV nitroglycerin or nicardipine	Nicardipine, 1-5 mg, +1-10 μg/kg/min
		Nitroglycerin, as above
Hypotension, tachycardia[†]	IV α-agonist	Phenylephrine, 25-100 μg
	Alter anesthetic regimen (e.g., lighten)	Norepinephrine, 2-4 μg
	IV nitroglycerin when normotensive	Nitroglycerin, as above
Hypotension, bradycardia	Lighten anesthesia	
	IV ephedrine	Ephedrine, 5-10 mg
	IV epinephrine	Epinephrine, 4-8 μg
	IV atropine	Atropine, 0.3-0.6 mg
	IV nitroglycerin when normotensive	Nitroglycerin, as above
Hypotension, normal heart rate	IV α-agonist/ephedrine	α-Agonist, as above
	IV epinephrine	Epinephrine, as above
	Alter anesthesia (e.g., lighten)	
	IV nitroglycerin when normotensive	Nitroglycerin, as above
No abnormality	IV nitroglycerin	Nitroglycerin, as above
	IV nicardipine	Nicardipine, as above

*Ensure adequacy of oxygenation, ventilation, and intravascular volume status and consider surgical factors, such as manipulation of heart of coronary grafts.
†Tachyarrhythmias (e.g., paroxysmal atrial tachycardia, atrial fibrillation) should be treated directly with synchronized cardioversion or specific pharmacologic agents.
‡Bolus doses (25-50 μg) and high infusion rate may be required initially.

13

Preoperatively, it is often used to treat patients with unstable angina or ischemic mitral regurgitation and to limit the size of an evolving myocardial infarction, reduce associated complications, and reverse segmental wall motion abnormalities. In the pre-CPB period and during OPCAB, nitroglycerin is used to treat signs of ischemia such as ST-segment depression, hypertension uncontrolled by the anesthetic technique, ventricular dysfunction, or coronary artery spasm (Box 13-4). During CPB, nitroglycerin can be used to control the mean arterial pressure; however, nitroglycerin is not always effective in controlling mean arterial pressure during CPB (approximately 60% of patients respond) because of alterations of the pharmacokinetics and pharmacodynamics of the drug with CPB. Factors contributing to the

---

BOX 13-4 *Profile for Intraoperative Use of Intravenous Nitroglycerin*

- Hypertension > 20% above control values
- Pulmonary capillary wedge pressure > 18 to 20 mm Hg
- AC and V waves > 20 mm Hg
- ST-segment changes > 1 mm
- New segmental wall motion abnormalities on transesophageal echocardiography
- Acute right ventricular or left ventricular dysfunction
- Coronary artery spasm

BOX 13-5 *Uses of Intravenous Nitroglycerin on Termination of Cardiopulmonary Bypass*

- Elevated pulmonary capillary wedge pressure
- Elevated systemic vascular resistance or pulmonary vascular resistance
- Infusion of oxygenator reservoir volume
- Incomplete revascularization
- Ischemia
- Intraoperative myocardial infarction
- Coronary artery spasm

---

reduction of its effectiveness include adsorption to the plastic in the CPB system, alterations in regional blood flow, hemodilution, and hypothermia. Different oxygenators and filters sequester up to 90% of circulating nitroglycerin during CPB. After revascularization, nitroglycerin is used to treat residual ischemia or coronary artery spasm and reduce preload and afterload, and it may be combined with vasopressors (e.g., phenylephrine) to increase the CPP when treating coronary air embolism (Box 13-5).

Intravenous nitroglycerin has been compared with other vasodilators such as nitroprusside and the calcium channel blockers during CABG and in other clinical situations. Kaplan demonstrated that nitroglycerin was preferable to nitroprusside during CABG. Both drugs were shown to control intraoperative hypertension and to decrease myocardial oxygen consumption; however, nitroglycerin improved ischemic changes on the ECG but nitroprusside did not. The lack of improvement in the ischemic ST segments with nitroprusside was thought to result from a decrease in CPP or the production of an intracoronary steal.

Calcium Channel Antagonists

Calcium antagonists have been found to be cardioprotective against reperfusion injury. This is due to their energy-saving actions of negative inotropy and chronotropy. These antagonists have also been shown to reduce reperfusion arrhythmias and attenuate myocardial stunning. In a review of methods to reduce ischemia during OPCAB, Kwak included the calcium antagonists along with newer drugs such as nitric oxide–releasing agents, free radical scavengers, and Na^+/H^+ exchange inhibitors in the management of ischemia-reperfusion injury.[23]

Nicardipine is a short-acting dihydropyridine calcium antagonist similar to nifedipine but possessing a tertiary amine structure in the ester side chain. Unlike other available dihydropyridines, nicardipine is stable as a parenteral solution and therefore can be administered intravenously. It has highly specific modes of action, which include coronary antispasmodic and vasodilatory effects and systemic vasodilation. Among the calcium antagonists, nicardipine is unique in its consistent augmentation of coronary blood flow and its ability to induce potent and more selective vasodilator responses in the coronary bed than in the systemic vascular bed. Other important hemodynamic effects include reductions in blood pressure and systemic vascular resistance and increases in myocardial contractility and cardiac output. Nicardipine also produces minimal myocardial depression and significant improvement in diastolic function in patients with ischemic heart disease. Intravenous doses of 5 to 10 mg of nicardipine administered to patients with CAD produce therapeutic plasma levels. Plasma concentrations decline in a biphasic manner, with an initial half-life of 14 minutes and a terminal half-life of 4.75 hours. Clearance of nicardipine results mainly from its metabolism by the liver, and excretion is primarily through bile and the feces. It undergoes rapid and extensive first-pass hepatic metabolism with the production of inactive metabolites. Nicardipine's rapid onset and cessation of action make it an attractive drug for the perioperative management of hypertension or myocardial ischemia. It has been administered to control hemodynamics during and after noncardiac vascular surgery and CABG.

Esmolol

Hypertension, tachycardia, arrhythmias, and myocardial ischemia from sympathetic stimulation are common occurrences in the perioperative period. Despite the benefits of early use of β-blockers in the treatment of myocardial ischemia, the relatively long half-life and prolonged duration of action of previously available β-blockers have limited their usefulness during surgery and the immediate postoperative period. The introduction of esmolol, an ultra-short-acting cardioselective β_1-blocker with a half-life of 9 minutes because of rapid esterase metabolism, provides a β-blocker that is extremely useful in the perioperative period. Esmolol has been shown to be effective in treating patients with acute unstable angina or during acute coronary occlusion. During percutaneous transluminal coronary angioplasty, esmolol was also found to reduce the amount of ST-segment elevation and the onset of segmental wall motion abnormalities. Esmolol has been used during CABG in a prophylactic manner to prevent hypertension, tachycardia, and myocardial ischemia. Before the introduction of newer stabilizing mechanical devices, it had been used frequently during OPCAB procedures to slow the heart rate during the surgical procedure. Esmolol has also been used to treat intraoperative hypertension, tachycardia, and myocardial ischemia. Bolus doses of 1.5 mg/kg have been found to be effective in treating ST-segment changes in patients with CAD. More commonly, a smaller bolus dose is used and is combined with an infusion of esmolol. Bolus doses ranging from 0.5 to 1.0 mg/kg have been used, followed by infusions of 50 to 300 μg/kg/min. These doses have been found to effectively treat increases in heart rate that occur during surgery and to block the β-adrenergic effects of catecholamines associated with surgical stress.

Coronary Artery and Arterial Conduit Spasm

Spasm has usually been associated with profound ST-segment elevation on the ECG, hypotension, severe dysfunction of the ventricles, and myocardial irritability. Many hypotheses have been put forward to explain the origin of coronary artery

13

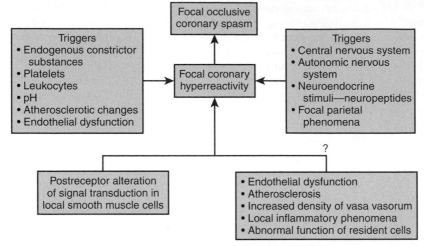

Figure 13-9 Schematic representation of the pathogenesis of coronary artery spasm.

spasm; some of the mechanisms that may play a role are demonstrated in Figure 13-9. The mechanism of postoperative spasm may or may not be the same as that underlying Prinzmetal's variant angina, but the same stimuli seem to be present and therapy is usually effective with a wide range of vasodilators such as nitroglycerin, calcium channel blockers, milrinone, or combinations of nitroglycerin and calcium channel blockers in both situations. Arterial grafts such as the internal mammary artery, and particularly radial artery grafts, are prone to spasm after revascularization and its prevention and recognition are crucial to prevent serious complications.

SUMMARY

IV

- The risk profile of the average patient presenting for CABG has increased with greater numbers of patients with triple-vessel disease, poor targets, reduced ventricular function, and reoperations.
- The pathophysiology of a myocardial infarction has been clarified, with an understanding that it is an acute obstruction of a coronary artery caused by an acute thrombosis in the lumen that often results from the rupture of a vulnerable arterial plaque. Inflammation plays a crucial role in development of the plaque, along with the deposits of lipoproteins.
- Preoperative ordering of premedication should include careful consideration of all of the patient's relevant antihypertensive, antianginal, and other medications.
- Preexisting abnormalities of ventricular function, wall motion, and ischemic mitral regurgitation, along with long ischemic time during CPB, are predictors of difficulty in weaning and postoperative low cardiac output states.
- Pulmonary artery catheterization may still be of particular benefit in patients with impaired ventricular function and major comorbidities who require postoperative cardiac output monitoring.
- The days of high-dose opioid anesthesia for CABG are over with nearly universal adoption of fast-tracking programs aimed at early extubation with reduced ICU and hospital stay.

- All contemporary inhalation agents have been shown to have potent ischemic preconditioning effects, and newer randomized trials have demonstrated reductions in postoperative troponin release and improved ventricular function relative to exclusively intravenous techniques.
- Intraoperative recall is a risk in all cardiac surgical procedures, although its incidence appears to have declined substantially with the increased continuous use of inhalation anesthetics associated with fast-tracking.
- Off-pump CABG is the greatest change in surgical revascularization technique in the past 2 decades.
- The hemodynamic changes associated with OPCAB include reduction in cardiac output, stroke volume, and mean arterial pressure.
- Intravenous nitroglycerin and short-acting β-blockers, such as esmolol, remain the mainstay of treatment for perioperative myocardial ischemia.

REFERENCES

1. Myles PS, Daly DJ, Djaiani G, et al: A systematic review of the safety and effectiveness of fast-track cardiac anesthesia. Anesthesiology 99:982, 2003
2. Cheng DC, Bainbridge D, Martin JE, et al: Does off-pump coronary artery bypass reduce mortality, morbidity, and resource utilization when compared with conventional coronary artery bypass? A meta-analysis of randomized trials. Anesthesiology 102:188, 2005
3. Chakravarthy M, Thimmangowda P, Krishnamurthy J, et al: Thoracic epidural anesthesia in cardiac surgical patients: A prospective audit of 2,113 cases. J Cardiothorac Vasc Anesth 19:44, 2005
4. Shroyer AL, Coombs LP, Peterson ED, et al: The Society of Thoracic Surgeons: 30-day operative mortality and morbidity risk models. Ann Thorac Surg 75:1856, 2003
5. Nashef SA, Roques F, Hammill BG, et al: Validation of European System for Cardiac Operative Risk Evaluation (EuroSCORE) in North American cardiac surgery. Eur J Cardiothorac Surg 22:101, 2002
6. Wei K, Kaul S: The coronary microcirculation in health and disease Cardiol Clin 22:221, 2004
7. Fuster V, Moreno PR, Fayad ZA, et al: Atherothrombosis and high-risk plaque. J Am Coll Cardiol 46:937, 2005
8. London MJ, Zaugg M, Schaub MC, et al: Perioperative beta-adrenergic receptor blockade: Physiologic foundations and clinical controversies. Anesthesiology 100:170, 2004
9. Ferguson TB Jr, Coombs LP, Peterson ED: Preoperative beta-blocker use and mortality and morbidity following CABG surgery in North America. JAMA 287:2221, 2002
10. Stein PD, Schunemann HJ, Dalen JE, et al: Antithrombotic therapy in patients with saphenous vein and internal mammary artery bypass grafts: The Seventh ACCP Conference on Antithrombotic and Thrombolytic Therapy. Chest 126:600S, 2004
11. O'Neil-Callahan K, Katsimaglis G, Tepper MR, et al: Statins decrease perioperative cardiac complications in patients undergoing noncardiac vascular surgery: The Statins for Risk Reduction in Surgery (StaRRS) study. J Am Coll Cardiol 45:336, 2005
12. Murphy GS, Vender JS: Is the pulmonary artery catheter dead? con position. J Cardiothorac Vasc Anesth 21:147, 2007
13. Minhaj M, Patel K, Muzic D, et al: The effect of routine intraoperative transesophageal echocardiography on surgical management. J Cardiothorac Vasc Anesth 21:800, 2007
14. Herr DL, Sum-Ping ST, England M: ICU sedation after coronary artery bypass graft surgery: Dexmedetomidine based versus propofol-based sedation regimens. J Cardiothorac Vasc Anesth 17:576, 2003
15. Zaugg M, Lucchinetti E, Garcia C, et al: Anaesthetics and cardiac preconditioning: II. Clinical implications. Br J Anaesth 91:566, 2003
16. De Hert SG, Van der Linden PJ, Cromheecke S, et al: Cardioprotective properties of sevoflurane in patients undergoing coronary surgery with cardiopulmonary bypass are related to the modalities of its administration. Anesthesiology 101:299, 2004
17. Piriou V, Chiari P, Gateau-Roesch O, et al: Desflurane-induced preconditioning alters calcium-induced mitochondrial permeability transition. Anesthesiology 100:581, 2004
18. Ranta SO, Herranen P, Hynynen M: Patients' conscious recollections from cardiac anesthesia. J Cardiothorac Vasc Anesth 16:426, 2002
19. Chakravarthy M, Thimmangowda P, Krishnamurthy J, et al: Thoracic epidural anesthesia in cardiac surgical patients: A prospective audit of 2,113 cases. J Cardiothorac Vasc Anesth 19:44, 2005
20. Hawkes CA, Dhileepan S, Foxcroft D: Early extubation for adult cardiac surgical patients. Cochrane Database Syst Rev 4:CD003587, 2003

13

21. Raja SG, Dreyfus GD: Off-pump coronary artery bypass surgery: To do or not to do? Current best available evidence. J Cardiothorac Vasc Anesth 18:486, 2004
22. Sellke FW, DiMaio JM, Caplan LR, et al: Comparing on-pump and off-pump coronary artery bypass grafting: Numerous studies but few conclusions: A scientific statement from the American Heart Association council on cardiovascular surgery and anesthesia in collaboration with the interdisciplinary working group on quality of care and outcomes research. Circulation 111:2858, 2005
23. Kwak YL: Reduction of ischemia during off-pump coronary artery bypass graft surgery. J Cardiothorac Vasc Anesth 19:667, 2005
24. Hannan EL, Wu C, Walford G, et al: Drug-eluting stents versus coronary-artery bypass grafting in multivessel coronary disease. N Engl J Med 358:331, 2008

IV

Chapter 14

Valvular Heart Disease: Replacement and Repair

David J. Cook, MD • Philippe R. Housmans, MD • Kent H. Rehfeldt, MD

Valve surgery is very different from coronary artery bypass grafting (CABG). Over the natural history of valvular heart disease (VHD), the physiologic characteristics change markedly and, in the operating room, physiologic and hemodynamic conditions are quite variable and are readily influenced by anesthetic interventions. For some types of valve lesions it can be relatively difficult to predict preoperatively how the heart will respond to the altered loading conditions associated with valve repair or replacement.

It is essential to understand the natural history of each of the major adult-acquired valve defects and how the pathophysiologic conditions evolve. Surgical decision making regarding valve repair or replacement must also be understood, because a valve operated on at the appropriate stage of its natural history will have a good and more predictable outcome than one operated on at a late stage, when the perioperative result can be quite poor. Because pathophysiologic conditions are dynamic and differ significantly among valve lesions, understanding the physiology and natural history of individual valve defects is the foundation of developing an anesthetic plan that includes various requirements for pacing rate and rhythm, use of inotropes (or negative inotropes), and use of vasodilators or vasoconstrictors to alter loading conditions.

Although valvular lesions impose various physiologic changes, all VHD is characterized by abnormalities of ventricular loading. The status of the ventricle changes over time as ventricular function and the valvular defect are influenced by the progression of volume or pressure overload. The clinical status of patients with VHD therefore can be complex and dynamic. It is possible to have clinical decompensation in the context of normal ventricular contractility or ventricular decompensation with normal ejection indices. The altered loading conditions characteristic of VHD may result in a divergence between the function of the heart as a systolic pump and the intrinsic inotropic state of the myocardium. This divergence between cardiac performance and inotropy occurs as a result of compensatory physiologic mechanisms specific to each of the ventricular loading abnormalities.

AORTIC STENOSIS

Clinical Features and Natural History

Aortic stenosis is the most common cardiac valve lesion in the United States. One to 2 percent of the population is born with a bicuspid aortic valve, which is prone to stenosis with aging. Calcific aortic stenosis has several features in common with coronary artery disease (CAD). Both conditions are more common in men, older people, and patients with hypercholesterolemia, and both result in part from an active inflammatory process. There is clinical evidence of an atherosclerotic hypothesis for the cellular mechanism of aortic valve stenosis. There is a clear association between clinical risk factors for atherosclerosis and the development of aortic stenosis: elevated lipoprotein levels, increased low-density lipoprotein (LDL) cholesterol, cigarette smoking, hypertension, diabetes mellitus, increased serum calcium and creatinine levels, and male gender.[1] The early lesion of aortic valve sclerosis may be associated with CAD and vascular atherosclerosis. Aortic valve calcification is an inflammatory process promoted by atherosclerotic risk factors.

The rate of progression is on average a decrease in aortic valve area (AVA) of 0.1 cm^2/yr, and the peak instantaneous gradient increases by 10 mmHg/yr. The rate of progression of aortic stenosis in men older than age 60 years is faster than in women, and it is faster in women older than age 75 years than in women 60 to 74 years old.

Angina, syncope, and congestive heart failure (CHF) are the classic symptoms of the disease, and their appearance is of serious prognostic significance, because postmortem studies indicate that symptomatic aortic stenosis is associated with a life expectancy of only 2 to 5 years. There is evidence that patients with moderate aortic stenosis (i.e., valve areas of 0.7 to 1.2 cm^2) are also at increased risk for the development of complications, with the appearance of symptoms further increasing their risk.

Angina is a frequent and classic symptom of the disease, occurring in approximately two thirds of patients with critical aortic stenosis; and about one half of symptomatic patients are found to have anatomically significant CAD.

The preoperative assessment of aortic stenosis with Doppler echocardiography includes measurement of the AVA and the transvalvular pressure gradient. The latter is calculated from the Doppler-quantified transvalvular velocity of blood flow, which is increased in the presence of aortic stenosis. This maximal velocity (v) is then inserted in the modified Bernoulli equation to determine the pressure gradient (PG) between the left ventricle and the aorta:

$$PG = P(\text{left ventricle}) - P(\text{aorta}) = 4(v^2)$$

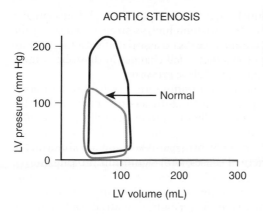

AORTIC STENOSIS

Figure 14-1 Pressure-volume loop in aortic stenosis. LV = left ventricular. (From Jackson JM, Thomas SJ, Lowenstein E: Anesthetic management of patients with valvular heart disease. Semin Anesth 1:239, 1982.)

Pathophysiology

The normal AVA is 2.6 to 3.5 cm², with hemodynamically significant obstruction usually occurring at cross-sectional valve areas of 1 cm² or less. Generally accepted criteria for critical outflow obstruction include a systolic pressure gradient greater than 50 mmHg, with a normal cardiac output and an AVA of less than 0.4 cm². In view of the ominous natural history of severe aortic stenosis (AVA < 0.7 cm²), symptomatic patients with this degree of aortic stenosis are generally referred for immediate aortic valve replacement. A simplification of the Gorlin equation to calculate the AVA is based on the cardiac output (CO) and the peak pressure gradient (PG) across the valve:

$$AVA\left(cm^2\right)= \frac{CO}{\sqrt{PG}}$$

An obvious corollary of the previously described relationship is that "minimal" pressure gradients may actually reflect critical degrees of outflow obstruction when the cardiac output is significantly reduced (i.e., the generation of a pressure gradient requires some finite amount of flow). Clinicians have long recognized this phenomenon as a "paradoxical" decline in the intensity of the murmur (i.e., minimal transvalvular flow) as the aortic stenosis worsens.

Stenosis at the level of the aortic valve results in a pressure gradient from the left ventricle to the aorta. The intracavitary systolic pressure generated to overcome this stenosis directly increases myocardial wall tension (σ) in accordance with Laplace's law:

$$\sigma = \frac{P\times R}{2h}$$

in which P is the intraventricular pressure, R is the inner radius, and h is the wall thickness.

This elevation of wall tension is believed to be the direct stimulus for the further parallel replication of sarcomeres, which produces the concentrically hypertrophied ventricle characteristic of chronic pressure overload. The consequences of this LV hypertrophy include alterations in diastolic compliance, potential imbalances in the myocardial oxygen supply and demand relationship, and possible deterioration of the intrinsic contractile performance of the myocardium.

Figure 14-1 shows a typical pressure-volume loop for a patient with aortic stenosis. Two differences from the normal curve are immediately apparent. First, the peak

14

pressure generated during systole is much higher because of the high transvalvular pressure gradient. Second, the slope of the diastolic limb is steeper, reflecting the reduced left ventricular (LV) diastolic compliance that is associated with the increase in chamber thickness. Clinically, this means that small changes in diastolic volume produce relatively large increases in ventricular filling pressure.

This increased chamber stiffness places a premium on the contribution of atrial systole to ventricular filling, which in patients with aortic stenosis may account for up to 40% of the LV end-diastolic volume (LVEDV), rather than the 15% to 20% characteristic of the normal left ventricle. Echocardiographic and radionuclide studies have documented that diastolic filling and ventricular relaxation are abnormal in patients with hypertrophy from a variety of causes, with significant prolongation of the isovolumic relaxation period being the most characteristic finding. This necessarily compromises the duration and amount of filling achieved during the early rapid diastolic filling phase and increases the relative contribution of atrial contraction to overall diastolic filling. A much higher mean left atrial (LA) pressure is necessary to distend the left ventricle in the absence of the sinus mechanism. One treatment of junctional rhythm is volume infusion.

The systolic limb of the pressure-volume loop shows preservation of pump function, as evidenced by maintenance of the stroke volume (SV) and ejection fraction (EF). It is likely that use of preload reserve and adequate LV hypertrophy are the principal compensatory mechanisms that maintain forward flow. Clinical studies have confirmed that ejection performance is preserved at the expense of myocardial hypertrophy, and the adequacy of the hypertrophic response has been related to the degree to which it achieves normalization of wall stress, in accordance with the Laplace relationship. LV hypertrophy can be viewed as a compensatory physiologic response; however, severe afterload stress and proportionately massive LV hypertrophy could decrease subendocardial perfusion and superimpose a component of ischemic contractile dysfunction.

In aortic stenosis, signs and symptoms of CHF usually develop when preload reserve is exhausted, not because contractility is intrinsically or permanently impaired. This contrasts to mitral and aortic regurgitation, in which irreversible myocardial dysfunction may develop before the onset of significant symptoms. The major threat to the hypertrophied ventricle is its exquisite sensitivity to ischemia. Ventricular hypertrophy directly elevates basal myocardial oxygen demand ($M\dot{v}o_2$). The other major determinants of overall $M\dot{v}o_2$ are heart rate, contractility, and, most important, wall tension. Increases in the latter occur as a direct consequence of Laplace's law in patients with relatively inadequate hypertrophy. The possibility of ischemic contractile dysfunction in the inadequately hypertrophied ventricle arises from increases in wall tension, which directly parallels the imbalance between the elevated peak systolic pressure and the degree of mural hypertrophy. Although there is considerable evidence for "supply-side" abnormalities in the myocardial supply and demand relationship in patients with aortic stenosis, clinical data also support increased $M\dot{v}o_2$ as important in the genesis of myocardial ischemia.

On the supply side, the higher LV end-diastolic pressure (LVEDP) of the poorly compliant ventricle inevitably narrows the diastolic coronary perfusion pressure (CPP) gradient. With severe outflow obstruction, decreases in SV and resultant systemic hypotension may critically compromise coronary perfusion. A vicious cycle may develop because ischemia-induced abnormalities of diastolic relaxation can aggravate the compliance problem and further narrow the CPP gradient. This sets the stage for ischemic contractile dysfunction, additional decreases in SV, and worsening hypotension.

Difficulty of Low-Gradient, Low-Output Aortic Stenosis

A subset of patients with severe aortic stenosis, LV dysfunction, and low transvalvular gradient suffers a high operative mortality rate and poor prognosis.[2] It is difficult to accurately assess the AVA in this low-flow, low-gradient aortic stenosis because the calculated valve area is proportional to forward SV and because the Gorlin constant varies in low-flow states. Some patients with low-flow, low-gradient aortic stenosis have a decreased AVA as a result of inadequate forward SV rather than anatomic stenosis. Surgical therapy is unlikely to benefit these patients because the underlying pathology is a weakly contractile myocardium. However, patients with severe anatomic aortic stenosis may benefit from valve replacement despite the increased operative risk associated with the low-flow, low-gradient hemodynamic state. Guidelines from the American College of Cardiology (ACC) and American Heart Association (AHA) call for a dobutamine echocardiography evaluation to distinguish patients with fixed anatomic aortic stenosis from those with flow-dependent aortic stenosis with LV dysfunction. Low-flow, low-gradient aortic stenosis is defined for a mean gradient of less than 30 mmHg and a calculated AVA less than 1.0 cm^2.

Timing of Intervention

In asymptomatic patients with aortic stenosis, it appears to be relatively safe to delay surgery until symptoms develop, but outcomes vary widely. The presence of moderate or severe valvular calcification along with a rapid increase in aortic-jet velocity identifies patients with a very poor prognosis. These patients should be considered for early valve replacement rather than delaying until symptoms develop.

Echocardiography and exercise testing may identify asymptomatic patients who are likely to benefit from surgery.[3] In a study of 58 asymptomatic patients, 21 had symptoms for the first time during exercise testing. Guidelines for AVR in patients with aortic stenosis are shown in Table 14-1.

Functional outcome after aortic valve replacement in patients older than 80 years is excellent, operative risk is limited, and late survival rates are good. In patients with

14

Table 14-1 Recommendations for the Use of Aortic Valve Replacement in Patients with Aortic Stenosis

Replacement Indicated
- Patients with severe aortic stenosis and any of its classic symptoms (e.g., angina, syncope, dyspnea)
- Patients with severe aortic stenosis who are undergoing coronary artery bypass surgery
- Patients with severe aortic stenosis who are undergoing surgery on the aorta or other heart valves

Replacement Possibly Indicated
- Patients with moderate aortic stenosis who require coronary artery bypass surgery or surgery on the aorta or heart valves
- Asymptomatic patients with severe aortic stenosis and at least one of the following: ejection fraction of no more than 0.50, hemodynamic instability during exercise (e.g., hypotension), ventricular tachycardia; not indicated to prevent sudden death in asymptomatic patients who have none of the findings listed

Adapted from the American Heart Association web site (www.americanheart.org).

BOX 14-1	*Aortic Stenosis*
Preload:	Increased
Afterload:	Increased
Goal:	Sinus rhythm
Avoid:	Hypotension, tachycardia, bradycardia

severe LV dysfunction and low transvalvular mean gradient, operative mortality is increased, but aortic valve replacement was associated with improved functional status. Postoperative survival was best in younger patients and with larger prosthetic valves, whereas medium-term survival was related to improved postoperative functional class.

Anesthetic Considerations

The foregoing pathophysiologic principles dictate that anesthetic management be based on the avoidance of systemic hypotension, maintenance of sinus rhythm and an adequate intravascular volume, and awareness of the potential for myocardial ischemia (Box 14-1). In the absence of CHF, adequate premedication may reduce the likelihood of undue preoperative excitement, tachycardia, and the resultant potential for exacerbating myocardial ischemia and the transvalvular pressure gradient. In patients with truly critical outflow tract obstruction, however, heavy premedication with an exaggerated venodilatory response can reduce the appropriately elevated LVEDV (and LVEDP) needed to overcome the systolic pressure gradient. In these patients in particular, the additional precaution of administering supplementary oxygen may provide worthwhile insurance.

Intraoperative monitoring should include a standard five-lead ECG system, including a V_5 lead, because of the left ventricle's vulnerability to ischemia. A practical constraint in terms of interpretation is that these patients usually exhibit ECG changes because of preoperative LV hypertrophy. The associated ST-segment abnormalities (i.e., strain pattern) may be indistinguishable from or at least very similar to those of myocardial ischemia, making the intraoperative interpretation difficult. Lead II should be readily obtainable for assessing the P-wave changes in the event of supraventricular arrhythmias.

Hemodynamic monitoring is controversial, and few prospective data are available on which to base an enlightened clinical decision. The central venous pressure (CVP) is a particularly poor estimate of LV filling when LV compliance is reduced. A normal CVP can significantly underestimate the LVEDP or pulmonary capillary wedge pressure (PCWP). The principal risks, although minimal, of using a pulmonary artery (PA) catheter in the patient with aortic stenosis are arrhythmia-induced hypotension and ischemia. Loss of synchronous atrial contraction or a supraventricular tachyarrhythmia can compromise diastolic filling of the poorly compliant left ventricle, resulting in hypotension and the potential for rapid hemodynamic deterioration. The threat of catheter-induced arrhythmias is significant for the patient with aortic stenosis. However, accepting a low-normal CVP as evidence of good ventricular function can lead to similarly catastrophic underfilling of the left ventricle on the basis of insufficient replenishment of surgical blood loss. To some extent, even the PCWP can underestimate the LVEDP (and LVEDV) when ventricular compliance is markedly reduced. Placement of a PA catheter also allows for measurement of cardiac output, derived hemodynamic parameters, mixed venous oxygen saturation $S\bar{v}o_2$, and possible transvenous pacing.

Intraoperative fluid management should be aimed at maintaining appropriately elevated left-sided filling pressures. This is one reason why many clinicians believe that the PA catheter is worth its small arrhythmogenic risk. Keeping up with intravascular volume losses is particularly important in noncardiovascular surgery.

Patients with symptomatic aortic stenosis are usually encountered only in the setting of cardiovascular surgery because of their ominous prognosis without aortic valve replacement. Few studies have specifically addressed the response of these patients to the standard intravenous and inhalation induction agents; however, the responses to narcotic and non-narcotic intravenous agents are apparently not dissimilar from those of patients with other forms of VHD. The principal benefit of a narcotic induction is the assurance of an adequate depth of anesthesia during intubation, which reliably blunts potentially deleterious reflex sympathetic responses capable of precipitating tachycardia and ischemia.

Many clinicians also prefer a pure narcotic technique for maintenance. The negative inotropy of the inhalation anesthetics is a theoretical disadvantage for a myocardium faced with the challenge of overcoming outflow tract obstruction. A more clinically relevant drawback may be the increased risk of arrhythmia-induced hypotension, particularly that associated with nodal rhythm and resultant loss of the atrium's critical contribution to filling of the hypertrophied ventricle.

Occasionally, surgical stimulation elicits a hypertensive response despite the impedance posed by the stenotic valve and a seemingly adequate depth of narcotic anesthesia. In such patients, a judicious trial of low concentrations of an inhalation agent, used purely for control of hypertension, may prove efficacious. The ability to concurrently monitor cardiac output is useful in this situation. The temptation to control intraoperative hypertension with vasodilators should be resisted in most cases. Given the risk of ischemia, nitroglycerin seems to be a particularly attractive drug. Its effectiveness in relieving subendocardial ischemia in patients with aortic stenosis is controversial; however, there is always the risk of even transient episodes of "overshoot." The hypertrophied ventricle's critical dependence on an adequate CPP may be very unforgiving of even a momentary dip in the systemic arterial pressure.

Intraoperative hypotension, regardless of the primary cause, should be treated immediately and aggressively with a direct α-adrenergic agonist such as phenylephrine. The goal should be to immediately restore the CPP and then to address the underlying problem (e.g., hypovolemia, arrhythmia). After the arterial pressure responds, treatment of the precipitating event should be equally aggressive, but rapid transfusion or cardioversion should not delay the administration of a direct-acting vasoconstrictor. Patients with severe aortic stenosis in whom objective signs of myocardial ischemia persist despite restoration of the blood pressure should be treated extremely aggressively. This may mean the immediate use of an inotropic agent or simply accelerating the institution of cardiopulmonary bypass (CPB).

HYPERTROPHIC CARDIOMYOPATHY

Hypertrophic cardiomyopathy (HCM, formerly known as hypertrophic obstructive cardiomyopathy) is a relatively common genetic malformation of the heart with a prevalence of approximately 1 in 500. The hypertrophy initially develops in the septum and extends to the free walls, often giving a picture of concentric hypertrophy. Asymmetric septal hypertrophy leads to a variable pressure gradient between the apical LV chamber and the LV outflow tract (LVOT). The LVOT obstruction leads to increases in LV pressure, which fuels a vicious cycle of further hypertrophy and increased LVOT obstruction.[4] Various treatment modalities include β-adrenoceptor antagonists, calcium channel blockers, and surgical myectomy of the septum. For more than 40 years, the traditional standard treatment has been the ventricular septal myotomy-myomectomy of Morrow, in which a small amount of muscle from the subaortic septum is resected. Two new treatment modalities have gained popularity in recent years: dual-chamber pacing and septal reduction (ablation) therapy with ethanol.

Clinical Features and Natural History

Patients vary widely in their clinical presentation. The contribution of echocardiography to the diagnosis has unquestionably increased the number of asymptomatic patients who carry the diagnosis. Most patients with HCM are asymptomatic and have been seen by the echocardiographer because of relatives having clinical disease. Follow-up remains an important problem for cardiologists because sudden death or cardiac arrest may occur as the presenting symptom in slightly more than one half of previously asymptomatic patients.[5]

Less dramatic frequently presenting complaints include dyspnea, angina, and syncope. The clinical picture is often similar to that of valvular aortic stenosis. The symptoms may share a similar pathophysiologic basis (e.g., poor diastolic compliance) in the two conditions. The prognostic implications of clinical disease, however, are less certain for patients with HCM. Although cardiac arrest may be an unheralded event, other patients may have a stable pattern of angina or intermittent syncopal episodes for many years. Palpitations are also frequently described and may be related to a variety of underlying arrhythmias.

Pathophysiology

In HCM, the principal pathophysiologic abnormality is myocardial hypertrophy. The hypertrophy is a primary event in these patients and occurs independently of outflow tract obstruction. Unlike aortic stenosis, the hypertrophy begets the pressure gradient, not the other way around. Histologically, the hypertrophy consists of myocardial fiber disarray, and, anatomically, there is usually disproportionate enlargement of the interventricular septum.

A consensus exists that the disease is characterized by a wide spectrum of the severity of obstruction. It is totally absent in some patients, may be variable in others, or may be critically severe. Its most distinctive qualities are its dynamic nature (depending on contractile state and loading conditions), its timing (begins early, peaks variably), and its subaortic location. Subaortic obstruction arises from the hypertrophied septum's encroachment on the systolic outflow tract, which is bounded anteriorly by the interventricular septum and posteriorly by the anterior leaflet of the mitral valve. In most patients with obstruction, exaggerated anterior (i.e., toward the septum) motion of the anterior mitral valve leaflet during systole accentuates the obstruction. The cause of this systolic anterior motion (SAM) is unclear. One possibility is that the mitral valve is pulled toward the septum by contraction of the papillary muscles, whose orientation is abnormal because of the hypertrophic process. Another theory is that vigorous contraction of the hypertrophied septum results in rapid acceleration of the blood through a simultaneously narrowed outflow tract. This could generate hydraulic forces consistent with a Venturi effect whereby the anterior leaflet of the mitral valve would be drawn close to or within actual contact with the interventricular septum (Fig. 14-2). This means that after the obstruction is triggered the mitral valve leaflet is forced against the septum by the pressure difference across the orifice.

IV

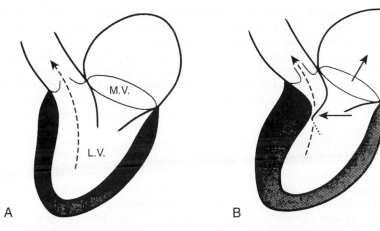

A   B

Figure 14-2   Proposed mechanism of systolic anterior motion (SAM) in hypertrophic cardiomyopathy (HCM). **A,** Normally, blood is ejected from the left ventricle through an unimpeded outflow tract. **B,** Thickening of the ventricular septum results in a restricted outflow tract, and this obstruction causes the blood to be ejected at a higher velocity, closer to the area of the anterior mitral valve leaflet. As a result of its proximity to this high-velocity fluid path, the anterior mitral valve leaflet is drawn toward the hypertrophied septum by a Venturi effect (*arrow*). M.V. = mitral valve; L.V. = left ventricle. (From Wigle ED, Sasson Z, Henderson MA, et al: Hypertrophic cardiomyopathy: The importance of the site and the extent of hypertrophy. A review. Prog Cardiovasc Dis 28:1, 1985.)

However, the pressure difference further decreases orifice size and further increases the pressure difference in a time-dependent amplifying feedback loop. This analysis is also consistent with observations that the measured gradient is directly correlated with the duration of mitral-septal contact. There appears to be good correlation between the degree of SAM and the magnitude of the pressure gradient. The SAM-septal contact also underlies the severe subaortic obstruction characteristic of HCM of the elderly, although the narrowing is usually more severe and the contribution of septal movement toward the mitral valve is usually greater.

In addition to SAM, approximately two thirds of patients exhibit a constellation of structural malformations of the mitral valve. These malformations include increased leaflet area and elongation of the leaflets or anomalous papillary muscle insertion directly into the anterior mitral valve leaflet. HCM is not a disease process confined to cardiac muscle alone, because these anatomic abnormalities of the mitral valve are unlikely to be acquired or secondary to mechanical factors.

Three basic mechanisms—increased contractility, decreased afterload, and decreased preload—exacerbate the degree of SAM-septal contact and produce the dynamic obstruction characteristic of patients with HCM. The common pathway is a reduction in ventricular volume (actively by increased contractility, directly or reflexly in response to vasodilation, or passively by reduced preload), which increases the proximity of the anterior mitral valve leaflet to the hypertrophied septum. Factors that usually impair contractile performance, such as myocardial depression, systemic vasoconstriction, and ventricular overdistention, characteristically improve systolic function in patients with HCM and outflow tract obstruction. Diagnostically, these paradoxes are exploited by quantifying the degree of subaortic obstruction after isoproterenol (e.g., increased inotropy, tachycardia, and decreased volume) and the Valsalva maneuver (e.g., decreased venous return and ventricular volume), both of which reliably elicit increases in the pressure gradient. In the operating room, catheter-induced ectopy or premature ventricular contractions resulting from cardiac manipulation may also

14

transiently exacerbate the gradient by increased inotropy from postextrasystolic potentiation. Therapeutically, volume loading, myocardial depression, and vasoconstriction should minimize obstruction and augment forward flow.

Poor diastolic compliance is the most clinically apparent manifestation of the relaxation abnormalities. LV filling pressures are markedly elevated despite enhanced systolic ejection and the normal or subnormal end-diastolic volume. This reduced ventricular volume reemphasizes the pivotal role played by the hypertrophied but intrinsically depressed myocardium. Reductions in afterload, mediated by hypertrophy, support the ventricle's systolic performance, resulting in increased emptying and a small diastolic volume. However, hypertrophy also impairs relaxation, resulting in poor diastolic compliance and an elevated ventricular filling pressure. The key point is that the high filling pressure does not reflect distention of a failing ventricle, even though stress-volume relationships suggest that its contractility is intrinsically depressed. This disease is characterized by systolic and diastolic dysfunction.

As in patients with valvular aortic stenosis, relatively high filling pressures reflect the LVEDV (i.e., degree of preload reserve) needed to overcome the outflow obstruction. Intervention with vasodilators is therefore inappropriate. The poor ventricular compliance also means that patients with HCM depend on a large intravascular volume and the maintenance of sinus rhythm for adequate diastolic filling. The atrial contribution to ventricular filling is even more important in HCM than in valvular aortic stenosis, and it may approach 75% of total SV.

Another similarity between HCM and valvular aortic stenosis is that the combination of myocardial hypertrophy, with or without LVOT obstruction, may precipitate imbalances in the myocardial oxygen supply and demand relationship. Angina-like discomfort is one of the classic symptoms of patients with HCM, and its pathogenesis has been attributed to increases in $M\dot{v}o_2$, specifically the increased overall muscle mass and the high systolic wall tension generated by the ventricle's ejection against the dynamic subaortic obstruction. However, as in patients with aortic stenosis, there is also evidence of a compromise in myocardial oxygen supply.

Hemodynamic derangements peculiar to the disease may aggravate the ventricle's anatomic vulnerability to ischemia. The increased LVEDP for any LVEDV (i.e., poor compliance) inevitably narrows the diastolic CPP gradient. This may precipitate subendocardial ischemia in some patients with HCM, particularly those faced with the increased oxygen demand of overcoming late-systolic obstruction. There is evidence that hypertrophy-induced myocardial ischemia may underlie the diastolic dysfunction characteristic of HCM. As in patients with valvular aortic stenosis, ischemia-induced abnormalities of diastolic calcium sequestration may further exacerbate relaxation abnormalities, initiating a vicious cycle.

β-Blockers and calcium channel blockers form the basis of medical therapy for HCM. β-Blockade is most useful for preventing sympathetically-mediated increases in the subaortic gradient and for the prevention of tachyarrhythmias, which can also exacerbate outflow obstruction. Disopyramide has also been used to reduce contractility and for its antiarrhythmic properties. Calcium channel blockers often prove clinically effective in patients with HCM regardless of the presence or absence of systolic obstruction. The mechanism of action involves improvement in diastolic relaxation, allowing an increase in LVEDV at a relatively lower LVEDP. The negative inotropy may attenuate the subaortic pressure gradient, although in selected patients, the gradient may worsen because of pronounced and unpredictable degrees of vasodilation.

Surgery—a septal myotomy or partial myomectomy by the aortic approach—is reserved for those patients who remain symptomatic despite maximal pharmacologic therapy. In a long-term retrospective study, the cumulative survival rate was significantly better in surgically than in pharmacologically treated patients. However, it is

IV

BOX 14-2	*Hypertrophic Cardiomyopathy*
Preload:	Increased
Afterload:	Increased
Goal:	Myocardial depression
Avoid:	Tachycardia, inotropes, vasodilators

quite likely that pharmacologic therapy may be more appropriate for the patient with a dynamic component to their degree of subaortic obstruction. Further improvement in the clinical outcome of surgically treated patients may be achieved with the addition of verapamil, presumably reflecting a two-pronged attack on the systolic (myomectomy) and diastolic (verapamil) components of the disease. Enthusiasm continues for the therapeutic use of dual-chamber pacing in this disease, with some patients demonstrating reductions in their subaortic gradients. It is not an option for patients in atrial fibrillation.

Anesthetic Considerations

Priorities in anesthetic management are to avoid aggravating the subaortic obstruction while remaining aware of the derangements in diastolic function that may be somewhat less amenable to direct pharmacologic manipulation (Box 14-2). It is therefore necessary to maintain an appropriate intravascular volume while avoiding direct or reflex increases in contractility or heart rate. The latter goals can be achieved with a deep level of general anesthesia and the associated direct myocardial depression. Regardless of the specific technique, the preservation of an adequate CPP, using vasoconstrictors rather than inotropes, is necessary to avoid myocardial ischemia. Heavy premedication is advisable with a view to avoiding anxiety-induced tachycardia or a reduction in ventricular filling. Chronic β-blockade or calcium channel blockade, or both, should be continued up to and including the day of surgery. These medications should be restarted immediately after surgery, particularly in those patients undergoing noncardiac surgery.

Intraoperative monitoring should include an ECG system with the capability of monitoring a V_5 lead and each of the six limb leads. Inspection of lead II may be helpful in the accurate diagnosis of supraventricular and junctional tachyarrhythmias, which may precipitate catastrophic hemodynamic deterioration due to the potential for inadequate ventricular filling resulting from the reduction in diastolic time or loss of the atrial contribution to ventricular filling. The latter may be crucial in patients with significantly reduced diastolic compliance. Abnormal Q waves have been described on the ECGs in 20% to 50% of patients with HCM. These waves should not raise concern about a previous myocardial infarction; instead, they probably represent accentuation of normal septal depolarization or delay in depolarization of electrophysiologically abnormal cells. Some patients exhibit a short PR interval with initial slurring of the QRS complex, and they may be at increased risk for supraventricular tachyarrhythmias on the basis of preexcitation. Although the specific predisposing factors are unknown, patients with HCM are at increased risk for any type of arrhythmia in the operative setting.

Given the pronounced abnormalities in LV diastolic compliance, the CVP is likely to be an inaccurate guide to changes in LV volume. However, a CVP catheter is extremely useful for the prompt administration of vasoactive drugs if they become necessary. As in valvular aortic stenosis, the information provided by insertion of a PA catheter is worth the small arrhythmogenic risk. The potential for

14

hypovolemia-induced exacerbation of outflow tract obstruction makes it crucial that the clinician have an accurate gauge of intravascular filling. The reduced diastolic compliance means that the PCWP will overestimate the patient's true volume status, and a reasonable clinical objective is to maintain the PCWP in the high-normal to elevated range. A PAC with pacing capability is ideal because atrial overdrive pacing can effect immediate hemodynamic improvement in the event of episodes of junctional rhythm. The absolute requirement of these patients for an adequate preload cannot be overemphasized, because even abrupt positioning changes have resulted in acute hemodynamic deterioration, including acute pulmonary edema.

Intraoperative arrhythmias require aggressive therapy. During cardiac surgery, insertion of the venous cannulae may precipitate atrial arrhythmias. Because the resultant hypotension may be severe, the surgeon should cannulate the aorta before any atrial manipulations. Supraventricular or junctional tachyarrhythmias may require immediate cardioversion if they precipitate catastrophic degrees of hypotension. Although verapamil is one drug of choice for paroxysmal atrial and junctional tachycardia, it has the potential of disastrously worsening the LVOT obstruction if it elicits excessive vasodilation or if it is used in the setting of severe hypotension. Cardioversion is preferable when the mean arterial pressure is already very low; the concurrent administration of phenylephrine is also advisable. This drug is almost always a low-risk, high-yield choice for the hypotensive patient with HCM. It augments perfusion, may ameliorate the pressure gradient, and often elicits a potentially beneficial vagal reflex when used to treat tachyarrhythmia-induced hypotension.

The inhalation anesthetics are commonly used for patients with HCM. Their dose-dependent myocardial depression is ideal because negative inotropy reduces the degree of SAM-septal contact, which results in LVOT obstruction. Hypotension is almost always the result of underlying hypovolemia, which is potentially exacerbated by anesthetic-induced vasodilation. Inotropes, β-adrenergic agonists, and calcium are all contraindicated because they worsen the systolic obstruction and perpetuate the hypotension. In most cases, a beneficial response can be obtained with aggressive replenishment of intravascular volume and concurrent infusion of phenylephrine.

AORTIC REGURGITATION

Clinical Features and Natural History

Aortic regurgitation may result from an abnormality of the valve itself or from bicuspid anatomy; there may be a rheumatic or infectious origin, or it may occur in association with any condition producing dilation of the aortic root and leaflet separation. Nonrheumatic valvular diseases commonly resulting in aortic regurgitation include infective endocarditis, trauma, and connective tissue disorders such as Marfan syndrome or cystic medionecrosis of the aortic valve. Aortic dissection from trauma, hypertension, or chronic degenerative processes can also result in dilatation of the root and functional incompetence.

The natural history of chronic aortic regurgitation is that of a long asymptomatic interval during which the valvular incompetence and secondary ventricular enlargement become progressively more severe. When symptoms do appear, they are usually those of CHF; and chest pain, if it occurs, is often nonexertional in origin. The life expectancy for patients with significant disease has historically been about 9 years, and in contrast to aortic stenosis, the onset of symptoms due to aortic regurgitation

IV

does not portend an immediately ominous prognosis. In the absence of surgery, early recognition of aortic regurgitation and chronic use of vasodilators appear to be prolonging life span in this patient population.

A relatively unique and problematic feature of chronic aortic regurgitation is that the severity of symptoms and their duration may correlate poorly with the degree of hemodynamic and contractile impairment. The issue in surgical decision making is that many patients can remain asymptomatic, during which time they are undergoing progressive deterioration in their myocardial contractility. Noninvasive diagnostic studies may facilitate the detection of early derangements in contractile function in relatively asymptomatic patients. This finding is important to the cardiologist when considering surgical referral, because patients with depressed preoperative LV function have a higher perioperative mortality rate and are at increased risk for persistent postoperative heart failure.

As in acute mitral regurgitation, the physiology of acute aortic regurgitation is quite different from chronic aortic regurgitation. Common causes include endocarditis, trauma, and acute aortic dissection. Because of a lack of chronic compensation, these patients usually present with pulmonary edema and heart failure refractory to optimal medical therapy. These patients are often hypotensive and clinically appear to be on the verge of cardiovascular collapse.

Pathophysiology

Left ventricular volume overload is the pathognomonic feature of chronic aortic regurgitation. The degree of volume overload is determined by the magnitude of the regurgitant flow, which is related to the size of the regurgitant orifice, the aorta-ventricular pressure gradient, and the diastolic time.

Chronically, aortic regurgitation results in a state of LV volume and pressure overload. Progressive volume overloading from aortic regurgitation increases end-diastolic wall tension (i.e., ventricular afterload) and stimulates the serial replication of sarcomeres, producing a pattern of eccentric ventricular hypertrophy.[6] This dilation of the ventricle, in accordance with Laplace's law, also elevates the systolic wall tension, stimulating some concentric hypertrophy. This process of eccentric hypertrophy results in the greatest absolute degrees of cardiomegaly seen in valve disease. End-diastolic volume may be three to four times normal, and very high cardiac outputs can be sustained.

Figure 14-3 shows the pressure-volume loops for acute and chronic aortic regurgitation. In the chronic form, the diastolic pressure-volume curve is shifted far to the right. This permits a tremendous increase in LVEDV with minimal change in filling pressure, a property frequently described as high diastolic compliance.

Because the increase in preload is compensated for by ventricular hypertrophy, cardiac output is maintained by the Frank-Starling mechanism, and cardiac failure is not seen. This is true despite probable decreases in contractility. There is virtually no isovolumic diastolic phase, because the ventricle is filling throughout diastole. The isovolumic phase of systole is also brief because of the low aortic diastolic pressure. This minimal impedance to the forward ejection of a large SV allows for the performance of maximal myocardial work at a minimum of oxygen consumption. Eventually, however, progressive volume overload increases ventricular end-diastolic volume to the point that compensatory hypertrophy is no longer sufficient to compensate, and a decline in systolic function occurs. As systolic function declines, end-systolic dimension increases further, LV wall stress increases, and LV function is further compromised by the excessive ventricular afterload. At this point, the decline of ventricular function is progressive and can be quite rapid.

14

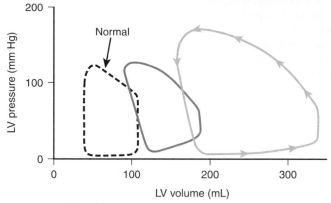

Figure 14-3   Pressure-volume loop in acute (*middle loop*) and chronic (*right loop*) aortic regurgitation. (Adapted from Jackson JM, Thomas SJ, Lowenstein E: Anesthetic management of patients with valvular heart disease. Semin Anesth 1:239, 1982.)

Despite the relatively normal $M\dot{v}o_2$, angina can occur in one third of patients with severe aortic regurgitation, even in the absence of CAD. Patients with chronic aortic regurgitation may be at risk for myocardial ischemia caused by hypertrophy-induced abnormalities of the coronary circulation. The increase in total myocardial mass can increase baseline $M\dot{v}o_2$, and there is evidence that total coronary blood flow (CBF), although increased, fails to keep pace with the increase in myocardial mass. Evidence suggests that the insidious development of contractile dysfunction may in part have an ischemic basis.

Intraoperatively, patients with chronic aortic regurgitation may be at risk for acute ischemia with episodes of significant bradycardia. Because bradycardia prolongs diastolic time, it increases regurgitant flow, and LV diastolic pressure and wall tension rise rapidly. Simultaneously, the CPP is decreased as aortic runoff occurs during diastole and diastolic ventricular pressure is increased. Under these conditions, myocardial perfusion pressure may be insufficient. Clinically, very rapid decompensation can occur. The ischemic ventricle can rapidly dilate such that progressively increased end-systolic dimensions are seen, and ischemia and ventricular failure become a positive feedback loop.

Acute Aortic Regurgitation

In acute aortic regurgitation, sudden diastolic volume overload of a nonadapted left ventricle results in a precipitous rise in the end-diastolic pressure because the ventricle is operating on the steepest portion of the diastolic pressure-volume curve. In severe acute aortic regurgitation, the LVEDP can equilibrate with aortic diastolic pressure and exceed the LA pressure in late diastole. This may be sufficient to cause closure of the mitral valve before atrial systole. This is an important echocardiographic finding indicative of severe aortic regurgitation. Although this phenomenon initially shields the pulmonary capillaries from the full force of the dramatically elevated LVEDP, the protection may be short-lived. Severe LV distention often follows and produces mitral annular enlargement and functional mitral regurgitation.

The inevitable fall in SV in acute decompensating aortic regurgitation elicits a reflex sympathetic response so that tachycardia and a high systemic vascular resistance

BOX 14-3 *Aortic Regurgitation*	
Preload:	Increased
Afterload:	Decreased
Goal:	Augmentation of forward flow
Avoid:	Bradycardia

(SVR) are common. Moderate tachycardia beneficially shortens the regurgitant time without reducing the transmitral filling volume. Vasoconstriction, however, preserves CPP at the expense of increasing the aorta-ventricular gradient and regurgitation.

As may be expected, patients with acute aortic regurgitation may be at greater risk for myocardial ischemia. As with chronic aortic regurgitation and bradycardia, coronary perfusion may be compromised by the combination of a low diastolic arterial pressure and the precipitously increased LVEDP. This narrowing of CPP may be so severe that the phasic epicardial blood flow may change to a predominantly systolic pattern with very severe acute aortic regurgitation. Dissection of the coronary ostia is rare but frequently causes fatality in patients with acute aortic regurgitation. In addition to the structural impediment to myocardial oxygen delivery, catastrophic hypotension and high LVEDP combine to cause accentuated ischemia and ventricular dilation. Immediate surgical correction is the only hope for salvaging these patients, who often prove refractory to inotropes and vasodilators. Attempts at stabilizing the ischemic component of their injury with the intra-aortic balloon are usually contraindicated, because augmenting the diastolic pressure worsens regurgitation.

Acute aortic regurgitation is most commonly caused by infective endocarditis or aortic dissection, and intraoperative transesophageal echocardiography (TEE) has assumed increasing importance in diagnosis of acute aortic regurgitation and in decisions regarding its surgical management. TEE studies are highly sensitive and specific for the diagnosis of infective endocarditis, and they are significantly more sensitive than transthoracic echocardiography (TTE). TEE has been particularly useful in the diagnosis of abscesses associated with endocarditis and may detect previously unsuspected abnormalities.

Anesthetic Considerations

Intraoperative monitoring should include an ECG system with the capability of monitoring a lateral precordial lead, because ischemia is a potential hazard (Box 14-3). For most valvular procedures, a PA catheter provides very useful information. A PA catheter allows determination of basal filling pressures and cardiac output, which is particularly useful in chronic aortic regurgitation given the potential unreliability of the clinical history and EF. Equally important is the ability to accurately monitor ventricular preload and cardiac output response to pharmacologic interventions. The aggressive use of vasodilators is often appropriate therapy perioperatively for the failing ventricle, but their use can compromise the preload to which the ventricle has chronically adjusted. Concurrent preload augmentation, guided by the pulmonary artery diastolic pressure or PCWP, may be crucial to optimize cardiac output when afterload is pharmacologically manipulated. The other requirement for a PA catheter is to allow for pacing when it is anticipated. The deleterious effects of significant bradycardia in aortic regurgitation have been described. In patients who arrive in the operating room with heart rates less than 70 or in patients for whom rapid epicardial pacing may be difficult to establish (e.g., redo operations), placement of a pacing wire is probably indicated. Typically, only a ventricular wire would be appropriate; it is

14

more reliable than atrial pacing and, in aortic regurgitation, the atrial contribution to ventricular diastolic volume usually is not essential. Capturing the ventricle with a PA-based transvenous wire can be difficult because of the very large ventricular cavity size in patients with chronic aortic regurgitation.

Because patients with aortic regurgitation may differ widely in their degree of myocardial dysfunction, anesthetic management must be appropriately individualized. The hemodynamic goals are a mild tachycardia, a positive inotropic state, and a controlled reduction in SVR. For cardiac surgery, dopamine or dobutamine, pancuronium, ketamine, and nitroprusside infusions are excellent choices. For the patient with acute aortic regurgitation, the goals are the same but urgency must be stressed. It is essential to try to rapidly reduce end-diastolic and end-systolic ventricular volumes with the very aggressive use of inotropes (e.g., epinephrine) and vasodilators. Positive inotropes should not be withheld from the patient whose condition deteriorates in the operating room because they may provide the precious additional minutes of hemodynamic stability needed to get on CPB. In acute and chronic forms of aortic regurgitation, serial measurements of cardiac output can indicate that ventricular size and cardiac output have been optimized, regardless of the systemic pressure. TEE is also useful to look at ventricular size, but probably maximizing cardiac output under these conditions gets closer to the therapeutic goal than looking at ventricular size alone. With acute aortic regurgitation and premature closure of the mitral valve, the PA pressures may grossly underestimate the LVEDP, which continues to rise under the influence of the diastolic regurgitant jet from the aorta.

The early and late phases of CPB can be a real problem in aortic regurgitation, particularly in repeat operations. Before cross-clamp placement, the ventricle is at risk for distention if it is not ejecting or being vented. If the ventricle dilates with aortic regurgitation during bypass, the intraventricular pressures may equilibrate with the aortic root pressures. Under these conditions, there is no coronary perfusion, and the ventricle may rapidly dilate and become profoundly ischemic. This can occur before cross-clamp placement with bradycardia, ventricular fibrillation, or tachycardia, or even with a rapid supraventricular rhythm that compromises organized mechanical activity. Correcting the rhythm, pacing, cross-clamping the aorta, or venting the ventricle addresses this problem. This can also occur in cardiac surgery for conditions other than aortic regurgitation. In patients with unknown or uncorrected aortic regurgitation, removal of the cross-clamp causes the same ventricular dilation and ischemia if a rhythm and ejection are not rapidly established. Ventricular venting or pacing may be essential until an organized, mechanically efficient rhythm is established. This problem must be considered in patients referred for coronary surgery alone, in those with mild or moderate aortic regurgitation not having aortic valve replacement, and in patients in whom intraoperative TEE is not used.

MITRAL REGURGITATION

Clinical Features and Natural History

Unlike mitral stenosis, which is almost always the result of rheumatic valve disease, mitral regurgitation may result from a variety of disease processes that affect the valve leaflets, the chordae tendineae, the papillary muscles, the valve annulus, or the left ventricle. Mitral regurgitation can be classified as organic or functional. Organic mitral regurgitation describes diseases that result in distortion, disruption, or destruction of the mitral leaflets or chordal structures. In Western countries, degenerative processes that lead to leaflet prolapse with or without chordal rupture represent the most common cause of mitral regurgitation. Other causes of organic mitral regurgitation include infective endocarditis, mitral annular calcification, rheumatic valve disease, and connective tissue disorders such as Marfan or Ehlers-Danlos syndrome. Much less common causes of organic mitral regurgitation include congenital mitral valve clefts, diet-drug or ergotamine toxicity, and carcinoid valve disease with metabolically active pulmonary tumors or right-to-left intracardiac shunting.

Functional mitral regurgitation describes cases in which mitral regurgitation occurs despite structurally normal leaflets and chordae tendineae. Resulting from altered function or geometry of the left ventricle or mitral annulus, functional mitral regurgitation often occurs in the setting of ischemic heart disease, and the term *ischemic mitral regurgitation* is sometimes used interchangeably with *functional mitral regurgitation*. However, the functional form can occur in patients without demonstrable CAD, such as those with idiopathic dilated cardiomyopathy and mitral annular dilatation.

Because it can be caused by a wide variety of disease processes, the natural history of mitral regurgitation is quite variable. Even among patients with acute-onset disease, the clinical course depends on the mechanism of regurgitation and the response to treatment. For instance, patients presenting with acute, severe mitral regurgitation due to a ruptured papillary muscle have a dismal outcome without surgery. However, the clinical course of acute mitral regurgitation due to endocarditis could be favorable if the patient responds well to antibiotic therapy. Although those with chronic mitral regurgitation usually enter an initial, often asymptomatic, compensated phase, the time course for progression to LV dysfunction and symptomatic heart failure is unpredictable. The literature reflects the wide variability in the natural history of mitral regurgitation, with published 5-year survival rates for patients with mitral regurgitation of 27% to 97%.[7]

Pathophysiology

Mitral regurgitation causes LV volume overload. The regurgitant volume combines with the normal LA volume and returns to the left ventricle during each diastolic period. This elevated preload leads to increased sarcomere stretch and, in the initial phases of the disease process, augmentation of LV ejection performance by the Frank-Starling mechanism. Systolic ejection into the relatively low-pressure left atrium further enhances the contractile appearance of the left ventricle.

The presentation of patients with mitral regurgitation varies depending on the pathophysiology of the specific condition, which is affected by the mechanism, severity, and acuity of the mitral regurgitation. In cases of acute, severe mitral regurgitation, such as patients with a ruptured papillary muscle after acute myocardial infarction, the sudden increase in preload enhances LV contractility by the Frank-Starling mechanism. Despite the increased preload, LV size is initially normal. Normal LV size combined with the ability to eject into a low-pressure circuit (i.e., the left atrium) results in decreased afterload in the acute setting. The measured LVEF in cases of sudden, severe mitral regurgitation may approach 75%, although forward SV is reduced. However, because the left atrium has not yet dilated in response to the large regurgitant volume, LA pressure rises acutely and may lead to pulmonary vascular congestion, pulmonary edema, and dyspnea.

Many patients with mitral regurgitation, particularly those whose valvular incompetence develops more slowly, may enter a chronic, compensated phase. In this phase, chronic volume overload triggers LV cavity enlargement by promoting eccentric hypertrophy. Elevated preload continues to augment LV systolic performance. At the same time, the left atrium dilates in response to the ongoing regurgitant volume. Although LA dilatation maintains a low-pressure circuit that facilitates LV systolic ejection, the increased radius of the LV cavity leads to increased wall tension.

14

With the eventual decline in LV systolic function, patients enter a decompensated phase. Progressive LV dilatation increases wall stress and afterload, causing further deterioration in LV performance, mitral annular dilatation, and worsening of the mitral regurgitation. LV end-systolic pressure increases. The increased LV filling pressures result in elevation of LA pressures and, given time, pulmonary vascular congestion, pulmonary hypertension, and RV dysfunction. In addition to fatigue and weakness, patients with decompensated, chronic mitral regurgitation may also report dyspnea and orthopnea. It is difficult to predict when a patient with mitral regurgitation is likely to decompensate clinically. The progression of disease in any given patient depends on the underlying cause of mitral regurgitation, its severity, the response of the left ventricle to volume overload, and possibly the effect of medical management.[8]

Surgical Decision Making

Just as progress in the understanding of the pathophysiology of mitral regurgitation has evolved, so too has the surgical approach to this disease process. A high operative mortality associated with the surgical correction of mitral regurgitation in the 1980s led many clinicians to manage patients conservatively. Because favorable loading conditions and high LA compliance allow even patients with significant mitral regurgitation to remain asymptomatic for long periods, it is likely that many patients did not undergo surgery until the onset of disabling symptoms. Studies show that more severe preoperative symptoms are associated with a lower EF and a higher incidence of postoperative CHF. Historically, poor outcomes after surgery for mitral regurgitation might have occurred because clinicians did not appreciate the true degree of LV dysfunction at the time of surgery in symptomatic patients. An EF of less than 60% in the setting of severe mitral regurgitation represents significant LV dysfunction and predicts a worse outcome with surgery or medical management. Surgical techniques common in the 1980s probably also contributed to unfavorable postoperative outcomes. For instance, although the mechanisms are incompletely understood, resection of the subvalvular apparatus contributes to decreased LV systolic performance after mitral replacement.

In part because of improved surgical techniques, the operative mortality rate for patients with organic mitral regurgitation who are younger than 75 years is about 1% in some centers. Besides preservation of the subvalvular apparatus, valve repair represents another surgical technique associated with improved postoperative outcome.[9] Although not applicable to all patients, such as those with advanced rheumatic disease, the popularity of valve repairs continues to grow. Studies indicate numerous benefits associated with mitral repair. For instance, after accounting for baseline characteristics, patients who undergo mitral repair instead of replacement experience lower operative mortality and better long-term survival largely because of improved postoperative LV function. The survival benefit that accompanies valve repair is also observed among patients undergoing combined valve and coronary artery surgery. Valve repair does not increase the likelihood of reoperation when compared with replacement. Although originally used most often for posterior leaflet disease, surgeons now routinely repair anterior mitral leaflets with good success. When repairing anterior leaflet prolapse, surgeons may insert artificial chordae. The approach to flail or prolapsing posterior mitral leaflet segments often involves resection of a portion of the leaflet. In addition to resecting a portion of the leaflet and plicating the redundant tissue, an annuloplasty ring is often placed to reduce mitral orifice size and return the annulus to a more anatomic shape. Some surgeons favor a flexible, partial, posterior annuloplasty band, which may allow improved systolic contraction of the posterior annulus and better postoperative LV function.

BOX 14-4 *Mitral Regurgitation*	
Preload:	Increased
Afterload:	Decreased
Goal:	Mild tachycardia, vasodilation
Avoid:	Myocardial depression

Anesthetic Considerations

Patients who present to the operating room with mitral regurgitation may differ significantly with respect to duration of disease, symptoms, hemodynamic stability, ventricular function, and involvement of the right heart and pulmonary circulation (Box 14-4). For instance, a patient presenting with severe mitral regurgitation due to acute papillary muscle rupture may enter the operating room in cardiogenic shock with pulmonary congestion requiring intra-aortic balloon pump (IABP) augmentation. Another patient with a newly diagnosed flail posterior mitral leaflet may enter the surgical suite with relatively preserved LV function and no symptoms whatsoever. In the latter patient, the compliance of the left atrium may have prevented pulmonary vascular congestion, pulmonary hypertension, and RV dysfunction. Despite the differences in presentation, the general management goals remain similar and include maintenance of forward cardiac output and reduction in the mitral regurgitant fraction. The anesthesiologist must also seek to optimize RV function, in part by avoiding increases in pulmonary vascular congestion and pulmonary hypertension. Various degrees of intervention are needed to achieve these hemodynamic management goals depending on the patient's presentation.

Invasive hemodynamic monitoring provides the anesthesiologist with a wealth of important information. Arterial catheters are essential for monitoring beat-to-beat changes in blood pressure that occur in response to a variety of surgical and anesthetic manipulations. PA catheters facilitate many aspects of intraoperative patient management. Intraoperative use of a PA catheter allows the anesthesiologist to more carefully optimize left-sided filling pressures. Although the PCWP and PA diastolic pressure depend on LA and LV compliance and filling, examination of intraoperative trends in these variables enhances the ability of the anesthesiologist to provide appropriate levels of preload while avoiding volume overload. Periodic determination of cardiac output allows a more objective assessment of the patient's response to interventions such as fluid administration or inotropic infusion. The presence or size of a V wave on a PCWP tracing does not reliably correlate with the severity of mitral regurgitation, because this finding depends on LA compliance. Just as in the management of patients with aortic valvular regurgitation, another benefit of PA catheter insertion is the ability to introduce a ventricular pacing wire to rapidly counteract hemodynamically significant bradycardia. In patients with RV compromise, monitoring trends in the CVP recording may also be helpful. Tricuspid regurgitation detected through analysis of the CVP tracing may suggest RV dilatation, which may be caused by pulmonary hypertension.

Intraoperative TEE provides invaluable information during the surgical correction of mitral regurgitation. It reliably identifies the mechanism of mitral regurgitation, thereby guiding the surgical approach,[10] and it objectively demonstrates the size and function of the cardiac chambers. TEE can readily identify the cause of hemodynamic derangements, facilitating proper intervention. For instance, the appearance of SAM of the mitral apparatus immediately after valve repair allows the anesthesiologist to intervene with volume infusion and medications such as esmolol or phenylephrine as appropriate. In rare circumstances when hemodynamically significant SAM persists

14

despite these interventions, the surgeon may elect to further repair or even replace the mitral valve. TEE also identifies concomitant pathology that may warrant surgical attention, such as atrial level shunts and additional valve disease.

The intraoperative management of patients with mitral regurgitation before the institution of CPB focuses on optimizing forward cardiac output, minimizing the mitral regurgitant volume, and preventing deleterious increases in pulmonary artery pressures. Maintaining adequate LV preload is essential. An enlarged left ventricle that operates on a higher portion of the Frank-Starling curve requires adequate filling. At the same time, excessive volume administration is to be avoided because it may cause unwanted dilatation of the mitral annulus and worsening of the mitral regurgitation. Excessive fluid administration may precipitate RV failure in patients with pulmonary vascular congestion and pulmonary hypertension. Optimization of preload is aided by analysis of data obtained from PA catheter measurements and TEE images. Because significant LV dysfunction is present in many patients with mitral regurgitation, anesthesiologists often select specific induction and maintenance regimens to avoid further depressing LV function. For this reason, large doses of narcotics have been popular in the past. Others have shown that smaller doses of narcotics combined with vasodilating inhalation anesthetics also produce acceptable intraoperative hemodynamics. By reducing the amount of narcotics administered, the addition of a vasodilating inhalation agent to the anesthetic regimen may allow for faster extubation of the trachea postoperatively. With the current trend toward early referral of asymptomatic patients for mitral repair, anesthetic regimens that reduce the duration of postoperative mechanical ventilation may be advantageous.

In patients with severe LV dysfunction, infusions of inotropic medications such as dopamine, dobutamine, or even epinephrine may be required to maintain an adequate cardiac output. Phosphodiesterase inhibitors such as milrinone may also augment systolic ventricular performance and reduce pulmonary and peripheral vascular resistances. By reducing pulmonary and peripheral vascular resistance, forward cardiac output is facilitated. Nitroglycerin and sodium nitroprusside represent two additional options for reducing the impedance to ventricular ejection. If patients prove refractory to inotropic and vasodilator therapy, insertion of an IABP should be strongly considered.

Manipulation of the heart rate may be necessary in some patients to optimize hemodynamics. Bradycardia should generally be avoided because slower heart rates allow for larger filling volumes, potentially resulting in LV distention and mitral annular dilatation. Regurgitant volumes may increase at slower heart rates. Slightly increased heart rates, especially when combined with increased LV contractility, favor a smaller mitral annular area and may decrease the regurgitant fraction. Sinus rhythm and preserved atrial contraction are less important in patients with mitral regurgitation compared with patients with stenotic valves. Mitral annular dilatation accompanies most cases of long-standing mitral regurgitation. Patients with pure mitral regurgitation generally have no impedance to LV filling, and atrial fibrillation is usually better tolerated than in patients with stenotic lesions.

Because severe mitral regurgitation may result in pulmonary hypertension and RV dysfunction, anesthesiologists should tailor their intraoperative management strategies accordingly. Hypercapnia, hypoxia, and acidosis elevate pulmonary artery pressures and should be avoided. Mild hyperventilation may be beneficial in some patients.

Patients with severe RV dysfunction after CPB can prove exceptionally difficult to manage. Besides avoiding the factors known to increase peripheral vascular resistance (PVR), only a few options exist for these patients. Inotropic agents with vasodilating properties such as dobutamine, isoproterenol, and milrinone augment RV systolic performance and decrease PVR, but their use is often confounded by systemic hypotension. Prostaglandin E_1 (PGE_1) reliably reduces PVR and undergoes extensive first-pass metabolism in the pulmonary circulation. Although PGE_1 reduces pulmonary artery pressures after CPB, systemic hypotension requiring infusions of vasoconstrictors through an LA catheter has also occurred. Inhaled nitric oxide represents another alternative available for the treatment of RV failure in the setting of pulmonary hypertension. Nitric oxide reliably relaxes the pulmonary vasculature and is then immediately bound to hemoglobin and inactivated. Studies indicate that systemic hypotension during nitric oxide therapy is unlikely.

LV dysfunction may also contribute to post-CPB hemodynamic instability. With mitral competence restored, the low-pressure outlet for LV ejection is removed. The enlarged left ventricle must then eject entirely into the aorta. Because LV enlargement leads to increased wall stress, a condition of elevated afterload often exists after CPB. At the same time, the preload augmentation inherent to mitral regurgitation is removed. It is therefore not surprising that the systolic performance of the left ventricle often declines after surgical correction of mitral regurgitation. Treatment options in the immediate post-CPB period include inotropic and vasodilator therapy and, if necessary, IABP augmentation.

MITRAL STENOSIS

Clinical Features and Natural History

Clinically significant mitral stenosis in adult patients usually is a result of rheumatic disease. Congenital abnormalities of the mitral valve represent a rare cause of mitral stenosis in younger patients. Other uncommon conditions that do not directly involve the mitral valve apparatus but may limit LV inflow and simulate the clinical findings of mitral stenosis include cor triatriatum, large LA neoplasms, and pulmonary vein obstruction.

A decades-long asymptomatic period characterizes the initial phase of rheumatic mitral stenosis. Symptoms rarely appear until the normal mitral valve area of 4 to 6 cm^2 (Fig. 14-4) has been reduced to 2.5 cm^2 or less. When the mitral valve area reaches 1.5 to 2.5 cm^2, symptoms usually occur only in association with exercise or other conditions, such as fever, pregnancy, or atrial fibrillation, that lead to an increase in heart rate or cardiac output. After the mitral valve area falls below 1.5 cm^2, symptoms may develop at rest. Some patients are able to remain asymptomatic for long periods by gradually reducing their level of activity. Patients with mitral stenosis commonly report dyspnea as their initial symptom, a finding reflective of elevated LA pressure and pulmonary congestion. In addition to dyspnea, patients may report palpitations that signal the onset of atrial fibrillation. Systemic thromboembolization occurs in 10% to 20% of patients with mitral stenosis and does not appear to be correlated with the mitral valve area or LA size. Chest pain that simulates angina is present in a small number of patients with mitral stenosis and may result from RV hypertrophy rather than CAD.

There has been a change in the typical age of presentation of patients with mitral stenosis. Previously, patients, often women, presented with mitral stenosis while in their 20s and 30s. In the past 15 years, perhaps because of more slowly progressive disease in the United States, patients have been presenting in their 40s and 50s. After symptoms develop, mitral stenosis remains a slow, progressive disease. Often, patients live 10 to 20 years with mild symptoms, such as dyspnea with exercise, before disabling NYHA class III and IV symptoms develop. The symptomatic state of the patient predicts the clinical outcome. For instance, the 10-year survival rate of patients with mild symptoms approaches 80% but the 10-year survival rate of patients with disabling symptoms is only 15% without surgery.

14

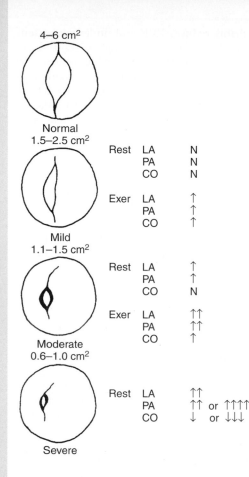

4–6 cm²

Normal
1.5–2.5 cm²

Mild
1.1–1.5 cm²

Moderate
0.6–1.0 cm²

Severe

Rest	LA	N
	PA	N
	CO	N
Exer	LA	↑
	PA	↑
	CO	↑

Rest	LA	↑
	PA	↑
	CO	N
Exer	LA	↑↑
	PA	↑↑
	CO	↑

Rest	LA	↑↑
	PA	↑↑ or ↑↑↑↑
	CO	↓ or ↓↓↓

Figure 14-4 Hemodynamic changes with progressive narrowing of the mitral valve. LA = left atrium; PA = pulmonary artery; CO = cardiac output. (From Rapaport E: Natural history of aortic and mitral valve disease. Am J Cardiol 35:221, 1971.)

IV

Pathophysiology

Rheumatic mitral stenosis results in valve leaflet thickening and fusion of the commissures. Later in the disease process, leaflet calcification and subvalvular chordal fusion may occur. These changes combine to reduce the effective mitral valve area and limit diastolic flow into the left ventricle. As a result of the fixed obstruction to LV inflow, LA pressures rise. Elevated LA pressures limit pulmonary venous drainage and result in elevated PA pressures. Over time, PA hypertrophy develops in response to chronically elevated pulmonary vascular pressures. Pulmonary hypertension may trigger increases in RV end-diastolic volume and pressure, and in some patients, signs of RV failure such as ascites or peripheral edema may appear. LA enlargement is an almost universal finding in patients with established mitral stenosis and is a risk factor for the development of atrial fibrillation.

Patients with mitral stenosis tolerate tachycardia particularly poorly. LV inflow, already limited by a mechanically abnormal valve, is further compromised by the disproportionate decline in the diastolic period that accompanies tachycardia. To maintain LV filling in a shorter diastolic period, the flow rate across the stenotic valve must increase. Because the valve area remains constant, the pressure gradient between the left atrium and left ventricle increases by the square of the increase in the flow rate, according to the Gorlin formula, in which PG is the transvalvular pressure gradient:

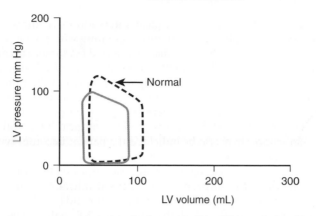

MITRAL STENOSIS

Figure 14-5   Pressure-volume loop in mitral stenosis. LV = left ventricular. (From Jackson JM, Thomas SJ, Lowenstein E: Anesthetic management of patients with valvular heart disease. Semin Anesth 1:239, 1982.)

$$\text{Value area} = \frac{\text{Flow}}{\sqrt{\text{PG}}}$$

Tachycardia necessitates a significant increase in the transvalvular pressure gradient and may precipitate feelings of breathlessness in awake patients. In patients with atrial fibrillation, it is the elevated ventricular rate that is most deleterious, rather than the loss of atrial contraction. Although coordinated atrial activity is always preferable, the primary goal in treating patients with mitral stenosis and atrial fibrillation should be control of the ventricular rate.

Mitral stenosis results in diminished LV preload reserve. As seen in the pressure-volume loop in Figure 14-5, LVEDV and LVEDP are reduced with an accompanying decline in SV. Controversy exists, however, regarding the contractile state of the left ventricle in these patients. Limited preload may contribute to a reduced EF in some of these patients. However, the observation that LV contractile impairment persists postoperatively in some patients suggests that other causes of LV dysfunction may exist. Rheumatic myocarditis has been reported, although its role in producing LV contractile dysfunction is uncertain.

Assessment of Mitral Stenosis

As for patients with mitral regurgitation, echocardiography represents the diagnostic modality of choice for patients with suspected mitral stenosis.[11] Two-dimensional and Doppler echocardiographic techniques are able to accurately and noninvasively measure the transvalvular pressure gradient and mitral valve area. Because the pressure gradient varies with the flow rate and diastolic period, the assessment of mitral stenosis severity ideally should be based on the measured or calculated mitral valve area. Echocardiographic methods used to obtain mitral valve area include the pressure half-time technique, the continuity equation, planimetry of the valve orifice, and Proximal Isovelocity Surface Area (PISA) analysis. Other invaluable information obtained during an echocardiographic study includes the size and function of the ventricles and an estimation of the pulmonary artery pressure.

14

Surgical Decision Making

Appropriate referral of patients for surgical intervention requires integration of clinical and echocardiographic data. Patients presenting with severe symptoms (i.e., NYHA class III and IV) should be immediately referred for surgery because their outcome is poor if treated medically. Patients with only mild mitral stenosis and few or no symptoms may be managed conservatively with periodic evaluation. Patients who are asymptomatic but have moderate mitral stenosis (i.e., mitral valve area between 1.0 and 1.5 cm^2) require careful assessment. If significant pulmonary hypertension (i.e., PA systolic pressure > 50 mmHg) is present, surgical intervention should be considered. Intervention may also be indicated if a patient becomes symptomatic or PA pressures increase significantly during exercise testing.

The surgical options for treating mitral stenosis continue to evolve. Closed commissurotomy, in which the surgeon fractures fused mitral commissures, was first performed in the 1920s. It became popular in the 1940s and is still used to treat mitral stenosis in developing countries. With the advent of CPB in the 1950s, techniques of open commissurotomy developed, allowing the surgeon to directly inspect the valve before splitting the commissures. The common goals of closed and open mitral commissurotomy include increasing the effective mitral valve area and decreasing the LA-to-LV pressure gradient with a resultant relief in the patient's symptoms.

Percutaneous mitral commissurotomy (PMC) allows a less invasive, catheter-based approach to mitral stenosis. First reported by Inoue in 1984,[12] clinicians worldwide perform PMC more than 10,000 times each year. The technique of PMC involves directing a balloon-tipped catheter across the stenotic mitral valve. Specifically designed balloons allow sequential inflation of the distal and proximal portions of the balloon, ensuring correct positioning across the mitral valve before the middle portion of the device is inflated to split the fused commissures. Patient selection for PMC requires careful echocardiographic evaluation.

Not all patients are candidates for surgical commissurotomy or PMC. For instance, those with heavily calcified valves or significant mitral regurgitation are likely to experience suboptimal results after commissurotomy. Mitral valve anatomy unsuitable for PMC is more commonly encountered in Western countries, where patients with mitral stenosis typically present at an older average age. Mitral valve replacement is commonly recommended for these patients. The risk of mitral valve replacement depends on patient characteristics such as age, functional status, and other comorbid conditions. Surgical risk in younger patients with few coexisting medical problems generally is less than 5%. Conversely, surgical risk in elderly patients with severe symptoms related to mitral stenosis and multiple comorbidities may be 10% to 20%.

Anesthetic Considerations

Several important goals should guide the anesthetic management of patients with significant mitral stenosis. First, the anesthesiologist should seek to prevent tachycardia and treat it promptly if it develops in the perioperative period (Box 14-5). Maintenance of LV preload without exacerbation of pulmonary vascular congestion represents a second management goal. Third, anesthesiologists should avoid factors that aggravate pulmonary hypertension and impair RV function.

Prevention and treatment of tachycardia are central to the perioperative management of these patients. Tachycardia shortens the diastolic filling period. To maintain LV preload with a shortened diastolic period, an elevation in transvalvular flow rate is required with a resultant increase in the LA-to-LV pressure gradient. Avoidance of

BOX 14-5	*Mitral Stenosis*
Preload:	Normal or increased
Afterload:	Normal
Goal:	Controlled ventricular response
Avoid:	Tachycardia, pulmonary vasoconstriction

tachycardia begins in the preoperative period. Anxiety-induced tachycardia may be treated with small doses of narcotics or benzodiazepines. However, excessive sedation is counterproductive because sedative-induced hypoventilation can result in hypoxemia or hypercarbia, potentially aggravating a patient's underlying pulmonary hypertension, and because large doses of premedication can jeopardize the patient's already limited LV preload. Appropriate monitoring and supplemental oxygen therapy should be considered for patients receiving preoperative narcotics or benzodiazepines. Medications taken by the patient preoperatively to control heart rate, such as digitalis, β-blockers, calcium receptor antagonists, or amiodarone, should be continued in the perioperative period. Additional doses of β-blockers and calcium-receptor antagonists may be required intraoperatively, particularly to control the ventricular rate in patients with atrial fibrillation. Control of the ventricular rate remains the primary goal in managing patients with atrial fibrillation, although cardioversion should not be withheld from patients with atrial tachyarrhythmias who become hemodynamically unstable. Narcotic-based anesthetics are often helpful in avoiding intraoperative tachycardia. However, clinicians should realize these patients may be receiving other vagotonic drugs and that profound bradycardia is possible in response to large doses of narcotics. The selection of a muscle relaxant such as pancuronium may help prevent the unwanted bradycardia associated with high-dose narcotics.

Maintenance of preload is another important goal for managing patients who have a fixed obstruction to LV filling. Appropriate replacement of blood loss and prevention of excessive anesthetic-induced venodilation help preserve hemodynamic stability intraoperatively. Invasive hemodynamic monitoring allows the anesthesiologist to maintain adequate preload while avoiding excessive fluid administration that could aggravate pulmonary vascular congestion. Placement of an arterial catheter facilitates timely recognition of hemodynamic derangements. PA catheters can be invaluable in the management of patients with significant mitral stenosis. Even though the PCWP overestimates LV filling and the pulmonary artery diastolic pressure may not accurately reflect left-sided heart volume in patients with pulmonary hypertension, examination of trends and responses to intervention can be more readily assessed. Tachycardia increases the pressure gradient between the left atrium and left ventricle. Elevated heart rates widen the discrepancy between the PCWP and the true LVEDP. Despite these limitations, the PA catheter remains a useful monitoring tool, providing information on cardiac output and pulmonary artery pressures. As anesthesiologists gain an increasing appreciation for the role of intraoperative TEE, this powerful imaging modality will no doubt be used more frequently to assess ventricular filling and function.

Many patients with mitral stenosis present with pulmonary hypertension. Anesthetic techniques that avoid increases in PVR are likely to benefit these patients and prevent additional RV embarrassment. Meticulous attention to arterial blood gas analysis results allows appropriate adjustment of ventilatory parameters. Vasodilator therapy in patients with pulmonary hypertension generally is ineffective as the venodilation produced further limits LV filling and does not improve cardiac output.

14

The only mitral stenosis patients who may benefit from vasodilator therapy are those with concomitant mitral regurgitation or those with severe pulmonary hypertension and RV dysfunction in whom pulmonary vasodilation can facilitate transpulmonary blood flow and improve LV filling. The treatment of RV dysfunction has been discussed in preceding sections.

TRICUSPID REGURGITATION

Clinical Features and Natural History

Surgical tricuspid disease is caused by a structural defect in the valve apparatus or is a functional lesion. Functional tricuspid regurgitation is far more common and usually results from RV overload and tricuspid annular dilation. Left-sided valvular disease, usually mitral regurgitation, is most commonly responsible. Functional tricuspid incompetence can also result from mitral stenosis, aortic regurgitation or stenosis, or from isolated pulmonary hypertension. When mitral regurgitation is severe enough to warrant valve repair or replacement, tricuspid regurgitation may be present in 30% to 50% of patients.[13]

Tricuspid regurgitation may also be caused by structural defects as in rheumatic valve disease, carcinoid syndrome, endocarditis, Epstein's anomaly, or trauma.[14] In rheumatic disease, histologic involvement of the tricuspid valve may occur in 46% of patients, but it is rarely clinically severe, and in these cases, the valve is usually also stenotic. Tricuspid regurgitation has also been described in association with CAD as a result of ischemia, infarction, or rupture of the RV papillary muscles.

Symptoms of isolated tricuspid insufficiency are usually minor in the absence of concurrent pulmonary hypertension. Intravenous drug abusers who develop tricuspid endocarditis are the classic example. In these patients, structural damage to the valve may be quite severe, but because they are free of other cardiac disease, they can tolerate complete excision of the tricuspid valve with few adverse effects. Excision of the tricuspid valve in endocarditis has been common because of the undesirability of placing a valve prosthesis in a region of infection. Surgical annuloplasty may be a better long-term option if the valve is structurally salvageable. Another factor that broadly favors tricuspid repair rather than replacement is the high incidence of thrombotic complications with a valve in this position.

In chronic tricuspid regurgitation due to RV dilation, the clinical scenario is often much different from that of isolated tricuspid disease. The major hemodynamic derangements are usually those of the associated mitral or aortic valve disease. The right ventricle dilates in the face of the afterload stress from long-standing pulmonary hypertension, and the resultant increase in end-diastolic fiber stretch (i.e., preload reserve) promotes increases in SV mediated by the Starling mechanism. These increases are negated by a concurrently rising RV afterload, however, because of relatively inadequate RV hypertrophy. Regurgitation through the tricuspid valve reduces RV wall tension at the price of a decrease in effective forward SV.

An important corollary of RV chamber enlargement is the possibility of a leftward shift of the interventricular septum and encroachment on the LV cavity. This phenomenon can reduce the LV chamber size and the slope of the LV diastolic pressure-volume curve, rendering the left ventricle less compliant. Septal encroachment may mask LV underfilling by decreasing LV compliance, thereby artificially elevating LVEDP. A failing right ventricle underloads the left side by reduced effective SV and anatomic (septal shift) mechanisms.

IV

Surgical Decision Making

In structural tricuspid insufficiency, the decision to repair or replace the valve is straightforward. The same cannot be said of functional tricuspid regurgitation. Because most functional cases are the consequence of left-sided valve lesions with RV overload, the tricuspid regurgitation usually improves significantly after the aortic or mitral valve is repaired or replaced, typically at least one grade. It can be unclear in the operating room whether addition of a tricuspid procedure to the left-sided valve surgery is indicated. In this situation, intraoperative TEE plays an essential role. If the tricuspid regurgitation is severe in the pre-CPB assessment, tricuspid valve surgery is almost always performed.[14] However, the evidence is less clear when the regurgitation is graded as moderate. Some surgeons choose to repair the tricuspid with moderate regurgitation, but others advocate observation.[15] It is common with moderate or moderate to severe tricuspid regurgitation, in the context of left-sided valve surgery, to complete the left-sided procedure and then reassess the tricuspid valve with TEE when the heart is full and ejecting. If the regurgitation remains more than moderate after the left-sided valve is fixed, many surgeons then do the tricuspid procedure. If the regurgitation is moderate or less, the appropriate surgical course may remain unclear. Some patients having left-sided valve procedures must return to the operating room in the future for tricuspid surgery. When this occurs, the morbidity and mortality rates are probably significantly increased over what would have been experienced were the tricuspid valve fixed at the time of the aortic or mitral valve procedure. Decision making in functional tricuspid regurgitation is made more complicated by the inability to rigorously quantify the severity of the regurgitation and RV dysfunction.

Anesthetic Considerations

Because most tricuspid surgery occurs in the context of significant aortic or mitral disease, anesthetic management is primarily determined by the left-sided valve lesion. The exception to this is when significant pulmonary hypertension and RV failure are present. Under these conditions, the primary impediment to hemodynamic stability after surgery will be RV failure rather than the left-sided process.

If RV dysfunction is predicted, it is useful to place a PA catheter, even if the tricuspid valve will be replaced. Even if the PA catheter has to be removed because of tricuspid valve replacement, it still can be helpful to obtain cardiac outputs and pulmonary artery pressures before CPB to get insight into RV function and anticipate the hemodynamic support that may be required. A PA catheter is also of greater use than a central venous catheter alone because the CVP is a poor index of intravascular filling and the degree of tricuspid regurgitation. This is true because the atrium and vena cavae are highly compliant and will accept large regurgitant volumes with relatively little change in pressure. A PA catheter is also useful even if intraoperative TEE is used. As in aortic insufficiency with the left ventricle, the right ventricle in chronic tricuspid regurgitation is volume overloaded and dilated and requires a large end-diastolic volume to maintain forward flow. At the same time, because of the unreliability of the CVP as an indicator of filling, it is possible to volume overload patients with tricuspid regurgitation and RV failure. Cardiac output in RV failure can often be augmented with the use of vasodilators; and even though RV dimensions can be followed intraoperatively with TEE, maximizing cardiac output (sometimes at the cost of systemic arterial pressure) is best done with serial cardiac output measurements (as in aortic regurgitation). Whenever there is significant RV distention, the possibility of septal shift and secondary deterioration of LV diastolic compliance should be carefully considered. Echocardiography is uniquely helpful for this assessment.

14

The post-CPB management of the patient undergoing an isolated tricuspid valve procedure is usually straightforward. These patients usually do not have significant RV failure or pulmonary hypertension and typically require only a brief period of CPB without aortic cross-clamping. A larger group of patients, particularly those with tricuspid regurgitation related to aortic stenosis, typically come off CPB with little need for support of the right ventricle. These patients often do well because the improvement in LV function after AVR for aortic stenosis is usually sufficient to reduce pulmonary artery pressures significantly and offload the right side of the heart. When the left-sided valve surgery is for mitral disease, the improvement is usually not as marked and greater degrees of inotropic support of the right ventricle are often indicated. The combination of a phosphodiesterase inhibitor with a vasodilator and a catecholamine infusion is useful. Serial cardiac output measurements to balance systemic pressure and RV output and filling are critical.

A few other practical points on tricuspid valve repair and replacement should be made. First, because right-sided pressures can be chronically elevated with tricuspid regurgitation, it is important to look for a patent foramen ovale and the potential for right-to-left shunting before initiation of CPB. Second, intravascular volume may be quite high in this patient population, and it is often practical to avoid red blood cell transfusion by hemofiltration during bypass. Third, if significant RV dysfunction is present or there is peripheral edema or ascites, there is the potential for a coagulopathy related to liver congestion, and the patient should be managed accordingly. Fourth, it is important to ensure that central venous catheters, particularly PA catheters, are not entrapped in right atrial suture lines.

INNOVATIONS IN VALVE REPAIR

Interventional cardiology has had a significant impact on the volume of CABG surgery, and it can be predicted that interventional cardiology will alter surgery for VHD over time. Multiple, less invasive approaches to mitral valve repair are being examined in animal or early clinical trials, and significant inroads have been made in percutaneous replacement of the aortic and pulmonic valves. Innovations in surgical valve repair are also being made. These include aortic valve repair and closed- and open-chamber procedures for mitral regurgitation.

Aortic Valve Repair

Over the past several years there has been a major shift from valve replacement to valve repair in degenerative mitral valve disease. The same has not been true of the aortic valve, in part because the valve disease is different in most patients, but also because the high flow and pressure conditions across the aortic valve might make repair more prone to failure. That said, aortic valve repair is being increasingly done as an appropriate patient population is being defined. Valve repair for aortic regurgitation has found broader use when regurgitation is associated with dissection or dilation of the aortic root, but isolated valve repair has been less common.[16] A growing body of data suggests that aortic valve repair may offer advantages over valve replacement in younger individuals with aortic insufficiency caused by bicuspid valves. In contrast to aortic valve replacement, this eliminates the need for anticoagulation for a mechanical valve and may delay the need for reoperation if a tissue valve has been placed. When regurgitation occurs with a bicuspid valve, the insufficiency is usually caused by retraction or prolapse of the conjoined cusp and repair consists of a triangular incision to shorten and elevate that cusp to improve apposition. Although very long-term follow-up has not been reported, in a large series from the Mayo Clinic with a mean follow-up of 4.2 years, late failure of the repair requiring reoperation occurred in 14 of 160 consecutive patients, with most of that failure occurring from repairs done in the first decade of the 15-year experience.

As a result of this experience, aortic valve repair is likely to find increasing application in this patient population. For this group anesthetic management is usually straightforward although the clinical indications for valve repair in aortic insufficiency are the same as those for AVR. The compelling issue for the anesthesiologist in these cases is TEE assessment of the valve for suitability of repair and the adequacy of the repair after the procedure.

Techniques for Mitral Valve Repair

Mitral regurgitation is frequently associated with CHF. In dilated and ischemic cardiomyopathy, enlargement of the mitral annulus results in a failure of coaptation of the mitral leaflets and valve incompetence. Although cardiac surgery is an effective treatment, morbidity can be high. Three different approaches have been developed to address mitral regurgitation occurring in the absence of structural mitral pathology. These approaches address the failure of leaflet coaptation at the level of the valve leaflets or the valve annulus or by altering the anatomic relationship of the septal and lateral walls of the left ventricle.

Mitral Leaflet Repair

Alfieri and associates showed that mitral regurgitation could be improved using an edge-to-edge technique by which mitral valve leaflets are brought together by a central suture. This surgical approach led to a catheter-based technology, which results in edge-to-edge repair by apposing the edges of a regurgitant mitral valve. The Evalve device consists of a catheter-mounted clip that is threaded using a femoral and transseptal approach.[17] With the use of general anesthesia and echocardiographic and fluoroscopic guidance, the clip is placed to achieve apposition of the central portion of the anterior and posterior leaflets. If the severity of mitral regurgitation is not reduced, the device can be opened and repositioned.

Percutaneous Mitral Annuloplasty

The second type of approach to functional mitral regurgitation is alteration of the mitral annulus, as might occur with a traditional open mitral repair; however, with the percutaneous approach the annulus is downsized by an extracardiac restraint.[18] With this technique, interventional cardiologists percutaneously thread a wire from the venous system into the right atrium and the coronary sinus. The relationship between the coronary sinus and posterior leaflet allows downsizing of the septal-lateral diameter from this position. Under echocardiographic guidance, tension is applied to cinch the mitral annulus smaller and an anchor is deployed to maintain position.

Altering Ventricular Anatomy to Reduce Mitral Regurgitation

The third approach to closed mitral valve repair consists of altering the geometry of the lateral and septal LV walls to bring the valve leaflets together. The commercial Coapsys device has entered clinical trials. This device consists of anterior and posterior epicardial pads connected by a cord. With an open chest, the cord is placed transventricularly in a subvalvular position and the tension on the cord is adjusted before the opposing epicardial pad is fixed in place.[19] This effectively brings the ventricular walls together and in doing so improves leaflet coaptation. TEE is used to optimize cord length and pad positioning. In contrast to the leaflet-based and

14

annular-based approaches, the Coapsys approach is surgical, requiring an open chest but not CPB. The position of the epicardial vessels and the relationship of the submitral apparatus could pose significant risk, but the device has been used successfully in animal models and preliminary clinical trials.

Percutaneous Valve Replacement

Although surgery, particularly for aortic valve disease, has expanded to include a much older population in recent years, there remains a subset of patients for whom cardiac surgery may entail unacceptable risks. For this population, less invasive techniques such as percutaneous aortic valve replacement are being developed, with the initial clinical experience with percutaneous replacement having been reported.[20]

The study population included patients with severe aortic stenosis and class IV heart failure who had been denied surgery because of excessive risk. The mean AVA was 0.49 cm^2, with a low transvalvular gradient reflecting ventricular decompensation. Patients had a mean EF of 24%. With the use of local anesthesia with sedation, the femoral vein was catheterized, and, using a transseptal approach, a balloon-tipped catheter was placed across the stenotic aortic valve. After valvuloplasty, the aortic valve stent (with incorporated leaflets) was seated at the native valve over a second balloon. In one patient, the valve was ejected into the ascending aorta on placement, and the patient died shortly thereafter. In two patients, hemodynamic collapse occurred during the initial valvuloplasty but both patients were resuscitated.

It is likely that many of these technologies will come to clinical trial and will demonstrate various degrees of efficacy. However, it is unclear what the long-term benefits of these less invasive interventions will be or how they will compare with each other or with traditional surgical approaches. Some may find use in high-risk patients as temporizing procedures, in place of reoperations, or in conjunction with percutaneous approaches for coronary disease.[21] These technologies will get better, and there will be pressure for clinical application. The most important factors will be case selection and long-term follow-up of outcomes; otherwise, these innovations and others like them will add markedly to the burden of health care costs without clear social benefit. For any of the percutaneous valves to succeed, they must demonstrate long-term successful clinical outcomes similar to the excellent results seen with mechanical or tissue valves for more than 10 to 15 years.[22]

IV

SUMMARY

- Although various valvular lesions generate different physiologic changes, all valvular heart disease is characterized by abnormalities of ventricular loading.
- The left ventricle normally compensates for increases in afterload by increases in preload. This increase in end-diastolic fiber stretch or radius further elevates wall tension in accordance with Laplace's law, resulting in a reciprocal decline in myocardial fiber shortening. The stroke volume is maintained because the contractile force is augmented at the higher preload level.
- Aortic stenosis is the most common valvular heart abnormality. Angina, syncope, and congestive heart failure are the classic symptoms and the indications for surgery.
- Treatment modalities for hypertrophic obstructive cardiomyopathy, a relatively common genetic malformation of the heart, include β-adrenoceptor antagonists, calcium channel blockers, and myectomy of the septum. Newer approaches include dual-chamber pacing and septal reduction (ablation) therapy with ethanol.

- The severity and duration of symptoms of aortic regurgitation may correlate poorly with the degree of hemodynamic and contractile impairment, delaying surgical treatment while patients are undergoing progressive deterioration.
- Mitral regurgitation causes left ventricular volume overload. Treatment depends on the underlying mechanism and includes angiotensin-converting enzyme inhibitors and surgical repair or replacement of the mitral valve.
- Rheumatic disease and congenital abnormalities of the mitral valve are the main causes of mitral stenosis, a slowly progressive disease. Surgical treatment options include closed and open commissurotomy and percutaneous mitral commissurotomy.
- Most tricuspid surgery occurs in the context of significant aortic or mitral disease, and anesthetic management is primarily determined by the left-sided valve lesion.
- Innovations in surgical valve repair include aortic valve repair and closed- and open-chamber procedures for mitral regurgitation.

REFERENCES

1. Rajamannan NM, Gersh B, Bonow RO: Calcific aortic stenosis: From bench to the bedside—emerging clinical and cellular concepts. Heart 89:801, 2003
2. Grayburn PA, Eichhorn EJ: Dobutamine challenge for low-gradient aortic stenosis. Circulation 106:763, 2002
3. Carabello BA: Clinical practice. Aortic stenosis. N Engl J Med 346:677, 2002
4. Roberts R, Sigwart U: New concepts in hypertrophic cardiomyopathies: II. Circulation 104:2249, 2001
5. Nishimura RA, Holmes DR: Hypertrophic obstructive cardiomyopathy. N Engl J Med 350:1320, 2004
6. Enriquez-Sarano M, Tajik AT: Clinical practice: Aortic regurgitation. N Engl J Med 351:1539, 2004
7. Enriquez-Sarano M, Avierinos JF, Messika-Zeitoun D, et al: Quantitative determinants of the outcome of asymptomatic mitral regurgitation. N Engl J Med 352:875, 2005
8. Carabello BA: The pathophysiology of mitral regurgitation. J Heart Valve Dis 9:600, 2000
9. Enriquez-Sarano M, Schaff HV, Orszulak TA, et al: Valve repair improves the outcome of surgery for mitral regurgitation: A multivariate analysis. Circulation 91:1022, 1995
10. Shapira Y, Vaturi M, Weisenberg D, et al: Impact of intraoperative transesophageal echocardiography in patients undergoing value replacement. Ann Thorac Surg 78:579, 2004
11. Popovic AD, Stewart M, Stewart M: Echocardiographic evaluation of valvular stenosis: The gold standard for the next millennium? Echocardiography 18:59, 2001
12. Iung B, Vahanian A: The long-term outcome of balloon valvuloplasty for mitral stenosis. Curr Cardiol Rep 4:118, 2002
13. Mueller XM, Tevaearai HT, Stumpe F, et al: Tricuspid valve involvement in combined mitral and aortic valve surgery. J Cardiovasc Surg 42:443, 2001
14. Messika-Zeitoun D, Thomson H, Bellamy M, et al: Medical and surgical outcome of tricuspid regurgitation caused by flail leaflets. J Thorac Cardiovasc Surg 128:296, 2004
15. Shatapathy P, Aggarwal BK, Kamath SG: Tricuspid valve repair: A rational alternative. J Heart Valve Dis 9:276, 2000
16. Minakata K, Schaff HV, Zehr KJ, et al: Is repair of aortic valve regurgitation a safe alternative to valve replacement? J Thorac Cardiovasc Surg 127:645, 2004
17. Block PC: Percutaneous mitral valve repair for mitral regurgitation. J Int Cardiol 16:93, 2003
18. Kaye DM, Byrne M, Alferness C, et al: Feasibility and short-term efficacy of percutaneous mitral annular reduction for the therapy of heart failure-induced mitral regurgitation. Circulation 108:1795, 2003
19. Inoue M, McCarthy PM, Popovic ZB, et al: The Coapsys device to treat functional mitral regurgitation: In vivo long-term canine study. J Thorac Cardiovasc Surg 127:1068-discussion 1076, 2004
20. Cribier A, Eltchaninoff H, Tron C, et al: Early experience with percutaneous transcatheter implantation of heart valve prosthesis for the treatment of end-stage inoperable patients with calcific aortic stenosis. J Am Coll Cardiol 43:698, 2004
21. Byrne JG, Leacche M, Unic D, et al: Staged initial percutaneous coronary intervention followed by valve surgery ("hybrid approach") for patients with complex coronary and valve disease. J Am Coll Cardiol 45:14, 2005
22. Rahimtoola SH: The year in valvular heart disease. J Am Coll Cardiol 47:427, 2006

14

Chapter 15

Minimally Invasive Cardiac Surgery

Marianne Coutu, MD • Lishan Aklog, MD • David Reich, MD

Since its early days, cardiac surgery has typically involved large incisions with complete access to the heart and great vessels. After the popularization of minimally invasive techniques in general surgery, cardiac surgeons began to experiment with less invasive procedures in the early 1990s. Although the goals of minimally invasive cardiac surgery (MICS) are fairly well established as decreased pain, shorter hospital stay, accelerated recuperation, and improved cosmesis, a strict definition of *minimally invasive cardiac surgery* has been more elusive. "Less invasive" is probably a more appropriate term, because these procedures span a wide spectrum from full sternotomy off-pump procedures to totally endoscopic procedures. There has been an ongoing debate within the specialty whether eliminating sternotomy or cardiopulmonary bypass (CPB) is a more fundamental component of MICS. Some have even argued that cardiac surgery will not be truly minimally invasive until general anesthesia itself is eliminated and a handful of centers have reported on various off-pump coronary artery bypass grafting (OPCAB) procedures performed with high thoracic epidural anesthesia alone.

This chapter focuses on the anesthetic implications of operations performed through an incision other than a full sternotomy or thoracotomy and does not address the various endovascular procedures under development. The common incisions used for these procedures are shown in Figure 15-1 and include partial sternotomies (upper vs. lower, unilateral vs. bilateral) and minithoracotomies (anterior vs. anterolateral vs. posterolateral, nonspreading vs. spreading) in addition to totally endoscopic procedures done exclusively through thoracoscopic ports (defined as < 15 mm).

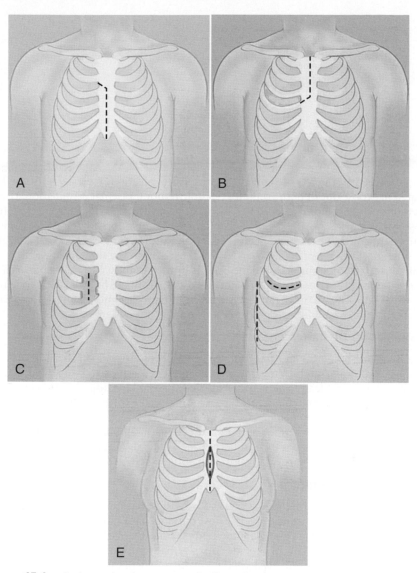

Figure 15-1 **A,** Lower hemisternotomy. **B,** Upper hemisternotomy. **C,** Parasternal incision. **D,** Anterolateral minithoracotomy. **E,** Full sternotomy with small skin incision.

GENERAL ANESTHETIC CONSIDERATIONS

Patient Setup

Position, Prepping, and Draping

Conventional cardiac surgery is almost always performed with the patient flat and supine, prepped, and draped with the sterile field extending from mid-neck to the ankles (Box 15-1). Many MICS procedures, however, require different positions and sterile field setups. For example, most procedures performed through anterior minithoracotomies or exclusively thoracoscopically are done with the patient's left or right side elevated approximately 30 degrees. Some thoracoscopic procedures

BOX 15-1   *Anesthetic Considerations*

- Position, prepping, and draping
- Temperature management
- Hemodynamic monitoring
- Airway management
- Anesthetic regimen
- Pain management

are performed in the left or right lateral decubitus position, typically with the hips rotated to expose one or both groins for possible femoral vascular cannulation. Unlike conventional sternotomy procedures, surgical access to remote areas (neck, lateral chest wall, groin) may be necessary for peripheral cannulation, placement of camera/instrument ports, or transcutaneous retraction sutures. This should be taken into consideration when placing ECG leads or other items on the skin during setup.

Because, by definition, access to the heart is limited in most MICS, *external defibrillator pads* should be considered mandatory. Again, care should be taken with placement and draping to ensure the current passes through the heart and that burns associated with seepage of prep solution or other liquids under the pads are avoided.

Temperature Management

Because nearly all MICS and all off-pump procedures are performed under normothermic conditions, careful temperature management is critical to avoid hypothermia, which not only can lead to ventricular fibrillation and bleeding but also can negate some of the potential benefits of MICS by prolonging the time to extubation. In addition to maintaining room temperature, one of a variety of *warming blankets* is usually required. Although conventional water or forced warm air blankets can suffice, more innovative solutions such as the Kimberly-Clark Patient Warming System (formerly the Arctic Sun) may be particularly advantageous in MICS.

Hemodynamic Monitoring

Hemodynamic monitoring requirements for MICS are typically not different from those of conventional cardiac surgery. Most patients have radial arterial and pulmonary artery (PA) catheters placed. Some centers limit themselves to a central venous pressure catheter, especially in patients with normal ventricular function undergoing MICS. Intraoperative *transesophageal echocardiography* (TEE) is the standard of care for all valvular surgery, and it can be critical in MICS cases to assess ventricular preload and pick up early changes in regional or global ventricular function, because visualization of the heart may be limited. In addition, TEE is helpful and often necessary to guide placement of various catheters, cannulae, and balloons. Because access to a ventricular wall for temporary pacing wire placement can be limited in some MICS approaches, a PA catheter with a pacing port can be helpful in valve procedures or other cases in which the need for temporary cardiac pacing may arise.

Anesthetic Technique

Airway

Many MICS procedures, including all minithoracotomy and thoracoscopic approaches, require at least some period of *one-lung ventilation*. Double-lumen endotracheal tubes are generally preferred because they are less likely to be dislodged during repositioning. It is critical to take the time to confirm proper placement and lung isolation before and just after positioning, because loss of lung isolation during an anastomosis or during some other critical stage of the procedure can be extremely dangerous.

Carbon dioxide insufflation of the hemithorax is frequently used during thoracoscopic MICS procedures, especially during robotic procedures. Insufflation to a pressure of 8 to 15 cm H_2O can dramatically increase the working space in the chest by shifting the mediastinal structures posteriorly and to the contralateral chest. Because there is always some obligatory leak around ports and incisions, the constant flow of CO_2 also clears smoke generated during electrocauterization of tissues. The intrathoracic pressure should be set to the minimal value necessary to achieve adequate exposure, and very careful monitoring of hemodynamics and gas exchange is essential, because the physiology is effectively that of a controlled tension pneumothorax. Although generally well tolerated, significant hypotension, hypercapnia, or hypoxia can occur if the pressure is set too high, particularly in patients with ventricular dysfunction or lung disease.[1]

Anesthetic Regimen

Because accelerated recovery and discharge are major goals of MICS, it is important to note that careful selection of the anesthetic agents is necessary to ensure that the patient obtains the full benefit from the minimally invasive approach. Most centers will use some sort of *"fast-track" anesthesia* regimen—typically very short-acting narcotics and muscle relaxants in conjunction with an inhalation agent.[2] Some have advocated precise pharmacokinetically *controlled total intravenous anesthesia* (TIVA) regimens. Routine intraoperative extubation of MICS patients is controversial. Although some centers have established protocols whereby nearly all patients are extubated at the completion of the procedure,[3] others have argued that a clinical or economic benefit is difficult to document unless the patient recovers in a postoperative acute care unit setting without an overnight stay in the intensive care unit.[4]

Pain Management

Aggressive pain management is another critical component of the care of patients undergoing MICS, without which it is difficult to obtain the full benefit of this approach. Successful pain management permits intraoperative or early postoperative extubation, early ambulation, and discharge. There is some evidence that the amount of pain in the early postoperative period may not be significantly less in many types of MICS and that it may actually be higher in some, particularly those involving rib-spreading thoracotomies. The pain, however, seems to dissipate more rapidly than with full sternotomy; most patients are off narcotic pain medicines within 1 or 2 weeks of surgery.[5]

Spinal/Epidural Anesthesia

Spinal and epidural anesthetics have been used as an adjunct to general anesthesia at many institutions practicing MICS. A single intrathecal dose of a long-acting narcotic can be beneficial in reducing intraoperative and postoperative parenteral or enteral narcotic requirements.[6] A thoracic epidural catheter with narcotic or local anesthetics can be administered continuously or with patient-controlled dosing.[7] The excellent pain control and potential cardioprotective benefits from this approach, however, are mitigated by the additional operative time, the small but finite additional risk from the epidural anesthesia, and its potential to delay the typically rapid mobilization and discharge of MICS patients.

15

> **BOX 15-2** *Cardiopulmonary Bypass Considerations*
>
> - Arterial cannulation
> - Venous cannulation
> - Aortic occlusion and cardioplegia
> - Cardiac decompression and de-airing

Local Anesthesia

Every effort should be made to supplement the pain management of MICS with local measures at the surgical site. This can include conventional methods such as direct infiltration of the wound with a long-acting local anesthetic such as bupivacaine or *intercostal rib blocks* extending a couple of interspaces above and below the incision.

GENERAL CARDIOPULMONARY BYPASS CONSIDERATIONS

Although nearly all minimally invasive coronary artery bypass surgery is performed on a beating heart, without the use of CPB, minimally invasive surgery of the cardiac valves and other intracardiac structures requires creative and innovative techniques to safely establish CPB (Box 15-2). There are a variety of approaches depending on the incision and access to cardiovascular structures. Some minimally invasive approaches permit direct, central cannulation similar to conventional cardiac surgery but typically with relatively small cannulae and vacuum-assisted venous drainage. On the other end of the spectrum, "Port-Access" techniques, pioneered by Heartport, Inc. (Redwood City, CA) in the early 1990s, sought to have all elements of the CPB circuit enter peripherally, preferably percutaneously, to allow procedures to be performed through very small incisions or totally endoscopically. The anesthesiologist plays a central role in all "Port-Access" procedures from insertion of certain cannulae to monitoring cannula position and function by TEE.[8]

Cannulation

IV

Arterial

Some MICS approaches, including most partial sternotomy incisions, permit direct cannulation of the ascending aorta in a fashion similar, if not identical, to conventional approaches. Some surgeons use aortic cannulae with tapered dilators designed to be inserted over a guidewire to facilitate direct cannulation through a limited incision. Through many MICS approaches, however, the ascending aorta cannot be safely cannulated and peripheral cannulation is necessary. The femoral approach is most commonly used. The axillary artery is a viable alternative but is not usually used in MICS because accessing it usually requires a cosmetically prominent 3- to 6-cm incision. TEE assessment of the descending aorta is important before considering femoral artery cannulation to rule out extensive atherosclerotic disease, which can lead to retrograde embolization and neurologic injury.

Femoral arterial cannulation can be achieved percutaneously but is usually performed through a very small transverse incision guided by the pulse or a Doppler signal. The cannulae can be short, with the tip sitting in the pelvis, or long, extending into the thoracic aorta with multiple side ports. Contraindications include significant peripheral vascular disease. Potential complications include retrograde dissection, embolization, and perforation with retroperitoneal hemorrhage.

Venous

Even though the right atrium (RA) is accessible in many MICS approaches, percutaneous femoral venous cannulation has become popular because it removes the venous cannulae from the operative field, enhancing exposure. The right femoral vein is usually used because the right common iliac vein joins the inferior vena cava (IVC) at a much straighter angle, facilitating advancement into the RA. Modern, highly efficient long venous cannulae as small as 20 to 21 Fr, coupled with vacuum-assisted venous drainage, can support full CPB flows even in large individuals. TEE is used to confirm guidewire and cannula position during percutaneous insertion.

A single cannula with the tip near the RA/superior vena cava (SVC) junction and side ports spanning the RA usually suffices for aortic valve operations. Situations in which surgical manipulation can interfere with SVC drainage must be considered to avoid complications due to upper body venous hypertension. In mitral valve operations, for example, retraction of the RA and septum can interfere with drainage. The Chitwood transthoracic aortic clamp, used commonly in videoscopic and robotic mitral valve surgery, passes over the SVC and can compress it. RA procedures (atrial septal defects [ASDs], tricuspid surgery) usually require separate IVC and SVC drainage. In these situations, improved drainage can be ensured by using a two-stage long venous cannula that can be advanced into the SVC itself. Another approach is to cannulate the right internal jugular vein percutaneously with a small cannula advanced into the SVC.

Aortic Occlusion and Cardioplegia

Intracardiac procedures usually require aortic occlusion and cardioplegic arrest. In direct-access MICS procedures, direct clamping of the aorta can be achieved with conventional, slightly streamlined, or articulating aortic clamps. Videoscopic and robotic procedures, however, require some type of remote aortic occlusion. The two most common options are the Chitwood transthoracic clamp and balloon occlusion. The Chitwood clamp has conventional jaws, but a long shaft, and is passed through a separate port in the right chest with the posterior jaw in the transverse sinus.

Balloon aortic occlusion is the centerpiece of most Port-Access approaches. A catheter with a large, low-pressure balloon is passed via the femoral artery and positioned with the balloon in the ascending aorta under echocardiographic guidance. The balloon is inflated until the pressure in the port distal to the balloon falls, confirming occlusion of the ascending aorta. The right and left radial artery pressures are monitored simultaneously to ensure the balloon is not impinging on the orifice of the innominate artery. Balloon migration can be an irritating problem early in the learning curve, but experienced centers report good results with routine use of this technique. However, all centers emphasize careful collaboration among the surgery, anesthesia, and perfusion teams. Continuous TEE monitoring of balloon position is important to prevent complications. The most dreaded complication of this technique is aortic dissection, and some reports indicate that the incidence may be higher than in conventional surgery.

Myocardial protection during MICS can be achieved via an anterograde, retrograde, or combined approach. In direct-access and videoscopic approaches, the anterograde cardioplegia catheter is usually directly inserted into the ascending aorta. In the Port-Access approach, the cardioplegic solution is infused through the distal port of the balloon catheter into the aortic root. In direct-access approaches, a retrograde catheter can be advanced into the coronary sinus, with or without echocardiographic guidance. The Port-Access system includes a percutaneous retrograde coronary sinus catheter that is inserted by the anesthesia team through the right internal jugular vein and advanced under echocardiographic guidance.

15

BOX 15-3 *Minimally Invasive Coronary Artery Surgery*

- Off-pump coronary artery bypass grafting (OPCAB) (see Chapter 13)
- Minimally invasive direct coronary artery bypass (MIDCAB)
  - Enhanced (robotic-assisted) MIDCAB
- Total endoscopic coronary artery revascularization (TECAB)
  - TECAB on the arrested heart
  - TECAB on the beating heart
- Multivessel small thoracotomy revascularization

Cardiac Decompression/De-airing

Limited visibility of and access to the cardiac chambers during MICS can make the critical steps of cardiac decompression and de-airing more difficult and requires special attention to avoid the potentially devastating complications arising from unsuspected sustained myocardial distention or air embolism.

The most vulnerable period for distention is during administration of antegrade cardioplegia and immediately after removing the cross-clamp before restoration of ventricular ejection. The ventricular dimensions on TEE and the pulmonary artery pressures should be monitored closely to ensure adequate ventricular decompression. Patients with thick, small-cavity ventricles may be particularly difficult to monitor because the ventricle may not appear particularly dilated on TEE despite an elevated cavitary pressure and because they are more susceptible to subendocardial ischemia. A left ventricular (LV) vent can be inserted through the right superior pulmonary vein in some patients undergoing direct-access MICS. The Port-Access system includes a percutaneous pulmonary artery vent that is advanced through the jugular vein and can maintain decompression. A terminal dose of warm blood in the aortic root can rouse the heart and initiate ventricular ejection before removing the cross-clamp, avoiding distention.

Because manual manipulation of the cardiac chambers is usually impossible with MICS, the best way to deal with intracardiac air is to prevent it from accumulating in the first place. Flooding the surgical field with CO_2 while the chambers are open can dramatically decrease the amount of air. Some de-airing is usually necessary, and manipulation of the table while ventilating and filling the heart usually facilitates this.

MINIMALLY INVASIVE CORONARY ARTERY BYPASS GRAFTING

The goals of minimally invasive coronary artery bypass grafting are to reduce the surgical trauma by minimizing access and to obviate the need for extracorporeal circulation (Box 15-3). These procedures encompass minimally invasive direct coronary artery bypass grafting (MIDCAB), totally endoscopic coronary artery bypass grafting on an arrested or beating heart, and multivessel small thoracotomy revascularization.

Minimally Invasive Direct Coronary Artery Bypass Grafting

MIDCAB is a coronary revascularization procedure through an anterolateral thoracotomy. Patients who should be considered for a MIDCAB are those with isolated left anterior descending (LAD) or right coronary artery (RCA) stenosis, patients with multivessel disease in which the lesion in the other vessels can be addressed percutaneously (hybrid procedure), and patients with multiple comorbidities.

The patient is positioned supine on the operating table. External defibrillator pads are placed allowing space for sternotomy access in the event of a conversion. A double-lumen endotracheal tube or a bronchial blocker is used to collapse the left lung. Standard monitoring for cardiac surgery is used, plus TEE to monitor cardiac filling and myocardial segmental wall motion abnormalities.

This procedure is performed through a small anterolateral thoracotomy. A 6- to 10-cm incision is made over the fourth intercostal space, the pleural space is opened, and the ribs are spread with a specialized left internal mammary artery (LIMA) retractor. The LIMA is harvested as a pedicle (length of about 15 cm) and prepared after systemic heparinization. The LAD is then identified, dissected, and opened after the heart has been stabilized. Finally, the LIMA is anastomosed to the LAD on a beating heart through the thoracic incision. This procedure can also be performed for a proximal high-grade RCA stenosis through a right anterolateral thoracotomy using the right internal mammary artery (RIMA).

The main advantages of the MIDCAB procedure are the avoidance of CPB and median sternotomy, potentially less postoperative pain, and faster recovery to normal activities. Studies showed good short-term patency rates of the LIMA-to-LAD anastomosis.[9]

Totally Endoscopic Coronary Artery Revascularization

It is the development of computer-enhanced telemanipulators that has enabled robotically assisted surgery and totally endoscopic coronary artery revascularization. The currently available system, the DaVinci Telemanipulation System (Intuitive Surgical, Inc., Sunnyvale, CA), provides a high-resolution three-dimensional videoscopic image and allows remote, tremor-free, and scaled control of endoscopic surgical instruments with 6 degrees of freedom. It consists of a master console for remote control of microinstruments mounted on a surgical cart with three arms (one stereoendoscope and two endothoracic end-effectors). This procedure can be done on the arrested heart and on the beating heart and is most often performed for single- or double-vessel coronary artery disease.

Totally Endoscopic Coronary Artery Bypass on the Arrested Heart

The most frequently performed procedure using this technique to date is revascularization of the LAD with the LIMA via a left-sided approach.[10] The RCA can also be grafted with the RIMA via a right-sided approach.

For robotically assisted LIMA harvest, patients are placed in a supine position with the left side of the chest elevated 30 to 40 degrees. Ventilation of the right lung is performed. A 30-degree scope angled up is inserted at the fourth intercostal space (ICS) in the left anterior axillary line. Continuous CO_2 insufflation (<10 mmHg) of the thoracic cavity is used to enhance exposure by increasing the available space between the heart and the sternum. Two endoscopic instruments used for LIMA harvesting are then placed under direct vision through ports in the third and seventh ICS in the midaxillary line. The LIMA is dissected as a pedicle from the subclavian artery to the bifurcation. After systemic heparinization, the LIMA is transected at its distal end. Femoral-femoral CPB is initiated by using the Port-Access system for closed-chest and antegrade cardioplegic cardiac arrest. The femoral venous cannula is positioned in the RA under echocardiographic guidance. After institution of CPB, the pericardium is opened, the target vessel is identified on the beating heart, and the epicardium over the anastomotic region is dissected. The heart is arrested using the endoaortic occlusion catheter and cardioplegia administration. The coronary anastomosis is performed end-to-side with a running suture (7-0 or 8-0 Prolene) or interrupted sutures (U-clips). After completion of the anastomosis, the endoaortic occlusion catheter is deflated and the patient is weaned from CPB.

Totally Endoscopic Coronary Artery Bypass Grafting on the Beating Heart

The development of endoscopic CABG on the beating heart required the development of endoscopic stabilizers and methods for temporary coronary occlusion. Vascular occlusion can be achieved by using vascular clamps or Silastic bands. For this procedure, the patient is prepared as described earlier. In addition to the three left-sided ports, an endoscopic epicardial stabilizer is inserted through a subxiphoid port after harvest and preparation of the LIMA. Endoscopic stabilizers use combined pressure and suction stabilization to facilitate the performance of the anastomosis. Because the heart is not decompressed with this technique, the space in the thoracic cavity is limited despite CO_2 insufflation. In this particular situation, CO_2 pressure may be increased above 12 mmHg if the heart is sufficiently filled and myocardial contractility is adequate. Compared with full-sternotomy beating heart surgery, the myocardial tolerance to ischemia in beating heart totally endoscopic coronary artery bypass grafting (TECAB) is reduced. After occlusion of the target vessel, if severe ST-segment elevation or multiple extrasystoles appear on the ECG, the conversion threshold to MIDCAB should be low.[11] The anastomosis is performed with a running suture (7-0 or 8-0 Prolene), interrupted sutures (U-clips), or distal anastomotic devices.

Even as progress has been made, as with all new technologies, a learning curve has to be overcome. Operating times are still long and conversions to open surgery are frequently necessary. A lot of steps occurring between IMA takedown and performance of the anastomosis are hampered by the lack of assistance, limited space, the lack of fine tactile feedback, and a limited number of instruments.

MINIMALLY INVASIVE VALVULAR SURGERY

Valvular procedures such as aortic valve replacement and mitral valve replacement and repair are now performed using different types of minimally invasive procedures (Box 15-4).

Minimally Invasive Aortic Valve Surgery

The goals of minimally invasive aortic valve surgery are to reduce the incision size and decrease the surgical trauma and pain, in addition to improving cosmetics, patient satisfaction, and recovery times. This must be realized without compromising the efficacy and the safety of the conventional aortic valve surgery.

BOX 15-4 *Minimally Invasive Valvular Surgery*

- Minimally invasive aortic valve surgery
- Minimally invasive mitral valve surgery (MIMVS)
- Direct-vision MIMVS
- Video-assisted and directed MIMVS
- Robot-directed MIMVS telemanipulation and computer-enhanced MIMVS

IV

Minimally invasive aortic valve surgery has been performed via several approaches such as a right parasternal incision, right anterolateral thoracotomy, and transverse sternotomy, but the most frequently performed approach is the partial upper sternotomy or "ministernotomy." This latter approach allows excellent exposure for aortic root procedures and aortic valve replacement or repair. It is particularly useful for reoperative valve surgery and has been reported to decrease blood loss, transfusion requirements, wound complications, and total operative times compared with a full sternotomy technique. Contraindications to this technique are its use in high-risk and elderly patients, with significant coronary artery disease that needs to be corrected, and in the presence of chest wall deformities, cardiac malposition, and morbid obesity.

For the ministernotomy, transcutaneous defibrillator pads, a PA catheter, and TEE are used, and the patient is prepped in a supine position. After a 6- to 10-cm skin incision, a longitudinal midsternal cut is made from the notch to the third or fifth ICS, deviating to the right. Care is taken not to injure the internal thoracic vessels. Right femoral venous cannulation is performed, and with echocardiographic guidance, the cannula is advanced into the RA. Direct venous cannulation in the RA can also be done but reduces the surgeon's exposure. Arterial cannulation is performed in the ascending aorta or in the femoral artery, and CPB is initiated. Both antegrade and retrograde cardioplegia are used for myocardial protection. After cross-clamping, antegrade cardioplegia is given either in the aortic root or directly into the coronary ostia and retrograde cardioplegia is delivered via a transjugular catheter directed into the coronary sinus. The aortic valve procedure is then performed as usual. After cross-clamp removal, intracardiac air is carefully monitored with TEE, the patient is weaned from CPB, and sternal closure is performed as usual.

The Brigham and Women's Hospital surgeons reported their series of more than 500 mini-invasive aortic valve replacements with an operative mortality of 2% and a freedom from reoperation at 6 years of 99%.[12]

Minimally Invasive Mitral Valve Surgery

Developments in minimally invasive mitral valve surgery (MIMVS) started in the mid-1990s. Within a few years, with technologic advancements in instrumentation, assisted vision, and CPB support, conventional mitral valve surgery through a full sternotomy evolved to a totally endoscopic operation. This surgical evolution led to four levels of surgical invasiveness: (1) mini-incision and direct vision; (2) video-assisted and directed; (3) robot-directed; and (4) telemanipulation and robotically enhanced operations. These procedures are currently performed in several centers in the United States and Europe. Most suitable candidates are patients with primary valve disease, reoperative mitral valve disease, and obesity. Contraindications to these techniques are highly calcified mitral annulus, prior right-sided chest surgery, or significant coronary artery disease and peripheral vascular disease. In addition to improved cosmetics, these procedures are associated with less perioperative blood loss, fewer blood transfusions, shorter intubation time and length of stay, and faster recovery.

Level 1: Direct-Vision Minimally Invasive Mitral Valve Surgery

Direct-vision MIMVS can be performed through a ministernotomy, a parasternal incision, or through a limited anterolateral thoracotomy. CPB is instituted in a standard fashion or using the Port-Access system. Arterial cannulation is done through the femoral artery in the parasternal and in the limited thoracotomy approaches, but it can sometimes be accomplished directly in the ascending aorta in the lower partial sternotomy approach. Venous cannulation is accomplished by direct cannulation of the SVC (with a right-angled cannula) through the incision. The IVC is cannulated with a small percutaneous transfemoral cannula advanced over a guidewire and under guidance of TEE. The aorta is usually clamped through the incision. Finally, the mitral valve is approached either directly (standard left atriotomy) or transseptally via the RA.

The Brigham group published their experience of 1000 minimally invasive valve operations.[12] They performed 474 mitral procedures through a lower sternotomy, a right parasternal, or a right thoracotomy incision. They reported excellent results with operative and late mortality rates of 0.2% and 3.0%, respectively, and freedom from reoperation at 6 years was 95%. Compared with patients who had a full sternotomy incision, those who had a minimally invasive approach had shorter CPB and cross-clamp times, fewer myocardial infarctions, fewer pacemaker insertions, and a shorter length of stay (2 days).

Level 2: Video-Assisted and Video-Directed Minimally Invasive Mitral Valve Surgery

Video-assisted mitral valve surgery was developed to allow smaller incisions without compromising the results of the procedure and the patient's safety. A telescope and a thoracoscopic camera are used to perform the surgery. The camera is manipulated by an assistant under the guidance of the surgeon. Mitral valve repair and replacement are performed using assisted vision through the thoracoscope.

Carpentier was the pioneer of video-assisted MIMVS. He and his group performed the first video-assisted mitral valve repair through a minithoracotomy using hypothermic ventricular fibrillation. Chitwood and his team modified the original technique, using a minithoracotomy, percutaneous transthoracic aortic occlusion, video assistance, and peripheral CPB.

Chitwood and colleagues reported their experience with 31 consecutive patients (20 mitral repairs and 11 replacements) with excellent results.[13] Thirty-day mortality was 3.2%. No stroke or aortic dissection was reported. Compared with patients who had conventional mitral valve surgery, these patients had significantly shorter hospitalization times, less perioperative pain, and faster recovery. In addition, hospital charges were reduced.

Level 3: Robot-Directed Minimally Invasive Mitral Valve Surgery

In robotically directed MIMVS, a voice-activated system (AESOP 3000; Computer Motion, Inc., Santa Barbara, CA) is attached to the thoracoscope. The motion of the robot is controlled by the surgeon with voice activation and one- or two-word commands. The overall performance of the procedure by allowing a full range of motion and a steady operative field and by decreasing the number of lens cleanings and, hence, operating times. Chitwood's group published their experience of robotically directed MIMVS with low mortality and morbidity. Seventy percent of the cases were repairs. They reported that the robotically directed technique showed significant decreases in blood loss, ventilator time, and hospitalization compared with sternotomy-based technique.[14]

Level 4: Telemanipulation and Computer-Enhanced Minimally Invasive Mitral Valve Surgery

Mitral valve surgery can now be done completely endoscopically using the DaVinci system (Intuitive Surgical, Inc., Sunnyvale, CA). This system has three components: (1) a surgeon console, (2) an instrument cart, and (3) a vision platform. The operative

IV

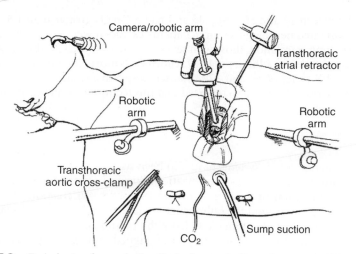

Camera/robotic arm

Transthoracic
atrial retractor

Robotic
arm

Robotic
arm

Transthoracic
aortic cross-clamp

CO_2

Sump suction

Figure 15-2   Typical setup for a robotic mitral valve repair. (From Kypson AP, Chitwood WR Jr: Robotic mitral valve surgery. Am J Surg 188[4A suppl]:83S, 2004. Copyright 2004, with permission from Excerpta Medica Inc.)

console is removed physically from the patient and allows the surgeon to sit comfortably. The surgeon's fingers and wrist movements are registered through sensors in computer motor banks, and then these actions are transferred to the instrument cart, which operates synchronous end-effector instruments. A three-dimensional digital visioning system enables natural depth perception with high-power magnification (Fig. 15-2).

Patients who are good candidates for this kind of procedure are those with isolated degenerative mitral valve disease. Exclusion criteria for robotic mitral valve surgery were described by Kypson and Chitwood and are as follows: previous right thoracotomy, renal failure, liver dysfunction, bleeding disorders, severe pulmonary hypertension (systolic PAP > 60 mmHg), significant aortic or tricuspid valve disease, coronary artery disease requiring surgery, recent myocardial infarction (<30 days), recent stroke (<30 days), and severely calcified mitral valve annulus.[15] Patients with poor lung function undergo pulmonary testing to make sure that they can tolerate one-lung ventilation. Should they not be able to tolerate it, CPB is instituted earlier for intrathoracic preparation.

OTHER MINIMALLY INVASIVE CARDIAC PROCEDURES

Congenital Heart Surgery

In pediatric cardiac surgery, current robotic systems have been used primarily to facilitate thoracoscopic pediatric procedures on extracardiac lesions, such as ligation of patent ductus arteriosus (PDA) and division of vascular rings.[16] With the present technology, patients weighing less than 15 kg cannot undergo a robotically-assisted surgery because the instruments are too big and occupy the entire ICS of most small infants.

Intracardiac lesion repair had been performed by robotically-assisted surgery in the adult population. Argenziano and associates reported a series of 17 patients (12 secundum-type ASDs and 5 patent foramen ovales [PFOs]). Patients included were aged between 18 and 80 years old and had a Qp:Qs greater than 1.5 or a PFO with a documented neurologic event.[17] Patients excluded were those who could not tolerate one-lung ventilation, those with severe peripheral vascular disease, and those with dense right pleural adhesions. They reported no mortality, median aortic cross-clamp and CPB times of 32 and 122 minutes, respectively, and a successful repair rate of 94% (16 of 17). They also reported that this technique hastened postoperative recovery and improved quality of life.[18]

Surgery for Atrial Fibrillation

Robotic telemanipulation systems have also been used to perform surgery for atrial fibrillation and ventricular resynchronization. Surgical treatment of atrial fibrillation allows elimination of the arrhythmia in two ways: (1) creation of a contiguous encircling lesion around the pulmonary veins that prohibits the propagation of current and future foci of automaticity from the pulmonary veins, and (2) creation of linear lesions in other parts of the atrium designed to interrupt potential macro-reentrant circuits.[19]

SUMMARY

- The goals of minimally invasive cardiac surgery are decreased pain, shorter hospital stays, accelerated recuperation, and improved cosmetics.
- These "less invasive" surgical procedures span a wide spectrum from full sternotomy off-pump surgery to totally endoscopic procedures done through small ports.
- Anesthetic management for minimally invasive cardiac surgery ranges from fast-track general anesthesia through awake patients under thoracic epidural anesthesia.
- Cardiopulmonary bypass may or may not be used in minimally invasive surgery. One approach for cardiopulmonary bypass is to use the "Port-Access" system developed by Heartport, Inc. (Redwood City, CA).
- Minimally invasive direct coronary artery bypass is a coronary revascularization procedure performed through a small anterolateral thoracotomy.
- The development of computer-enhanced telemanipulators has enabled the development of robotically assisted cardiac surgery and totally endoscopic coronary artery revascularization.
- Totally endoscopic coronary artery revascularization procedures can be performed on the arrested heart or on the beating heart.
- Valvular procedures such as aortic valve replacement and mitral valve replacement or repair can now be performed using minimally invasive procedures.
- Other minimally invasive cardiac procedures include congenital heart surgery, arrhythmia surgery, and ventricular resynchronization procedures.

REFERENCES

1. Vassiliades TA Jr: The cardiopulmonary effects of single-lung ventilation and carbon dioxide insufflation during thoracoscopic internal mammary artery harvesting. Heart Surg Forum 5:22, 2002
2. Myles PS, McIlroy D: Fast-track cardiac anesthesia: Choice of anesthetic agents and techniques. Semin Cardiothorac Vasc Anesth 9:5, 2005
3. Lee TW, Jacobsohn E: Pro: Tracheal extubation should occur routinely in the operating room after cardiac surgery. J Cardiothorac Vasc Anesth 14:603, 2000

4. Peragallo RA, Cheng DC: Con: tracheal extubation should not occur routinely in the operating room after cardiac surgery. J Cardiothorac Vasc Anesth 14:611, 2000
5. Niinami H, Ogasawara H, Suda Y, et al: Single-vessel revascularization with minimally invasive direct coronary artery bypass: Minithoracotomy or ministernotomy? Chest 127:47, 2005
6. Parlow JL, Steele RG, O'Reilly D: Low dose intrathecal morphine facilitates early extubation after cardiac surgery: Results of a retrospective continuous quality improvement audit. Can J Anaesth 52:94, 2005
7. Kessler P, Aybek T, Neidhart G, et al: Comparison of three anesthetic techniques for off-pump coronary artery bypass grafting: General anesthesia, combined general and high thoracic epidural anesthesia, or high thoracic epidural anesthesia alone. J Cardiothorac Vasc Anesth 19:32, 2005
8. Ceriana P, Pagnin A, Locatelli A, et al: Monitoring aspects during Port-Access cardiac surgery. J Cardiovasc Surg (Torino) 41:579, 2000
9. Mack MJ, Magovern JA, Acuff TA, et al: Results of graft patency by immediate angiography in minimally invasive coronary artery surgery. Ann Thorac Surg 68:383; discussion 389, 1999
10. Wimmer-Greinecker G, Deschka H, Aybek T, et al: Current status of robotically assisted coronary revascularization. Am J Surg 188(4A suppl):76S, 2004
11. Mierdl S, Byhahn C, Lischke V, et al: Segmental wall motion abnormalities during minimally invasive and endoscopic coronary artery bypass grafting. Anesth Analg 100:306, 2005
12. Mihaljevic T, Cohn LH, Unic D, et al: One thousand minimally invasive valve operations: Early and late results. Ann Surg 240:529; discussion 534, 2004
13. Chitwood WR Jr, Wixon CL, Elbeery JR, et al: Video-assisted minimally invasive mitral valve surgery. J Thorac Cardiovasc Surg 114:773; discussion 780, 1997
14. Felger JE, Chitwood WR Jr, Nifong LW, et al: Evolution of mitral valve surgery: Toward a totally endoscopic approach. Ann Thorac Surg 72:1203; discussion 1208, 2001
15. Kypson AP, Chitwood WR Jr: Robotic mitral valve surgery. Am J Surg 188(4A suppl):83S, 2004
16. Suematsu Y, del Nido PJ: Robotic pediatric cardiac surgery. Present and future perspectives. Am J Surg 188(4A suppl):98S, 2004
17. Argenziano M, Oz MC, Kohmoto T, et al: Totally endoscopic atrial septal defect repair with robotic assistance. Circulation 108(suppl II):II–191, 2003
18. Morgan JA, Peacock JC, Kohmoto T, et al: Robotic techniques improve quality of life in patients undergoing atrial septal defect repair. Ann Thorac Surg 77:1328, 2004
19. Garrido MJ, Williams M, Argenziano M: Minimally invasive surgery for atrial fibrillation: Toward a totally endoscopic, beating heart approach. J Card Surg 19:216, 2004

15

Chapter 16

Congenital Heart Disease in Adults

Victor C. Baum, MD

Advances in perioperative care for children with congenital heart disease (CHD) over the past several decades has resulted in an ever-increasing number of these children reaching adulthood with their cardiac lesions palliated or repaired. The first paper on adult CHD was published in 1973; the field has grown such that there is now a text devoted to it, and even a specialty society dedicated to it, the International Society for Adult Congenital Cardiac Disease (http://www.isaccd.org).[1] There are estimated to be about 32,000 new cases of CHD each year in the United States and 1.5 million worldwide. More than 85% of infants born with CHD are expected to grow to adulthood. It is estimated that there are more than 500,000 adults in the United States with CHD; 55% of these adults remain at moderate to high risk, and more than 115,000 have complex disease.[2,3] There are as many adults with CHD as there are children, and the number of adults will only continue to increase. These patients can be seen by anesthesiologists for primary cardiac repair, repair after a prior palliation, revision of repair due to failure or lack of growth of prosthetic material, or conversion of a suboptimal repair to a more modern operation (Box 16-1). In addition, these adults with CHD will be seen for all the other ailments of aging and trauma that require surgical intervention. Although it has been suggested that teenagers and adults can have repair of congenital cardiac defects with morbidity and mortality approaching that of surgery done during childhood, these data are limited and may reflect only a relatively young and acyanotic sampling.[4] Other data suggest that, in general, adults older than 50 years of age represent an excessive proportion of the early postoperative mortality encountered, and the number of previous operations and cyanosis are both risk factors. Risk factors for noncardiac surgery include heart failure, pulmonary hypertension, and cyanosis.[5]

These patients bring with them anatomic and physiologic complexities of which physicians accustomed to caring for adults may be unaware and medical problems

> ### BOX 16-1   *Indications for Cardiac Surgery in Adults with Congenital Heart Disease*
>
> - Primary repair
> - Total correction following palliation
> - Revision of total correction
> - Conversion of suboptimal obsolescent operation into more modern repair

associated with aging or pregnancy that might not be familiar to physicians used to caring for children. This problem has led to the establishment of the growing subspecialty of adult CHD. An informed anesthesiologist is a critical member of the team required to care optimally for these patients. A specific recommendation is that noncardiac surgery on adult patients with moderate to complex CHD be done at an adult congenital heart center (regional centers) with the consultation of an anesthesiologist experienced with adult CHD. In fact, one of the founding fathers of the subspecialty wrote: "A cardiac anesthesiologist with experience in CHD is pivotal. The cardiac anesthesiologist and the attending cardiologist are more important than the noncardiac surgeon."[2] Centers may find it helpful to delegate one attending anesthesiologist to be the liaison with the cardiology service to centralize preoperative evaluations and triage of patients to an anesthesiologist with specific expertise in managing patients with CHD, rather than random consultations with generalist anesthesiologists.

GENERAL NONCARDIAC ISSUES WITH LONG-STANDING CONGENITAL HEART DISEASE

A variety of organ systems can be affected by long-standing CHD; these are summarized in Table 16-1. Because congenital cardiac disease can be one manifestation of a multiorgan genetic or dysmorphic syndrome, all patients require a full review of systems and examination.[6,7]

CARDIAC ISSUES

The basic hemodynamic effects of an anatomic cardiac lesion can be modified by time and by the superimposed effects of chronic cyanosis, pulmonary disease, or the effects of aging. Although surgical cure is the goal, true universal cure, without residua, sequelae, or complications, is uncommon on a population-wide basis. Exceptions include closure of a nonpulmonary hypertensive patent ductus arteriosus (PDA) or atrial septal defect (ASD), probably in childhood. Although there have been reports of series of surgeries on adults with CHD, the wide variety of defects and sequelae from prior surgery make generalizations difficult, if not impossible. Poor myocardial function can be inherent in the CHD but can also be affected by long-standing cyanosis or superimposed surgical injury, including inadequate intraoperative myocardial protection. This is particularly true of adults who had their cardiac repair several decades ago when myocardial protection may not have been as good and when repair was undertaken at an older age. Postoperative arrhythmias are common, particularly when surgery entailed long atrial suture lines. Thrombi can be found in these atria,

16

Table 16-1 Potential Noncardiac Organ Involvement in Patients with Congenital Heart Disease

Potential Respiratory Implications

- Decreased compliance (with increased pulmonary blood flow or impediment to pulmonary venous drainage)
- Compression of airways by large, hypertensive pulmonary arteries
- Compression of bronchioles
- Scoliosis
- Hemoptysis (with end-stage Eisenmenger's syndrome)
- Phrenic nerve injury (prior thoracic surgery)
- Recurrent laryngeal nerve injury (prior thoracic surgery; very rarely from encroachment of cardiac structures)
- Blunted ventilatory response to hypoxemia (with cyanosis)
- Underestimation of $Paco_2$ by capnometry in cyanotic patients

Potential Hematologic Implications

- Symptomatic hyperviscosity
- Bleeding diathesis
- Abnormal von Willebrand factor
- Artifactually elevated prothrombin/partial thromboplastin times with erythrocytic blood
- Artifactual thrombocytopenia with erythrocytic blood
- Gallstones

Potential Renal Implication

- Hyperuricemia and arthralgias (with cyanosis)

Potential Neurologic Implications

- Paradoxic emboli
- Brain abscess (with right-to-left shunts)
- Seizure (from old brain abscess focus)
- Intrathoracic nerve injury (iatrogenic phrenic, recurrent laryngeal, or sympathetic trunk injury)

precluding immediate cardioversion. Bradyarrhythmias can be secondary to surgical injury to the sinus node or conducting tissue or can be a component of the cardiac defect.

The number of cardiac lesions and subtypes, together with the large number of contemporary and obsolescent palliative and corrective surgical procedures, makes a complete discussion of all CHD impossible. The reader is referred to one of the current texts on pediatric cardiac anesthesia for more detailed descriptions of these lesions, the available surgical repairs, and the anesthetic implications during primary repair.[8,9] Some general perioperative guidelines to caring for these patients are offered in Table 16-2.

Aortic Stenosis

Most aortic stenosis in adults is due to a congenitally bicuspid valve that does not become problematic until late middle age or later, although endocarditis risk is lifelong. Once symptoms (angina, syncope, near-syncope, heart failure) develop, survival is markedly shortened. Median survival is 5 years after the development of angina, 3 years after syncope, and 2 years after heart failure. Anesthetic management of aortic stenosis does not vary whether the stenosis is congenital (most common) or acquired.

Table 16-2 General Approaches to Anesthesia for Patients with Congenital Heart Disease

General

The best care for both cardiac and noncardiac surgery in adult patients with CHD is afforded in a center with a multidisciplinary team experienced in the care of adults with CHD and knowledgeable about both the anatomy and physiology of CHD and also the manifestations and considerations specific to adults with CHD.

Preoperative

- Review most recent laboratory data, catheterization, and echocardiogram and other imaging data. The most recent office letter from the cardiologist is often most helpful. Obtain and review these in advance.
- Drawing a diagram of the heart with saturations, pressures, and direction of blood flow often clarifies complex and superficially unfamiliar anatomy and physiology.
- Avoid prolonged fast if patient is erythrocytotic to avoid hemoconcentration.
- No generalized contraindication to preoperative sedation.

Intraoperative

- Large-bore intravenous access for repeat sternotomy and cyanotic patients.
- Avoid air bubbles in all intravenous catheters. There can be transient right-to-left shunting even in lesions with predominant left-to-right shunting (filters are available but will severely restrict ability to give volume and blood).
- Apply external defibrillator pads for repeat sternotomies and patients with poor cardiac function.
- Use appropriate endocarditis prophylaxis (orally or intravenously before skin incision).
- Consider antifibrinolytic therapy, especially for patients with prior sternotomy.
- Transesophageal echocardiography for cardiac operations.
- Modulate pulmonary and systemic vascular resistances as appropriate pharmacologically and by modifications in ventilation.

Postoperative

- Appropriate pain control (cyanotic patients have normal ventilatory response to hypercarbia and narcotics).
- Maintain hematocrit appropriate for arterial saturation.
- Maintain central venous and left atrial pressures appropriate for altered ventricular diastolic compliance or presence of beneficial atrial level shunting.
- Pao_2 may not increase significantly with the application of supplemental oxygen in the presence of right-to-left shunting.

16

Aortopulmonary Shunts

Depending on their age, adult patients may have had one or more of several aortopulmonary shunts to palliate cyanosis during childhood. These are shown in Figure 16-1. Although life saving, there were considerable shortcomings of these shunts in the long term. All were inherently inefficient, because some of the oxygenated blood returning through the pulmonary veins to the left atrium and ventricle would then return to the lungs through the shunt, thus volume loading the ventricle. It was difficult to quantify the size of the earlier shunts such as the Waterston (side-to-side ascending aorta to right pulmonary artery) and Potts (side-to-side descending aorta to left pulmonary artery). If too small, the patient was left excessively cyanotic; if too large, there was pulmonary overcirculation with the risk of developing pulmonary vascular disease. The Waterston, in fact, could on occasion result in a hyperperfused, hypertensive ipsilateral pulmonary artery and a hypoperfused contralateral pulmonary artery as it could direct flow to the ipsilateral side. There were also

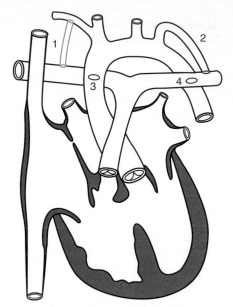

Figure 16-1 The various aortopulmonary anastomoses. The illustrated heart shows tetralogy of Fallot. The anastomoses are 1, modified Blalock-Taussig; 2, classic Blalock-Taussig; 3, Waterston (Waterston-Cooley); and 4, Potts. (Reprinted with permission from Baum VC: The adult with congenital heart disease. J Cardiothorac Vasc Anesth 10:261, 1996.)

Table 16-3 **Aortopulmonary Shunts**		
Waterston	Ascending aorta → right pulmonary artery	No longer done
Potts	Descending aorta → left pulmonary artery	No longer done
Classic Blalock-Taussig	Subclavian artery → ipsilateral pulmonary artery	No longer done
Modified Blalock-Taussig	Gore-Tex tube subclavian artery → ipsilateral pulmonary artery	Current
Central shunt	Gore-Tex tube ascending aorta → main pulmonary artery	Current

IV

surgical issues when complete repair became possible. Takedown of Waterston shunts often required a pulmonary arterioplasty to correct deformity of the pulmonary artery at the site of the anastomosis, and the posteriorly located Potts anastomoses could not be taken down from a median sternotomy. Patients with a classic Blalock-Taussig shunt almost always lack palpable pulses on the side of the shunt. Even if there is a palpable pulse (from collateral flow around the shoulder), blood pressure obtained from that arm will be artifactually low. Even after a modified Blalock-Taussig shunt (using a piece of Gore-Tex tubing instead of an end-to-side anastomosis of the subclavian and pulmonary arteries), there can be a blood pressure disparity between the arms. To ensure a valid measurement, preoperative blood pressure should be measured in both arms (Table 16-3).

> **BOX 16-2** *Complications of Atrial Septal Defect in Adulthood*
>
> - Paradoxic emboli
> - Effort dyspnea
> - Atrial tachyarrhythmias
> - Right-sided failure with pregnancy
> - Pulmonary hypertension
> - ↑ Right-sided failure with ↓ left ventricular compliance with aging
> - Mitral insufficiency

Atrial Septal Defect and Partial Anomalous Pulmonary Venous Return

There are several anatomic types of ASD. The most common type, and if otherwise undefined the presumptive type, is the secundum type located in the midseptum. The primum type at the lower end of the atrial septum is a component of the endocardial cushion defects, the most primitive of which is the common atrioventricular canal. The sinus venosus type, high in the septum near the entry of the superior vena cava, is almost always associated with partial anomalous pulmonary venous return, most frequently drainage of the right upper pulmonary vein to the low superior vena cava. An uncommon atrial septal-type defect is when blood passes from the left atrium to the right via an unroofed coronary sinus. Only secundum defects are considered, although the natural histories of all of the defects are similar (Box 16-2).

Because the symptoms and clinical findings of an ASD can be quite subtle and patients often remain asymptomatic until adulthood, ASDs represent approximately one third of all CHD discovered in adults. Although asymptomatic survival to adulthood is common, significant shunts ($\dot{Q}p/\dot{Q}s > 1.5:1$) will probably cause symptoms over time, and paradoxic emboli can occur through defects with smaller shunts. Effort dyspnea occurs in 30% by the third decade, and atrial flutter or fibrillation in about 10% by age 40. The avoidance of complications developing in adulthood provides the rationale for surgical repair of asymptomatic children. The mortality for a patient with an uncorrected ASD is 6% per year over 40 years of age, and essentially all patients over 60 years of age are symptomatic. Large nonrepaired defects can cause death from atrial tachyarrhythmias or right ventricular failure in 30- to 40-year-old patients. With the decreased left ventricular diastolic compliance accompanying the systemic hypertension or coronary artery disease that is common with aging, left-to-right shunting increases with age. Pulmonary vascular disease typically does not develop until after the age of 40, unlike ventricular or ductal level shunts, which can lead to it in early childhood. Mitral insufficiency can be found in adult patients and is significant in about 15% of adult patients. Paradoxic emboli remain a lifelong risk.

Late closure of the defect, after 5 years of age, has been associated with incomplete resolution of right ventricular dilation. Left ventricular dysfunction has been reported in some patients having defect closure in adulthood, and closure particularly in middle age may not prevent the development of atrial tachyarrhythmias or stroke.[10] Survival of patients without pulmonary vascular disease has been reported to be best if operated on before 24 years of age, intermediate if operated on between 25 and 41 years of age, and worst if operated on thereafter. However, more recent series have shown that even at ages over 40, surgical repair provides an overall survival and complication-free benefit compared with medical management.[11] Surgical morbidity in these patients is primarily atrial fibrillation, atrial flutter, or junctional rhythm.

Current practice is to close these defects in adults in the catheterization laboratory via transvascular devices if anatomically practical (Fig. 16-2). For example, there needs to be an adequate rim of septum around the defect to which the device can attach. Device closure is inappropriate if the defect is associated with anomalous pulmonary venous drainage. The indications for closure are the same as for surgical closure.[12]

An otherwise uncomplicated secundum ASD, unlike most congenital cardiac defects, is not associated with an increased endocarditis risk. Presumably this is because the shunt, although potentially large, is low pressure and unassociated with jet lesions of the endocardium.

Although some discussion is given to onset times with intravenous or inhalation induction agents, clinical differences are hard to notice with modern low-solubility volatile agents. Thermodilution cardiac output reflects pulmonary blood flow, which will be in excess of systemic blood flow. Pulmonary arterial catheters are not

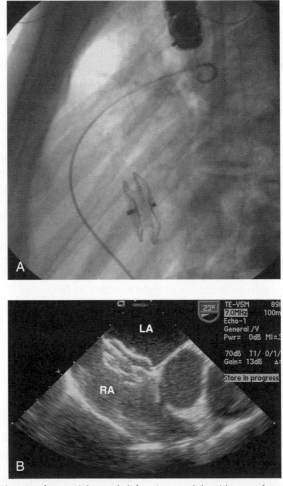

Figure 16-2 Closure of an atrial septal defect in an adult with use of a transvascular device (the Amplatzer septal occluder). **A,** Radiograph. **B,** Transesophageal echocardiogram. The device is clearly visualized spanning and occluding the atrial septal defect. RA = right atrium; LA = left atrium. (Courtesy of Dr. Scott Lim.)

routinely indicated. Patients generally do tolerate any appropriate anesthetic; however, particular care should be taken in patients with pulmonary arterial hypertension or right-sided failure.

Coarctation of the Aorta

Nonrepaired coarctation of the aorta in the adult brings with it significant morbidity and mortality. Mortality is 25% by age 20, 50% by age 30, 75% by age 50, and 90% by age 60. Left ventricular aneurysm, rupture of cerebral aneurysms, and dissection of a postcoarctation aneurysm all contribute to the excessive mortality. Left ventricular failure can occur in patients over 40 with nonrepaired lesions. If repair is not undertaken early, there is incremental risk for the development of premature coronary atherosclerosis. Even with surgery, coronary artery disease remains the leading cause of death 11 to 25 years after surgery. Coarctation is accompanied by a bicuspid aortic valve in the majority of patients. Although endocarditis of this abnormal valve is a lifelong risk, these valves often do not become stenotic until middle age or later. Coarctation can also be associated with mitral valve abnormalities (Box 16-3).

Aneurysms at the site of coarctation repair can develop years later, and restenosis as well can develop in adolescence or adulthood. Repair includes resection of the coarctation and end-to-end reanastomosis. Because this sometimes resulted in recoarctation when done in infancy, for many years a common repair was the Waldhausen or subclavian flap operation, in which the left subclavian artery is ligated and the proximal segment opened and rotated as a flap to open the area of the coarctation. Aneurysms in the area of repair are a particular concern in adolescents and adults after coarctectomy. Persistent systemic hypertension is common after coarctation repair. Adult patients require continued periodic follow-up for hypertension. A pressure gradient of 20 mmHg or more (less in the presence of extensive collaterals) is an indication for treatment. Recoarctation can be treated surgically or by balloon angioplasty with stenting.[13] Surgical repair of recoarctation or aneurysm in adults is associated with increased mortality and can be associated with significant intraoperative bleeding. It requires lung isolation for optimal surgical exposure and placement of an arterial catheter in the right arm.

Half of patients operated on after age 40 have persistent hypertension, and many of the remainder have an abnormal hypertensive response to surgery. Long-term survival is worse for patients having repair later in life. Patients older than 40 having repair have a 15-year survival of only 50%.

Blood pressure should be obtained in the right arm unless pressures in the left arm or legs are known to be unaffected by residual or recurrent coarctation. Postoperative hypertension is common after repair of coarctation and often requires treatment for some months. Postoperative ileus is also common, and patients should be maintained NPO for about 2 days.

16

BOX 16-3 *Complications of Aortic Coarctation in Adulthood*

- Left ventricular failure
- Premature coronary atherosclerosis
- Rupture of cerebral aneurysm
- Aneurysm at site of coarctation repair
- Complications of associated bicuspid aortic valve
- Exacerbation of hypertension during pregnancy

Eisenmenger's Syndrome

Eisenmenger described a particular type of large VSD with dextroposition of the aorta. In a general way, the term *Eisenmenger's syndrome* has come to describe the clinical setting in which a large left-to-right cardiac shunt results in the development of pulmonary vascular disease. Although early on the pulmonary vasculature remains reactive, with continued insult pulmonary hypertension becomes fixed and does not respond to pulmonary vasodilators. Ultimately, the level of pulmonary vascular resistance is so high that the shunt reverses and becomes right-to-left. The development of pulmonary vascular disease is dependent on shear rate. Lesions with high shear rates, such as a large VSD or a large PDA, can result in pulmonary hypertension in early childhood. Lesions such as an ASD with high pulmonary blood flow but low pressure may not result in pulmonary vascular disease until late middle age. Pulmonary vascular disease progression is also accelerated in patients living at altitude.

Eisenmenger physiology is compatible with survival into adulthood. However, reported rates of survival after diagnosis vary, probably based on the relatively long life expectancy and variability in the time of diagnosis. Cantor and coworkers reported median survival to 53 years but with wide variation. Others reported survival of 80% at 10 years after diagnosis and 42% at 25 years; or survival of 77% at 5 years and 58% at 10 years. Syncope, increased central venous pressure, and arterial desaturation to less than 85% are all associated with poor short-term outcome.[14,15] Most deaths are sudden cardiac deaths. Other causes of death include heart failure, hemoptysis, brain abscess, thromboembolism, and complications of pregnancy and noncardiac surgery. These patients face potentially significant perioperative risks. Findings of Eisenmenger's syndrome are summarized in Table 16-4.

Surgical closure of cardiac defects with fixed pulmonary vascular hypertension is associated with very high mortality. Lung or heart-lung transplantation is a surgical alternative. Although there are several surgical series reporting survival after heart-lung or single- or double-lung transplantation performed for primary pulmonary hypertension, it is unclear if this cohort of patients is similar to patients with Eisenmenger physiology.

Fixed pulmonary vascular resistance precludes rapid adaptation to perioperative hemodynamic changes. Changes in systemic vascular resistance are mirrored by changes in intracardiac shunting. A decrease in systemic vascular resistance is accompanied by increased right-to-left shunting and a decrease in systemic oxygen saturation. Systemic

---

Table 16-4 Findings in Eisenmenger's Syndrome

- *Physical examination:* loud pulmonic component of the second heart sound, single or narrowly split second heart sound, Graham Steell murmur of pulmonary insufficiency, pulmonic ejection sound ("click")
- *Chest radiography:* decreased peripheral pulmonary arterial markings with prominent central pulmonary vessels ("pruning")
- *ECG:* Right ventricular hypertrophy
- Impaired exercise tolerance
- Exertional dyspnea
- Palpitations (often due to atrial fibrillation or flutter)
- Complications from erythrocytosis/hyperviscosity
- Hemoptysis from pulmonary infarction, rupture of pulmonary vessels or aortopulmonary collateral vessels
- Complications from paradoxical embolization
- Syncope from inadequate cardiac output or arrhythmias
- Heart failure (usually end stage)

vasodilators, including regional anesthesia, need to be used with caution, and close assessment of intravascular volume is important. Epidural analgesia has been used successfully in patients with Eisenmenger physiology, but the local anesthetic needs to be delivered slowly and incrementally with close observation of blood pressure and oxygen saturation. Postoperative postural hypotension can also increase the degree of right-to-left shunting, and these patients should change position slowly.

Placement of pulmonary artery catheters in these patients is problematic for a variety of reasons and of less utility than might be expected. Pulmonary arterial hypertension is a risk factor for pulmonary artery rupture from a pulmonary artery catheter. Rupture is particularly worrisome in these cyanotic patients who can also have hemostatic deficits associated with erythrocytosis. Abnormal intracardiac anatomy and right-to-left shunting can make successful passage into the pulmonary artery difficult without fluoroscopy. Relative resistances of the pulmonary and systemic beds are reflected in the systemic oxygen saturation, readily measured by pulse oximetry, so measures of pulmonary artery pressure are not required. In addition, in the presence of right-to-left shunting, thermodilution cardiac outputs do not accurately reflect systemic output. Thus, the value of pulmonary artery catheters in these patients is minimal at best, and they essentially are never indicated. The one potential exception is the patient with an ASD who is at risk to develop right ventricular failure if suprasystemic right ventricular pressure develops.

Fixed pulmonary vascular resistance is by definition unresponsive to pharmacologic manipulation. That said, it would seem prudent to avoid factors known to increase pulmonary vascular resistance, including cold, hypercarbia, acidosis, hypoxia, and α-adrenergic agonists. Although the last of these is commonly listed to be avoided, it seems that in the presence of pulmonary vascular disease due to intracardiac shunting, the systemic vasoconstrictive effects predominate and systemic oxygen saturation increases.

Nerve blocks offer an attractive alternative to general anesthesia if otherwise appropriate. If patients have general anesthesia, consideration should be given to postoperative observation in an intensive or intermediate care unit. Because of the increased perioperative risk, patients should be observed overnight, particularly if they have not had recent surgery or anesthesia, because their responses will be unknown. Ambulatory surgery is possible for patients having uncomplicated minor surgery with sedation or nerve block.

16

Patent Ductus Arteriosus

Beyond the neonatal period, spontaneous closure of a PDA is uncommon. The risk of a long-standing moderate to large PDA is volume overloading of the left atrium and left ventricle with the risk of development of pulmonary vascular disease. With time, the ductus can become calcified or aneurysmally dilated with a risk of rupture. Ductal calcification or aneurysm increases the risk of surgery, which rarely requires cardiopulmonary bypass. Nonrepaired, the natural history is for one third of patients to die of heart failure, pulmonary hypertension, or endocarditis by 40 years of age and two thirds by age 60. Although small PDAs are of no hemodynamic consequence, even small PDAs carry relatively high endocarditis risk. Surgical closure should be considered for all adults with PDA, and transvascular closure by means of one of several devices is possible.[16]

Tetralogy of Fallot

The classic description of tetralogy of Fallot includes (1) a large, nonrestrictive malaligned VSD, with (2) an overriding aorta, (3) infundibular pulmonic stenosis, and (4) consequent right ventricular hypertrophy, all derived from an embryonic anterocephalad deviation of the outlet septum. However, there is a spectrum of disease, with more severe defects including stenosis of the pulmonary valve, stenosis of the pulmonary valve annulus, or stenosis and hypoplasia of the pulmonary arteries in the most severe cases. Pentalogy of Fallot refers to the addition of an ASD. With advances in genetics, up to one third or more of cases of tetralogy have been ascribed to one of several genetic abnormalities, including trisomy 21, the 22q11 microdeletion, the genes *NKX 2.5* and *FOG 2.4*, and others. Tetralogy of Fallot is the most common cyanotic lesion encountered in the adult population. Nonrepaired or nonpalliated, approximately 25% of patients survive to adolescence, after which the mortality is 6.6% per year. Only 3% survive to age 40.[17] Unlike children, teenagers and adults with tetralogy do not develop "tet spells." Long-term survival with a good quality of life is expected after repair. The 32- to 36-year survival has been reported to be 85% to 86%, although symptoms, primarily arrhythmias and decreased exercise tolerance, occur in 10% to 15% at 20 years after the primary repair (Box 16-4).

It is uncommon to encounter an adolescent or adult with nonrepaired tetralogy. However, it can be encountered in immigrants or in patients whose anatomic variation was considered to be inoperable when they were children. In tetralogy, the right ventricle "sees" the obstruction from the pulmonic stenosis. Pulmonary vascular resistance is typically normal to low. Right-to-left shunting is unaffected by attempts at modulating pulmonary vascular resistance. Shunting is minimized, however, by pharmacologically increasing systemic vascular resistance. Increases in the inotropic state of the heart increase the dynamic obstruction at the right ventricular infundibulum and worsen right-to-left shunting. β-Blockers are often used to decrease inotropy. Although halothane was the historic anesthetic of choice in children with tetralogy due to its myocardial depressant effects and ability to maintain systemic vascular resistance, current practice is to use sevoflurane, without undue consequence from a reduction in systemic vascular resistance. Anesthetic induction in adults can easily be achieved with narcotics.[18]

Patients require closure of the VSD and resolution of the pulmonic stenosis. Although current practice is to repair the VSD through the right atrium in an effort to maintain competence of the pulmonary valve and limit any ventriculotomy, older patients will likely have had repair via a right ventriculotomy. A large right ventriculotomy increases the risks of arrhythmias and sudden death. Patients who have had a right ventriculotomy will have an obligate right bundle-branch block pattern on the ECG. However, unlike the more usual bundle-branch block in adults, this represents disruption of the His-Purkinje system only in the right ventricular outflow, in the area of the right ventricular incision. Because the vast majority of His-Purkinje conduction is intact, it does not carry increased risk for the development of complete heart block. These patients can have an abnormal response to exercise.

IV

BOX 16-4 *Risk Factors for Sudden Death after Repair of Tetralogy of Fallot*

- Repair requiring ventriculotomy
- Older age at repair
- Severe left ventricular dysfunction
- Postoperative right ventricular hypertension (residual outflow tract obstruction)
- Wide-open pulmonary insufficiency
- Prolongation of the QRS

Some patients require repair of pulmonic stenosis by placement of a transannular patch, with obligate residual pulmonary insufficiency. Isolated mild to moderate pulmonary insufficiency is generally well tolerated, but in the long term it can contribute to right ventricular dysfunction with a risk of ventricular tachycardia and sudden death. Atrial tachyarrhythmias occur in about one third of adults late after repair and can contribute to late morbidity.[19] The development of atrial flutter or atrial reentrant tachycardia is often a harbinger of hemodynamic compromise. The substrate is usually an atrial surgical scar and the trigger is atrial dilation, such as from tricuspid insufficiency with right ventricular dysfunction. The mechanism for the development of ventricular arrhythmias is presumably the same, namely dilation superimposed on surgical scar.

In some cases, the right ventricular outflow tract patch needs to be extended onto the branch pulmonary arteries to relieve obstruction. Patients with abnormal coronary arteries may have required repair using a right ventricle-to-pulmonary-artery conduit to avoid doing a right ventriculotomy in the area of the coronary artery. Repair at a younger age (<12 years) results in better postoperative right ventricular function. Because there is an unrestrictive VSD, in the nonrepaired adult systemic hypertension developing in adult life imposes an additional load on both ventricles, not just the left. The increase in systemic vascular resistance decreases right-to-left shunting and diminishes cyanosis but at the expense of right ventricular or biventricular failure.

Sudden death or ventricular tachycardia requiring treatment can occur in up to 5.5% of postoperative patients over 30 years, often years postoperatively. The foci for these arrhythmias are typically in the right ventricular outflow tract in the area that has had surgery, and they can be ablated in the catheterization laboratory. Older age at repair, severe left ventricular dysfunction, postoperative right ventricular hypertension from residual or recurrent outflow tract obstruction, wide-open pulmonary insufficiency, and prolongation of the QRS are all predictors of sudden death.[20] Premature ventricular contractions and even nonsustained ventricular tachycardia are not rare but do not seem to be associated with sudden death, making appropriate treatment options difficult. It has been suggested that QRS prolongation to longer than 180 milliseconds is a risk factor. This marker, although highly sensitive, has a low positive predictive value. The impact of this risk factor in the current group of younger patients who have not had ventriculotomies is unclear, as their initial postoperative QRS durations are shorter than in patients who had a right ventriculotomy.

Although for many years it was thought that moderate to severe pulmonary insufficiency in these patients was well tolerated, it has become apparent from a number of series that right ventricular dysfunction and both atrial and ventricular arrhythmias can be common long-term sequelae. For this reason, patients with symptomatic pulmonary insufficiency from a transannular patch or aneurysm formation at the site of a right ventricular outflow tract patch can require reoperation to replace a widely incompetent pulmonary valve with a bioprosthetic valve with or without a tricuspid annuloplasty. Interestingly, the incidence of atrial arrhythmias may not be diminished when adult patients have a pulmonary valve placed, although the incidence of ventricular arrhythmias is decreased. Right ventricular dysfunction improves in a variable number of adults, suggesting that pulmonary valve placement be done sooner rather than later. There is very early experience with a pulmonary valve that can be inserted transvenously in the catheterization laboratory, although currently it is appropriate only for a limited range of pulmonary artery sizes.

Additional possible late-term complications include residual VSD, patch dehiscence, progressive aortic insufficiency, left ventricular dysfunction from surgical injury to an anomalous coronary artery or long-standing preoperative cyanosis, and heart block from VSD closure (uncommon today). Because patients who have had repairs using a conduit require multiple sternotomies and the valved conduit tends to lie immediately behind and in close proximity to the sternum, sternotomy carries with it significant potential risk for laceration of the conduit. On occasion, the femoral vessels are cannulated for bypass prior to sternotomy.

Most adult patients require reoperation to repair the right ventricular outflow tract or to insert or replace a valve in the pulmonic position. Other reasons for reoperation include repair of an outflow tract aneurysm at the site of a patch, repair of a residual VSD, or repair of an incompetent tricuspid valve. These patients often have diminished right ventricular diastolic compliance and require higher-than-normal central venous pressure. Postoperative management includes minimizing pulmonary vascular resistance and maintaining central venous pressure. Patients often require treatment post-bypass with an inotrope and afterload reduction.[21]

Transposition of the Great Arteries (D-Transposition)

In D-transposition of the great arteries, there is a discordant connection of the ventricles and the great arteries. The aorta (with the coronary arteries) arises from the right ventricle, and the pulmonary artery arises from the left ventricle. Thus, the two circulations are separate. Postnatal survival requires interchange of blood between the two circulations, typically via a patent foramen ovale and/or a PDA. With a 1-year mortality approximating 100%, all adults with D-transposition have had some type of surgical intervention. Adults will have had atrial-type repairs (Mustard or Senning), whereas children born after the mid-1980s will have had repair by arterial switch (the Jantene operation). Some will also have had repair of D-transposition with a moderate to large VSD by means of a Rastelli operation.

Atrial repairs function by redirecting systemic venous blood to the left ventricle (and thence to the transposed pulmonary artery) and pulmonary venous blood to the right ventricle (and thence to the aorta). The Mustard operation uses an intra-atrial conduit of native pericardium, whereas the Senning operation uses native atrial tissue to fashion the conduit. The arterial switch operation transposes transected aorta and pulmonary artery such that they now arise above the appropriate ventricle. This operation also requires transposing the coronary arteries from the aorta to the pulmonary root, which, following the procedure, becomes the aortic root. The Rastelli procedure closes the VSD on a bias such that the left ventricle empties into the aorta and connects the right ventricle to the pulmonary artery by means of a valved conduit.

Atrial repairs result in a systemic right ventricle, and these patients consistently have abnormal right ventricular function that can be progressive with a right ventricular ejection fraction of about 40%. Mild tricuspid insufficiency is common, but severe tricuspid insufficiency suggests the development of severe right ventricular dysfunction. There is an 85% to 90% 10-year survival with these operations, but by 20 years survival is less than 80%. Over 25 years, about half develop moderate right ventricular dysfunction and one third develop severe tricuspid insufficiency. Although it always remains abnormal, it has been suggested that earlier surgery minimizes right ventricular dysfunction. Because of the incidence of right ventricular dysfunction, some patients with atrial repairs have been converted to an arterial switch, following preparation of the left ventricle by a pulmonary artery band to prepare it to tolerate systemic arterial pressure.

Atrial repairs bring an incidence of late electrophysiologic sequelae including sinus node dysfunction (bradycardia), junctional escape rhythms, atrioventricular block, and supraventricular arrhythmias. Atrial flutter occurs in 20% of patients by age 20 with half having progressive sinus node dysfunction by that time. On occasion these tachyarrhythmias can result in sudden death, presumably from 1:1 conduction producing ventricular fibrillation. The loss of sinus rhythm in the face of right ventricular (the systemic ventricle) dysfunction can also contribute to late sudden death. The risk of late death after an atrial repair is almost three times higher if there is an associated VSD. The incidence of tachyarrhythmias does decrease, however, after the tenth postoperative year.

An arterial switch operation can be done after a failed atrial repair in adults, but the outcome is generally poor. It is suggested that younger patients do better.

Very-long-term outcome after the arterial switch procedure is still not known. It does appear that there is essentially no mortality after 5 years postoperatively, and late surgical reintervention is mostly due to supravalvular pulmonic stenosis.[22] Although many of these children have abnormal resting myocardial perfusion, up to 9% can have evidence of exercise-induced myocardial ischemia. The implication for the development of premature coronary artery disease in adulthood is not known, and there is also some concern about the ultimate function of the neoaortic valve.

After an atrial or a Rastelli repair, pregnancy and delivery are generally well tolerated, although right ventricular failure and deterioration in functional capacity can occur. There is an increased incidence of prematurity and small-for-date infants in these women.

Ventricular Septal Defects

More than 75% of small and moderate VSDs close spontaneously during childhood by a gradual ingrowth of surrounding septum. Of those that close spontaneously, almost all have closed by 10 years of age. Other mechanisms for natural closure include closure by tricuspid valve tissue, closure by prolapsed aortic leaflet, and closure by endocarditis. Some VSDs result in the development of aortic insufficiency in adults from prolapse of the aortic valve into the defect. Although the risk of endocarditis is ongoing, there is no hemodynamic risk of a small VSD in the adult. If pulmonary vascular disease is present, it can progress if closure of a large VSD is delayed.

Although some studies have reported possible ventricular dysfunction years after surgical repair, these are older reports and patients were operated on later than by current standards. It does appear, though, that the ventricle successfully remodels from chronic volume overload if surgical correction is done by 5 years of age and perhaps up to 10 to 12 years of age.

Although some discussion is given to onset times with intravenous or inhalation induction agents, clinical differences are hard to notice with modern low-solubility volatile agents. Thermodilution cardiac output reflects pulmonary blood flow, which will be in excess of systemic blood flow. Pulmonary arterial catheters are not routinely indicated. In the patient with a moderate or large left-to-right shunt, low inspired oxygen and moderate hypercarbia avoid intraoperative decreases in pulmonary vascular resistance with pulmonary overcirculation and left ventricular dilation. However, unlike children, it would be rare to encounter adults with large left-to-right shunts. Adults with nonrepaired lesions would have either small shunts or would have had large shunts that caused Eisenmenger physiology.

SUMMARY

- Due to surgical successes in treating congenital cardiac lesions, there are currently as many or more adults than children with congenital heart disease (CHD).
- These patients may require cardiac surgical intervention for primary cardiac repair, repair after prior palliation, revision of repair due to failure or lack of growth of prosthetic material, or conversion of a suboptimal repair to a more modern operation.

16

- These patients will be encountered by noncardiac anesthesiologists for a vast array of ailments and injuries requiring surgery.
- If at all possible, noncardiac surgery on adult patients with moderate to complex CHD should be done at an adult congenital heart center with the consultation of an anesthesiologist experienced with adult CHD.
- Delegation of one anesthesiologist as the liaison with the cardiology service for preoperative evaluation and triage of adult CHD patients will be helpful.
- All relevant cardiac tests and evaluations should be reviewed in advance.
- Sketching out the anatomy and path(s) of blood flow is often an easy and enlightening aid in simplifying apparently very complex lesions.

REFERENCES

1. Gatzoulis M, Webb GD, Daubeney PEF: Diagnosis and Management of Adult Congenital Heart Disease, Philadelphia, Churchill Livingstone, 2003
2. Perloff JK, Warnes CA: Challenges posed by adults with repaired congenital heart disease. Circulation 103:2637, 2001
3. Warnes CA, Liberthson R, Danielson GK, et al: Task force 1: The changing profile of congenital heart disease in adult life. J Am Coll Cardiol 37:1170, 2001
4. Andropoulos DB, Stayer SA, Skjonsby BS, et al: Anesthetic and perioperative outcome of teenagers and adults with congenital heart disease. J Cardiothorac Vasc Anesth 16:731, 2002
5. Warnes CA: The adult with congenital heart disease: Born to be bad? J Am Coll Cardiol 46:1-8, 2005
6. Kamphuis M, Ottenkamp J, Vliegen HW, et al: Health-related quality of life and health status in adult survivors with previously operated complex congenital heart disease. Heart 87:356, 2002
7. Vonder Muhll I, Cumming G, Gatzoulis MA: Risky business: Insuring adults with congenital heart disease. Eur Heart J 24:1595, 2003
8. Lake CL, Booker PD: Pediatric Cardiac Anesthesia, 4th edition. Philadelphia, Lippincott-Williams and Wilkins, 2004
9. Andropoulos DB, Stayer SA, Russell IA: Anesthesia for Congenital Heart Disease. Armonk, NY, Futura, 2004
10. Gatzoulis MA, Freeman MA, Siu SC, et al: Atrial arrhythmia after surgical closure of atrial septal defects in adults. N Engl J Med 340:839, 1999
11. Attie F, Rosas M, Granados N, et al: Surgical treatment for secundum atrial septal defects in patients >40 years old. A randomized clinical trial. J Am Coll Cardiol 38:2035, 2001
12. Du ZD, Hijazi ZM, Kleinman CS, et al: Comparison between transcatheter and surgical closure of secundum atrial septal defect in children and adults: Results of a multicenter nonrandomized trial. J Am Coll Cardiol 39:1836, 2002
13. Hamdan MA, Maheshwari S, Fahey JT, Hellenbrand WE: Endovascular stents for coarctation of the aorta: Initial results and intermediate-term follow-up. J Am Coll Cardiol 38:1518, 2001
14. Vongpatanasin W, Brickner ME, Hillis LD, Lange RA: The Eisenmenger syndrome in adults. Ann Intern Med 128:745, 1998
15. Cantor WJ, Harrison DA, Moussadji JS, et al: Determinants of survival and length of survival in adults with Eisenmenger syndrome. Am J Cardiol 84:677, 1999
16. Fisher RG, Moodie DS, Sterba R, Gill CC: Patent ductus arteriosus in adults-long-term follow-up: Nonsurgical versus surgical treatment. J Am Coll Cardiol 8:280, 1986
17. Nollert G, Fischlein T, Bouterwek S, et al: Long-term survival in patients with repair of tetralogy of Fallot: 36-Year follow-up of 490 survivors of the first year after surgical repair. J Am Coll Cardiol 30:1374, 1997
18. Russell IA, Miller Hance WC, Gregory G, et al: The safety and efficacy of sevoflurane anesthesia in infants and children with congenital heart disease. Anesth Analg 92:1152, 2001
19. Harrison DA, Siu SC, Hussain F, et al: Sustained atrial arrhythmias in adults late after repair of tetralogy of Fallot. Am J Cardiol 87:584, 2001
20. Abd El Rahman MY, Abdul-Khaliq H, Vogel M, et al: Relation between right ventricular enlargement, QRS duration, and right ventricular function in patients with tetralogy of Fallot and pulmonary regurgitation after surgical repair. Heart 84:416, 2000
21. Heggie J, Poirer N, Williams RG, Karski J: Anesthetic considerations for adult cardiac surgery patients with congenital heart disease. Semin Cardiothorac Vasc Anesth 7:141, 2003
22. Losay J, Touchot A, Serraf A, et al: Late outcome after arterial switch operation for transposition of the great arteries. Circulation 104:I-121, 2001

Chapter 17

Thoracic Aortic Disease

Enrique J. Pantin, MD • Albert T. Cheung, MD

Thoracic aortic diseases are generally surgical problems and require surgical treatment (Table 17-1). Acute aortic dissections, rupturing aortic aneurysms, and traumatic aortic injuries are surgical emergencies. Subacute aortic dissection and expanding aortic aneurysms require urgent surgical intervention. Stable thoracic or thoracoabdominal aortic aneurysms (TAAAs), aortic coarctation, or atheromatous disease causing embolization may be considered for elective surgical repair. Increased public awareness of thoracic aortic disease, early recognition of acute aortic syndromes by emergency medical personnel, improved diagnostic imaging technology for the diagnosis of thoracic aortic disease, and an aging population all contribute to the increased number of patients requiring aortic surgery. Furthermore, improvements in the surgical treatment of thoracic aortic diseases combined with increased treatment options such as endovascular stent repair have led to an increased number of patient referrals to centers specializing in the management of patients with thoracic aortic diseases. Improved treatment and survival after aortic surgical procedures often provide a cure for the original disease but have created new and unique problems. An increasing number of patients who have had prior aortic surgical procedures require reoperation for long-term complications of aortic surgery such as bioprosthetic valve or graft failure,

Table 17-1	Diseases of the Thoracic Aorta That Are Amenable to Surgical Treatment

Aneurysm
Congenital or developmental
   Marfan syndrome, Ehlers-Danlos syndrome
Degenerative
   Cystic medial degeneration
   Annuloaortic ectasia
   Atherosclerotic
Traumatic
   Blunt and penetrating trauma
Inflammatory
   Takayasu's arteritis, Behçet's syndrome, Kawasaki disease
Microvascular diseases (polyarteritis)
Infectious (mycotic)
   Bacterial, fungal, spirochetal, viral
Mechanical
   Post-stenotic, associated with an arteriovenous fistula
   Anastomotic (post arteriotomy)
Pseudoaneurysm
Aortic dissection
   Stanford type A
   Stanford type B
Intramural hematoma
Penetrating atherosclerotic ulcer
Atherosclerotic disease
Traumatic aortic injury
Aortic coarctation

Adapted from Kouchoukos NT, Dougenis D: Surgery of the aorta. N Engl J Med 336:1876, 1997.

aortic pseudoaneurysm at old vascular graft anastomosis, endocarditis, or progression of the original disease process into native segments of the thoracic aorta.

The anesthetic management of surgical patients requiring aortic surgery presents some distinctive medical problems in addition to the usual considerations associated with major thoracic or thoracoabdominal operations. The process of repairing or replacing a portion of the thoracic aorta usually requires the temporary interruption of blood flow, creating the potential for ischemia or infarction of almost any major organ system in the body. Strategies to provide organ perfusion, to protect organs from the consequences of hypoperfusion, and to monitor and treat end-organ ischemia during aortic operations are critical aspects of the anesthetic management for thoracic aortic diseases and contribute importantly to the overall success of operations. Some of the procedures performed and managed by surgeons and anesthesiologists for organ protection during thoracic aortic operations, such as partial left-sided heart bypass for distal aortic perfusion, deep hypothermic circulatory arrest (DHCA), selective antegrade or retrograde cerebral perfusion (ACP or RCP), and lumbar cerebrospinal fluid (CSF) drainage, are practiced routinely in no other area of medicine.

GENERAL CONSIDERATIONS FOR THE PERIOPERATIVE CARE OF AORTIC SURGICAL PATIENTS

Patients undergoing thoracic aortic operations of any type share common considerations for the safe conduct of anesthesia and perioperative care (Table 17-2).

IV

Table 17-2 General Considerations for the Anesthetic Care of Thoracic Aortic Surgical Patients

Preanesthetic Assessment

Urgency of the operation (emergent, urgent, or elective)
Pathology and anatomic extent of the disease
Median sternotomy vs. thoracotomy vs. endovascular approach
Mediastinal mass effect
Airway compression or deviation

Preexisting or Associated Medical Conditions

Aortic valve disease
Cardiac tamponade
Coronary artery stenosis
Cardiomyopathy
Cerebrovascular disease
Pulmonary disease
Renal insufficiency
Esophageal disease (contraindications to TEE)
Coagulopathy
Prior aortic operations

Preoperative Medications

Warfarin (Coumadin)
Antiplatelet therapy
Antihypertensive therapy

Anesthetic Management

Hemodynamic monitoring
   Proximal aortic pressure
   Distal aortic pressure
   Central venous pressure
   Pulmonary artery pressure and cardiac output
   Transesophageal echocardiography
Neurophysiologic monitoring
   Electroencephalography (EEG)
   Somatosensory evoked potentials (SSEPs)
   Motor evoked potentials (MEPs)
   Jugular venous oxygen saturation
   Lumbar cerebrospinal fluid pressure
   Body temperature
Single-lung ventilation for thoracotomy
   Double-lumen endobronchial tube
   Endobronchial blocker
Potential for bleeding
   Large-bore intravenous access
   Blood product availability
   Antifibrinolytic therapy
Antibiotic prophylaxis

Postoperative Care Considerations and Complications

Hypothermia
Hypotension
Hypertension
Bleeding
Spinal cord ischemia
Stroke
Renal insufficiency
Respiratory insufficiency
Phrenic nerve injury
Diaphragmatic dysfunction
Recurrent laryngeal nerve injury
Pain management

17

Preanesthetic Assessment

It is important to determine the operative diagnosis because both the anesthetic management and surgical approach are dictated by the anatomic extent of the lesion and the physiologic consequences of the disease. Diseases involving the aortic root, ascending aorta, and proximal aortic arch are generally approached through a median sternotomy, whereas diseases of the distal aortic arch or descending thoracic aorta are approached through a left thoracotomy or thoracoabdominal incision. Sometimes, the operative diagnosis can be established in advance. Other times, a presumptive diagnosis has been made based on patient symptoms or available reports and the definitive diagnosis needs to be verified after patient arrival into the operating room by direct review of the diagnostic studies or by intraoperative transesophageal echocardiography. In either case it is important to discuss the anesthetic and operative plan with the surgical team to be properly prepared for all possible contingencies. Direct review of the actual diagnostic imaging studies such as the angiogram, computed tomographic scan, magnetic resonance image, or echocardiogram not only verifies the operative diagnosis but also provides important information that determines the surgical options. Knowing the size and anatomic extent of aortic pathology provides information about the physiologic impact and consequences of the lesion, permitting the anesthesiologist to anticipate potential difficulties associated with anesthetic procedures, problems related to the surgical repair, and postoperative complications.

Anesthetic Management

Considered as a group, any operative procedure involving the aorta from endovascular stent repairs to open repair of TAAAs is associated with the potential for catastrophic bleeding and cardiovascular collapse. For this reason, continuous diagnostic ECG monitoring, intra-arterial blood pressure monitoring, large-bore vascular access for rapid volume expansion, and ensuring the immediate availability of packed red blood cells can be justified in virtually every patient. Central venous access for monitoring the right atrial pressure and the administration of vasoactive drug therapy to control the circulation can also be justified in almost all cases. Pulmonary artery catheterization to measure pulmonary artery pressures, cardiac output, and mixed venous oxygen saturation is useful for operations involving cardiopulmonary bypass (CPB), DHCA, partial left-sided heart bypass, or cross-clamping of the thoracic aorta. Routine availability and use of intraoperative TEE provide both diagnostic information and the ability to assess ventricular function.

Arguments can be made for using either the left or right radial artery for intra-arterial blood pressure monitoring. A right radial arterial catheter can detect partial occlusion or obstruction of flow into the innominate artery caused by inadvertent placement of the aortic cross-clamp too near to the origin of the innominate artery during the course of operations involving the ascending aorta or aortic arch. A right radial arterial catheter also permits monitoring of blood pressure during repair of the proximal thoracic aorta or distal aortic arch if the left subclavian artery has to be clamped. A left radial arterial catheter must be used for selective ACP via the right axillary artery. Sometimes bilateral radial arterial catheters are necessary. A femoral arterial catheter is necessary to monitor distal aortic pressure when partial left-sided heart bypass is used to provide distal aortic perfusion.

Large-bore peripheral intravenous catheters that are 16 gauge or larger provide satisfactory sites for rapid intravascular volume expansion. An intravenous administration set integrated with a fluid warming unit is desirable, particularly for the rapid administration of blood products. Often, patients coming to the operating room from other areas of the hospital already have established intravascular access with small-bore intravenous catheters at the site of large veins. One approach in this scenario is to exchange the small-bore catheter with a commercially available 7.5- to 8.5-Fr large-bore rapid infusion catheter over a sterile guidewire. The only precaution in the use of these catheters is to ensure that the vein is large enough to accept the larger-diameter catheter. Alternatively, a large-bore central venous catheter, usually an 8.5-Fr introducer sheath, 9-Fr introducer/multiple-access catheter, or hemodialysis catheter, placed in the internal jugular, subclavian, or femoral vein can be used for volume expansion. When a pulmonary artery catheter is necessary, a second introducer sheath for volume expansion can be placed also into the right internal jugular vein. For this procedure, both guidewires should be placed with at least 2 cm of separation between them. Central venous cannulation can be achieved by either anatomic landmark guidance or ultrasound guidance. Ultrasound guidance may increase both the speed and safety of venous cannulation, which is particularly advantageous in emergency operations or when the patient is hemodynamically unstable. A urinary catheter with a temperature probe to measure core temperature, together with a nasopharyngeal temperature probe, is necessary to monitor both the absolute temperature and rate of change of body temperature during deliberate hypothermia and subsequent rewarming. The temperature probe of the pulmonary artery catheter can provide core temperature monitoring, and a rectal temperature probe can be used to monitor shell temperature.

The hemodynamic condition of the patient should be reassessed immediately before the induction of general anesthesia. The decrease in arterial pressure in response to anesthetic drugs and subsequent increase in response to tracheal intubation should be anticipated. Both vasopressor drugs and vasodilator drugs should be immediately available to provide precise control of the blood pressure. Intravenous vasodilator drugs being infused to treat preoperative hypertension often need to be reduced in dose or discontinued on induction of general anesthesia. Etomidate is a useful induction agent for patients in cardiogenic shock because it does not attenuate sympathetic nervous system responses and has no direct actions on myocardial contractility or vascular tone. In hemodynamically unstable patients, a narcotic such as fentanyl in combination with a benzodiazepine such as midazolam can be subsequently titrated incrementally to maintain general anesthesia after induction with etomidate. In elective cases, general anesthesia can be induced with routine intravenous hypnotic drugs followed by a narcotic to attenuate the hypertensive responses to tracheal intubation and skin incision. Antibiotic prophylaxis administration should optimally be completed at least 30 minutes before skin incision to achieve adequate bactericidal levels in tissue. Antifibrinolytic therapy, if used, should be administered before full anticoagulation for extracorporeal circulation.

The maintenance of general anesthesia can usually be accomplished with a combination of narcotic analgesics, benzodiazepine sedative hypnotics, an inhaled general anesthetic, and a nondepolarizing muscle relaxant. Anesthetics can be reduced in response to moderate hypothermia in the range of 30°C and then discontinued during deep hypothermia at 18°C and resumed on rewarming. When electroencephalographic (EEG) or somatosensory evoked potential (SSEP) monitoring is required during surgery, barbiturates or bolus doses of propofol are avoided and the dose of the inhaled anesthetic is reduced to 0.5 MAC and kept constant to prevent anesthetic-induced changes in the monitored signals. Propofol, narcotics, and neuromuscular blocking drugs can be used during SSEP monitoring. When intraoperative motor evoked potential (MEP) monitoring is required, total intravenous anesthesia with

17

propofol in combination with remifentanil or similar narcotic without neuromuscular blockade is necessary to ensure consistent reproducible recordings and a good-quality signal. In the majority of cases, the duration of general anesthesia is designed to persist for 1 to 2 hours after patient transfer to the intensive care unit (ICU) to permit a gradual and controlled emergence from general anesthesia. If epidural analgesia is used intraoperatively, a dilute solution of local anesthetic and narcotic is preferred to prevent hypotension caused by sympathetic nervous system blockade and to prevent complete motor or sensory blockade to permit neurologic assessment of lower extremity function.[1]

The potential for blood loss and bleeding is always a consideration in operations on the thoracic aorta. The presence of intrinsic disease of the vessel wall, construction of numerous vascular anastomoses in large conducting vessels, need for extracorporeal circulation, and application of deliberate hypothermia all combine to create a situation in which blood loss and transfusion therapy are commonplace. Because blood loss can occur rapidly and unpredictably and be difficult to control, it is often prudent to have fresh frozen plasma and platelets available to provide ongoing replacement of coagulation factors during transfusion of packed red blood cells. The time delay required for laboratory testing to verify the depletion of platelets and clotting factors in the setting of ongoing blood loss is often too long to be useful as a guide for transfusion therapy. Strategies to decrease the risk of bleeding and to conserve blood include discontinuation of anticoagulation and antiplatelet therapy before surgery, antifibrinolytic therapy, the routine use of intraoperative cell salvage, biologic glue, and precise control of arterial pressure and prevention of hypertensive episodes in the perioperative period. The antifibrinolytic agents, ε-aminocaproic acid or tranexamic acid, have been safely used in the setting of thoracic aortic surgery with DHCA. The infusion of an antifibrinolytic agent should be discontinued during the period of DHCA and resumed on reperfusion. Recombinant activated factor VIIa is a synthetic hemostatic agent that promotes hemostasis by binding with tissue factor at the site of tissue injury to promote clot formation. Although experience with this agent has been limited, dramatic responses to this drug have been observed in response to coagulopathic bleeding refractory to conventional therapy in the setting of trauma, cardiac, and aortic surgery.[2] In the surgical setting, recombinant activated factor VIIa has been administered intravenously in doses up to 90 µg/kg and repeated once after 2 hours. Recombinant activated factor VIIa has an estimated plasma half-life of 2.6 hours and causes a rapid decrease in the prothrombin time.

Postoperative Care

After completion of the operation, the patient should be transported directly from the operating room into the ICU or postanesthetic care unit for recovery. Transfer of information to the critical care team in advance of receiving the patient is necessary to ensure an uninterrupted transition of care. Immediate application of forced-air warming prevents further temperature drift and restores normothermia even in the moderately hypothermic patient. In the absence of complications and when the medical condition of the patient is stable, the patient can be allowed to emerge from the effects of general anesthesia. Early emergence from general anesthesia is preferable because it permits early postoperative assessment of neurologic function. If the physiologic condition of the patient does not permit safe emergence from general anesthesia, sedation and analgesia can be provided in combination with mechanical ventilatory or circulatory support until the condition of the patient improves.

Common early complications include hypothermia, bleeding, hypertension, hypotension, ischemia, embolism, stroke, agitation and confusion, respiratory failure, and renal failure. Hyperglycemia, anemia, coagulopathy, electrolyte disturbances, and acid-base abnormalities are also common. Frequent hemodynamic assessment is important to control the circulation with short-acting vasoactive drug therapy and to detect cardiac arrhythmias. Arterial blood gas analysis and respiratory assessment are necessary to adjust the level of mechanical ventilatory support and determine the optimal time for safe extubation of the trachea. Laboratory testing to measure electrolyte concentration, hematologic parameters, and coagulation profile is necessary to institute immediate corrective measures. Maintaining glucose concentrations within the normal physiologic range is considered important because hyperglycemia has been associated with increased risk of infection, increased mortality in the ICU, and adverse neurologic outcome. The chest roentgenogram is obtained to verify the proper position of the endotracheal tube and the position of intravascular catheters and to diagnose pneumothorax, atelectasis, pleural effusions, or pulmonary edema. Perioperative antibiotic prophylaxis is typically continued for 48 hours after surgery to decrease the risk of wound and endovascular infections.

THORACIC AORTIC ANEURYSM

An aortic aneurysm is a dilatation of the aorta containing all three layers of the vessel wall that has a diameter of at least 1.5 times that of the expected normal diameter of that given aortic segment. Thoracic aortic aneurysms are common, are detected in 10% of autopsies, have an incidence of 5.9 per 100,000 person-years, and are the most common reason for thoracic aortic surgery. The median age at the time of diagnosis is 65 years, and this lesion occurs two to four times more frequently in males. Common risk factors for thoracic aortic aneurysms include hypertension, hypercholesterolemia, prior tobacco use, collagen vascular disease, and family history of aortic disease. Thoracic aortic aneurysms are classified by their location, size, shape, and etiology. Among thoracic aortic aneurysms, descending thoracic aortic aneurysms are most common, followed by ascending aortic aneurysms, and less often by aortic arch aneurysms.

The anatomic location of the aneurysm and its extent determine its pathophysiologic consequences, operative approaches, and postoperative complications. Aneurysms involving the aortic root and ascending aorta are commonly associated with bicuspid aortic valve or aortic regurgitation (AR). Aneurysms extending into or involving the aortic arch require temporary interruption of cerebral blood flow to accomplish the operative repair. Endovascular stent repair is an option for aneurysms isolated to the descending thoracic aorta ending above the diaphragm. Repair of descending TAAAs requires the sacrifice of some or all of the segmental intercostal arteries branches and is associated with a risk of postoperative paraplegia from spinal cord ischemia or infarction. Aneurysmal disease of the thoracic aorta is often a diffuse process affecting multiple segments of the aorta and producing vessel tortuosity and often coexists in combination with isolated aneurysms of the abdominal aorta.

Most thoracic aortic aneurysms are asymptomatic and discovered incidentally through screening or as a consequence of medical workup for other cardiovascular disease (Box 17-1). The most common initial symptoms of thoracic aortic aneurysm are chest or back pain caused by aneurysmal expansion, rupture, or bony erosion. The mass effect of the aneurysm can cause hoarseness from stretching or compression

17

BOX 17-1	*Potential Complications of Thoracic Aortic Aneurysms*

- Rupture
- Aortic regurgitation
- Trachea or left main stem bronchial compression
- Right pulmonary artery or right ventricular outflow tract obstruction
- Esophageal compression

of the recurrent laryngeal nerve, atelectasis from compression of the left lung, superior vena cava syndrome from compression of the superior vena cava or innominate vein, dysphagia from compression of the esophagus, or dyspnea from compression of the trachea, main stem bronchus, or pulmonary artery. Other symptoms include wheezing, cough, hemoptysis, or hematemesis. Aneurysm of the aortic root causing AR may present as dyspnea on exertion, heart failure, or pulmonary edema. Atherosclerotic aneurysms with mural thrombus may present as embolism, stroke, mesenteric ischemia, renal insufficiency, or limb ischemia.

Leakage or rupture of thoracic aortic aneurysms should be treated as a surgical emergency. Expansion and impending rupture are often heralded by the development of new or worsening pain, often of sudden onset. Rupture is accompanied by the dramatic onset of excruciating pain and hypotension. Rupture of an ascending aortic aneurysm into the pericardial sac causes cardiac tamponade. Rupture of a descending aortic aneurysm may cause hemothorax, aortobronchial fistula, or aortoesophageal fistula. If surrounding tissue does not contain a ruptured aortic aneurysm, the patient will exsanguinate and die.

General Surgical Considerations for Thoracic Aortic Aneurysms

The objective of surgical repair is to replace the aneurysmal segment of aorta with a tube graft to prevent morbidity and mortality as a consequence of aneurysm rupture. Indications for operative repair include the presence of symptoms refractory to medical management, evidence of rupture, an aneurysm diameter of 5.0 to 5.5 cm for an ascending aortic aneurysm, an aneurysm diameter of 6.0 to 7.0 cm for a descending thoracic aneurysm, or an increase in aneurysm diameter greater than or equal to 10 mm/yr. Earlier surgical intervention may be justified in patients with Marfan syndrome, a family history of aortic disease, or dissection. In several series, 1-, 3-, and 5-year survival was as high as 65%, 36%, and 20% for medically treated patients with thoracic aortic aneurysms, respectively. Aneurysm rupture may account for up to 32% to 47% of deaths.[3]

An important factor that dictates how the surgical repair is performed is the location and extent of the thoracic aortic aneurysm. Thoracic aortic aneurysms of the ascending aorta and aortic arch are approached from a median sternotomy incision. Standard CPB can be used for the repair of aneurysms limited to the aortic root and ascending aorta that do not extend into the aortic arch by cannulating the distal ascending aorta or proximal aortic arch and applying an aortic cross-clamp between the aortic cannula and the aneurysm. Aneurysms that involve the aortic arch require CPB with temporary interruption of cerebral perfusion. Neuroprotection strategies that involve a combination of deliberate hypothermia, selective ACP, and RCP are important to protect the brain from ischemic injury during reconstruction of the aortic arch. Aortic aneurysms that involve the descending thoracic aorta are approached from a lateral thoracotomy or thoracoabdominal incision. Reconstruction of the descending thoracic aorta can be accomplished without extracorporeal circulation by cross-clamping the thoracic aorta or with extracorporeal circulation using partial left-sided heart bypass to provide distal aortic perfusion. Partial left-sided heart bypass is accomplished through cannulation of the left atrium via a left pulmonary vein and cannulation of the distal aorta, internal iliac artery, or femoral artery. If the descending thoracic aortic aneurysm extends into the distal aortic arch, DHCA may be necessary to construct the proximal aortic anastomosis. Operations for descending thoracic aortic aneurysms require consideration of strategies to protect the mesenteric organs, spinal cord, and lower extremities from ischemia as a consequence of temporary interruption of organ blood flow or the sacrifice of collateral vessels to accomplish the repair.

Surgical Repair of Ascending Aortic and Arch Aneurysms

The surgical options for repair of ascending aortic aneurysms depend on the presence of aortic valve disease, aneurysm of the sinuses of Valsalva, and distal extension of the aneurysm into the aortic arch. Intraoperative TEE is useful for evaluating the aortic valve to determine if a valve-sparing surgery is feasible, to determine the aortic valve annular diameter in relation to the diameter of the sinotubular junction to assess aneurysmal dilation of the aortic root, and to detect and quantify the presence of AR after valve repair. The most common aortic valve diseases associated with ascending aortic aneurysm are bicuspid aortic valve or AR caused by dilation of the aortic root (Fig. 17-1). If the aortic valve and aortic root are normal, a simple tube graft can be used to replace the ascending aorta. If the aortic valve is diseased but the sinuses of Valsalva are normal, an aortic valve replacement combined with a tube graft for the ascending aorta without need for re-implantation of the coronary arteries can be performed. If disease involves the aortic valve, aortic root, and ascending aorta, the options include tube graft of the ascending aorta in combination with aortic valve repair, reconstruction of the aortic root with sparing or repair of the aortic valve, bioprosthetic aortic root replacement, composite valve/graft conduit aortic root replacement (Bentall procedure), or replacement of the aortic root with a pulmonary autograft (Ross procedure). Replacement of the aortic root requires re-implantation of the coronary arteries or aortocoronary bypass grafting (Cabrol technique). If there is evidence of significant coronary artery disease, a combined ascending aortic aneurysm repair and coronary artery bypass grafting (CABG) may be necessary.

Anesthetic Management for Ascending Aorta and Arch Aneurysms

The conduct of general anesthesia for repair of ascending aortic aneurysms requires attention to a number of specific concerns. A large ascending aortic aneurysm can cause a mediastinal mass effect. Computed tomographic or magnetic resonance imaging studies should be reviewed to assess for aneurysm compression of the right pulmonary artery, right ventricular outflow tract, trachea, or left main stem bronchus. A right radial arterial catheter is preferred for most cases. If arterial cannulation of the right axillary, subclavian, or innominate artery is planned for CPB or selective cerebral perfusion, bilateral radial arterial catheters are often necessary to measure cerebral and

17

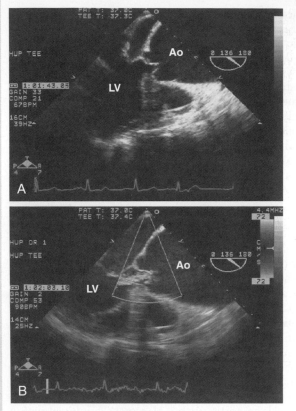

Figure 17-1   A, TEE midesophageal long-axis image of the aortic valve demonstrating aneurysmal dilation of the aortic root and ascending aorta. **B,** Doppler color flow imaging demonstrating severe aortic regurgitation caused by outward tethering of the aortic valve cusps by the aortic aneurysm. LV = left ventricle; Ao = aorta.

systemic perfusion pressures. Nasopharyngeal, tympanic, and bladder temperatures are important for estimating brain and core temperatures for monitoring the conduct of deliberate hypothermia and DHCA. EEG, SSEP, or oximetric jugular bulb venous oxygen saturation monitoring is sometimes useful for assessing cerebral metabolic activity for the conduct of DHCA. Control of the arterial pressure and prevention of hypertension are important to decrease left ventricular afterload in patients with AR and to decrease the risk of aneurysm rupture or expansion during induction of general anesthesia and surgical exposure. In patients with AR, antihypertensive drugs that decrease heart rate or myocardial contractility should be used cautiously to avoid heart failure. Intraoperative TEE is useful for evaluating the aortic valve and aortic root to determine the need for aortic root replacement or the feasibility of aortic valve repair. In patients with AR, a left ventricular vent is necessary to prevent ventricular distention during CPB. Patients with AR also require direct coronary cannulation for delivery of antegrade cardioplegic solution or a coronary sinus catheter to provide retrograde cardioplegia.

Neuroprotection Strategies for Temporary Interruption of Cerebral Blood Flow

Thoracic aortic surgery requiring temporary interruption of cerebral perfusion has been associated with the highest incidence of brain injury in comparison to other cardiac operations. Many reports assessing the incidence of neurologic injury were based

---

BOX 17-2 *Brain Protection for Aortic Arch Reconstruction*

- Deep systemic hypothermia
- Topical cerebral cooling
- Retrograde cerebral perfusion
- Selective antegrade cerebral perfusion
- Prevent cerebral hyperthermia during rewarming

---

on retrospective data collection or clinically diagnosed stroke. These reports suggest an incidence of stroke in the range of 7% to 9%. Studies that included a more detailed neurologic assessment and neuropsychological testing have found that neurologic deficits were more frequent in older patients and those subjected to DHCA for >25 minutes.[4]

Two major mechanisms are believed to explain the high incidence of stroke and neurocognitive dysfunction related to thoracic aortic operations. The first is cerebral ischemia or infarction caused by hypoperfusion or the need for temporary circulatory arrest during reconstruction of the aortic arch. The second is cerebral ischemia or infarction caused by cerebral embolization as a consequence of extracorporeal circulation or intrinsic vascular disease. Arterial emboli causing stroke can originate from multiple sources during thoracic aortic operations and include air introduced into the circulation from open cardiac chambers, vascular cannulation sites, or arterial anastomosis. Atherosclerotic or particulate debris may be released during clamping and unclamping of the aorta, the creation of anastomoses in the ascending aorta and aortic arch, or the excision of severely calcified and diseased cardiac valves. CPB may result in the generation of platelet aggregates, fat particles, and other microparticulate debris. The turbulent high-velocity blood flow out of the aortic cannula employed for CPB may also dislodge atherosclerotic debris within the aorta. Retrograde blood flow through a diseased descending thoracic aorta as a consequence of CPB conducted with femoral artery cannulation may cause retrograde cerebral embolization. For all these reasons, strategies to provide neurologic protection are important in the conduct of thoracic aortic operations (Box 17-2).

Deep Hypothermic Circulatory Arrest

The brain is exquisitely susceptible to ischemic injury within minutes after the onset of circulatory arrest because it has a high metabolic rate, continuous requirement for metabolic substrate, and limited reserves of high-energy phosphates. In the 1970s, deep hypothermia and circulatory arrest were introduced to protect the brain from ischemic injury for operations on the aortic arch requiring temporary interruption of cerebral blood flow. The physiologic basis for deep hypothermia as a neuroprotection strategy is to decrease cerebral metabolic rate and oxygen demands to increase the period of time that the brain can tolerate circulatory arrest. Existing evidence indicates that autoregulation of cerebral blood flow is maintained during deliberate hypothermia with alpha-stat blood gas management. In adults, a 10°C decrease in body temperature decreases cerebral metabolic rate by an average factor of 2.6, a factor commonly referred to as the Q_{10} ratio. Assuming an ischemic tolerance of 3 to 5 minutes under normothermic conditions, a Q_{10} ratio of 2.6 predicts an ischemic tolerance in the range of 20 to 34 minutes at a brain temperature of 17°C or 53 to 88 minutes at a brain temperature of 7°C. More recent estimations of cerebral metabolism in adults undergoing DHCA suggest an ischemic tolerance of 30 minutes at 15°C and 40 minutes at 10°C.[5] Direct measurement of cerebral metabolites and brainstem electrical activity in adults undergoing DHCA with RCP at 14°C indicated the onset of cerebral ischemia after only 18 to 20 minutes. It is also possible that hypothermia provides brain protection through mechanisms other than the reduction in cerebral metabolic rate. Despite an incomplete understanding of the mechanism and efficacy of hypothermia for cerebral protection, the large body of experimental evidence and clinical experience with the deliberate hypothermia suggest that it is the single most important intervention for preventing neurologic injury in response to circulatory arrest.

Despite the proven efficacy of hypothermia for operations that require circulatory arrest, no consensus exists on an optimal protocol for the conduct of deliberate hypothermia for circulatory arrest. The average nasopharyngeal temperature used for DHCA in several reported clinical series was 18°C, but the optimal temperature for DHCA has not been established. One problem with establishing the optimal temperature for DHCA is the inability to measure directly the brain temperature. In a study using EEG monitoring to establish physiologic criteria for cerebral metabolic suppression in response to hypothermia, the median nasopharyngeal temperature that electrocortical silence was achieved was 18°C, but a nasopharyngeal temperature of 12.5°C was necessary to ensure that 99.5% of patients achieved electrocortical silence.

The conduct of DHCA has several potential adverse sequelae. Lowering the target brain temperature extends the duration of CPB necessary for cooling and rewarming and all the problems inherent with prolongation of CPB such as injury to blood elements and the potential for cerebral embolization. Rewarming increases cerebral metabolic rate and has the potential to make the brain more vulnerable to ischemic injury, particularly during reperfusion after circulatory arrest. For these reasons, strategies to decrease the risk of brain injury during rewarming include delaying the start of rewarming by a period of hypothermic reperfusion, maintaining a temperature gradient of no more than 10°C in the heat exchanger, preventing the nasopharyngeal temperature from exceeding 37.5°C, or incomplete rewarming. Systemic hypothermia has commonly been associated with coagulopathy and increased risk of bleeding, but it has not been firmly established whether hypothermia is the underlying etiology of coagulopathy and bleeding. It is possible that systemic bleeding is a consequence of prolonged surgery, blood transfusion therapy, and intravascular volume expansion.

Retrograde Cerebral Perfusion

In 1990, RCP was reported as a means to deliver metabolic substrate to the brain during operations involving the aortic arch that required the interruption of ACP. RCP is performed by infusing cold oxygenated blood into the superior vena cava cannula at a temperature of 8°C to 14°C via the CPB machine. The internal jugular venous pressure is maintained at less than or equal to 25 mmHg to prevent cerebral edema. Internal jugular venous pressure is measured from the introducer port of the internal jugular venous cannula at a site proximal to the superior vena cava perfusion cannula and zeroed at the level of the ear. The patient is positioned in 10 degrees of Trendelenburg to decrease the risk of cerebral air embolism and prevent trapping of air within the cerebral circulation in the presence of an open aortic arch. RCP flow rates of 200 to 600 mL/min can usually be achieved. The potential benefits of RCP for neuroprotection include prolonging the safe period of DHCA by providing some metabolic substrate delivery to the brain, flushing embolic material from the cerebral arterial vasculature to decrease the risk of cerebral embolization on resuming ACP, and providing a means to maintain cerebral hypothermia during DHCA.[6,7]

Pharmacologic Neuroprotection Strategies for Deep Hypothermic Circulatory Arrest

There are no proven pharmacologic regimens that have demonstrated effectiveness for decreasing the risk or severity of neurologic injury in the setting of thoracic aortic operations. Barbiturates or other central nervous system depressants decrease

IV

cerebral oxygen consumption and in theory offer the potential for cerebral protection in the setting of incomplete ischemia. Experimental studies and several clinical series support the administration of high-dose glucocorticoid to protect against cerebral and end-organ injury in the setting of DHCA, leading to the routine intravenous administration of methylprednisolone, 1 g, or dexamethasone, 100 mg, to patients undergoing thoracic aortic operations that require DHCA at many centers. Other unproved pharmacologic adjuncts that are routinely administered intravenously in an effort to provide organ protection in the setting of thoracic aortic operations requiring DHCA include magnesium sulfate, 1 to 2 g, lidocaine, 200 mg, or mannitol, 25 g. In general, the existing evidence suggests that pharmacologic neuroprotection is unreliable and should not be considered a substitute for hypothermia to protect against cerebral ischemia in the setting of hypoperfusion.

DESCENDING THORACIC AND THORACOABDOMINAL AORTIC ANEURYSMS

The objective of surgical repair for descending thoracic aortic aneurysms or TAAAs is to replace the diseased portion of the aorta with a prosthetic tube graft. The surgical approach to repair is through a lateral thoracotomy or thoracoabdominal incision. Despite technologic improvements, major challenges remain in the surgical management of patients with TAAA. The major etiology of this disease is atherosclerosis, and the typical patient requiring surgery often is elderly with coexisting peripheral vascular disease, cerebral vascular disease, renal vascular disease, coronary artery disease, and frequently chronic obstructive pulmonary disease from a history of tobacco use. Patients are particularly susceptible to renal, mesenteric, and lower extremity ischemia as a consequence of thromboembolic disease, the temporary interruption of blood flow to these organs, reperfusion injury, and difficulties encountered in the reconstruction of branch vessel anastomosis during the course of surgical repair. The need for a thoracoabdominal incision, division of the diaphragm, and surgical dissection in the proximity of the phrenic nerve, recurrent laryngeal nerve, and the esophagus represents major physiologic trespasses that increase the risk of postoperative wound dehiscence, respiratory failure, and dysphagia and is associated with a prolonged convalescence in many patients. Finally, the inability to identify or reattach all intercostal arteries to accomplish the repair decreases the vascular collateral supply to the spinal cord, making postoperative paraplegia a recognized complication of these operations. As a consequence of these medical, physiologic, and surgical challenges, repair of TAAA is considered a high-risk procedure and associated with high morbidity and mortality that vary depending on the hospital volume and surgical experience. In a nationwide sample of 1542 patients, the overall average mortality rate associated with TAAA repair was 22.3% with a cardiac complication rate of 14.8%, pulmonary complication rate of 19%, and acute renal failure rate of 14.2%.

Thoracic aortic aneurysms and TAAAs are classified according to the anatomic extent of the aneurysmal segment. The most commonly used classification scheme is that described by Crawford that categorizes aneurysm extent into four major groups (Fig. 17-2). Extent I TAAA involves the entire descending thoracic aorta from the origin of the left subclavian artery down to the level of the diaphragm ending above the renal arteries. Extent II TAAA involves the entire descending thoracic aorta with extension across the diaphragm into and through the abdominal aorta all the way to the aortic bifurcation. Extent III TAAA involves the distal half of the descending thoracic aorta, crosses the diaphragm, and involves most of the abdominal aorta. Extent IV TAAA is confined to the upper abdominal aorta.

17

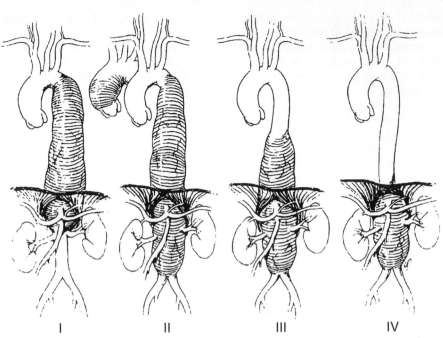

I   II   III   IV

Figure 17-2　Crawford classification of extent of thoracoabdominal aortic aneurysm. (From Coselli JS: Descending thoracoabdominal aortic aneurysms. In Edmunds LH [ed]: Cardiac Surgery in the Adult. New York, McGraw-Hill, 1997, p 1232.)

Surgical repair of TAAA with an interposition tube graft can be accomplished by three major techniques that are used in varying degrees at different centers. The original technique for repair was accomplished by cross-clamping the thoracic aorta proximal to the aneurysm. The simple cross-clamp technique was subsequently refined by the application of arterial shunting (Gott shunt) or partial left-sided heart bypass using extracorporeal circulation to provide distal aortic perfusion while the proximal descending thoracic aorta was cross-clamped. The third technique is to perform the repair using DHCA alone or in combination with retrograde perfusion or selective antegrade perfusion of the brain or mesenteric organs. With all of the techniques, an attempt is usually made to reattach intercostal, lumbar, and sacral arteries to the graft to decrease the risk of spinal cord ischemia. Endovascular stent repair is now the fourth option, and clinical trials to assess its safety and efficacy are well under way.

Simple Aortic Cross-Clamp Technique

In 1965, Crawford developed the technique of aortic cross-clamping for TAAA repair and subsequently reported a mortality rate of 8.9% in more than 600 TAAA cases repaired with the simple cross-clamp technique. Mortality and paraplegia were related to the position and length of the resected aorta, the condition of the patient at the time of presentation, and the duration of time that the aorta was cross-clamped. A major disadvantage of the simple cross-clamp technique is the obligatory ischemic period to the body and organs distal to the aortic cross-clamp. For this reason, when the simple cross-clamp technique is used, the surgeon must clamp and sew as quickly as possible to limit ischemia time to the spinal cord and distal aortic territory. The incidence of paraplegia and renal failure has been observed to correlate with the

Table 17-3	**Advantages and Disadvantages of Distal Perfusion Techniques for Thoracic or Thoracoabdominal Aortic Reconstruction**

Potential Advantages

- Control of proximal hypertension
- Decrease left ventricular afterload
- Less hemodynamic perturbations with aortic clamping and unclamping
- Decrease duration of mesenteric ischemia
- Decrease risk of paraplegia from spinal cord ischemia
- Ability to control systemic temperature with heat exchanger
- Vascular access for rapid volume expansion
- Ability to oxygenate blood with extracorporeal oxygenator
- Capability to selectively perfuse mesenteric organs or aortic branch vessels
- Maintain lower extremity SSEPs and MEPs for neurophysiologic monitoring

Potential Disadvantages

- Require greater level of systemic anticoagulation
- Increase risk of vascular injury at cannulation sites
- Increase risk of thromboembolic events
- Require perfusion team
- Need to monitor and control upper- and lower-body arterial pressure and flow
- Increase technical complexity of operation

duration of the aortic cross-clamp time and was increased significantly for aortic cross-clamp times greater than 30 minutes. Other disadvantages associated with cross-clamping the descending thoracic aorta include proximal aortic hypertension, bleeding from arterial collaterals, and hemodynamic instability on reperfusion. Proximal aortic hypertension during the period that the aorta is cross-clamped may be poorly tolerated in patients with abnormal left ventricular function, regurgitant cardiac valve disease, or ischemic coronary artery disease. Blood loss as a result of bleeding from arterial collateral vessels can be minimized by the use of intraoperative red blood cell salvaging. Hemodynamic instability during release of the aortic cross-clamp and reperfusion often has to be managed with correction of metabolic acidosis, rapid intravascular volume expansion, vasopressor therapy, or the intermittent reapplication and gradual release of the aortic cross-clamp. Adjuncts to protect end-organ function from ischemia during aortic cross-clamping include mild deliberate hypothermia and selective cooling of the spinal cord. Despite the physiologic consequences, the aortic cross-clamp technique remains a relatively simple technique with proven clinical outcomes and is still favored by many surgeons (Table 17-3).

Gott Shunt

Passive shunting of blood from the proximal to distal aorta has been used to provide distal aortic perfusion during aortic cross-clamping for TAAA repair. A Gott shunt is a tapered heparin-coated tube designed so that both ends can serve as arterial cannulas. The ascending aorta or aortic arch can serve as the proximal cannulation site for the Gott shunt. The distal descending thoracic aorta, iliac artery, or femoral artery can serve as the distal cannulation site for the Gott shunt. Blood flow from the proximal to distal aorta through the Gott shunt is variable and governed by the proximal aortic pressure, diameter and length of the shunt, and distal aortic pressure. Monitoring the distal aortic pressure through a femoral arterial catheter can be used to assess distal aortic perfusion and shunt flow. Advantages of the Gott shunt are that it is simple, inexpensive, requires only partial anticoagulation, and does not require perfusion personnel. Disadvantages of the Gott shunt include technical difficulty with cannulation in some patients, vessel injury, dislodgment, bleeding from the cannulation site, embolic stroke, and unproven efficacy for the prevention of paraplegia and end-organ dysfunction. An alternative technique to provide passive distal aortic perfusion is to perform an axillofemoral bypass before aortic cross-clamping.

Partial Left-Sided Heart Bypass

Partial left-sided heart bypass with extracorporeal circulation is a method of controlling both proximal aortic and distal aortic perfusion during aortic cross-clamping for TAAA repair. The technique of partial left-sided heart bypass involves cannulation of the left atrium from a left thoracotomy incision usually via a left pulmonary vein. Oxygenated blood from the left atrium is directed through the extracorporeal circuit with a centrifugal pump and into an arterial cannula placed in either the distal aorta, iliac artery, or femoral artery.[8] The extracorporeal circuit used to provide partial left-sided heart bypass can be modified in a number of ways to include or not include a heat exchanger, membrane oxygenator, or venous reservoir. Heparin requirements for partial left-sided heart bypass range from minimal to no heparin when heparin-coated circuits without oxygenators are used to full systemic anticoagulation with activated coagulation time greater than 400 seconds when circuits with membrane oxygenators and heat exchangers are used. During partial left-sided heart bypass, the mean arterial pressure in the proximal aorta monitored by a radial arterial catheter is generally maintained in the range of 90 mmHg. Bypass flow rates in the range of 1.5 to 2.5 L/min are usually necessary to maintain a distal aortic mean arterial pressure in the range of 60 to 70 mm Hg measured through a femoral arterial catheter.[9] Sequential advancement of the distal aortic cross-clamp during partial left-sided heart bypass after successive reattachment of intercostal arteries, mesenteric artery, and the renal arteries to the graft permits segmental reconstruction of the thoracoabdominal aorta to decrease end-organ ischemia. Advantages of partial left-sided heart bypass include the ability to control proximal aortic and distal aortic perfusion pressures, control systemic temperature with a heat exchanger, provide reliable perfusion to the lower body and mesenteric organs, permit selective cannulation and antegrade perfusion of mesenteric branch vessels, and preserve lower extremity somatosensory and motor nerve function for intraoperative neurophysiologic monitoring. Two contemporary clinical series have suggested that use of partial left-sided heart bypass was protective against postoperative paraplegia.[10] Disadvantages to partial left-sided heart bypass include increased expense, increased complexity, and requirement for systemic anticoagulation (see Table 17-3).

Cardiopulmonary Bypass and Deep Hypothermic Circulatory Arrest

Full CPB and DHCA has been described for TAAA repair with acceptable morbidity.[11] DHCA is necessary for construction of the proximal graft anastomosis if the aneurysm extends into the distal aortic arch or if the proximal descending aorta cannot be cross-clamped because the aorta is heavily calcified or cross-clamping compromises flow in the left common carotid artery. DHCA has also been advocated as an alternative method to protect the spinal cord and mesenteric organs from ischemia before the reattachment of branch vessels. If full CPB and DHCA are planned for TAAA repair through a left thoracotomy incision, preoperative echocardiography or intraoperative TEE is necessary to evaluate for the presence of AR so that a left ventricular vent can be inserted during surgery to prevent overdistention of the left ventricle with the onset of asystole during deliberate hypothermia. DHCA has the advantage of providing a bloodless surgical field for open anastomosis. Potential disadvantages of CPB and DHCA is the limited safe period for circulatory arrest, risk of stroke from cerebral embolization caused by retrograde perfusion of the aortic arch through a diseased descending thoracic aorta, increased duration of CPB for deliberate hypothermia and rewarming, and possibly increased risk of bleeding from hypothermia.

Endovascular Stent Graft Repair of Thoracic Aortic Aneurysms

Endovascular stent grafts are fabric or synthetic tube grafts reinforced by a wire frame that can be collapsed within a catheter for delivery and deployment within the aortic lumen. The endovascular stent graft is designed to be deployed within the aorta to span the length of the aneurysm and exclude blood flow into the aneurysm cavity. Endovascular stent graft repair for thoracic aortic aneurysms has been reported for the repair of isolated descending thoracic aortic aneurysms, repair of distal aortic arch aneurysms with partial arch reconstruction, and a few cases of transverse aortic arch aneurysms with dissection.[12] Endovascular stent repair requires the existence of a 1-cm-long nontapered region of aorta on either end of the aneurysm, often called the aneurysm neck, to provide a landing zone for each end of the graft. Furthermore, aneurysms that span essential aortic branch vessels require extra-anatomic bypass of those vessels before endovascular stent grafting.

Long-term results and efficacy of endovascular stent repair of thoracic aortic aneurysms remain to be determined. Problems that have been encountered with endovascular stent graft repair include vessel injury caused by the delivery catheter, intravascular migration of the graft, strut fracture of the stent frame, postoperative paraplegia, and endovascular leak at the graft ends, between graft segments, or from segmental arteries within the aneurysm cavity.

Anesthetic Management for Thoracoabdominal Aortic Aneurysm Repair

The anesthetic management of patients undergoing TAAA repair requires several special considerations. Selective one-lung ventilation is required for left thoracotomy or thoracoabdominal incision. Paraplegia is a major complication of the procedure, and an important aspect of the anesthetic management is directed toward strategies to decrease the risk of postoperative paraplegia from spinal cord ischemia in high-risk patients. A right radial arterial catheter is preferred to monitor proximal aortic pressure if the aortic cross-clamp has to be applied across the left subclavian artery or if the left brachial artery has to be accessed for endovascular stent graft deployment. A femoral artery or distal aortic cannula is necessary to measure distal aortic perfusion pressure for partial left-sided heart bypass or when a Gott shunt is used. Hemodynamic monitoring of the central venous pressure, pulmonary artery pressure, and cardiac output is useful for managing the circulation during proximal aortic cross-clamping, distal aortic reperfusion, partial left-sided heart bypass, or partial CPB. Intraoperative neurophysiologic monitoring with SSEPs or MEPs for the detection of spinal cord ischemia requires specific attention to the types and doses of anesthetic agents used for the operation. Perioperative renal insufficiency from mesenteric ischemia may complicate intravascular fluid and electrolyte management and require adjustment in the dose of drugs cleared by renal excretion. Left thoracotomy, thoracoabdominal incision, division

17

of the diaphragm, and dissection near the recurrent laryngeal and phrenic nerve increase the risk of postoperative respiratory failure and aspiration pneumonia. Postoperative pain is also an important concern, and effective postoperative pain management by intravenous analgesics or epidural analgesia may improve pulmonary function.

Lung Isolation Techniques

Selective right lung ventilation is required for left thoracotomy or left thoracoabdominal approach to TAAA repair. Selective ventilation of the right lung and collapsing the left lung during TAAA repair improves surgical exposure and decreases the risk of pulmonary contusion or torsion of the left lung. One-lung ventilation also serves to protect the right lung in the event of hemoptysis or bleeding from the left lung. Although it is possible to accomplish TAAA repair with a single-lumen endotracheal tube and lung retraction, anesthetic techniques to provide one-lung ventilation are always preferable.

Two major techniques are available to provide one-lung ventilation. The first is selective endobronchial intubation with a double-lumen endobronchial tube. The second is the use of a bronchial blocker. The routine use of fiberoptic bronchoscopic guidance has increased the reliability of achieving satisfactory lung isolation with either of the techniques. Although a right or left endobronchial double-lumen endotracheal tube can be used for lung isolation, a left-sided endobronchial tube is used most commonly. The increased length of the left main stem bronchus makes it easier to properly position the endobronchial lumen of a left-sided double-lumen tube and makes it less prone to dislodgment or malposition during surgery. Commercially available integrated airway devices (Arndt blocker, Cohen blocker, or Univent tube) to accomplish endobronchial blockade has also improved the ease and reliability of this technique compared with improvisation using a Fogarty balloon-tipped catheter. Wire-guided endobronchial blocking catheters permit the balloon-tipped catheter to be guided and positioned precisely in the left main stem bronchus with a fiberoptic bronchoscope.

Paraplegia after Thoracoabdominal Aortic Aneurysm Repair

The most devastating complication of TAAA repair is postoperative paraplegia caused by spinal cord ischemia and infarction. Although the exact pathophysiology and clinical events that lead to paraplegia after TAAA repair are incompletely understood, temporary interruption of distal aortic perfusion and sacrifice of intercostal and segmental arteries to accomplish TAAA repair are central events that predispose the spinal cord to ischemia and subsequent infarction. The incidence of paraplegia or paraparesis after TAAA repair based on clinical series reported in the literature varies widely and ranges from 2.9% to 32%. Factors believed to contribute or influence the risk of postoperative paraplegia include the extent of the TAAA, acute presentation, aneurysm rupture, the duration of ischemia as a consequence of aortic cross-clamping, the loss of critical intercostal arteries, the presence of dissection, the surgical technique used to accomplish the repair, and the use of techniques to protect the spinal cord.[13] The extent of the neurologic deficit in paraplegia or paraparesis varies from patient to patient but typically extends from the lumbosacral cord to the mid- to high thoracic level. Postoperative paraplegia is particularly poorly tolerated in elderly patients, is associated with respiratory insufficiency, and has a mortality rate that ranges from 63% to 100% depending on the length of follow-up. Although controversial, it is likely that perioperative

Table 17-4	Strategies to Decrease the Risk of Paraplegia from Spinal Cord Ischemia after Thoracic or Thoracoabdominal Aortic Procedures

Minimize Aortic Cross-Clamp Time

Distal aortic perfusion
Passive shunt (Gott)
Partial left-sided heart bypass
Partial cardiopulmonary bypass

Deliberate Hypothermia

Mild-to-moderate systemic hypothermia (32°C to 35°C)
Deep hypothermic circulatory arrest (14°C to 18°C)
Selective spinal cord hypothermia (epidural cooling, 25°C)

Increase Spinal Cord Perfusion Pressure

Re-implantation of critical intercostal and segmental arterial branches
Lumbar cerebrospinal fluid drainage (CSF pressure ≤ 10 mmHg)
Arterial pressure augmentation (MAP ≥ 85 mmHg)

Intraoperative Monitoring of Lower Extremity Neurophysiologic Function

Somatosensory evoked potentials (SSEPs)
Motor evoked potentials (MEPs)

Postoperative Neurologic Assessment for Early Detection of Delayed-Onset Paraplegia

Serial neurologic examinations

Pharmacologic Neuroprotection

Glucocorticoid
Barbiturate or central nervous system depressants
Magnesium sulfate
Mannitol
Naloxone
Lidocaine
Intrathecal papaverine

management strategies directed at the detection and treatment of spinal cord ischemia have the potential to decrease the risk of paraplegia after TAAA repair (Table 17-4).

The anatomic distribution of arteries that supply the spinal cord provides a partial explanation of the risk and clinical features of postoperative paraplegia after TAAA repair. The anterior spinal artery supplies the anterior two thirds of the spinal cord, and a pair of posterior spinal arteries supplies the posterior third of the spinal cord. Branches from each vertebral artery join to form the anterior spinal artery that descends along the midline of the anterior surface of the spinal cord. As it descends, the anterior spinal artery is sometimes discontinuous and fed in a variable extent by radicular arteries derived from ascending cervical, deep cervical, intercostal, lumbar, and sacral segmental arteries. The paired posterior spinal arteries also branch off the vertebral arteries and receive flow to a varying extent from posterior radicular arteries. The terminal region of the spinal cord and the caudal extent of the anterior and posterior spinal arteries are supplied by radicular arteries that arise from the internal iliac, lateral sacral, iliolumbar, and middle sacral arteries. The thoracic and lumbosacral regions of the spinal cord often receive blood supplied from more than one arterial source and are particularly vulnerable to ischemia if suddenly deprived of blood from one of the sources. In these watershed regions, blood supply from one or several large radicular arteries may be crucial. In some

---

BOX 17-3 *Techniques to Decrease the Risk of Intraoperative Spinal Cord Ischemia*

- Mild systemic hypothermia
- Lumbar cerebrospinal fluid drainage
- Selective spinal cord cooling
- Distal aortic perfusion
- Intraoperative motor or somatosensory evoked potential monitoring
- Arterial pressure augmentation

IV

patients, a particularly large radicular artery arising from an intercostal artery between T9 and T12 in 75% of patients, T8 to L3 in 15%, and L1 to L2 in 10%, often called the arteria magna or artery of Adamkiewicz, can be identified. Based on the anatomic distribution of vessels supplying the spinal cord, temporary or permanent disruption of flow to the segmental arteries arising from the descending thoracic aorta can make the spinal cord vulnerable to ischemia and subsequent infarction.

Postoperative paraplegia can be subdivided into those with immediate-onset paraplegia and those with delayed-onset paraplegia. Delayed-onset paraplegia accounts for 30% to 70% of patients with postoperative paraplegia or paraparesis. The extent of the neurologic deficit often varies among patients. In patients with postoperative neurologic deficits, the incidence of paraplegia and paraparesis is equally divided. Infarction in the territory of the anterior spinal artery classically causes motor paralysis with preservation of proprioception or some sensory function, but clinical experience has demonstrated that the pattern of paraplegia and paraparesis after TAAA is variable and often asymmetric and can affect either or both motor and sensory function.

In immediate-onset paraplegia, the patient is paraplegic on emergence from general anesthesia after TAAA repair. Immediate-onset paraplegia is likely a consequence of spinal cord ischemia leading to infarction that occurred at some time during surgery while the patient was under general anesthesia. In contrast to delayed-onset paraplegia, recovery or response to treatment in immediate-onset paraplegia has not been consistently demonstrated. The lack of improvement in response to measures to improve spinal cord perfusion in immediate-onset paraplegia indicate that irreversible injury had already occurred by the time paraplegia was diagnosed. For this reason, strategies to prevent immediate-onset paraplegia are directed toward protection of the spinal cord from ischemia and infarction during surgery (Box 17-3). Intraoperative efforts to protect the spinal cord from ischemia include augmentation of the arterial pressure, lumbar CSF drainage, provision of distal aortic perfusion with partial left-sided heart bypass, minimization of the ischemic time, deliberate hypothermia, segmental reconstruction of the aorta, re-implantation of intercostal arteries, or pharmacologic neuroprotection. The objective of using intraoperative neurophysiologic monitoring during general anesthesia is to detect spinal cord ischemia to permit immediate interventions to improve spinal cord perfusion during general anesthesia. Distal aortic perfusion maintains spinal cord function during aortic cross-clamping and improves the ability to monitor spinal cord integrity during surgery with SSEPs or MEPs.

Delayed-onset paraplegia or paraparesis is the onset of spinal cord ischemia several hours or days after TAAA repair in a patient who awakes after surgery without

---

BOX 17-4 *Prevention and Treatment of Delayed-Onset Spinal Cord Ischemia*

- Maintain mean arterial pressure ≥85 mmHg
- Serial neurologic assessment for lower extremity weakness or sensory loss
- Immediate treatment to augment spinal cord perfusion pressure
- Arterial pressure augmentation with vasopressor therapy
- Lumbar cerebrospinal fluid drainage
- Prevent hypotension

---

evidence of neurologic dysfunction. The syndrome of delayed-onset paraplegia indicates that the spinal cord was successfully protected during TAAA repair but remains vulnerable to ischemia and infarction in the early postoperative period. The abrupt onset of paraplegia or paraparesis in a patient with an initially intact neurologic examination after surgery suggests that immediate interventions to improve spinal cord perfusion may be effective for reversing spinal cord ischemia and preventing or limiting the extent of subsequent infarction. The clinical presentation of delayed-onset paraplegia or paraparesis can be variable and include progressive loss of lower extremity motor strength or sensation. Findings are sometimes asymmetric, affecting one side more than the other. The cause or events provoking delayed-onset paraplegia are not fully understood, but a number of reports suggest that it is often preceded by hypotension. Strategies to prevent and treat delayed-onset paraplegia are directed at preventing hypotension after TAAA repair, early recovery from general anesthesia to permit neurologic assessment and detection of delayed-onset paraplegia, serial monitoring of lower extremity motor and sensory function, and lumbar CSF drainage for the initial 24 to 72 hours after surgery if a lumbar CSF catheter was placed during surgery (Box 17-4). Success in the treatment of delayed-onset paraplegia or paraparesis has been reported in response to immediate interventions directed at increasing the spinal cord perfusion pressure. Full or partial recovery of neurologic function after delayed-onset paraplegia has been reported in response to lumbar CSF drainage, arterial pressure augmentation, and intravenous naloxone used alone or in combination. Reports suggested that early or immediate implementation of treatment at the onset of symptoms was more effective.[14] Considering the morbidity and mortality associated with permanent paraplegia after TAAA repair, all reasonable attempts to treat delayed-onset paraplegia can be justified.

Lumbar Cerebrospinal Fluid Drainage

Lumbar CSF drainage is a recognized adjunct for the prevention and treatment of paraplegia caused by spinal cord ischemia after TAAA repair. The physiologic rationale for lumbar CSF drainage is that reduction of lumbar CSF pressure improves spinal cord perfusion pressure. It is also believed that CSF drainage counters an abnormal increase in lumbar CSF pressure in response to aortic cross-clamping, reperfusion, increased central venous pressure, or spinal cord edema. Interpreting the contribution of CSF drainage for the prevention and treatment of postoperative paraplegia has been difficult because any incremental benefit of lumbar CSF drainage must be considered in the context of heterogeneous patient populations, differences in the surgical technique, and lack of control of the arterial pressure. A randomized, controlled trial of 150 patients undergoing extent I and extent II TAAA repair using a uniform surgical technique employing distal aortic perfusion with partial left-sided heart bypass demonstrated that lumbar CSF drainage was associated with an 80% risk reduction of postoperative paraplegia. Two clinical series suggest that lumbar CSF drainage used in combination with arterial pressure augmentation to increase spinal cord perfusion pressure was effective for the treatment of delayed-onset paraplegia when the intervention was employed immediately after the onset of symptoms.[9,14]

Lumbar CSF drainage is performed by the insertion of a silicon elastomer ventriculostomy catheter via a 14-gauge Tuohy needle at the L3-L4 vertebral interspace. The catheter is usually advanced 10 to 15 cm into the subarachnoid space and securely fastened to the skin to prevent catheter movement while the patient is anticoagulated. The open end of the catheter is attached to a sterile reservoir, and CSF is allowed to drain when the lumbar CSF pressure exceeds 10 mmHg. The lumbar CSF pressure is measured with a pressure transducer zero-referenced to the midline of the brain. At present, the best strategy to manage a traumatic lumbar puncture or the drainage of blood-tinged CSF has not been determined. For surgery, the lumbar CSF drainage catheter is inserted before or at the time of surgery and CSF drainage is continued typically for the first 24 hours after surgery. The lumbar drainage catheter can then be capped and left in place for the next 24 hours and then removed if the patient demonstrates a normal neurologic examination and coagulation function is satisfactory. Some clinicians use the catheter up to 72 hours after surgery.

The potential complications of lumbar CSF drainage include epidural hematoma, intradural hematoma, catheter fracture, meningitis, intracranial hypotension, and post–lumbar puncture headache. The potential for hemorrhagic complications as a consequence of dural puncture with a large-bore needle for insertion of the lumbar CSF drainage catheter in patients subjected to subsequent systemic anticoagulation during surgery remains an important concern. Despite the perceived risks of hemorrhagic complications of lumbar CSF drainage in aortic surgical patients, there are few reports in the literature to support this concern. Precautions to minimize the risk of hemorrhagic complications include avoiding the procedure in the presence of coagulopathy, allowing a delay of several hours after placement of the lumbar drainage catheter before administration of systemic anticoagulation, and ensuring adequate coagulation function on removal of the CSF drainage catheter. Intracranial hypotension as a consequence of excessive CSF drainage may cause brain herniation or subdural hematoma from stretching and rupture of the bridging dural veins. The risk of intracranial hypotension may be reduced by monitoring the lumbar CSF pressure during and after surgery with a pressure transducer not attached to a pressurized flush apparatus. For routine use, CSF should only be drained, using a closed circuit reservoir, when the lumbar CSF pressure exceeds 10 mmHg. The risk of meningitis increases with the duration of lumbar CSF drainage and has been reported as high as 4.2% in a neurosurgical patient population. Meningitis should be suspected in patients with high fever and altered mentation. Lumbar puncture demonstrating CSF pleocytosis or bacteria is diagnostic for meningitis. The risk of catheter fracture can be reduced by attention to patient position during catheter removal to prevent the catheter from being trapped between the posterior spinal processes.

Arterial Pressure Augmentation

The importance of arterial pressure augmentation for the prevention and treatment of spinal cord ischemia after TAAA repair has been recognized. The basis for arterial pressure augmentation to prevent and treat postoperative paraplegia is loss of segmental arteries as a consequence of TAAA repair makes the spinal cord vulnerable to hypotensive infarction. Furthermore, hypotension has been observed to precede or possibly trigger the onset of postoperative paraplegia and controlling the arterial pressure is an important component in combination with CSF drainage to support

IV

spinal cord perfusion pressure. Spinal cord perfusion pressure can be estimated as the mean arterial pressure minus the lumbar CSF pressure. In general, the spinal cord perfusion pressure should be maintained above 70 mmHg after TAAA repair.

Intraoperative Neurophysiologic Monitoring

The objective of intraoperative neurophysiologic monitoring is to permit the detection of spinal cord ischemia during surgery while the patient is under general anesthesia. The ability to detect intraoperative spinal cord ischemia may permit immediate interventions to improve spinal cord perfusion and prevent immediate-onset postoperative paraplegia. Two neurophysiologic monitoring techniques have been used to detect intraoperative spinal cord ischemia during TAAA repair. SSEP monitoring is performed by applying electrical stimuli to peripheral nerves and recording the evoked potential that is generated at the level of the peripheral nerves, spinal cord, brainstem, thalamus, and cerebral cortex. MEP monitoring is performed by applying paired stimuli to the scalp and recording the evoked potential that is generated in the anterior tibialis muscle.[15] Paraplegia caused by spinal cord ischemia causes a decrease in amplitude or disappearance of lower extremity evoked potentials compared with the upper extremity evoked potentials. Comparing the lower to the upper extremity evoked potentials during surgery is useful to distinguish changes caused by spinal cord ischemia from changes caused by the systemic effects of anesthetic agents, hypothermia, or electrical interference. SSEP monitoring can usually be accomplished using a balanced anesthetic technique with narcotic, muscle relaxant, benzodiazepine, and/or propofol and by keeping the inhaled anesthetic concentration less than 0.5 MAC. MEP monitoring requires total intravenous anesthesia without neuromuscular blockade.

Selective Spinal Cord Cooling

In addition to deep hypothermia and moderate systemic hypothermia, selective cooling of the spinal cord by the infusion of cold saline into the epidural space has been described as a technique to protect the spinal cord from ischemia during TAAA repair. The original technique for selective spinal cord cooling described the infusion of 4°C saline at flow rates up to 33 mL/min through a standard 4-Fr epidural catheter inserted at the T11-T12 vertebral interspace. A second 4-Fr thermister-tipped catheter inserted 4 cm into the subarachnoid space at the L3-L4 vertebral interspace was used to measure CSF temperature, measure CSF pressure, and act as a conduit for CSF drainage. A CSF temperature of around 26°C was achieved after the infusion of an average of 489 mL of iced saline into the epidural space over 50 minutes. CSF hypothermia was maintained by the additional infusion of 347 mL of iced saline into the epidural space while the aorta was cross-clamped. CSF was intermittently drained from the subarachnoid catheter to maintain a mean arterial to CSF pressure gradient of 30 to 50 mmHg to ensure spinal cord perfusion. The technique of selective spinal cord cooling is predominantly used in combination with the clamp-and-sew technique but has also been described for use in cases performed with CPB.[16] The clinical experience with selective spinal cord cooling has been limited to only a few institutions. A case series of 170 patients undergoing TAAA repair with this technique reported a postoperative paraparesis or paraplegia rate of 7%. A potential problem with the technique was excessive CSF pressures in response to epidural infusion that may have contributed to the development of a proximal cord compression syndrome in two individual patients.

Pharmacologic Protection of the Spinal Cord

Various pharmacologic adjuncts have been described in an attempt to prevent and treat spinal cord ischemia as a consequence of TAAA repair. Glucocorticoids such as methylprednisolone, 1 gr to 30 mg/kg, thiopental, 0.5 to 1.5 g, mannitol, 12.5 to 25 g,

17

or magnesium, 1.0 to 2.0 g, are commonly administered intravenously alone or together as part of a multimodal clinical intervention strategy in an effort to protect the spinal cord from ischemia, but it is difficult to determine the individual contribution of each agent to overall clinical outcomes.

Postoperative Analgesia after Thoracoabdominal Aortic Aneurysm Repair

It is well recognized that thoracotomy and thoracoabdominal incision is very painful and may cause respiratory splinting and retention of airway secretions that may contribute to the development of postoperative respiratory failure. Epidural analgesia is a proven method of providing postoperative pain relief for thoracotomy, laparotomy, and other surgical incisions that span the regions innervated by the spinal nerves. Although the clinical efficacy of epidural analgesia for postoperative pain relief has not been specifically tested in patients undergoing TAAA repair, an effort is usually made to supplement systemic opioid analgesia with epidural analgesia to achieve patient comfort during convalescence. Furthermore, providing effective postoperative analgesia may permit patients to awake earlier after surgery for assessment and monitoring of neurologic function.

The usual management of epidural anesthesia and analgesia may need to be modified when applied to the patient undergoing TAAA repair because the complications of epidural analgesia are difficult to distinguish from postoperative paraplegia caused by spinal cord ischemia.[17] The epidural analgesia regimen should be formulated to minimize interference with the ability to monitor lower extremity neurologic function and not cause sympathetic blockade that may contribute to postoperative hypotension. For example, bupivacaine 0.05% combined with fentanyl, 2 µg/mL, can be administered via a patient-controlled epidural analgesia infusion pump at a basal rate of 4 to 8 mL/hr initiated after surgery and after the patient exhibits normal neurologic function. Bolus administration of concentrated local anesthetic through the epidural catheter should be discouraged to avoid sympathetic blockade and associated hypotension. The epidural catheter can be inserted before, at the time of surgery, or in the postoperative period. Hemorrhagic complications attributed to epidural catheter insertion or removal have been rare, but care should be exercised to verify that the patient is not being treated with antiplatelet or anticoagulant drugs and that coagulation parameters are satisfactory before insertion and during removal of the epidural catheter.

AORTIC DISSECTION

Aortic dissection is caused by a tear in the intima of the aorta, exposing the underlying diseased medial layer to the pulsatile pressure of the blood within the aortic lumen. Blood exiting the true lumen of the aorta into the medial layer of the vessel through the intimal tear causes the intima to separate or dissect circumferentially and longitudinally within the aorta, creating a true and false lumen contained by the adventitia.[18] The aortic dissection may remain localized to an isolated segment of the aorta at the primary entry site at the original intimal tear. Often, the aortic dissection extends distally along the length of the aorta starting at the primary entry site, but it can also propagate proximally or in a retrograde direction. As the dissection propagates along the length of the vessel, the dissection can extend into the aortic branch vessels, cause occlusion of branch vessels resulting in malperfusion syndromes, or the intima may shear at the site of branch vessels creating multiple fenestrations.

IV

Table 17-5   Classification of Acute Aortic Dissection

DeBakey Classification

Type I: Involvement of entire aorta (ascending, arch, and descending)
Type II: Confined to the ascending aorta
Type III: Intimal tear originating in the descending aorta with either distal or retrograde extension
Type IIIA: Intimal tear originating in the descending aorta with extension distally to the diaphragm or proximally into the aortic arch
Type IIIB: Intimal tear originating in the descending aorta with extension below the diaphragm or proximally into the aortic arch

Stanford Classification

Type A: Involvement of the ascending aorta or aortic arch regardless of the site of origin or distal extent
Type B: Confined to the descending aorta distal to the origin of the left subclavian artery

Propagation of the dissection into the aortic root can cause AR. The development of a false lumen and weakening of the aortic wall caused by the dissection is often accompanied by dilation and expansion in the diameter of the aorta.

Thoracic aortic dissections can be classified according to the location and extent of the aortic dissection. There are two generally accepted classification schemes for thoracic aortic dissections (Table 17-5).

Type A Aortic Dissection

Aortic dissections that involve the ascending aorta (Stanford type A) are considered surgical emergencies. From 60% to 70% of patients presenting with aortic dissection will have a Stanford type A dissection. According to an international registry for acute aortic dissection, mortality rates for patients with Stanford type A aortic dissection managed without surgery were estimated to be 1% to 2% per hour after the initial symptom onset and 1% per hour thereafter for the first 48 hours, 60% by day 6, 74% by 2 weeks, and 91% by 6 months.[19] When managed with surgery, the mortality rate for type A aortic dissection was 26%. The causes of death and morbidity attributed to type A aortic dissection included rupture of the ascending aorta causing cardiac tamponade, myocardial ischemia or infarction when the dissection involves the coronary ostia, heart failure caused by acute AR, stroke caused by malperfusion of the aortic arch branch vessels, mesenteric malperfusion causing renal failure or ischemic bowel, or limb ischemia.[20] Aortic dissection can also rupture into the right atrium, the right ventricle, or the left atrium causing intracardiac shunting with congestive heart failure. An aortic dissection can be considered chronic after 2 weeks, because mortality tends to level off at that time. Late complications of type A aortic dissection include worsening AR, aneurysm formation, or aortic rupture.

Type B Aortic Dissection

Aortic dissections that are confined to the descending thoracic aorta (Stanford type B) are considered surgical emergencies only if there is evidence of a life-threatening complication such as malperfusion or aortic rupture. Patients with type B aortic dissection are generally older, with an average age of 66 years. Mortality in patients with acute type B aortic dissection managed surgically was 31.4% at 30 days compared with a mortality rate of 10.7% at 30 days in the medically managed patients. The high surgical mortality in type B aortic dissection may be attributed to the presence of complications such as aortic rupture or visceral ischemia that required emergent surgery in addition to the severity of the operation. Other clinical series have also reported high surgical mortality rates that range from 21% to 45% for patients with acute type B aortic dissection. Late complications of type B aortic dissection include aneurysm formation, aortic rupture, extension of the original dissection, or new dissection at a secondary site.

Anesthetic Management for Aortic Dissection

Acute aortic dissection is a medical emergency, and the medical management and diagnostic evaluation of a patient with suspected aortic dissection should proceed simultaneously. Time is of the essence because an initial mortality of 3% when surgery is expedited increases to as high as 20% when preoperative preparation is prolonged and diagnostic testing delays the start of surgery. Diagnostic studies are directed to verify the diagnosis of aortic dissection, identify patients with type A aortic dissections that require emergent surgery, and detect complications associated with aortic dissection. Patients who are unstable with a high likelihood of aortic dissection based on clinical evaluation and existing diagnostic studies should be transported immediately to the operating room where TEE can be performed to verify the diagnosis and surgery can proceed immediately thereafter. Acute medical management is directed at treatment of pain and decreasing the arterial pressure with antihypertensive agents to prevent aortic rupture or extension of the aortic dissection. In general, the anesthetic preparation and management of patients with type A aortic dissection is similar to the requirements for the management of patients with ascending aortic aneurysm that require DHCA. The anesthetic preparation and management of patients with type B aortic dissections who require emergent surgery are similar to the requirements for the management of patients undergoing TAAA repair.

The induction of general anesthesia in hemodynamically stable patients with aortic dissection should proceed in a cautious manner. The dose of intravenous antihypertensive drugs may need to be reduced at the time of anesthetic induction to prevent severe hypotension when combined with anesthetic drugs. Hypotension may also occur on anesthetic induction in response to the attenuation of sympathetic nervous system tone or decreased cardiac preload caused by venodilation and positive-pressure ventilation in patients with preexisting concentric left ventricular hypertrophy. The hypertensive response to endotracheal intubation, TEE probe insertion, and sternotomy should be anticipated and attenuated with narcotic analgesics.

Surgical Treatment of Stanford Type A Aortic Dissection

Surgical therapy for type A aortic dissection is superior to medical management. The objective of surgical repair for type A aortic dissection is to prevent death caused by AR, cardiac tamponade caused by rupture of the ascending aorta, myocardial infarction caused by dissection into the coronary ostia, and stroke caused by dissection into the aortic arch branch vessels. Intraoperative TEE is useful for detecting AR, identifying the mechanism of AR to assess the feasibility of aortic valve repair, and assessing the function of the aortic valve after completion of a valve-sparing aortic root replacement. Intraoperative TEE is also useful for evaluating right and left ventricular function to assess the need for CABG.

IV

CPB is accomplished by cannulating the femoral artery and inserting a venous cannula into the right atrium. Selective cannulation of the inferior vena cava and superior vena cava is necessary for RCP. On institution of CPB, flow through the true lumen of the aorta can be verified with intraoperative TEE. Acute cerebral malperfusion upon institution of CPB via the femoral artery is rare but can be detected by the acute decrease in EEG frequency and amplitude if EEG monitoring is used. Alternatively, duplex vascular ultrasound imaging of the carotid arteries in the neck can also be used to detect extension of the dissection into the carotid arteries or an acute decrease in carotid artery blood flow. Acute malperfusion can be treated by immediately discontinuing CPB if there is a perfusing cardiac rhythm and cannulating the contralateral femoral artery. In the absence of a cardiac rhythm, fenestrating the intimal flap within the aorta through a transverse incision in the vessel may be necessary.

Operations that are performed to treat type A aortic dissection include composite aortic root replacement with re-implantation of the coronary arteries, bioprosthetic aortic root replacement with re-implantation of the coronary arteries, aortic valve-sparing aortic root replacement, ascending aortic interposition tube graft, or aortic valve replacement and ascending aortic graft. Repair or replacement of the aortic root is typically performed in combination with graft repair of the ascending aorta and aortic arch. Partial or transverse aortic arch reconstruction requires temporary interruption of ACP. CABG is sometimes necessary for aortic dissections that involve the coronary ostia.

SUMMARY

- Deliberate hypothermia is the most important therapeutic intervention to prevent cerebral ischemia during temporary interruption of cerebral perfusion during aortic arch reconstruction.
- Selective antegrade cerebral perfusion should be considered if the anticipated duration of deep hypothermic circulatory arrest is greater than 30 to 45 minutes.
- Early detection and interventions to increase spinal cord perfusion pressure are effective for the treatment of delayed-onset spinal cord ischemia after thoracic or thoracoabdominal aortic aneurysm repair.
- Stanford type A aortic dissection involving the ascending aorta and aortic arch is a surgical emergency.
- Stanford type B aortic dissection confined to the descending thoracic or abdominal aorta should be managed medically when possible.
- Thoracic aortic aneurysms can cause compression of the trachea, left main stem bronchus, right ventricular outflow tract, right pulmonary artery, or esophagus.
- Intraoperative transesophageal echocardiography can be used to diagnose type A aortic dissection or traumatic aortic injuries that require emergency operation.
- Intraoperative transesophageal echocardiography and ultrasound imaging of the carotid arteries are useful for the diagnosis of aortic regurgitation, cardiac tamponade, myocardial ischemia, or cerebral malperfusion complicating type A aortic dissection.
- Severe atheromatous disease or thrombus in the thoracic or descending aorta is a risk factor for stroke.
- Distal aortic perfusion pressure should be maintained to prevent spinal cord ischemia in patients with aortic coarctation.

17

REFERENCES

1. Horlocker TT, Wedel DJ, Benzon H, et al: Regional anesthesia in the anticoagulated patient: Defining the risk. Reg Anesth Pain Med 29(suppl 1):1, 2004
2. Stratmann G, Russell IA, Merrick SH: Use of recombinant factor VIIa as a rescue treatment for intractable bleeding following repeat aortic arch repair. Ann Thorac Surg 76:2094, 2003
3. Nienaber CA, Eagle KA: Aortic dissection: New frontiers in diagnosis and management: II. Therapeutic management and follow-up. Circulation 108:772, 2003
4. Harrington DK, Bonser M, Moss A, et al: Neuropsychometric outcome following aortic arch surgery: A prospective randomized trial of retrograde cerebral perfusion. J Thorac Cardiovasc Surg 126:638, 2003
5. McCullough JN, Zhang N, Reich DL, et al: Cerebral metabolic suppression during hypothermic circulatory arrest in humans. Ann Thorac Surg 67:1895, 1999
6. Pochettino A, Cheung AT: Pro: Retrograde cerebral perfusion is useful for deep hypothermic circulatory arrest. J Cardiothorac Vasc Anesth 17:764, 2003
7. Reich DL, Uysal S: Con: Retrograde cerebral perfusion is not an optimal method of neuroprotection in thoracic aortic surgery. J Cardiothorac Vasc Anesth 17:768, 2003
8. O'Connor CJ, Rothenberg DM: Anesthetic considerations for descending thoracic aortic surgery: II. J Cardiothorac Vasc Anesth 9:734, 1995
9. Cheung AT, Weiss SJ, McGarvey ML, et al: Interventions for reversing delayed-onset postoperative paraplegia after thoracic aortic reconstruction. Ann Thorac Surg 74:413, 2002
10. Estrera AL, Miller CC 3rd, Huynh TT, et al: Neurologic outcome after thoracic and thoracoabdominal aortic aneurysm repair. Ann Thorac Surg 72:1225, 2001
11. Kouchoukos NT, Masetti P, Rokkas CK, et al: Hypothermic cardiopulmonary bypass and circulatory arrest for operations on the descending thoracic and thoracoabdominal aorta. Ann Thorac Surg 74:S1885, 2002
12. Dietl CA, Kasirajan K, Pett SB, et al: Off-pump management of aortic arch aneurysm by using an endovascular thoracic stent graft. J Thorac Cardiovasc Surg 126:1181, 2003
13. LeMaire SA, Miller CC 3rd, Conklin LD, et al: Estimating group mortality and paraplegia rates after thoracoabdominal aortic aneurysm repair. Ann Thorac Surg 75:508, 2003
14. Ackerman LL, Traynelis VC: Treatment of delayed-onset neurological deficit after aortic surgery with lumbar cerebrospinal fluid drainage. Neurosurgery 51:1414, 2002
15. Jacobs MJ, Elenbaas TW, Schurink GW, et al: Assessment of spinal cord integrity during thoracoabdominal aortic aneurysm repair. Ann Thorac Surg 74:1864, 2002
16. Motoyoshi N, Takahashi G, Sakurai M, et al: Safety and efficacy of epidural cooling for regional spinal cord hypothermia during thoracoabdominal aneurysm repair. Eur J Cardiothorac Surg 25:139, 2004
17. Bong CL, Samuel M, Ng JM, et al: Effects of preemptive epidural analgesia on post-thoracotomy pain. J Cardiothorac Vasc Anesth 19:786, 2006
18. Nienaber CA, Eagle KA: Aortic dissection: New frontiers in diagnosis and management: I. From etiology to diagnostic strategies. Circulation 108:628, 2003
19. Hagan PG, Nienaber CA, Isselbacher EM, et al: The international registry of acute aortic dissection (IRAD): New insights into an old disease. JAMA 283:897, 2000
20. Ehrlich M, Schillinger M, Grabenwoger M, et al: Predictors of outcome and transient neurologic dysfunction following surgical treatment of acute type A dissections. Circulation 108(suppl II):II, 2003

IV

Chapter 18

Uncommon Cardiac Diseases

William C. Oliver, Jr., MD • Gregory A. Nuttall, MD

Each subsection includes a general overview of the disease or condition and emphasizes anesthetic management of the coexistent disease in the setting of cardiac surgery. It is important that the anesthesiologist understand the pathology and pathophysiology of coexisting diseases, how they are affected by anesthesia, and how they affect the underlying cardiac problem.

CARDIAC TUMORS

Cardiac tumors are increasingly diagnosed before autopsy due to advancements in imaging, especially metastatic tumors of the heart and pericardium, which account for a majority of cardiac tumors. Data pooled from 22 large autopsy series show the prevalence of adult primary cardiac tumors as only about 0.02%, yet they are responsible for significant morbidity and mortality. Malignant tumors encompass about 20% of primary tumors in adults.[1] Diagnosis can be elusive because these tumors may be associated with nonspecific symptoms mimicking other disease entities. Two-dimensional echocardiography (echo) modalities and magnetic resonance

415

imaging (MRI) have allowed earlier, more frequent, and more complete assessment of cardiac tumors.

Primary cardiac tumors may originate from any cardiac tissue. Myxoma is the most common cardiac neoplasm, accounting for nearly 50% of tumors in adults. Less frequently observed benign tumors that may require surgery include rhabdomyoma, fibroma, papillary fibroelastoma, lipoma, and angioma. In contrast, malignant primary cardiac tumors are rare, with sarcomas comprising 95% of these tumors, followed by lymphomas. Sarcomas include angiosarcoma, rhabdomyosarcoma, and acquired immunodeficiency syndrome (AIDS)-related sarcomas. Surgery, radiation therapy, and chemotherapy may slow a tumor's encroachment on intracavitary spaces or relieve obstruction.

The incidence of metastatic cardiac tumors has increased from 0.2% to 10% as a result of improved survival. Metastatic cardiac tumors are much more common than primary cardiac tumors. Adenocarcinomas of the lung and breast, lymphomas that are commonly associated with AIDS or transplant immunosuppression, and melanoma are the most frequent metastatic cardiac tumors. Melanoma has a special tendency for metastasis to the heart and pericardium. However, metastasis of these tumors is rarely limited to the heart. The advent of arrhythmias or congestive heart failure (CHF) in patients with carcinomas suggests cardiac metastasis, but more than 90% of metastatic lesions to the heart are clinically silent.

Transthoracic echocardiography is excellent for identifying intracavitary tumors because it is noninvasive, identifies tumor type, and permits complete visualization of each cardiac chamber. It is the predominant imaging modality for screening. Often performed intraoperatively before initiation of cardiopulmonary bypass (CPB), transesophageal echocardiography (TEE) increases the diagnostic potential as the nature of the tumor according to location, dimensions, number of masses, and echogenic pattern is better identified.

The most effective treatment of primary tumors is generally surgical resection, and recurrence is rare (<5%). However, overall early mortality for primary cardiac tumors is 5%. Orthotopic cardiac transplantation has been recommended for unresectable tumors, but the benefit is indeterminate. Although more infrequent, the surgical risk and outcome for malignant tumor resection compared with benign tumor resection are significantly worse.

Myxoma

Often a diagnostic challenge, myxoma, a benign, solitary neoplasm that is slowly and microscopically proliferating, resembles an organized clot, which often obscures its identity as a primary cardiac tumor. The pedunculated mass is believed to arise from undifferentiated cells in the fossa ovalis and adjoining endocardium, projecting into the left atrium (LA) and right atrium (RA) 75% and 20% of the time, respectively. However, myxomas appear in other locations of the heart, even occupying more than one chamber. The undifferentiated cells of a myxoma develop along a variety of cell lines, accounting for the multiple presentations and pathologic conditions observed. Any age group can be affected. Myxomas predominate in the 30- to 60-year-old age range, with more than 75% of the affected patients being women.

Rarely discovered by incidental echocardiography examination, myxomas may manifest a variety of symptoms. The classic triad includes embolism, intracardiac obstruction, and constitutional symptoms. Approximately 80% of individuals present with one component of the triad, yet up to 10% may be asymptomatic even with mitral myxomas, arising from both atrial and ventricular sides of the anterior mitral leaflet. The most common initial symptom, dyspnea on exertion, reflects mitral valve obstruction usually present with LA myxomas (Fig. 18-1). Because of the

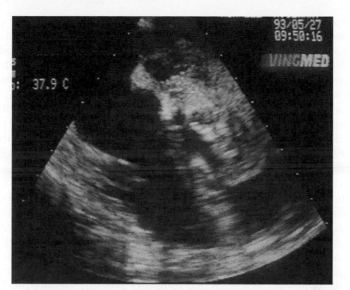

Figure 18-1   Transesophageal echocardiogram showing a left atrial myxoma prolapsing across and obstructing the mitral valve. (Reprinted with permission from Shapiro LM: General cardiology cardiac tumors: Diagnosis and management. Heart 85:219, 2001. Reproduced with permission from the BMJ Publishing Group.)

pedunculated nature of some myxomas, temporary obstruction of blood flow may cause hemolysis, hypotension, syncope, or sudden death. Other symptoms of mitral obstruction similar to mitral stenosis such as hemoptysis, systemic embolization, fever, and weight loss may also occur. The persistence of sinus rhythm in the presence of such symptoms may help distinguish atrial myxoma from mitral stenosis. Severe pulmonary hypertension without significant mitral valve involvement suggests obstruction of the tricuspid valve and recurrent pulmonary emboli known to occur with a myxoma in the RA or right ventricle (RV). Before echocardiography, angiography was used to identify all myxomas, but now it is only useful to confirm the diagnosis or determine coronary anatomy if considered necessary. TEE is 100% sensitive for diagnosis of myxoma. Specifically, it yields morphologic detail in the evaluation of cardiac tumors, including points of tumor attachment and degree of mobility. Computed tomography (CT) and MRI can help delineate the extent of the tumor and its relationships to surrounding cardiac and thoracic structures. MRI is especially valuable in the diagnosis of myxoma when masses are equivocal or suboptimal on echocardiography or if the tumor is atypical in presentation. Difficulty may arise in differentiating thrombus from myxoma because both are so heterogeneous.[2]

The first surgical resection of an atrial myxoma was performed in 1954. Subsequently, surgical resection has been recommended even if the myxoma is discovered incidentally, primarily because of the risk of embolization. Generally, the time interval between onset of symptoms and surgical resection is about 4 months, but surgery has been delayed for 10 years. Surgery is associated with a mortality rate of 0% to 3%.

Anesthetic Considerations for Myxoma

Tumor location has a strong influence on anesthetic management. LA myxomas most likely cause mitral valve obstruction, often in conjunction with pulmonary artery hypertension (PAH) and pulmonary venous hypertension. Anesthetic management closely resembles that for a patient with mitral stenosis. In contrast, RA myxomas may produce signs of right-sided heart failure corresponding to tricuspid

18

valve obstruction. Positioning of the patient for surgery must be carefully performed to detect severe restriction of venous return that is often followed quickly by profound hypotension and arrhythmias. A large tumor increases the likelihood of hemodynamic instability. Perioperative arrhythmias, especially atrial fibrillation or flutter, may arise in 25% of these patients, requiring immediate treatment. Hemodynamic instability with low cardiac output (CO) and arrhythmias are common.

Intraoperative TEE monitoring can aid in recognizing and avoiding tumor embolization. Consideration for not placing a pulmonary artery (PA) catheter as well as avoiding the RA completely should include the risk of tumor embolization. Evidence of postoperative neurologic injury should be carefully sought because of the likelihood of cerebral embolization and hemorrhage.

Median sternotomy is recommended for resection of atrial myxoma, although anterior thoracotomy and minimally invasive techniques may be possible in some benign tumors. Femoral cannulation for initiation of CPB may minimize the risk of dislodgment or fragmentation of the tumor. Subsequently, a venous cannula can be placed high in the superior vena cava, because a biatrial approach to an atrial septal tumor is necessary. Moderate systemic hypothermia, deep topical cooling, and cardioplegic arrest are often used, while circulatory arrest is reserved for malignant tumors with significant extension. To minimize systemic embolization of tumor fragments, the heart should not eject during CPB. Electrically induced ventricular fibrillation has been used to prevent ejection of blood after initiation of CPB. Wide excision of the septal base of the myxoma with Dacron or pericardial patching of the resulting defect is the preferred operation. Mitral valve replacement may be necessary in large tumors, ventricular side tumors, or tumors with other manifestations besides a propensity to embolize. Less-extensive operations risk a greater incidence of tumor recurrence because of incomplete tumor excision or a second tumor originating in susceptible atrial tissue. The recurrence rate after complete excision of a sporadic cardiac myxoma is low. Postoperatively, the most common complication is a 25% incidence of transient arrhythmias, mostly supraventricular in nature.

Tumors with Systemic Cardiac Manifestations

Carcinoid tumors are metastasizing tumors that arise primarily from the small bowel, occurring in 1 to 2 per 100,000 people in the population. Fewer than 5% of individuals with carcinoid tumors develop carcinoid syndrome, which is characterized by vasomotor symptoms, bronchospasm, and right-sided heart disease attributed to the release of serotonin, histamine, bradykinins, and prostaglandins, often in response to manipulation or pharmacologic stimulation. Manifestations of carcinoid syndrome occur primarily in patients with liver metastasis that impairs the ability of the liver to inactivate large amounts of vasoactive substances.

Initially described in 1952, carcinoid heart disease develops in more than 50% of patients with carcinoid syndrome and may be the initial feature. The prognosis has improved in the past 20 years for individuals with malignant carcinoid tumors, but carcinoid heart disease still causes considerable morbidity and mortality. Circulating serotonin levels have been found to be more than twice as high in persons with carcinoid syndrome who develop carcinoid heart disease. Carcinoid heart disease characteristically involves tricuspid regurgitation and pulmonic stenosis, resulting in severe right-sided heart failure. The left heart is usually spared involvement in carcinoid heart disease, possibly due to inactivation of serotonin in the lungs, but it may exist with the presence of a bronchial carcinoid or an interatrial shunt.

Without treatment, survival with carcinoid heart disease rarely exceeds 3 years. Surgery to replace both tricuspid and pulmonary valves with either bioprosthetic or mechanical valves is the only viable therapeutic option. The optimal timing to operate is uncertain, but consideration should be given to when signs of RV failure appear, in combination with steady follow-up. Perioperative mortality has been reported as high as 35%, but more recent data suggest it is below 10%. Despite surgery, RV dysfunction persists.

Anesthetic Considerations

Patients who have carcinoid heart disease and require cardiac surgery pose an anesthetic challenge.[3] A carcinoid crisis with vasoactive mediator release can be provoked by stress, physical stimulation, or medications such as meperidine, morphine, or histamine-releasing muscle relaxants (atracurium). Preoperative control of carcinoid activity is a critical aspect of perioperative management, made considerably easier with the administration of octreotide, a synthetic analog of somatostatin that inhibits the vasoactive compounds that produce carcinoid syndrome. It reduces the occurrence of symptoms in more than 70% of patients. The longer half-life of octreotide than somatostatin allows subcutaneous injection of 150 μg three times daily to control symptoms. Intermittent intravenous doses of 50 to 200 μg or continuous infusions are given to stop severe hypotension and prevent further carcinoid symptoms. Severe hyperglycemia may occur with octreotide due to its inhibition of insulin secretion.

Preoperative medication to reduce anxiety is strongly recommended for these patients. Individuals with more active carcinoid disease experience greater reductions in systolic blood pressure with induction of anesthesia. Sudden intraoperative hypotension should be regarded as a carcinoid crisis and intravenous octreotide administered until hemodynamic stability returns. Careful attention should be paid to physiologic parameters such as airway pressures as early warning signs of impending carcinoid crisis and treated before the onset of severe hypotension. Previously, certain catecholamines (epinephrine, norepinephrine, dopamine, and isoproterenol) were considered to provoke mediator release in carcinoid syndrome; consequently, phosphodiesterase-3 inhibitors became the preferred inotrope for cardiac surgery with carcinoid heart disease. More recently, 84 patients with carcinoid heart disease who underwent cardiac surgery did not display any deleterious effects or adverse outcomes with dopamine and epinephrine. A test dose of epinephrine may still be prudent to ensure that carcinoid crisis will not occur, but the use of dopamine and epinephrine may be considered in patients with carcinoid heart disease.

The use of an antifibrinolytic is routine in many centers to reduce blood loss and transfusion requirements associated with CPB and cardiac surgery. Because patients with carcinoid heart disease often require surgery involving several valves in association with liver metastasis, coagulopathy and excessive hemorrhage after CPB are more likely. Compared with other commonly used synthetic antifibrinolytic agents (tranexamic acid and aminocaproic acid), aprotinin has the dual properties of antifibrinolysis and anti-inflammation. Consequently, the use of aprotinin in this group of patients may be especially advantageous. However, to achieve inhibition of bradykinin and kallikrein, sufficient dosing is necessary to achieve aprotinin levels of 250 KIU/mL.

CARDIOMYOPATHY

In 1995, the World Health Organization/International Society of Cardiology (WHO/ISC) redefined the cardiomyopathies according to dominant pathophysiology or, if possible, by "etiologic/pathogenetic factors." Cardiomyopathies are now defined as "diseases of the myocardium associated with cardiac dysfunction." The original cardiomyopathies classified as dilated cardiomyopathy (DCM), restrictive cardiomyopathy (RCM), and hypertrophic cardiomyopathy (HCM) were preserved, and arrhythmogenic RV cardiomyopathy (ARVC) was added.

The annual incidence of cardiomyopathy in adults is 8.7 cases per 100,000 person-years. General characteristics of all four cardiomyopathies are displayed in Table 18-1.

Dilated Cardiomyopathy

DCM is by far the most common of the four cardiomyopathies in adults (60%). It is a condition of diverse etiologies such as viral, inflammatory, toxic, or familial/genetic and is associated with many cardiac and systemic disorders that influence the prognosis.

DCM is characterized morphologically by enlargement of RV and LV cavities without an appropriate increase in the ventricular septal or free wall thickness, giving an almost spherical shape to the heart. The valve leaflets may be normal, yet dilation of the heart may cause a regurgitant lesion secondary to displacement of the papillary muscle.

Table 18-1   Characteristics of Cardiomyopathies

	Hypertrophic Cardio-myopathy	Dilated Cardio-myopathy	Arrhythmogenic Right Ventricular Cardiomyopathy	Restrictive Cardiomyopathy
Clinical				
Heart failure	Occasional (LV)	Frequent (LV or BV)	Frequent (RV)	Frequent (BV)
Arrhythmias	Atrial and ventricular arrhythmias	Atrial and ventricular arrhythmias, conduction defects	Ventricular tachycardia (RV), conduction defects	Atrial fibrillation
Sudden death	0.7% to 11% per year	Frequent (ND)	Frequent (ND)	1% to 5% per year
Hemodynamic				
Systolic function	Hyperdynamic, outflow tract obstruction (occasionally)	Reduced	Normal-reduced	Near normal
Diastolic function	Reduced	Reduced	Reduced	Severely reduced
Morphologic				
Cavity size				
Ventricle	Reduced (LV)	Enlarged (LV or BV)	Enlarged (RV)	Normal or reduced (BV)
Atrium	Normal-enlarged (LA)	Enlarged (LA or BA)	Enlarged (RA)	Enlarged (BA)
Wall thickness	Enlarged, asymmetric (LV)	Normal-reduced (LV or BV)	Normal-reduced (RV)	Normal (BV)

LV = left ventricle; BV = both ventricles; RV = right ventricle; ND = not determined; BA = both atria; LA = left atrium; RA = right atrium.
From Franz WM, Müller OJ, Katus HA: Cardiomyopathies: From genetics to the prospect of treatment. Lancet 358:1628, 2001.

With DCM, there is more impairment of systolic function even though diastolic function is affected. As contractile function diminishes, stroke volume is initially maintained by augmentation of end-diastolic volume. Despite a severely decreased ejection fraction, stroke volume may be almost normal. Eventually, increased wall stress due to marked LV dilation and normal or thin LV wall thickness, combined with probable valvular regurgitation, compromises the metabolic capabilities of heart muscle and produces overt circulatory failure. Compensatory mechanisms may allow symptoms of myocardial dysfunction to go unnoticed for an extended period of time.

Management of acute decompensated CHF continues to evolve, but the onset of overt CHF is a poor prognostic indicator for patients with DCM. Treatment revolves around management of symptoms and progression of DCM, whereas other measures are designed to prevent complications such as pulmonary thromboembolism and arrhythmias. The mainstay of therapy for DCM is vasodilators combined with digoxin and diuretics.[4] All patients receive angiotensin-converting enzyme inhibitors (ACEIs) to reduce symptoms, improve exercise tolerance, and reduce cardiovascular mortality without a direct myocardial effect. Perhaps more important than the hemodynamic effects, ACEIs suppress ventricular remodeling and endothelial dysfunction, accounting for the improvement in mortality noted with this medication in DCM. Other afterload-reducing agents, such as selective phosphodiesterase-3 inhibitors like milrinone, may improve quality of life but do not affect mortality, so they are rarely administered in chronic situations. Spironolactone has assumed a greater role in treatment as mortality was reduced by 30% from all causes in patients receiving standard ACEIs for DCM with the addition of spironolactone in a large double-blind randomized trial. The use of β-blockers in DCM has provided not only symptomatic improvement but also substantial reductions in sudden death and progressive death in patients with New York Heart Association (NYHA) class II and III heart failure. This is especially significant because almost 50% of deaths are sudden. High-grade ventricular arrhythmias are common with DCM. Approximately 12% of all patients with DCM die suddenly, but overall prediction of sudden death in an individual with DCM is poor. The best predictor of sudden death remains the degree of LV dysfunction. Patients who have sustained ventricular tachycardia or out-of-hospital ventricular fibrillation are at increased risk for sudden death, but more than 70% of patients with DCM have nonsustained ventricular tachycardia during ambulatory monitoring. Antiarrhythmic medications are hazardous in patients with poor ventricular function owing to their negative inotropic and sometimes proarrhythmic properties. Amiodarone is the preferred antiarrhythmic agent in DCM because its negative inotropic effect is less than that of other antiarrhythmic medications and its proarrhythmic potential is lowest. Implantable defibrillators reduce the risk of sudden death as well as reducing mortality. Evidence has indicated that with previous cardiac arrest or sustained ventricular tachycardia, more benefit was gained from use of an implantable defibrillator. This was based on a 27% reduction in the relative risk of death attributed to a 50% reduction in arrhythmia-related mortality compared with treatment with amiodarone.

Patients who are resistant to pharmacologic therapy for CHF may derive benefit from dual-chamber pacing, cardiomyoplasty, or LV assist devices. Placement of LV assist devices has improved patients sufficiently to avoid heart transplantation or enable later transplantation. Transplantation can substantially prolong survival in patients with DCM, with a 5-year survival of 78% in adults.

Anesthetic Considerations

The most common cardiac procedures for patients with DCM are correction of atrioventricular valve insufficiency, placement of an implantable cardioverter/defibrillator (ICD) for refractory ventricular arrhythmias, and LV assist device placement or

18

allograft transplantation. Anesthetic management is formulated on afterload reduction, optimal preload, and minimal myocardial depression.

Individuals with DCM are extremely sensitive to cardiodepressant anesthetic drugs. Intravenously administered anesthetic agents such as fentanyl (30 μg/kg) provide excellent anesthesia and hemodynamics in patients with ejection fractions less than 0.3 but contribute to prolonged respiratory depression, delaying extubation. Etomidate has been shown to have little effect on the contractility of the cardiac muscle in patients undergoing cardiac transplantation. Ketamine has been recommended for induction in critically ill patients due to its cardiovascular actions attributed mainly to a sympathomimetic effect from the central nervous system. Ketamine is a positive inotrope in the isolated rat papillary muscle and, more important, in a model of cardiomyopathic hamsters, did not display a negative inotropic effect. This makes ketamine an excellent choice to use in combination with fentanyl for induction in patients with severe myocardial dysfunction secondary to cardiomyopathy.

Hypertrophic Cardiomyopathy

Referred to as idiopathic hypertrophic subaortic stenosis, hypertrophic obstructive cardiomyopathy, and asymmetric septal hypertrophy, among other names, the accepted term is now *hypertrophic cardiomyopathy*.[5] In the past 40 years, advancements regarding the hemodynamics, systolic and diastolic abnormalities, electrophysiology, genetics, and clinical care of HCM have contributed to a greater understanding of this disease. HCM is the most common genetic cardiac disease, with marked heterogeneity in clinical expression, pathophysiology, and prognosis. The overall prevalence for adults in the general population is 0.2%, affecting men and women equally.

HCM is a primary myocardial abnormality with sarcomeric disarray and asymmetric LV hypertrophy. The extent of sarcomeric disarray distinguishes HCM from other conditions. The hypertrophied muscle is composed of muscle cells with bizarre shapes and multiple intercellular connections arranged in a chaotic pattern. Increased connective tissue combined with markedly disorganized and hypertrophied myocytes contributes to the diastolic abnormalities of HCM that manifest as increased chamber stiffness, impaired prolonged relaxation, and an unstable EP substrate that causes complex arrhythmias and sudden death. Diastolic abnormalities are more a function of impaired relaxation than of decreased compliance. Impaired relaxation produces a reduced rate of volume during rapid ventricular filling, with an increase in atrial systolic filling associated with atrial dilation. As the abnormal diastolic properties affect ventricular filling, the clinical manifestations of HCM become evident. In contrast to the diastolic function, systolic function in HCM is usually normal, with an increased ejection fraction that eventually diminishes in the later stages of the disease.

Besides diastolic dysfunction, the other major abnormality and fundamental characteristic of HCM is myocardial hypertrophy unrelated to increased systemic vascular resistance (SVR). This nonuniform, asymmetric hypertrophy is marked in the basal anterior ventricular septum, with a disproportionate increase in the thickness of the ventricular wall relative to the posterior free wall. The LV wall thickness is the most extensive of all cardiac conditions. Heart size may be deceptive because it may vary from normal to more than 100% enlarged. However, chamber enlargement is not responsible for the increase in ventricular mass but rather increases in wall thickness.

Symptoms of HCM are nonspecific and include chest pain, palpitations, dyspnea, and syncope. Dyspnea occurs in 90% of patients secondary to diastolic abnormalities that increase filling pressures, causing pulmonary congestion. Syncope occurs in only 20% of patients, but 50% may have presyncopal symptoms.

Two-dimensional echocardiography establishes the diagnosis of HCM easily and reliably. Classic echocardiography features are thickening of the entire ventricular septum from base to apex disproportional to that of the posterior wall, poor septal motion, and anterior displacement of the mitral valve without LV dilation (Fig. 18-2). Echocardiography has reduced the need for invasive catheterization procedures, unless coronary artery disease (CAD) or severe mitral valve disease is suspected or diagnostic problems are present. MRI has been useful in cases in which echocardiography is technically inadequate.

Two thirds of individuals with LV outflow tract obstruction become severely symptomatic and 10% die within 4 years of diagnosis. The outflow tract is narrowed from septal hypertrophy and anterior displacement of the papillary muscles and mitral leaflets, creating a dynamic LV outflow obstruction (see Fig. 18-2). Elongation of the mitral leaflets results in coaptation of the body of the leaflets instead of the tips. The part of the anterior leaflet distal to the coaptation is subjected to strong Venturi forces that provoke systolic anterior motion (SAM), mitral septal contact, and

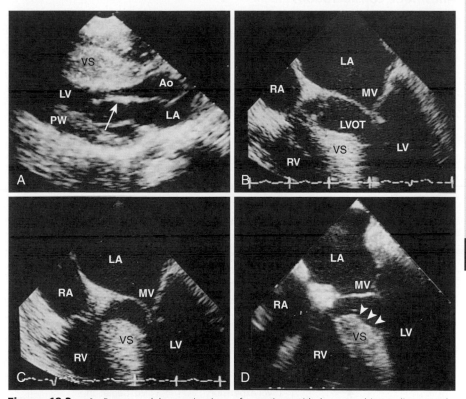

Figure 18-2   **A,** Parasternal long-axis view of a patient with hypertrophic cardiomyopathy (HCM). There is increased thickness of the septum from the base to the apex as well as the anterior free wall. The left ventricular cavity size is normal here. **B,** Transesophageal echocardiography in a patient with HCM for myectomy-myotomy. Early systole, demonstrating septal hypertrophy and narrowing of the left ventricular outflow tract (LVOT). **C,** Same patient in late systole. Systolic anterior motion of the mitral leaflets produced by a Venturi effect in the LVOT created by the high blood velocity. **D,** After myectomy-myotomy, the *arrowheads* point to the area of myocardium removed and the widened LVOT. LA = left atrium; RA = right atrium; LV = left ventricle; RV = right ventricle; VS = ventricular septum; MV = mitral valve; Ao = aorta; PW = posterior wall. (**A,** reprinted with permission from Giuliani ER, Fuster V, Gersh BJ, et al: Cardiology: Fundamentals and Practice. St. Louis, Mosby, 1991; **B, C,** and **D** courtesy of Martin D. Abel, MD, Mayo Clinic, Rochester, MN.)

ultimately LV outflow obstruction. SAM of the anterior leaflet may also cause mitral regurgitation. The onset and duration of mitral leaflet-septal contact determine the magnitude of the gradient and the degree of mitral regurgitation. The pressure gradient between the aorta and LV is worsened by decreased end-diastolic volume, increased contractility, or decreased aortic outflow resistance (Fig. 18-3).

Surgical correction of HCM is directed primarily at relieving symptoms of LV obstruction in the 5% of patients who are refractory to medication.[6] In general, these are individuals with subaortic gradients more than 50 mmHg and frequently associated with severe CHF. A myotomy-myectomy through a transaortic approach relieves the obstruction. The muscle is excised from the proximal septum extending just beyond the mitral valve leaflets to widen the LV outflow tract. This is a technically challenging operation due to the limited exposure and precise area to excise the muscle. It is usually reserved for centers with considerable experience. When myectomy is successful, the outflow tract of the LV is widened and SAM, mitral regurgitation, and outflow gradient are all decreased.

Anesthetic Considerations

Anesthetic management of individuals with HCM is based on similar principles for those having cardiac or noncardiac surgery. The characteristic diastolic dysfunction makes the heart sensitive to changes in volume, contractility, and SVR. Because of this diastolic dysfunction, an acute rise in the pulmonary artery pressure (PAP) may warn of the rapid onset of pulmonary congestion and edema. If the patient has LV outflow obstruction, anesthetic management should minimize or prevent any exacerbation of obstruction and the corresponding increase in the intraventricular gradient that will affect systolic blood pressure. Induction of anesthesia is a hazardous period because the preoperative fast reduces preload combined with a rapid fall in the

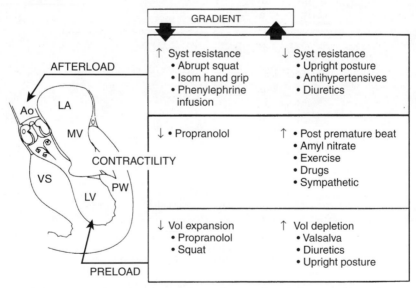

Figure 18-3 Interventions that change the outflow gradient in hypertrophic cardiomyopathy (HCM), with resultant change in intensity of the systolic murmur in HCM. Outflow gradient is affected by changes in afterload, preload, and contractility. Ao = aorta; LA = left atrium; MV = mitral valve; VS = ventricular septum; LV = left ventricle; PW = posterior wall. (Reprinted with permission from Giuliani ER, Fuster V, Gersh BJ, et al: Cardiology: Fundamentals and Practice. St. Louis, Mosby, 1991. By permission of Mayo Foundation.)

venous tone, provoking an increase in LV outflow obstruction. Central venous pressure (CVP) monitoring is recommended to optimize and maintain preload. Hypotension may be treated temporarily with positioning (Trendelenburg), volume replacement, and/or vasoconstriction. Vasoconstrictors rather than inotropes are preferred to maintain SVR. After induction of anesthesia and intubation, TEE can complement CVP monitoring to guide intraoperative volume status. Intravenously administered agents, such as narcotics, have been used successfully in HCM for induction of anesthesia. For shorter surgical procedures, propofol is popular, but its effect on hemodynamics has not been fully established. The systolic blood pressure often decreases significantly with propofol during induction of anesthesia. The mechanism of this fall in blood pressure is unknown, but it is likely an interaction of baroreflex activity, direct peripheral vasodilation, blunting of the sympathetic nervous outflow, and possibly a decrease in the myocardial contractility.

For anesthesia maintenance, the volatile agent halothane is advantageous because it decreases contractility and heart rate, but it is rarely used today. Halothane, in comparison with enflurane and isoflurane, has the least effect on SVR and heart rate. Vecuronium is the preferred muscle relaxant because it does not have histamine-releasing properties or hemodynamic effects.

Restrictive Cardiomyopathy

Restrictive cardiomyopathy (RCM) has included such entities as amyloidosis and eosinophilic endomyocardial disease. The 1995 WHO guidelines defined RCM as "restrictive filling and reduced diastolic volume of either or both ventricles with normal or near-normal systolic function and wall thickness." Instead of being classified according to morphologic criteria, as are HCM and DCM, RCM is characterized by function. It may appear in the final stages of other cardiac conditions.

RCM may be classified as myocardial (infiltrative, noninfiltrative, and storage) or endomyocardial (Box 18-1) according to etiology. RCM may be associated with another disease entity except pericardial disease. Restrictive myocardial disorders are characteristically atypical in presentation and hemodynamics at times, complicating perioperative management.

Because one or both ventricles may be involved, symptoms may predominate as right or left sided. The elevated filling pressures that occur in early diastole of both ventricles lead to symptoms of right-sided failure manifested by elevated venous pressures and peripheral edema and ascites or of left-sided failure manifested by CHF and progressive dyspnea and orthopnea. Both groups of symptoms may occur separately or together.

Anesthetic Considerations

Adults with RCM rarely require cardiac surgery for reasons other than transplantation or mitral or tricuspid valve replacement. Occasionally, anesthesia is administered for a scheduled pericardiectomy only to find RCM instead of constrictive pericarditis. Despite essentially normal ventricular systolic function, diastolic dysfunction and filling abnormalities result in a poor CO and systemic perfusion. Aggressive preoperative diuretic therapy may contribute to the difficulty of maintaining adequate circulating blood volume. Elevated airway pressures from pulmonary congestion may further impair oxygen delivery to the tissues.[7]

For induction of anesthesia, medications associated with decreased venous return, bradycardia, or myocardial depression should be avoided. Fentanyl (30 µg/kg) or sufentanil (5 µg/kg) provides stable hemodynamics for induction and maintenance in patients with poor myocardial function. These anesthetics maintain stable hemodynamics in patients undergoing cardiac surgery for valvular disease who have

> **BOX 18-1** *Classification of Types of Restrictive Cardiomyopathy According to Cause*
>
> **Myocardial**
>
> *Noninfiltrative*
> - Idiopathic cardiomyopathy*
> - Familial cardiomyopathy
> - Hypertrophic cardiomyopathy
> - Scleroderma
> - Pseudoxanthoma elasticum
> - Diabetic cardiomyopathy
>
> *Infiltrative*
> - Amyloidosis*
> - Sarcoidosis*
> - Gaucher's disease
> - Hurler's disease
> - Fatty infiltration
>
> **Storage Diseases**
> - Hemochromatosis
> - Fabry's disease
> - Glycogen storage disease
>
> **Endomyocardial**
> - Endomyocardial fibrosis*
> - Hypereosinophilic syndrome
> - Carcinoid heart disease
> - Metastatic cancers
> - Radiation*
> - Toxic effects of anthracycline*
> - Drugs causing fibrous endocarditis (serotonin, methysergide, ergotamine, mercurial agents, busulfan)
>
> ---
>
> *This condition is more likely than the others to be encountered in clinical practice.
> From Kushwaha SS, Fallon JT, Fuster V: Medical progress: Restrictive cardiomyopathy. N Engl J Med 336:268, 1997.

severely impaired preexisting volume or pressure loads on the heart and induce minimal hemodynamic fluctuation. Etomidate is an excellent alternative to fentanyl as an induction agent because it has minimal effect on contractility of the cardiac muscle, as demonstrated in patients undergoing cardiac transplantation. Similarly, ketamine has been advocated for induction in patients with cardiac tamponade or constrictive pericarditis because sympathetic activity is preserved. Ketamine is an excellent choice to use with fentanyl for induction in patients with severe myocardial dysfunction due to cardiomyopathy. Concerns of exacerbating PAH with ketamine are unfounded if ventilation is maintained. Propofol may have no direct myocardial depression, but indirect inhibition of sympathetic activity and a vasodilatory property may cause hemodynamic instability in patients with RCM. The use of sevoflurane and desflurane has also been shown not to adversely affect the ability of the LV to respond to increased work despite their negative inotropic properties in patients undergoing CPB and cardiac surgery, making them attractive agents for maintenance of anesthesia in this population.

Arrhythmogenic Right Ventricular Cardiomyopathy

Formerly called arrhythmogenic right ventricular dysplasia, ARVC is defined by the 1995 WHO as "progressive fibrofatty replacement of RV myocardium, initially with typical regional and later global RV and some LV involvement, with relative sparing of the septum." Evidence of a more progressive involvement of not only the RV but also the LV with long-term follow-up convinced the WHO to classify ARVC as a "disease of the myocardium" that incorporates the many different clinical presentations and aspects of this condition.

It presents as the onset of arrhythmias ranging from premature ventricular contractions to ventricular fibrillation originating from the RV. Diagnosis has been rare in the early stages but not at autopsy. Identifying symptoms are absent even though structural changes exist in the myocardium. Postmortem examination reveals diffuse or segmental loss of myocardium, primarily in the RV, replaced with fat and fibrous tissue. The replacement of myocardium with fat and fibrous tissue creates an excellent environment for a fatal arrhythmia, possibly the first sign of ARVC. Sudden death occurs in up to 75% of patients, although it is difficult to accurately state in view of the extent of missed diagnosis. Sudden death occurs most often during sports-related exercise, primarily from ventricular tachycardia/fibrillation. Twenty percent of patients die as a result of CHF.

Anesthetic Considerations

During the course of ARVC, arrhythmias may occur at any time. Presently, there are no guidelines for arrhythmia prevention. A family history of sudden death or syncope at an early age should heighten the awareness of ARVC.[8] With ARVC, arrhythmias are more likely in the perioperative period. During or after anesthesia, the patient should be carefully observed to avoid noxious stimuli, hypovolemia, hypercarbia, and light anesthesia. Acidosis may be especially detrimental due to its effect on arrhythmia generation and myocardial function. General anesthesia alone does not appear to be arrhythmogenic because reports describe multiple exposures to general anesthesia without arrhythmias. More than 200 patients with ARVC had undergone general anesthesia without a single cardiac arrest. Nonetheless, any family history of sudden death elicited during preoperative assessment merits further investigation. Anesthesia has been successfully conducted with propofol, midazolam, and alfentanil. Amiodarone is the first line of antiarrhythmic medication during anesthesia.

18

MITRAL VALVE PROLAPSE

Mitral valve prolapse (MVP), often referred to as Barlow's syndrome, is a structural and functional disorder affecting 2.5% to 5% of the population. As the most commonly diagnosed cardiac valve abnormality, it occurs in adults who are otherwise healthy or in association with many pathologic conditions (Box 18-2). Women, representing two thirds of adults with MVP, are more frequently affected during the third, fourth, and fifth decades of life but account for a decreasing prevalence beyond the third decade. The incidence of MVP in men is unrelated to age. MVP may be characterized as anatomic or functional (syndrome). Anatomic MVP includes individuals with a broad range of valvular abnormalities corresponding to symptoms of progressive mitral valve regurgitation. MVP syndrome consists of MVP with various symptoms reflecting a neuroendocrine or an autonomic basis. Approximately 80% of patients with MVP experience MVP syndrome instead of anatomic MVP.

| BOX 18-2 | *Conditions Associated with Mitral Valve Prolapse* |

Connective Tissue Disorders: Genetic

- Mitral valve prolapse: isolated
- Marfan syndrome
- Ehlers-Danlos syndrome: types I and II, IV
- Pseudoxanthoma elasticum
- Osteogenesis imperfecta
- Polycystic kidneys

Other Genetic Disorders

- Duchenne's muscular dystrophy
- Myotonic dystrophy
- Fragile X syndrome
- Mucopolysaccharidoses

Acquired Collagen Vascular Disorders

- Systemic lupus erythematosus
- Relapsing polychondritis
- Rheumatic endocarditis
- Polyarteritis nodosa

Other Associated Disorders

- Atrial septal defect, secundum
- Hypertrophic obstructive cardiomyopathy
- Wolff-Parkinson-White syndrome
- Papillary muscle dysfunction
- Ischemic heart disease
- Myocarditis
- Cardiac trauma
- Post–mitral valve surgery
- von Willebrand's disease

From O'Rourke RA (ed): Current Problems in Cardiology, May 1991, p 333.

Anatomic MVP, inherited in an autosomal dominant manner, is believed to result from myxomatous degeneration of the mitral valve, elongation and thinning of the chordae tendineae, and the presence of redundant and excessive valve tissue. The posterior leaflet is affected more frequently than the anterior leaflet. Changes are often observed at the site of chordal insertion, leading to rupture of the chordae and tethering of the valve leaflet. The degenerative changes of the mitral valve that are responsible for progression from an asymptomatic condition with murmurs and systolic clicks to dyspnea with severe mitral regurgitation occur over an average of 25 years. With the onset of severe mitral regurgitation, PAH, left atrial enlargement, and atrial fibrillation frequently emerge. Subsequently, mitral valve repair or replacement is usually necessary within 1 year.[9]

MVP syndrome is the more benign form of MVP in that the mitral valve annulus and LV size are essentially responsible for abnormal coaptation of the mitral leaflets during systole. Mitral valve leaflets normally close just before ventricular systole, thus preventing regurgitation of blood into the LA. Normal mitral valve leaflets may billow slightly with closure; but in MVP, redundant mitral leaflets prolapse into the LA during mid-to-late systole as the ventricle is emptied. Superior arching of the mitral leaflets above the level of the atrioventricular ring is diagnostic for MVP. Distortion or malfunction of any of the component structures of the mitral valve may cause prolapse and generate audible clicks or regurgitation associated with a murmur. If the chordae tendineae are lengthened, the valves may billow even more and progress to prolapse when valve leaflets fail to appose each other.

Severe mitral regurgitation develops in 2% to 4% of patients with MVP, two thirds of whom are male. MVP is the most common cause of severe mitral regurgitation, and its onset signals the need for therapeutic intervention. Once dyspnea occurs secondary to mitral regurgitation, surgery is imminent. Mitral valve repair or replacement is effective and safe for mitral regurgitation due to MVP. Mitral valve repair is preferred for prolapse of a degenerative mitral posterior leaflet, but 10% of patients need mitral valve replacement instead. Mitral valve repair confers a significantly improved operative as well as 5- and 10-year survival compared with mitral valve replacement. Early repair is recommended to preserve LV function and reduce the likelihood of atrial fibrillation.

The association of arrhythmias and sudden death with MVP is a long-held observation. Premature atrial and ventricular beats, atrioventricular block, and supraventricular or ventricular tachyarrhythmias are common during ambulatory monitoring in adults with MVP. Mechanisms that have been proposed for arrhythmias include ventricular enlargement, hyperadrenergic states, electrolyte imbalances, and mechanical irritation of the ventricle due to traction of the chordae tendineae. Arrhythmias may be secondary to mitral regurgitation, not MVP. According to a study of individuals with nonischemic mitral regurgitation, complex arrhythmias were common and equally prevalent regardless of whether the patient had MVP. Ventricular tachycardia occurred in 35% of those subjects with mitral regurgitation, in contrast to only 5% of participants with MVP alone. Similarly, the risk of sudden death for patients with MVP may be related to mitral regurgitation in view of a reduction in ventricular arrhythmias that occurred with mitral valve repair or replacement.

Anesthetic Considerations

It is important to distinguish between MVP syndrome and anatomic MVP regarding anesthetic considerations. Most individuals with MVP have an uncomplicated general anesthetic because they have MVP syndrome. These patients are usually younger than 45 years of age with few risk factors for anesthesia. Invasive monitoring is usually unnecessary. Patients may be taking β-blockers. Preoperative sedation is useful to suppress an increased sensitivity to catecholamines. Painful stimuli may exacerbate the autonomic system, possibly causing arrhythmias. Significant decreases in LV end-diastolic volume and SVR, or increased contractility and tachycardia, should be avoided because MVP may be enhanced by decreasing CO and coronary perfusion. Intraoperative arrhythmias usually resolve spontaneously or respond to standard therapy. If an arrhythmia occurs, adequate oxygenation should be confirmed and other causes of intraoperative arrhythmias investigated. If β-blockers are required perioperatively, the use of esmolol avoids the potential for prolonged blockade that might cause hemodynamically significant bradycardia. Digoxin may worsen MVP.

Anticholinergic preoperative medications are best avoided despite an increased vagal tone. A moderate anesthetic depth is desirable to minimize catecholamine levels and potential arrhythmias. Ketamine or drugs that have sympathomimetic effects must be administered with caution. These patients with MVP syndrome have been shown to possess good LV function if mitral regurgitation or CAD is absent; myocardial depression from volatile agents will be well tolerated. Narcotics such as fentanyl block sympathetic responses and promote hemodynamic stability; however, prolonged postoperative respiratory depression is a disadvantage. Shorter-acting narcotics such as alfentanil and remifentanil, as well as other intravenous agents such as propofol, are available to facilitate rapid extubation. Hypercapnia, hypoxia, and electrolyte disturbances increase ventricular excitability and should be corrected. If muscle relaxation is desired, vecuronium is an excellent choice because it does not cause tachycardia.

Patients with anatomic MVP warrant a different anesthetic approach compared with those with MVP syndrome. Patients with anatomic MVP are often in CHF and generally require cardiac surgery and CPB. The severity of mitral regurgitation strongly influences anesthetic decisions. Routine monitoring for patients undergoing cardiac surgery should be provided. TEE is placed after induction. Opioid agents provide excellent hemodynamic stability without depressing myocardial function.

ACUTE PULMONARY EMBOLISM

Pulmonary embolism (PE) has an incidence in the United States of 1 per 1000 and a mortality rate of more than 15% at 3 months after diagnosis.[10] Approximately two thirds of deaths occur within the first hour of a PE, and many of the remaining occur within 4 to 6 hours. Because 5% of patients present in cardiogenic shock, treatment involves not only prevention of a recurrence but also hemodynamic support. Because a correct diagnosis can alter the outcome of PE measurably, it is unfortunate that 60% to 80% of cases of fatal PE in the hospital setting are clinically unsuspected.

Formation of thrombus involves stasis, activation of coagulation, and vascular injury. Asymptomatic venous thrombus, originating primarily from proximal deep veins, is the source of pulmonary emboli in 80% of patients with documented PE. The potent fibrinolytic capacity of the lung dissolves most emboli spontaneously, rendering them clinically silent. Although the likelihood of a genetic predisposition for venous thrombosis is now more evident, well-known risk factors for a clinically recognizable PE include advanced age, previous venous thromboembolism, prolonged immobility or paralysis, malignancy, CHF, use of oral contraceptives, obesity, prolonged mechanical ventilation, and surgery that involves extensive pelvic or abdominal dissection. Compared with community residents, hospitalized individuals are 100 times more likely to develop venous thromboembolism and PE. Immobility has been noted in more than 50% of patients within 3 months of a PE. In most cases, immobility after surgery was less than 2 weeks.

A diagnosis of PE has always been problematic. A high index of suspicion is necessary to diagnose PE because symptoms are so nonspecific. Dyspnea, pleuritic chest pain, and hemoptysis are characteristic of a mild PE. Dyspnea is the most common symptom, occurring in 73% of patients with PE, followed by pleuritic chest pain (66%) and hemoptysis (13%). Dyspnea, chest pain, or tachypnea occurs in 97% of documented cases. However, symptoms or signs of venous thrombosis in the lower extremities appear in fewer than 25% of patients with documented PE. Thirty percent of patients may be asymptomatic. Even if classic signs and symptoms are present, a subsequent pulmonary angiogram may be negative.

The most widely used technique to evaluate suspected PE is the technetium-xenon lung scan. As a cornerstone of diagnosis for PE, it is least affected by preexisting cardiac or pulmonary disease. A negative scan essentially eliminates a PE, and a high-probability scan has a positive predictability of 85%. A corroborating clinical history increases the predictive ability of a lung scan.

Pulmonary angiography is still the gold standard as it detects about 98% of all clinically significant PE. It may actually be underused because fewer than 15% of patients with nondiagnostic ventilation-perfusion scans undergo angiography.

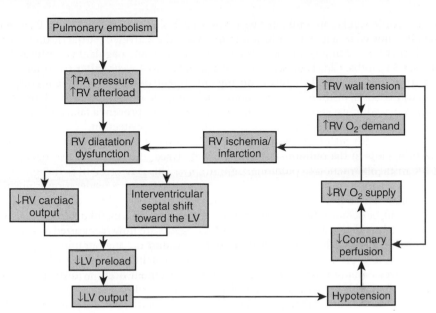

Figure 18-4 Pathophysiology of right ventricular dysfunction, ischemia, and infarction after acute pulmonary embolism. PA = pulmonary artery; RV = right ventricle; LV = left ventricle; O_2 = oxygen. (Reprinted with permission from Lualdi JC, Goldhaber SZ: Right ventricular dysfunction after acute pulmonary embolism: Pathophysiologic factors, detection, and therapeutic implications. Am Heart J 130:1276, 1995.)

Massive PE represents 5% of cardiac arrests, with more than 60% of those noted to be pulseless electrical activity. Symptoms include severe dyspnea, cyanosis, tachycardia, and elevated CVP. Massive PE is defined as 50% obstruction of pulmonary blood flow that usually leads to RV failure. On mechanical obstruction, humoral mediators are released, augmenting pulmonary vasoconstriction and PAH. This sudden increase in RV afterload results in RV dilation and dysfunction that displaces the interventricular septum, causing underfilling of the LV (Fig. 18-4). Low CO and severe hypotension follow, ultimately leading to circulatory collapse and death. Increased RV pressure also compresses the right coronary artery, causing RV ischemia and contributing to RV failure. Mortality is 40% to 80% within 2 hours of the onset of a PE.

Massive PE should be considered with the onset of unexplainable severe and sudden hypoxia and hypotension. The diagnosis is strengthened if LV function is relatively maintained in the midst of profound RV dysfunction. The differential diagnosis is cardiac tamponade, myocardial infarction, aortic dissection, and severe mitral regurgitation. Interventions that improve RV function should receive priority because they may greatly benefit the patient. Excessive fluid administration to correct hypotension must be avoided to prevent further RV dilation.

A major goal of treating PE is the prevention of new thrombi and death. Recurrence of PE is a major risk and is associated with a very high mortality. Frequently, the initial clot of a PE is small and symptoms are few or nonspecific, but a subsequent clot may significantly increase PVR and compromise hemodynamics without a clear warning. Prevention of recurrence may include one or more of the following: anticoagulation, thrombolysis, mechanical interruption (vena caval filters), and embolectomy.

Anticoagulation lessens morbidity, mortality, and recurrence of PE by addressing venous thromboembolism. In general, if a patient has a high-probability ventilation-perfusion scan and there is strong clinical suspicion, anticoagulation is begun. Anticoagulation is initiated with a heparin bolus of 10,000 to 20,000 U, immediately followed by a heparin infusion to maintain the activated partial thromboplastin time at 1.5 to 2 times control. Subsequently, an oral anticoagulant is continued for *at least* 3 months. Clot is present in most patients 1 to 4 weeks after treatment with anticoagulation alone. If PE recurs during anticoagulation, a continuing predisposition to PE exists, or there is a contraindication to anticoagulation, then a Greenfield filter is placed transvenously in the inferior vena cava to prevent a fatal embolus. It is effective in 98% of cases but does not provide absolute protection.

With the advent of fibrinolytic agents that convert circulating plasminogen to plasmin, clots in the pulmonary arteries can be lysed, thus removing or decreasing mechanical obstruction to pulmonary blood flow. This is referred to as thrombolytic therapy. There is no absolute indication for it with PE, but consideration is given if pulmonary blood flow is reduced by 40% to 50% with severe hypoxia or right-sided failure and/or deteriorating hemodynamics are present. Successful thrombolysis may reverse right-sided heart failure. Thrombolytic agents are now recognized as superior to heparin therapy alone for correcting defects found on angiographic and perfusion scans and for correcting hemodynamic abnormalities including RV dysfunction. Fewer complications and more rapid improvement occur with thrombolytic therapy than with heparin alone. There is also a reduced incidence of recurrent PE compared with heparin therapy, in part due to a resolution of the probable underlying venous thrombus and less RV hypokinesis. Nonetheless, anticoagulation with heparin should be started simultaneously with thrombolytic therapy.

Beyond thrombolysis, pulmonary embolectomy remains an option for massive PE if pharmacologic thrombolysis has been unsuccessful. Echocardiography is particularly valuable in the triage of patients to either thrombolysis, catheter embolectomy, or surgical embolectomy. As previously noted, RV function after PE is a major determinant of outcome, so aggressive efforts to reverse RV dysfunction should be pursued early after the onset of PE.

Anesthesia Considerations for Pulmonary Embolectomy and Pulmonary Embolism

The first surgical embolectomy without CPB was described by Trendelenburg in 1908, and the first with CPB was described by Cooley in 1961. Its frequency has decreased, partly due to the success of thrombolytic measures for massive PE; however, thrombolysis is unsuccessful in 15% to 30% of cases. Of 3000 patients with documented PE over a 20-year period, 3% underwent pulmonary embolectomy.[11] In general, it has been reserved for patients with PE and refractory circulatory compromise, failed medical management, or contraindications to thrombolysis. Contraindication to thrombolysis accounts for more than one third of embolectomies. The overall mortality of pulmonary embolectomy varies between 20% and 90%. The patient's preoperative status is predictive of survival. Preoperative cardiac arrest increases operative mortality by more than 50%. Age older than 60 years and a long history of dyspnea also increase the mortality of embolectomy. Echocardiography has greatly decreased the time to surgery by enabling a rapid and reliable diagnosis to be made without angiography. This has improved not only initial survival rate of embolectomy but also long-term survival.

Induction of anesthesia is a very hazardous period in the presence of PE and RV dysfunction that has precipitated cardiac arrest. Intraoperative monitoring should include an arterial catheter, ECG, pulse oximeter, capnograph, and CVP catheter or PA catheter. An inotrope may also be needed before induction. Individuals with massive PE have more of a "fixed" CO, which makes them extremely susceptible to decreases in volume and SVR. Cannulation of the femoral vessels under local anesthetic to initiate CPB may be advisable if the administration of anesthesia is judged too hazardous. Once the cannula is in place, positioning, skin cleansing, and draping should proceed while the patient is awake and breathing oxygen. After the patient is placed in a slightly head-down position to prevent venous pooling, an intravenous induction is performed. Anesthetic agents that increase PVR must be used cautiously in this setting. Ketamine is well known as an anesthetic agent for use in critically ill patients to maintain hemodynamics. Concerns about ketamine and increased PVR are unfounded if ventilation is maintained.

Embolectomy via right or left thoracotomy may be performed without CPB through venous inflow occlusion while clamping the proximal portion of the involved pulmonary artery to allow clot removal. Rapid institution of CPB by femoral cannulation percutaneously may be lifesaving in patients with cardiovascular collapse. If embolectomy is performed on CPB, the patient remains normothermic, the aorta is not cross-clamped, and cardioplegia is not administered. Maintenance of higher perfusion pressures reduces RV stunning. The CPB time is usually less than 30 minutes for embolectomy. Reperfusion bleeding may occur when reestablishment of pulmonary blood flow causes severely damaged capillaries of the pulmonary parenchyma to rupture. Large amounts of blood may be aspirated from the endotracheal tube (ETT). Large-bore intravenous catheters are necessary for embolectomy because rapid and massive blood loss can occur through reperfusion pulmonary hemorrhage.

PULMONARY ARTERY HYPERTENSION

Pulmonary artery hypertension, according to the 2004 WHO classification, is defined as a group of diseases characterized by virtually identical obstructive pathologic changes of the pulmonary microcirculation and by a favorable response to the long-term administration of prostacyclin.[12] The WHO classifies PAH into the following groups:

I: Primary PAH and PAH associated with such conditions as collagen vascular disease, portal hypertension, and left-to-right shunting
II: Pulmonary venous hypertension
III: Pulmonary disease with hypoxemia
IV: Thromboembolic disease
V: Miscellaneous

When no demonstrable cause for a sustained increase in PAP can be identified, the diagnosis is primary PAH. Regardless of the primary pathologic mechanisms, once PAH exists, the effects on the right heart and pulmonary arteries are similar.

Primary Pulmonary Hypertension

The essential characteristic of primary PAH is increased PVR that results in increased PAP, hypoxemia, elevated RV pressure, right-sided heart failure, and death. The National Institutes of Health registry's criteria for primary PAH include a PAP of more than 25 mmHg at rest or more than 30 mmHg with exercise and exclusion of the causes of secondary PAH. It is a rare disorder, occurring in one or two individuals per 1 million people per year, primarily women in their third decade. The diagnosis is often delayed an average of 2 years owing to the nonspecific nature of the symptoms.

18

Previously, even an early diagnosis yielded a median survival of 2.8 years. The introduction of intravenous epoprostenol (synthetic salt of prostacyclin) in the 1990s improved hemodynamics, functional capacity, and survival in patients with primary PAH in NYHA functional class III or IV. Treatment options have expanded as a new generation of drugs is being developed to address the pathologic arms of primary PAH.

Therapy for primary PAH is evolving but mostly remains empirical and nonspecific. Conventional therapy includes restricted activity, diuretics, anticoagulation, digoxin, and pulmonary vasodilators. For years, calcium channel blockers have been useful to lower PAP 10% to 20% if vasoreactivity testing was positive. Otherwise, they may precipitate right-sided heart failure and even death in those with primary PAH. Pulmonary vasodilators are administered to decrease PVR, PAP, and RV afterload. Many pulmonary vasodilators have been tried, with unreliable and short-term benefit. Continuous prostaglandin therapy was found to improve hemodynamics and exercise to tolerance and to prolong survival. Because prostaglandin therapy requires continuous intravenous administration to be efficacious, alternate forms have been created: oral (beraprost), subcutaneous (treprostinil), and inhaled (iloprost). Prostaglandin therapy contains valuable anti-inflammatory properties that represent treatment for PAH directed at the various pathologic mechanisms considered responsible for PAH besides pulmonary vasodilation. Newer agents targeting thromboxane inhibition (terbogrel) and endothelin-receptor antagonism (bosentan, sitaxsentan, and ambrisentan) have been developed. A new pulmonary vasodilator, sildenafil, may act synergistically with other vasodilators by inactivating the phosphodiesterase enzymes that inactivate the second messengers for the vasodilating signals cyclic adenosine monophosphate and cyclic guanosine monophosphate in lung tissues.

Secondary Pulmonary Hypertension

In most patients, PAH is secondary to cardiac or pulmonary disease. The term "secondary" PAH is being used less because of the many therapies for PAH regardless of etiology. Secondary PAH is more common than primary PAH. Often, the underlying disease overshadows the clinical manifestations of PAH. The natural history, prognosis, and appropriate treatment of patients with secondary PAH depend on the underlying condition. Secondary PAH may be reversible. Once the etiology of PAH is identified, treatment should begin immediately because it is most effective if instituted before the onset of right-sided heart failure. Unfortunately, at the time of diagnosis, PAH has often progressed to the point that the value of any treatment is limited to palliation of incapacitating symptoms.

Anesthetic management of individuals with PAH is challenging because perioperative increases in PVR readily occur and may provoke right-sided heart failure, resulting in death. The tolerance of the RV is a major concern. The RV is acutely sensitive to increases in PVR (afterload). Factors that increase PVR, such as hypoxia, acidosis, hypercapnia, hypothermia, and α-adrenergic stimulation, should be minimized. Furthermore, a decrease in blood pressure or increase in RV pressure impairs coronary perfusion of the right side of the heart. A PA catheter allows perioperative detection and monitoring of PVR and therapy, enabling hyperventilation to reduce PVR. In general, intravenous anesthetics have less effect on hypoxic pulmonary vasoconstriction, PVR, and oxygenation than do volatile agents. Nitrous oxide has been reported to increase PVR, but it is not contraindicated in these patients. Isoflurane may be beneficial by decreasing PAP and has been frequently used during noncardiac procedures. Fentanyl may be given as an adjunct or a primary anesthetic agent in these patients because it causes little myocardial depression and excellent circulatory stability.[13]

Pulmonary endarterectomy (PEA) is the accepted treatment today for chronic thromboembolic pulmonary hypertension. The operation is not an embolectomy but rather a true endarterectomy, removing the fibrosis obstructive tissue from the pulmonary arteries. Extracorporeal circulation and periods of circulatory arrest under deep hypothermia are essential for successful endarterectomy.[14]

PERICARDIAL HEART DISEASE

Anesthetic Considerations for Pericardial Disease

Pericardiectomy is performed for recurrent pericardial effusion and constrictive pericarditis. Pericardial dissection for effusive pericarditis is straightforward; however, pericardiectomy for constrictive pericarditis is a surgical challenge with a mortality of 5% to 15% and 5-year survival of 78%. Persistent low CO immediately after pericardiectomy is the primary cause of morbidity and mortality. In contrast to patients with cardiac tamponade, who usually improve clinically once the pericardium is opened, improvement is not always apparent initially after pericardiectomy. Instead, noticeable improvement in cardiac function may take weeks. Yet, 90% of patients ultimately experience relief of symptoms with surgery.

Median sternotomy provides excellent exposure and access for pericardiectomy, but thoracotomy in the left anterolateral position is also used. Opinions vary regarding the extent of pericardial resection for alleviation of cardiac constriction and the use of CPB. Good results have been obtained with and without CPB. Removal of adherent and scarred pericardium to release both the RV and LV involves extensive manipulation of the heart. Some have advocated routine CPB for pericardiectomy because a more complete pericardial excision and hemodynamic stability were thought possible. Yet, heparinization and CPB may exacerbate blood loss from exposed cardiac surfaces. Furthermore, prolonged CPB in debilitated patients contributes to early mortality associated with pericardiectomy.

Anesthetic goals for managing patients with constrictive pericarditis who require pericardiectomy include minimizing bradycardia and myocardial depression and minimizing decreases in afterload or preload. Monitoring considerations include arterial and central venous pressures. A dorsalis pedis or femoral arterial catheter in patients with uremic pericarditis may preserve future potential arteriovenous fistula sites in the upper extremities. One groin site should be reserved in case femoral cannulation is necessary to emergently initiate CPB. PA catheter monitoring is recommended due to the occurrence of postoperative low CO syndrome. Low CO, hypotension, and arrhythmias (atrial and ventricular) are common during chest dissection. Due to limited ventricular diastolic filling, CO is rate dependent. If myocardial function or heart rate is depressed, β-agonists or pacing improve CO. Lidocaine infusion may partially suppress arrhythmias during dissection. Catastrophic hemorrhage can occur suddenly if the atrium or ventricle is perforated, so sufficient venous access is necessary. Damage to coronary arteries may also occur during dissection; careful monitoring of the ECG for signs of ischemia is prudent. Pericardiectomy via left anterior thoracotomy requires close monitoring of oxygenation because the left lung is severely compressed during dissection. Anesthetic technique is based on achieving early extubation; however, patients who undergo pericardiectomy for constrictive pericarditis benefit from remaining intubated for at least 6 to 12 hours to assess bleeding and CO.

Cardiac Tamponade

Tamponade exists when fluid accumulation in the pericardial sac limits filling of the heart. Hemodynamic manifestations are mainly due to atrial rather than ventricular compression. Initially, with mild tamponade, diastolic filling is limited, causing reduced stroke volume that stimulates sympathetic reflexes to increase heart rate and contractility to maintain CO.[15] The rising RA pressure reflexly stimulates tachycardia and peripheral vasoconstriction. Blood pressure is supported by vasoconstriction, but CO begins to fall as pericardial fluid continues to increase. Subsequently, diastolic filling begins to disappear so the jugular venous pulse has no prominent Y-descent but a prominent X-descent. Eventually, the pericardial pressure-volume curve becomes almost vertical so any additional fluid greatly restricts cardiac filling and reduces diastolic compliance. Ultimately, the RA pressure, pulmonary artery diastolic pressure, and pulmonary capillary wedge pressure equilibrate. Equilibration of pressures (within 5 mmHg of each other) merits immediate action to rule out acute tamponade. Once the blood pressure begins to fall, it is a precipitous drop that reduces coronary artery blood flow, leading to ischemia, especially subendocardially.

The classic diagnostic triad of acute tamponade consists of (1) decreasing arterial pressure, (2) increasing venous pressure, and (3) a small, quiet heart. Pulsus paradoxus may be present; this is a fall in systolic blood pressure of more than 12 mmHg during inspiration caused by reduced LV stroke volume generated by increased filling of the right heart during inspiration. It is not specific for tamponade, because it may be present in patients with obstructive pulmonary disease, RV infarction, or constrictive pericarditis. It may be absent if there is LV dysfunction, positive-pressure breathing, atrial septal defect, or severe aortic regurgitation. ECG changes with tamponade include low-voltage QRS complex, electrical alternans, and T-wave abnormalities. Sinus rhythm is usually present in tamponade. Echocardiography is the most reliable noninvasive method to detect pericardial effusion and exclude tamponade; echocardiography usually reveals an exaggerated motion of the heart within the pericardial sac in conjunction with atrial and ventricular collapse. Additionally, echocardiography is used to guide needle or catheter aspiration of pericardial effusion.

After cardiac surgery, tamponade due to hemorrhage requires immediate mediastinal exploration to determine bleeding site and stabilize hemodynamics. The numerous causes of hypotension in the postoperative cardiac surgical patient make tamponade more difficult to diagnose. Persistent poor CO with increased and equalized RA and LA pressures strongly suggests tamponade, but classic signs are often missing in the postoperative cardiac surgical patient. Arterial hypotension, pulsus paradoxus, and raised jugular venous pressures were absent in one series of cardiac surgical patients by 30%, 40%, and 50%, respectively. Although echocardiography is capable of identifying the size of pericardial effusions postoperatively, it does not necessarily reflect its likelihood to cause tamponade. Late cardiac tamponade occurs in 0.1% to 6% of patients after cardiac surgery. A delay in diagnosis contributes greatly to mortality in late cardiac tamponade.

Pericardiocentesis is indicated for life-threatening cardiac tamponade in conjunction with a fluid infusion to maintain filling pressures. Hemodynamics improve immediately after pericardiocentesis. Although it does provide immediate relief of the symptoms of tamponade, definitive therapy requires drainage of the pericardial space. Major complications of pericardiocentesis include coronary laceration, cardiac puncture, and pneumothorax. Surgical management of pericardial tamponade includes subxiphoid pericardiotomy, pericardial window through a left anterior thoracotomy, and pericardiectomy.

Anesthesia Considerations for Cardiac Tamponade

Severe hypotension or cardiac arrest has followed induction of general anesthesia in patients with tamponade. The causes include further myocardial depression, sympatholysis, decreased venous return, and changes in heart rate. Resuscitation requires immediate drainage of pericardial fluid. Pericardiotomy via a subxiphoid incision with only local anesthetic infiltration or light sedation is an option. If intrapericardial injury is confirmed, general anesthesia can be induced after decompression of the pericardial space. Ketamine (0.5 mg/kg) and 100% oxygen have been used with local anesthetic infiltration of the preexisting sternotomy to drain severe pericardial tamponade. Spontaneous respiration instead of positive-pressure ventilation supports CO more effectively until tamponade is relieved. Volume expansion and correction of metabolic acidosis are mandatory. Catecholamine infusions or pacing may be used to avoid bradycardia.

CARDIAC SURGERY DURING PREGNANCY

The incidence of maternal cardiac disease in North America has decreased by nearly 50% in the past 25 years to 1.5% to 2%. Rheumatic heart disease accounts for nearly three fourths of it. Native valve disease and prosthetic valve dysfunction comprise most of the operations during pregnancy in addition to dissecting or traumatic rupture of the aorta, pulmonary embolism, closure of foramen ovale, and cardiac tumors representing only a small percentage of cases. Heart disease is the leading cause of maternal and fetal death during pregnancy. Nonpregnant women with well-compensated cardiac disease may acutely or gradually decompensate as cardiac demands increase during pregnancy. Delaying surgery until after delivery carries a higher maternal mortality than does proceeding with the operation. Extensive exposure to radiation may also limit therapeutic invasive catheterization procedures. If nonsurgical therapy is not possible or conflicts with fetal interests, cardiac surgery with CPB is the only option. Since 1958 when Leyse and associates described the first cardiac operation requiring CPB in a pregnant patient, maternal morbidity has fallen from 5% to less than 1.0%. Remarkably, pregnancy does not increase the risk of complications or mortality from cardiac surgical procedures for the mother but fetal mortality is high, ranging from 16% to 33%. CPB exposes the fetus to many undesirable effects that may have unpredictable consequences. Anesthetic management demands an appreciation for the cardiovascular changes of pregnancy and their impact on the corresponding heart disease and well-being of the fetus.

The nonphysiologic nature of CPB combines with the changes of pregnancy for an unpredictable response and tolerance by mother and fetus.[16] Initiation of CPB activates a whole-body inflammatory response, with multiple effects on coagulation, autoregulation, release of vasoactive substances, hemodilution, and other physiologic processes that may adversely affect the fetus and mother. Maternal blood pressure may fall immediately after or within 5 minutes of initiation of CPB, lowering placental perfusion secondary to low SVR, hemodilution, and release of vasoactive agents. Fetal heart rate variability is often lost and fetal bradycardia (<80 beats per minute) also may occur at this time. Because uterine blood flow is not autoregulated and relies on maternal blood flow, decreases in maternal blood pressure cause fetal hypoxia and bradycardia. Increasing CPB flows (>2.5 L/min/m^2) or perfusion pressure (>70 mmHg) will raise maternal blood flow and usually returns the heart rate to 120 beats per minute. A compensatory catecholamine-driven tachycardia (170 beats per minute) may ensue

18

that suggests an oxygen debt existed. Nonetheless, increasing CPB flow and mean arterial pressure does not always correct fetal bradycardia; if not, other causes must be considered. Problems with venous return or other mechanical aspects of extracorporeal circulation may also limit systemic flow, causing reduced placental perfusion. If acidosis persists throughout CPB, other factors may be responsible for it, such as maternal hypothermia, uterine contractions, or medications that are transferable to the fetus, rather than low maternal blood pressure. Monitoring the fetal heart rate is important to assess fetal viability and subsequent therapeutic initiatives. It partially reduces fetal mortality by early recognition of problems.

Hypothermia has been used for years in cardiac surgery. There are reports of fetal survival with maternal core temperatures of 23° to 25°C, and fetal survival is even documented after 37 minutes of hypothermic (19°C) circulatory arrest. However, when hypothermic versus normothermic CPB was examined retrospectively hypothermia was associated with an embryo-fetal mortality of 24% compared with 0% for normothermia. Maternal mortality was not influenced by differences in CPB temperature. Consequently, hypothermic CPB is no longer advocated. The fetus appears to maintain autoregulation of the heart rate with mild hypothermia, but most functions are reduced with severe hypothermia. Beyond the effect of hypothermia on acid-base status, coagulation, and arrhythmias, it may precipitate uterine contractions that limit placental perfusion and risk fetal ischemia. The explanation for hypothermia-induced contractions may be related to the severe dilution of CPB that lowers progesterone levels, thus activating uterine contractions. Contractions are more likely to occur at greater gestational age of the fetus. Accordingly, uterine monitoring is strongly recommended if CPB is required during pregnancy.

If uterine contractions should begin during CPB, it is vitally important for fetal survival to stop them. Treatment includes ethanol infusion, magnesium sulfate, terbutaline, or ritodrine. Many of these tocolytic agents have potential side effects and toxicities that can be especially detrimental to patients with heart disease, but tocolytic agents may be necessary if the contractions are associated with marked fetal decelerations indicative of severe oxygen deficit. Infants have died from protracted contractions. Prophylactic measures to prevent contractions, such as progesterone, have been of indeterminate benefit.

RENAL INSUFFICIENCY AND CARDIAC SURGERY

The number of individuals with chronic renal failure (CRF) undergoing cardiac surgery has increased to 2% to 3% of the cardiac surgical population. These patients with CRF may not necessarily be dialysis dependent before surgery but are more likely to develop worsening renal function after CPB than are those with normal preoperative renal function. Morbidity and mortality are especially high in long-term dialysis patients undergoing cardiac surgery and CPB. Regardless of whether the CRF patient is dialysis dependent, the patient is a significant anesthetic challenge, especially in regard to fluid management, electrolyte status, and hemostasis. The capacity to avoid dialysis in the non–dialysis-dependent CRF patient is even more important in regard to long-term mortality. A collaborative effort by cardiac surgeon, anesthesiologist, nephrologist, and cardiologist is instrumental in the care of these patients. Unfortunately, long-term survival is still appreciably diminished even with minimal perioperative morbidity.

Patients with CRF are more prone to fluid overload, hyponatremia, hyperkalemia, and metabolic acidosis. Optimal hemodynamic and fluid status before surgery is important. Hemodialysis should be strongly considered the day before surgery, especially in those who are strictly dialysis dependent. Chronic dialysis patients tend to arrive for surgery with worsened LV function, possibly from inefficient waste and toxin removal. CHF can occur as a result of hypervolemia and poor cardiac function, manifesting as pulmonary edema and respiratory distress. Dialysis and medical therapy directed at improving cardiac function may be required to correct this before surgery. Chronic medications should be carefully reviewed to ensure that antihypertensive agents were given. The importance of preoperative preparation for patients with CRF is evident by the significantly higher mortality associated with urgent surgery.

Beyond the increased perioperative mortality of patients with CRF undergoing cardiac surgery, several factors further increase mortality. A preoperative creatinine value of 2.5 mg/dL increases the mortality even in those patients with non–dialysis-dependent CRF. Late mortality may range from 8.3% to 55% if dialysis is ongoing for more than 60 months. Pulmonary dysfunction also increases the perioperative mortality of CRF patients.

Patients with CRF differ from those with normal renal function in a variety of ways that influence anesthesia management. A normochromic, normocytic anemia is common, primarily due to decreased or absent erythropoietin secretion, because the kidney is the predominant source of erythropoietin. Anemia is now treated with recombinant human erythropoietin therapy instead of blood. The cardiovascular benefits are especially noticeable with correction of anemia. However, treatment is costly and requires multiple injections weeks before surgery, which may not be possible in many cases.

Anesthesia Considerations

CRF affects dosing of medications that have a large volume of distribution. Decreased serum protein concentration diminishes plasma binding, leading to higher levels of free drug to bind with receptors. Many patients with CRF are hypoalbuminemic. In general, anesthetic induction agents and benzodiazepines are safe to use in patients with CRF. A common induction agent, thiopental, is highly protein bound so the dose should be reduced accordingly. Medications that rely totally on renal excretion have a limited role. Fentanyl and sufentanil may be more effective for pain management because excretion is not as renally dependent as morphine sulfate. Currently used volatile anesthetic agents rarely cause any additional renal dysfunction even with underlying CRF unless severely prolonged duration of anesthesia occurs. Muscle relaxants and agents for antagonism of muscle paralysis have varying degrees of renal excretion.

A rapid-sequence induction with cricoid pressure is recommended in those with CRF in response to the likelihood of delayed gastric emptying. Significant extracellular volume contraction may also be present before induction of anesthesia due to a 6- to 8-hour fast before surgery and dialysis within 24 hours of surgery that may lead to hypotension on induction. Because fluid requirements are usually significant with CPB, a PA catheter is especially useful to manage fluid requirements. TEE may complement fluid management by assessment of LV volume and function. Before the initiation of CPB, fluid administration should be limited, especially if the patient is dialysis dependent. Otherwise, fluid should be given to maintain adequate urine output but avoid excessive cardiovascular filling pressures risking pulmonary edema. However, restricting fluids too aggressively in these patients may lead to acute renal failure superimposed on CRF. Low-dose dopamine has been recommended for patients with CRF, but its value is

18

indeterminate. Fenoldopam, a new dopamine-1-receptor agonist, may reduce the incidence of renal dysfunction in patients with multiple risk factors for renal failure undergoing CPB. Patients with preoperative creatinine levels above 1.5 mg/dL were given renal-dose dopamine or fenoldopam perioperatively.[17] Postoperative parameters were only improved in those receiving fenoldopam, suggesting a renal protective effect.

In general, CRF worsens after CPB in part owing to a combination of nonpulsatile flow, low renal perfusion, and hypothermia. Renal perfusion is lowered as CPB is initiated, increasing the chance for ischemia of the renal cortex. Mean arterial pressure should be kept above 80 mmHg. The stress of surgery and hypothermia may impair autoregulation so that renal vasoconstriction reduces renal blood flow. The fluid required to initiate CPB may significantly reduce the hemoglobin (Hb) and oxygen-carrying capacity in view of the preexisting anemia of CRF without the addition of red blood cells (RBCs) to the priming volume or immediately on initiation of CPB. A hematocrit of 25% should be maintained during CPB. Washed RBCs are recommended for RBC transfusion to lessen excessive potassium and glucose levels intraoperatively. Potassium plasma levels should be checked periodically. Mannitol and furosemide may prevent early oliguric renal failure. Patients with CRF often have glucose intolerance from an abnormal insulin response, so more frequent determination of serum glucose levels is advisable.

The anephric patient poorly tolerates post-CPB hypervolemia that often follows prolonged duration of CPB. Dialysis can be performed during CPB and is technically easy and effective because small molecules (uremic solutes, electrolytes) are removed. Instead of dialysis during CPB, hemofiltration (ultrafiltration) is more frequently performed, effectively clearing excess water without the hemodynamic instability of dialysis. Circulating blood passes through the hollow fibers of the hemoconcentrators that have a smaller pore size than albumin (55,000 Da), which remove water and solutes. These midsize molecules (inflammatory molecules) are small enough to pass through the pores to concentrate the blood. Potassium is eliminated, helping reduce excessive potassium concentration commonly associated with cardioplegia administration. Hemofiltration during CPB may not achieve a net reduction in the overall total fluid balance of the patient, in part because a minimum volume of fluid must be maintained in the venous reservoir of the extracorporeal circuit.

Excessive bleeding after CPB is not uncommon in those with CRF, in part due to preoperative platelet dysfunction. Antifibrinolytic medications are pharmacologic measures used to successfully reduce excessive bleeding and transfusion requirements associated with cardiac surgery. Tranexamic acid, an inexpensive, synthetic antifibrinolytic, is excreted primarily through the kidneys, so a dose reduction is required based on the preoperative creatinine level. Aprotinin, a serine protease inhibitor with anti-inflammatory as well as antifibrinolytic properties, is concentrated in the proximal renal tubules and leads to a clinically important increase in the postoperative creatinine levels. If renal insufficiency without dialysis dependence is present with a corresponding serum creatinine level greater than 2.5 mg/dL, aprotinin is contraindicated.

HEMATOLOGIC PROBLEMS IN PATIENTS UNDERGOING CARDIAC SURGERY

Anesthetic concerns for patients with hematologic problems who undergo cardiac surgery are further complicated by the stress CPB places on coagulation and oxygen-carrying systems. Hemophilia, cold agglutinins, sickle cell disease, antithrombin deficiency, and von Willebrand's disease are a few of the hematologic disorders that may require special consideration if CPB is needed.

Antithrombin

Antithrombin (AT) and protein C are two primary inhibitors of coagulation. A delicate balance exists between the procoagulant system and the inhibitors of coagulation. AT is the most abundant and important of the coagulation pathway inhibitors. Deficiencies of AT increase the risk of thromboembolism and impact patients requiring CPB.

AT or AT III is an α_2-globulin that is produced primarily in the liver. It binds thrombin, as well as other serine proteases, factors IX, X, XI, and XII, kallikrein, and plasmin, irreversibly, which neutralizes their activity. However, only inhibition of thrombin and factor Xa by AT has physiologic and clinical significance. AT activity of less than 50% is clinically important. AT deficiency may occur as a congenital deficiency or as an acquired deficiency secondary to increased AT consumption, loss of AT from the intravascular compartment (renal failure, nephrotic syndrome), or liver disease (cirrhosis). Acquired deficiency is often associated with trauma, sepsis, and shock. Although AT deficiency may be acquired, cause and effect are difficult to prove because many factors may exist simultaneously to account for abnormal clotting.

Anticoagulation for CPB depends on AT to inhibit clotting because heparin alone has no effect on coagulation. Heparin catalyzes AT inhibition of thrombin by binding to a lysine residue on AT and altering its conformation. Thrombin actually attacks AT, disabling it, but in the process attaches AT to thrombin, forming the AT and thrombin complex. This complex has no activity and is rapidly removed. Thirty percent of AT is consumed during this process, so AT levels are reduced. AT deficiency may occur with cardiac and noncardiac operations. The "adequacy" of anticoagulation with heparin may be monitored with the activated coagulation time (ACT). If an individual has a reduced response to heparin, it is referred to as heparin resistance, which can lead to thrombus formation and serious complications.

Heparin exposure before CPB is increasingly common in cardiac surgical practice today, resulting in more cases of heparin resistance. The incidence varies among hospitals, but in 2270 cardiac cases, 3.7% were identified as heparin resistant. Although 50% more heparin may be required with heparin resistance, 30% of patients do not reach adequate ACT values despite having received 800 U/kg of heparin. Heparin anticoagulation for CPB causes further lowering of AT levels that were most likely low before surgery. AT activity falls an additional 25% to 50% with initiation of CPB, in part owing to dilution and elimination of the AT and thrombin complex. AT-deficient patients are at risk for major thrombosis if exposed to CPB, and clotting has been reported. Therefore, AT-deficient patients who require CPB should be treated aggressively. Once AT levels reach more than 80%, thrombosis is less likely. Postoperatively, AT levels continue to decline at a rate dependent on the extent of tissue disruption and hemorrhage. The nadir occurs on the third day and preoperative levels return by the fifth day.

Various blood products have been tried as an alternative to fresh frozen plasma (FFP) to rapidly raise the AT level. Cryoprecipitate and FFP have similar amounts of AT, but the infectious risk is greater for cryoprecipitate. AT concentrate preparations are derived from human plasma pools but are subjected to fractionation procedures and heating to inactivate viral contaminants. This process does not reduce biologic activity and viral transmission has not been reported. One bottle of AT contains approximately 500 units or the equivalent of 2 units of FFP and can be safely administered over 10 to 20 minutes. The baseline AT activity of the heparin-resistant patients was 56 ± 25%, which improved to 75 ± 31% after administration of AT concentrate.[18]

Cold Agglutinins

Cold agglutinins (CAs) are common but rarely clinically important. CAs form a complement antigen-antibody reaction on the surface of the RBC membrane that causes lysis. The degree of hemolysis is related to the circulating titer and thermal amplitude of the CAs. Thermal amplitude, the blood temperature below which the CAs react, is the key factor influencing clinical relevance. The titer and thermal amplitude are determined at various temperatures in the serum by an indirect hemagglutination test. Most people have cold autoantibodies that react at 4°C but in very low titers. Accelerated destruction of RBCs primarily occurs if the thermal amplitude is above 30°C. The higher is the thermal amplitude of the CAs, the more pathologic. Pathologic cold autoantibodies also have much higher titers at 30°C. However, thermal amplitude is more important than titer. With pathologic CAs, vascular occlusion occurs due to RBC clumping, injuring the myocardium, liver, and kidney. Microscopic RBC clumping may erroneously be attributed to other causes during hypothermic CPB unless agglutination is observed. Increasing temperature rapidly inactivates CAs.

Blood banks routinely screen for the presence of autoantibodies at 37°C, but cold antibodies, only reactive at lower temperatures, are not detected. The significance of CAs is determined by evaluating agglutination of RBCs in 20°C saline and 30°C albumin. If there is no agglutination, significant hemolysis is unlikely. Before initiation of CPB, the titer and thermal amplitude of CAs must be determined to avoid a temperature during CPB that would cause hemolysis. Intraoperatively, low-thermal-amplitude CAs can be determined by mixing cold cardioplegia with some of the patient's blood to check for separation of cells. If there is concern about CAs after routine testing, the sample can also be diluted to simulate CPB, cooled, and inspected for RBC agglutination. The hemodilution commonly associated with CPB may weaken agglutination and hemolysis in a patient with high reactivity and titer of CAs exposed to hypothermia.

The actions of CA may be difficult to diagnose because there are many other causes for hemolysis with CPB, so some cardiac surgeons avoid hypothermia if CAs are suspected or identified preoperatively. Despite normothermic CPB, cold cardioplegia may cause RBC agglutination in small myocardial vessels. Nevertheless, hypothermic myocardial protection has been used successfully in patients with CAs. A review of 832 patients scheduled to undergo surgery and CPB identified only seven cases of CAs that were strongly positive at 4°C. The authors concluded that asymptomatic patients with nonspecific, low-titer, and low-thermal-amplitude CAs may undergo hypothermia and CPB without serious detectable sequelae. However, the possibility of subtle end-organ damage exists.

If hypothermic CPB is necessary despite the presence of CAs, the choices are preoperative plasmapheresis, standard hemodilution, and maintenance of CPB temperature above the CA thermal amplitude.[19] Cold cardioplegia may be used without first undergoing plasmapheresis if normothermic CPB is used and 37°C cardioplegic solution is injected before administration of 4°C cardioplegic solution, clearing all potentially reactive cells. The risk of hemolysis is still high in patients with high-thermal-amplitude CAs. If CAs are particularly malignant, all of the patient's blood from the venous reservoir is drained and discarded. It is replaced entirely by donor blood, unfortunately exposing the patient to allogeneic blood products. Today, normothermic CPB and antegrade or retrograde warm blood cardioplegia may be the best option. If CAs should go undetected, postoperative end-organ damage or low CO may occur. Subsequently, plasma exchange, corticosteroids, elevated urine output, and maintenance of a good CO are the best treatments.

SUMMARY

- Carcinoid heart disease is a very serious condition that requires cardiac surgery. Optimal anesthetic management continues to evolve.
- In 1995, the World Health Organization/International Society of Cardiology redefined the cardiomyopathies.
- The emergence of technology to better diagnose pulmonary embolism and of echocardiography to assess the risk of mortality during acute pulmonary embolism continues to improve the treatment and management from both medical and surgical aspects.
- The introduction of intravenous epoprostenol (synthetic salt of prostacyclin) in the 1990s improved hemodynamics, functional capacity, and survival in patients with primary pulmonary hypertension, as have treatment options that include a new generation of drugs developed to address the pathologic arms of primary pulmonary hypertension.
- The definitive approach to a patient with both carotid and coronary artery disease requires a large multicenter, randomized trial.
- Heart disease continues to be the leading cause of maternal and fetal death during pregnancy.
- Individuals with chronic renal failure, not necessarily dialysis dependent, are more frequently undergoing cardiac surgery and are likely to develop worsening renal function after cardiopulmonary bypass.
- Anesthetic concerns for patients with hematologic problems who undergo cardiac surgery are further complicated by the stress that cardiopulmonary bypass places on coagulation and oxygen-carrying systems, and special considerations and techniques are required.

REFERENCES

1. Bakaeen FG, Reardon MJ, Coselli JS, et al: Surgical outcome in 85 patients with primary cardiac tumors. Am J Surg 186:641, 2003
2. Amano J, Kono T, Wada Y, et al: Cardiac myxoma: Its origin and tumor characteristics. Ann Thorac Cardiovasc Surg 9:215, 2003
3. Weingarten TN, Abel MD, Connolly HM, et al: Anesthetic management for cardiac surgery in carcinoid heart disease: A review of 84 patients. Anesth Analg 96:SCA 138, 2003
4. Tang WH, Francis GS: Novel pharmacological treatments for heart failure. Exp Opin Investig Drugs 12:1791, 2003
5. Maron BJ, McKenna WJ, Danielson GK, et al: American College of Cardiology/European Society of Cardiology clinical expert consensus document on hypertrophic cardiomyopathy. A report of the American College of Cardiology Foundation Task Force on Clinical Expert Consensus Documents and the European Society of Cardiology Committee for Practice Guidelines. J Am Coll Cardiol 42:1687, 2003
6. Roberts R, Sigwart U: New concepts in hypertrophic cardiomyopathies: II. Circulation 104:2249, 2001
7. Chatterjee K, Alpert J: Constrictive pericarditis and restrictive cardiomyopathy: Similarities and differences. Heart Failure Monit 3:118, 2003
8. Fontaine G, Gallais Y, Fornes P, et al: Arrhythmogenic right ventricular dysplasia/cardiomyopathy. Anesthesiology 95:250, 2001
9. Hanson EW, Neerhut RK, Lynch C 3rd: Mitral valve prolapse. Anesthesiology 85:178, 1996
10. Goldhaber SZ, Elliott CG: Acute pulmonary embolism: I. Epidemiology, pathophysiology, and diagnosis. Circulation 108:2726, 2003
11. Aklog L, Williams CS, Byrne JG, et al: Acute pulmonary embolectomy: A contemporary approach. Circulation 105:1416, 2002

18

12. Simonneau G, Galie N, Rubin LJ, et al: Clinical classification of pulmonary hypertension. J Am Coll Cardiol 43(suppl S):55, 2004
13. Fischer LG, Van Aken H, Burkle H: Management of pulmonary hypertension: Physiological and pharmacological considerations for anesthesiologists. Anesth Analg 96:1603, 2003
14. Manecke GR, Wilson W, Auger WR, et al: Anesthesia for pulmonary thromboendarterectomy. Semin Cardiothorac Vasc Anesth 9:189-204, 2005
15. Maisch B, Ristic AD: The classification of pericardial disease in the age of modern medicine. Curr Cardiol Rep 4:13, 2002
16. Mahli A, Izdes S, Coskun D: Cardiac operations during pregnancy: Review of factors influencing fetal outcome. Ann Thorac Surg 69:1622, 2000
17. Landoni G, Zoccai G, Marino G, et al: Fenoldopam reduces the need for renal replacement therapy and in-hospital death in cardiovascular surgery: A meta-analysis. J Cardiothorac Vasc Anesth 22:27, 2008
18. Lemmer JH Jr, Despotis GJ: Antithrombin III concentrate to treat heparin resistance in patients undergoing cardiac surgery, J Thorac Cardiovasc Surg 123:213, 2002
19. Agarwal SK, Ghosh PK, Gupta D: Cardiac surgery and cold-reactive proteins. Ann Thorac Surg 60:1143, 1995

IV

Chapter 19

Cardiac Pacing and Defibrillation

Marc A. Rozner, MD • Mark Trankina, MD

PACEMAKERS

Battery-operated, implantable pacing devices were first introduced in 1958, just 4 years after the invention of the transistor. The complexity, calculation, and data storage abilities of these devices have grown in a manner similar to that seen within the computer industry. The natural progression of pacemaker developments led to the invention of the implanted cardioverter-defibrillator (ICD) around 1980. As this technology has advanced, the divisions between these devices have become less clear. For example, every ICD currently implanted has anti-bradycardia pacing capability, and patients, news media, and even physicians often misidentify an implanted defibrillator as a pacemaker. The consequence of mistaking an ICD for a conventional pacemaker can lead to patient harm, either due to electromagnetic interference (EMI) issues resulting in inappropriate ICD therapy or the unintentional disabling of ICD therapies in some ICDs that can be permanently disabled by magnet placement. Figure 19-1 shows a three-lead defibrillation system and identifies the right ventricular shock coil, which differentiates an ICD system from a conventional pacemaking system. The complexity of cardiac pulse generators, as well as the multitude of programmable parameters, limits the number of sweeping generalizations that can be made about the perioperative care of the patient with an implanted pulse generator. Population aging, continued enhancements in implantable technology, and new indications for implantation will lead to growing

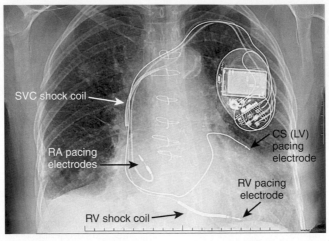

Figure 19-1 A defibrillator system with biventricular (BiV) anti-bradycardia pacemaker capability. Note that three leads are placed: a conventional, bipolar lead to the right atrium, a tripolar lead to the right ventricle (RV), and a unipolar lead to the coronary sinus (CS). This system is designed to provide "resynchronization biventricular-pacing therapy" in the setting of a dilated cardiomyopathy with a prolonged QRS (and frequently with a prolonged PR interval as well). The bipolar lead in the right atrium performs both sensing and pacing function. In the RV, the tip electrode functions as the cathode for pacing and sensing functions. The presence of a "shock" conductor (termed *shock coil*) on the RV lead in the RV distinguishes a defibrillation system from a conventional pacemaking system. In this particular patient, the RV shock coil also functions as the pacing and sensing anode (this is called an *integrated bipolar defibrillator lead*; true bipolar leads have a ring electrode between the tip electrode and the shock coil). The lead in the CS depolarizes the left ventricle, and the typical current pathway includes the anode in the right ventricle. Because of the typically wide QRS complex in a left bundle-branch pattern, failure to capture the left ventricle can lead to ventricular oversensing (and inappropriate anti-tachycardia therapy) in an implanted cardioverter-defibrillator (ICD) system. Many defibrillation systems also have a shock coil in the superior vena cava, which is electrically identical to the defibrillator case (called the "can"). When the defibrillation circuit includes the ICD case, it is called "active can configuration." Incidental findings on this chest radiograph include the presence of sternal wires from prior sternotomy and the lung carcinoma seen in the right upper lobe.

IV

numbers of patients with these devices. Both the American College of Cardiology (ACC) and the North American Society for Pacing and Electrophysiology-The Heart Rhythm Society (HRS-NASPE)* have taken note of these issues, and guidelines have been published regarding the care of the perioperative patient with such a device.[1] The American Society of Anesthesiology (ASA) has issued a practice advisory.[2]

Pacemaker Overview

Pacemaker manufacturers (more than 26 companies) have produced over 2000 models to date. More than 220,000 adults and children in the United States undergo new pacemaker placement each year, and nearly 3 million patients have pacemakers today. Many factors can lead to confusion regarding the behavior of a device and the perioperative care of a patient with a device.[3] An understanding of pulse generators and their likely idiosyncrasies in the operating or procedure room is needed. Whether the patient with a pacemaker is at increased perioperative risk remains unknown, but

---

*The North American Society of Pacing and Electrophysiology changed its name to the Heart Rhythm Society. In order to avoid confusion in this chapter, the abbreviation HRS-NASPE is used.

Table 19-1 NASPE/BPEG Revised (2002) Generic Paemaker Code (NBG)

Position I Pacing Chamber(s)	Position II Sensing Chamber(s)	Position III Response(s) to Sensing	Position IV Programmability	Position V Multisite Pacing
O = None	O = None	O = None	O = None	O = None
A = Atrium	A = Atrium	I = Inhibited	R = Rate Modulation	A = Atrium
V = Ventricle	V = Ventricle	T = Triggered		V = Ventricle
D = Dual (A + V)	D = Dual (A + V)	D = Dual (T + I)		D = Dual (A + V)

BOX 19-1 *Pacemaker Indications*

- Symptomatic sinus node disease
- Symptomatic atrioventricular node disease
- Long QT syndrome
- Hypertrophic obstructive cardiomyopathy*
- Dilated cardiomyopathy*

*See text and Pacemaker Programming for special precautions.

---

reports suggest that these patients deserve extra perioperative attention. No discussion of pacemakers can take place without an understanding of the generic pacemaker code, which has been published by the HRS-NASPE and The British Pacing and Electrophysiology Group (BPEG). This code, initially published in 1983, was revised in February 2002. Shown in Table 19-1, the code (NBG) describes the basic behavior of the pacing device.[4]

Pacemaker Indications

Indications for permanent pacing are shown in Box 19-1. Devices have also been approved by the U.S. Food and Drug Administration (FDA) for three-chamber pacing (right atrium, both ventricles) to treat dilated cardiomyopathy (DCM) (also called biventricular pacing [Bi-V] or cardiac resynchronization therapy [CRT]).[5] Also, specially programmed devices are used to treat hypertrophic cardiomyopathy (HCM) in both adults and children. Bi-V and HCM indications require careful attention to pacemaker programming, because effective pacing in these patients often requires a pacing rate greater than native sinus or junctional escape rate (often accomplished with drugs) and an atrioventricular (AV) delay shorter than the native PR interval so that the ventricle is paced 100% of the time. Inhibition or loss of pacing (e.g., from native conduction, atrial irregularity, ventricular irregularity, development of junctional rhythm, or EMI) can lead to deteriorating hemodynamics in these patients. Bi-V pacing can lengthen the QT interval in some patients, producing torsades de pointes.

BOX 19-2 *Pacemaker Magnet Behavior*

- No apparent rhythm or rate change
- No magnet sensor (some pre-1985 Cordis, Telectronics models)
- Magnet mode disabled (possible with CPI, Pacesetter, Telectronics, Vitatron models)
- EGM mode enabled (CPI, others)
- Program rate pacing in already paced patient (many CPI, Intermedics, Telectronics, Vitatron, others)
- Improper monitor settings (pace filter on)
- Brief (10 to 100 beats) asynchronous pacing, then return to program values (most Intermedics, some Biotronik models)
- Continuous or transient loss of pacing
- Discharged battery (some pre-1990 devices)
- Pacer enters diagnostic "Threshold Test Mode" (some Siemens, Intermedics, Medtronic, others)
- Asynchronous pacing without rate responsiveness using parameters possibly not in patient's best interest

*See text and Pacemaker Programming for special precautions.

Pacemaker Magnets

Despite often-repeated folklore, most pacemaker manufacturers warn that magnets were never intended to treat pacemaker emergencies or prevent EMI effects. Rather, magnet-activated switches were incorporated to produce pacing behavior that demonstrates remaining battery life and, sometimes, pacing threshold safety factors. Some pacemakers also demonstrate the detection of a problem during a telephone check, which should result in a call from the telephone center to the patient's pacemaker physician.

Placement of a magnet over a generator might produce no change in pacing because NOT ALL PACEMAKERS SWITCH TO A CONTINUOUS ASYNCHRONOUS MODE WHEN A MAGNET IS PLACED. Also, not all models from a given company behave the same way. Although most pacemakers have "high-rate" (80 to 100 beats per minute) asynchronous pacing with a magnet some still switch to asynchronous pacing at program rate, and some will respond with a brief (10 to 64 beats) asynchronous pacing event before reverting to original programmed behavior. Possible effects of magnet placement are shown in Box 19-2. In some devices, magnet behavior can be altered via programming. Also, any pacemaker from CPI-Guidant ignores magnet placement after any electrical reset, which is a possibility in the presence of strong EMI. For all generators, calling the manufacturer remains the most reliable method for determining magnet response and using this response to predict remaining battery life. For generators with programmable magnet behavior (Biotronik, CPI-Guidant, Pacesetter, and St. Jude Medical), only an interrogation with a programmer can reveal current settings. Most manufacturers publish a reference guide, although not all of these guides list all magnet idiosyncrasies. A telephone call can also alert the clinician to any recalls or alerts, which are not uncommon with these devices.

PREANESTHETIC EVALUATION AND PACEMAKER REPROGRAMMING

Preoperative management of the patient with a pacemaker includes evaluation and optimization of coexisting disease(s). No special laboratory tests or radiographs (chest radiographs are remarkably insensitive for determination of lead problems) are needed

> **BOX 19-3** *Preanesthetic Pulse Generator (Pacemaker, Implanted Cardioverter-Defibrillator) Evaluation*
>
> - Determine the indication for and date of initial device placement.
> - Identify the number and types of leads.
> - Determine the last generator test date and battery status.
> - Obtain a history of generator events (if any).
> - Obtain the current program information (device interrogation).
> - Ensure that pacing discharges become mechanical systoles with adequate safety margins.
> - Ensure that magnet detection is enabled if magnet use is planned.
> - Determine whether the pacing mode should be reprogrammed.
> - Determine if any recalls or alerts have been published.

for the patient with a pacemaker. Such testing should be dictated by the patient's underlying disease(s), medication(s), and planned intervention. For programmable devices, interrogation with a programmer remains the only reliable method for evaluating lead performance and obtaining current program information. A chest radiograph might be useful to document the position of the coronary sinus (CS) lead in a patient with a Bi-V pacemaker or defibrillator, especially if central venous catheter placement is planned, because spontaneous CS lead dislodgment was found in more than 11% of patients in early studies. A chest radiograph is certainly indicated for the patient with a device problem discovered during his or her pacemaker evaluation.

The prudent anesthesiologist reviews the patient's pacemaker history and follow-up schedule. Under the name NASPE, the HRS has published a consensus statement suggesting that pacemakers should be routinely evaluated with telephone checks for battery condition at least every 3 months. NASPE also recommends a comprehensive evaluation (interrogation) at least once per year. There are additional checks for devices implanted less than 6 or more than 48 (dual-chamber) or 72 (single-chamber) months. Rozner and associates reported a 2-year retrospective review of follow-up intervals in patients who presented for an anesthetic, and they found that more than 32% of 172 patients presenting for an anesthetic at their hospital did not meet the HRS-NASPE guideline for comprehensive evaluation.[6] They also reported that 5% of the patients presented for their anesthetic with a pacemaker in need of replacement for battery depletion and that nearly 10% of patients had less-than-optimal pacing settings. Note that a recent, preoperative interrogation is now part of the ASA Pacemaker Advisory and the ACC guidelines.[1,2]

Important features of the preanesthetic device evaluation are shown in Box 19-3. Determining dependency on the pacemaker function might require temporary reprogramming to a VVI mode with a low rate. In patients from countries where pacemakers might be reused, battery performance might not be related to length of implantation in the current patient. It should also be noted that in a registry of 345 pacemaker generator failures, 7% of failures were not related to battery depletion.[7]

Appropriate reprogramming (Box 19-4) might be the safest way to avoid intraoperative problems, especially if monopolar "Bovie" electrocautery will be used. For lithotripsy, consideration should be given to programming the pacing function out of an atrial-paced mode, because some lithotriptors are designed to fire on the R wave and the atrial pacing stimulus could be misinterpreted as the contraction of the ventricle. All of the manufacturers stand ready to assist with this task. Reprogramming a pacemaker to asynchronous pacing at a rate greater than the patient's underlying rate usually ensures that no oversensing or undersensing during EMI will take place, thus protecting the patient. Reprogramming a device *will not* protect it from internal damage or reset caused by EMI.

19

> ### BOX 19-4 *Pacemaker Reprogramming Probably Needed*
>
> - Any rate-responsive device: see text (problems are well known, problems have been misinterpreted with potential for patient injury, and the U.S. FDA has issued an alert regarding devices with minute ventilation sensors).
> - Special pacing indication (hypertrophic obstructive cardiomyopathy, dilated cardiomyopathy, pediatric patient)
> - Pacemaker-dependent patient
> - Major procedure in the chest or abdomen
> - Special procedures (see Box 19-5)

Experts do not agree on the appropriate reprogramming for the pacemaker-dependent patient. Setting a device to asynchronous mode to prevent inappropriate oversensing and ventricular output suppression can cause the pacemaker to ignore premature atrial or ventricular systoles, which could have the potential to create a malignant rhythm in the patient with significant structural compromise of the myocardium. Reviews demonstrate inappropriate R-on-T pacing with the development of a malignant ventricular rhythm.

In general, rate responsiveness and other "enhancements" (hysteresis, sleep rate, AV search, etc.) should be disabled by programming. Note that for many CPI devices, the Guidant Corporation recommends increasing the pacing voltage to "5 volts or higher" in any case in which the monopolar electrosurgical unit (ESU) will be used. Rozner and associates reported increases in both atrial and ventricular thresholds in 6 of 141 consecutive operations involving pacemaker cases in which the monopolar ESU was used, large volume and blood shifts were observed, or both.[6] Although many of the operations were thoracic explorations, no pacing threshold changes were noted for these cases. No cardiopulmonary bypass cases were included in this cohort. Special attention must be given to any device with a minute ventilation (bioimpedance) sensor, because inappropriate tachycardia has been observed secondary to mechanical ventilation, monopolar "Bovie" ESU, and connection to an ECG monitor with respiratory rate monitoring.

Intraoperative (or Procedure) Management

No special monitoring or anesthetic technique is required for the patient with a pacemaker. However, ECG monitoring of the patient must include the ability to detect pacemaker discharges. Often, noise filtering on the ECG monitor must be changed to permit demonstration of the pacemaker pulse, and devices such as a nerve stimulator can interfere with detection and display of the pacemaker pulses.

In addition, patient monitoring must include the ability to ensure that myocardial electrical activity is converted to mechanical systoles. Mechanical systoles are best evaluated by pulse oximetry, plethysmography, or arterial waveform display. Some patients might need an increased pacing rate during the perioperative period to meet an increased oxygen demand. A pulmonary artery catheter, an esophageal Doppler monitor, or a transesophageal echocardiogram can be used to evaluate pacing frequency and its relationship to cardiac output. In addition to blood pressure and systemic vascular resistance, the monitoring of acid-base status might be needed to determine adequacy of cardiac output.

BOX 19-5 *Special Procedures in Patients with Implantable Generators*

- Lithotripsy: acceptable with precautions to protect the generator and, possibly, programming out of an atrial pacing mode
- Transurethral resection (bladder, prostate) and uterine hysteroscopy: procedures using monopolar electrocautery that can be easily accomplished after device reprogramming
- Magnetic resonance imaging (MRI): absolutely contraindicated by most generator manufacturers, and deaths have been reported. However, a report suggests that appropriate patients can safely undergo MRI but not without appropriate precautions.
- Electroconvulsive therapy: requires asynchronous (nonsensing) mode
- Nerve stimulator testing/therapy: inappropriate detection of transcutaneous electrical nerve stimulation, neuromuscular, and chiropractic electrical muscle stimulation because ventricular tachycardia or fibrillation has been reported

---

With respect to anesthetic technique, no studies have championed one over another. Nevertheless, a number of reports of prolongation of the QT interval with the use of isoflurane, desflurane, or sevoflurane have been published, whereas halothane appears to reduce this interval.[8] No interactions have been reported for enflurane.

Monopolar "Bovie" electrocautery (ESU) use remains the principal intraoperative issue for the patient with a pacemaker. Between 1984 and 1997, the U.S. FDA was notified of 456 adverse events with pulse generators, 255 from electrocautery, and a "significant number" of device failures.[9] Monopolar ESU is more likely to cause problems than is bipolar ESU, and patients with unipolar electrode configuration are more sensitive to EMI than are those with bipolar configurations. Coagulation ESU will likely cause more problems than nonblended "cutting" ESU. Magnet placement during electrocautery might allow reprogramming of an older (pre-1990) generator; however, newer generators are relatively immune to such effects. In fact, most devices from CPI-Guidant as well as St. Jude cannot be reprogrammed in the presence of a magnet. Note, however, that strong EMI can produce an electrical reset or improper detection of battery depletion, which might change the programming mode, rate, or both. If monopolar electrocautery is to be used, then the current return pad should be placed to ensure that the electrocautery current path does not cross the pacemaking system. For cases such as head and neck surgery, the pad might be best placed on the shoulder contralateral to the implanted device. For breast and axillary cases, the pad might need to be placed on the ipsilateral arm with the wire prepped into the field by sterile plastic cover. Procedures with special pacing ramifications are shown in Box 19-5.

The use of an ultrasonic cutting device, commonly called a "harmonic scalpel," has been championed to prevent EMI while providing the surgeon with the ability to both cut and coagulate tissue. There are a number of case reports demonstrating successful surgery without EMI issues in these patients.

Magnetic resonance imaging (MRI) deserves special mention. In general, MRI has been contraindicated in pacemaker and ICD patients. However, reports suggests that MRI is probably safe for some patients with newer devices, as well as any patient who will be wide awake in the MRI tunnel, who is not dependent on his or her pacemaker for heart rhythm or survival, who will not need medication to undergo the MRI, and who can communicate regularly with the MRI care team. Nevertheless, not all MRI sequences and energy levels have been studied, and caution is advised.[10]

Pacemaker Failure

Pacemaker failure has three causes: (1) failure of capture, (2) lead failure, and (3) generator failure. Failure of capture owing to a defect at the level of the myocardium (i.e., the generator continues to fire but no myocardial depolarization takes place) remains the most difficult problem to treat. Myocardial changes that result in noncapture include myocardial ischemia/infarction, acid-base disturbance, electrolyte abnormalities, or abnormal levels of antiarrhythmic drug(s). Temporary pacing (transvenous, transcutaneous, transthoracic, or transesophageal) might inhibit pacemaker output at voltages that will not produce myocardial capture. Sympathomimetic drugs generally lower pacing threshold. Outright generator or lead failure is rare.

TEMPORARY PACEMAKERS

There are several techniques available to the anesthesiologist to establish reliable temporary pacing during the perioperative period or in the intensive care unit. Cardiovascular anesthesiologists are more likely than generalists to routinely use temporary transvenous or epicardial pacing in their practices. Temporary cardiac pacing can serve as definitive therapy for transient bradyarrhythmias or as a bridge to permanent generator placement.

The various forms of temporary pacing include many transvenous catheter systems, transcutaneous pads, transthoracic wires, and esophageal pacing techniques. This section reviews the indications for temporary cardiac pacing and discusses the techniques available to the anesthesiologist. Table 19-2 summarizes these techniques.

Indications for Temporary Pacing

Temporary pacemakers are commonly used postoperatively after cardiac surgery, in the treatment of drug toxicity resulting in arrhythmias, with certain arrhythmias complicating myocardial infarction, and for intraoperative bradycardia due to β-blocker use. The placement of a temporary pacing system can assist in the hemodynamic management in the perioperative period. Abnormal electrolytes, preoperative β-blocker use, and many of the intraoperative drugs have the potential to aggravate bradycardia and bradycardia-dependent arrhythmias. Because drugs used to treat bradyarrhythmias have a number of important disadvantages compared with temporary pacing, hemodynamically unstable perioperative bradyarrhythmias should be considered an indication for temporary pacing (Table 19-3). If the patient already has epicardial wires or a pacing catheter or wires, or transesophageal pacing is feasible, pacing is preferred to pharmacologic therapy. However, transcutaneous and ventricular-only transvenous pacing, even if feasible, may exacerbate hemodynamic problems in patients with heart disease because these pacing modalities do not preserve AV synchrony (i.e., produces ventricular or global activation).

Nearly every indication for a permanent pacemaker is an indication for temporary pacing in patients without a pacemaker who, due to circumstances (e.g., emergency surgery, critical illness), cannot have elective permanent pacemaker implantation. Temporary pacing may also be needed before implantation of a permanent pacemaker to stabilize patients with hemodynamically significant bradycardia.

Temporary pacing is also indicated if a patient with a myocardial infarction complicated by second- or third-degree heart block is scheduled for emergency surgery. Bifascicular block in an asymptomatic patient is not reason enough for temporary

Table 19-2 Comparison of Temporary Pacing Techniques

Temporary Pacing Method	Time to Initiate	Chambers Paced	Advantages	Disadvantages	Uses
Transcutaneous	1 to 2 min	Right ventricle	Simple, rapid, safe	Variable capture, chest wall movement, patient discomfort	Arrest, intraoperative, prophylactic
Transesophageal	Minutes	Left atrium	Reliable atrial capture, safe, simple	Requires special generator	Prophylactic atrial pacing, overdrive pacing for SVT, monitoring atrial electrogram
Transvenous semirigid	3 to 20 min	Atrium and/or ventricle	Most reliable, well tolerated	Invasive, time-consuming, potential complications	Arrest, prophylactic, maintenance
Transvenous flow directed	3 to 20 min	Right ventricle	Simple, does not require fluoroscopy	Invasive, stability questions, less readily available	Arrest, intraoperative, prophylactic, maintenance
Pacing pulmonary (PA) artery catheter	Minutes (if PA catheter in place)	Atrium and/or ventricle	Reliable ventricular capture, well tolerated	Requires specific PA catheter, which must be placed first	Arrest, intraoperative, prophylactic, maintenance
Epicardial pacing wires	<1 min	Atrium and/or ventricle	Reliable short term	Postoperative only, early lead failure	Arrest, prophylactic, maintenance
Transthoracic	10 to 60 s	Ventricle	Rapid and simple	Many potential complications	Arrest only

SVT = supraventricular tachycardia.

19

Table 19-3　Temporary Pacing Indications

Patient Condition	Event Requiring Temporary Pacing
AMI	Symptomatic bradycardia, medically refractory
	New bundle-branch block with transient complete heart block
	Complete heart block
	Postoperative complete heart block
	Symptomatic congenital heart block
	Mobitz II with AMI
	New bifascicular block
	Bilateral bundle-branch block and first-degree AV block
	Symptomatic alternating Wenckebach block
	Symptomatic alternating bundle-branch block
Tachycardia treatment or prevention	Bradycardia-dependent VT
	Torsades de pointes
	Long QT syndrome
	Treatment of recurrent SVT or VT
Prophylactic	Pulmonary artery catheter placement with left bundle-branch block (controversial)
	New AV block or bundle-branch block in acute endocarditis
	Cardioversion with sick sinus syndrome
	Post–defibrillation bradycardia
	Counteract perioperative pharmacologic treatment causing hemodynamically significant bradycardia
	AF prophylaxis post–cardiac surgery
	Post–orthotopic heart transplantation

AF = atrial fibrillation; AMI = acute myocardial infarction; AV = atrioventricular; SVT = supraventricular tachycardia; VT = ventricular tachycardia.

pacing preoperatively. The development of a new bifascicular block immediately postoperatively, however, suggests perioperative myocardial ischemia or infarction, and temporary pacing might be required. Surgical resection of neck and carotid sinus tumors may give rise to bradyarrhythmias requiring temporary cardiac pacing during surgical manipulation. Neurosurgical procedures involving the brainstem may also be associated with significant bradycardia.

Relative contraindications to transvenous ventricular pacing include digitalis toxicity with ventricular tachycardia (VT), tricuspid valve prostheses, or the presence of a coagulopathy. Pacing in the setting of severe hypothermia might induce ventricular fibrillation (VF) or alter the normal compensatory physiologic mechanisms to the hypothermia. Atrial fibrillation, multifocal atrial tachycardia, and significant AV conduction system disease are relative contraindications to transvenous *atrial* pacing.

Transvenous Temporary Pacing

Transvenous cardiac pacing provides the most reliable means of temporary pacing. Temporary transvenous pacing is dependable and well tolerated by patients. With a device that can provide both atrial and ventricular pacing, transvenous pacing can maintain AV synchrony and improve cardiac output. Disadvantages include the need for practitioner experience, time to appropriately place the wire(s) to provide capture, the potential complications of catheter placement and manipulation, and the need for fluoroscopy in many cases.

Rapid catheter position is most easily obtained by using the right internal jugular vein, even without fluoroscopy. The left subclavian vein is also easily used in emergent situations. Other sites are often impassable without fluoroscopy. In addition, brachial and femoral routes can increase the frequency of lead dislodgment during motion of the extremities.

Once central access is obtained, the lead is guided into position using hemodynamic data (not possible with the simple bipolar lead) or by fluoroscopic guidance. ECG guidance is less desirable. The right atrial appendage and right ventricular apex provide the most stable catheter positions. Techniques for placement into these positions are part of cardiology training and likely are foreign to most anesthesiologists. When fluoroscopy is unavailable or in emergency situations, a flow-directed catheter can be attempted using ECG and pressure guidance. Once the right ventricle is entered, the balloon is deflated, if used, and the catheter gently advanced until electrical capture is noted. Flow-directed catheters and a right internal jugular approach afford the shortest insertion times. The reported incidence of successful capture in urgent situations without fluoroscopy ranges from 30% to 90%.

Once catheters are positioned, pacing is initiated using the distal electrode as the cathode and the proximal electrode as the anode. Ideally, the capture thresholds should be less than 1 mA and generator output should be maintained at three times threshold as a safety margin. In dual-chamber pacing, AV delays of between 100 and 200 ms are used. Many patients are sensitive to this parameter. Cardiac output optimization with echocardiography and/or mixed venous oxygen saturation can be used to maximize hemodynamics by adjusting AV delay.[11] AV sequential pacing is clearly beneficial in many patients, but it should be remembered that emergency pacing starts with ventricular capture alone. There is a potential risk of interference of external pacemaker generators by walkie-talkies and digital cellular phones. Clinicians should also be aware of all complications related to transvenous lead placement.

Pacing Pulmonary Artery Catheters

The pulmonary artery AV pacing thermodilution (TD) catheter allows for AV sequential pacing via electrodes attached to the outside of the catheter, as well as routine pulmonary artery (PA) catheter functions. Combination of the two functions into one catheter eliminates the need for separate insertion of temporary transvenous pacing electrodes. However, several potential disadvantages exist with this catheter, including (1) varying success in initiating and maintaining capture, (2) external electrode displacement from the catheter, and (3) relatively high cost compared to standard pacing PA catheters. The Paceport PA catheter provides ventricular pacing with a separate bipolar pacing lead (Chandler probe), which allows for more stable ventricular pacing as well as hemodynamic measurements. This catheter has been used for successful resuscitation after cardiac arrest during closed-chest cardiac massage when attempts to capture with transcutaneous and transvenous flow-directed bipolar pacing catheters had failed. However, this unit does not provide the potential advantages associated with atrial pacing capability. The newer pulmonary artery A-V Paceport adds a sixth lumen to the older Paceport to allow placement of an atrial J-wire, flexible-tip bipolar pacing lead. Both of these Paceport catheters are placed by transducing the right ventricular pressure port to ensure correct positioning of the port 1 to 2 cm distal to the tricuspid valve. This position usually guides the ventricular wire (Chandler probe) to the apex where adequate capture should occur with minimal current requirements. Although ventricular capture is easily obtained, atrial capture

19

can be more difficult and less reliable.[11] This catheter has been used successfully after cardiac surgery. The atrial wire can be used to diagnose supraventricular tachycardia (SVT) by atrial electrograms and to overdrive atrial flutter and reentrant SVT.

Transcutaneous Pacing

Transcutaneous pacing is readily available and can be rapidly implemented in emergency situations. Capture rate is variable and the technique may cause pain in awake patients, but usually it is tolerated until temporary transvenous pacing can be instituted. It may be effective even when endocardial pacing fails. It is now considered by many to be the method of choice for prophylactic and emergent applications.

The large patches typically are placed anteriorly (negative electrode or cathode) over the palpable cardiac apex (or V_3 lead location) and posteriorly (positive electrode or anode) at the inferior aspect of the scapula. The anode has also been placed on the anterior right chest with success in healthy volunteers. The skin should be cleansed with alcohol (but not abraded) to reduce capture threshold and improve patient comfort. Abraded skin can cause more discomfort. Typical thresholds are 20 to 120 mA, but pacing may require up to 200 mA at long pulse durations of 20 to 40 ms.[12] Transcutaneous pacing appears to capture the right ventricle followed by near-simultaneous activation of the entire left ventricle. The hemodynamic response is similar to that of right ventricular endocardial pacing. Both methods can cause reductions in left ventricular systolic pressure, a decrease in stroke volume, and an increase in right-sided pressures due to AV dyssynchrony. Capture should be confirmed by palpation or display of a peripheral pulse. Maintenance current is set 5 to 10 mA above threshold as tolerated by the patient. Success rates appear to be highest when the system is used prophylactically or early after arrest—upward of 90%.

Coughing and discomfort from cutaneous stimulation are the most frequent problems. The technique poses no electrical threat to medical personnel, and complications are rare. There have been no reports of significant damage to myocardium, skeletal muscle, skin, or lungs in humans despite continuous pacing up to 108 hours and intermittent pacing up to 17 days. Several commercially available defibrillators include transcutaneous pacing generators as standard equipment.

Esophageal Pacing

The newest technique available to anesthesiologists is esophageal pacing, and it has been shown to be quite reliable.[13] Significant bradycardia, secondary to underlying pathology or pharmacologic effects, can occur during anesthesia. The response to pharmacologic therapy for significant bradycardia with vagolytic drugs can be unpredictable and difficult to sustain accurately. Chronotropic drugs may have little effect and can lead to tachyarrhythmias and/or myocardial ischemia. Esophageal pacing is relatively noninvasive and well tolerated even in the majority of awake patients, and it appears to be devoid of serious complications. This modality is useful for heart rate support of cardiac output, for overdrive suppression of reentrant SVT, and for diagnostic atrial electrograms. Ventricular capture must be excluded before attempts at rapid atrial pacing for overdrive suppression to prevent potential VT or VF.

Problems with esophageal pacing include (1) the necessity for special generators that must provide 20 to 30 mA of current with wide pulse widths of 10 to 20 ms and (2) the ability to pace only the left atrium reliably and not the left ventricle, which can be a significant problem in emergency situations. By comparison, typical temporary generators designed for endocardial pacing have a maximum output of 20 mA with pulse width durations of only 1 to 2 ms.

IV

The pacing stimulus is delivered through a modified esophageal stethoscope. Pacing is initiated by connecting the system and placing the esophageal stethoscope to a depth of 30 to 40 cm from the teeth. Capture should be confirmed using the peripheral pulse (i.e., from the pulse oximeter plethysmogram or an invasive hemodynamic monitor), because the pacing stimulus often is large relative to the QRS and frequently fools the ECG counting algorithm on the monitor. Atrial capture is obtained in virtually all patients using outputs of 8 to 20 mA, and the output should be set to two to three times the threshold for capture. Thresholds are not influenced by weight, age, atrial size, or previous cardiac surgery. Because there is no sensing element involved, esophageal pacing is AOO mode pacing. In general, transesophageal pacing requires reprogramming of a permanent pacemaker or ICD. It is contraindicated in these patients without expert assistance.

POSTANESTHESIA PACEMAKER EVALUATION

Any pacemaker that was reprogrammed for the perioperative period should be reset appropriately. For non-reprogrammed devices, most manufacturers recommend interrogation to ensure proper functioning and remaining battery life if any electrocautery was used. ACC guidelines recommend a postprocedure interrogation.

IMPLANTED CARDIOVERTER-DEFIBRILLATORS

The development of an implantable, battery-powered device able to deliver sufficient energy to terminate VT or VF has represented a major medical breakthrough for patients with a history of ventricular tachyarrhythmias. These devices prevent death in the setting of malignant ventricular tachyarrhythmias, and they clearly remain superior to antiarrhythmic drug therapy. Initially approved by the U.S. FDA in 1985, more than 80,000 devices will be placed this year, and industry sources report that more than 240,000 patients have these devices today.

A significant number of technologic advances have occurred since the first ICD was placed, including considerable miniaturization (pectoral pocket placement with transvenous leads is the norm) and battery improvements that permit permanent pacing with these devices. Thus, a pectoral ICD could easily be confused with a pacemaker. Like pacemakers, ICDs have a generic code to indicate lead placement and function, which is shown in Table 19-4.

Table 19-4 **North American Society for Pacing and Electrophysiology/The British Pacing and Electrophysiology Group Generic Defibrillator Code (NBD)**

Position I Shock Chambers(s)	Position II Anti-tachycardia Pacing Chamber(s)	Position III Tachycardia Detection	Position IV Anti-bradycardia Pacing Chamber(s)
O = None	O = None	E = Electrogram	O = None
A = Atrium	A = Atrium	H = Hemodynamic	A = Atrium
V = Ventricle	V = Ventricle		V = Ventricle
D = Dual (A + V)	D = Dual (A + V)		D = Dual (A + V)

Newer ICDs (since 1993) have many programmable features, but essentially they measure each cardiac RR interval and categorize the rate as normal, too fast (short RR interval), or too slow (long RR interval). When the device detects a sufficient number of short RR intervals within a period of time (all programmable), it begins an antitachycardia event. The internal computer decides to choose antitachycardia pacing (less energy use, better tolerated by patient) or shock, depending on the presentation and device programming. If shock is chosen, an internal capacitor is charged. Most newer devices are programmed to reconfirm VT or VF after charging in order to prevent inappropriate shock therapy. Typically, ICDs have six therapies available for each type of event (VT, fast VT, VF), and some of these therapies can be repeated before moving to the next higher energy sequence. Thus, ICDs can deliver 6 to 18 shocks per event. In an ICD with antitachycardia pacing, once a shock is delivered, no further antitachycardia pacing can take place.

Twenty to 40 percent of shocks are for rhythms other than VT or VF despite reconfirmation. SVT remains the most common cause of inappropriate shock therapy. Advances in ICDs to include dual-chamber detection might be able to lower the inappropriate shock rate, although it is still reported as high as 17%.[14] Whether inappropriate shocks injure patients remains a subject of considerable debate, but a significant number of patients who receive an inappropriate shock demonstrate elevated troponin levels in the absence of an ischemic event.

Programmable features in current ICDs to differentiate VT from a tachycardia of supraventricular origin (SVT) include the following:

1. Onset criteria: in general, onset of VT is abrupt whereas onset of SVT has sequentially shortening RR intervals.
2. Stability criteria: in general, the RR interval of VT is relatively constant, whereas the RR interval of atrial fibrillation with rapid ventricular response is quite variable.
3. QRS width criteria: in general, the QRS width in SVT is narrow (<110 ms), whereas the QRS width in VT is wide (>120 ms).
4. "Intelligence" in dual-chamber devices attempts to associate atrial activity with ventricular activity.
5. Morphology waveform analysis with comparison to stored historic templates.

Note that once the RR interval becomes sufficiently short for VF detection, the ICD begins a shock sequence. As noted, once the device delivers any shock therapy, no further anti-tachycardia pacing takes place. An ICD with anti-bradycardia pacing capability will begin pacing when the RR interval is too long. In July 1997, the U.S. FDA– approved devices with sophisticated dual-chamber pacing modes and rate-responsive behavior for ICD patients who need permanent pacing (about 20% of ICD patients).

Indications

Initially, ICDs were placed for hemodynamically significant VT or VF. Newer indications associated with sudden death include long QT syndrome, Brugada syndrome (right bundle-branch block, ST-segment elevation in leads V_1 to V_3), and arrhythmogenic right ventricular dysplasia. Studies suggest that ICDs can be used for primary prevention of sudden death (i.e., before the first episode of VT or VF) in young patients with hypertrophic cardiomyopathy, and data from the second Multicenter Automatic Defibrillator Intervention Trial (MADIT II) suggest that any patient after myocardial infarction with an ejection fraction less than 30% should undergo prophylactic implantation of an ICD.[15]

IV

BOX 19-6 *Implanted Cardioverter-Defibrillator Indications*

- Ventricular tachycardia
- Ventricular fibrillation
- Brugada syndrome (right bundle-branch block, ST-segment elevation V_1 to V_3)
- Arrhythmogenic right ventricular dysplasia
- Long QT syndrome
- Hypertrophic cardiomyopathy
- Prophylactic use after myocardial infarction, ejection fraction < 30%

Trials are under way for the cardiomyopathy patient with nonischemic cardiomyopathy as well. The Sudden Cardiac Death-Heart Failure Trial (SCD-HeFT) results and the previously published Defibrillators In Non-Ischemic Cardiomyopathy Treatment Evaluation (DEFINITE) study suggest that ICD placement will result in lower mortality in any patient with an ejection fraction less than 35% regardless of the cause of the cardiomyopathy. The DEFINITE results are important, because the patients in this study were randomized only after initiation of β-blockade and angiotensin-converting enzyme inhibitor therapy, which form the backbone of medical therapy for cardiomyopathy. The SCD-HeFT results showed ICDs reduced mortality by 23%. Based on these results, Medicare expanded its ICD coverage.[16,17]

Box 19-6 reviews ICD indications.

Dilated Cardiomyopathy

With the advent of Bi-V pacing for the patient with a DCM and prolonged QRS interval, and the approval of ICDs with Bi-V capability, the presence of a defibrillator with Bi-V pacing will become more common. About 550,000 new diagnoses of congestive heart failure are made in the United States every year, and the prevalence of this disease includes nearly 5 million patients. Significant risk factors for the development of congestive heart failure include ischemic heart disease and/or hypertension. These data, combined with the results from SCD-HeFT and MADIT II trials (ICD is indicated in any patient with cardiomyopathy and ejection fraction < 30% to 35%), suggest that the number of patients eligible to receive a defibrillator to include Bi-V pacing will increase dramatically. Whether any country's economy can absorb this economic burden remains to be seen. At present, Bi-V pacing without defibrillation capability improves functional status and quality of life and was shown to reduce mortality.[5,18]

Implanted Cardioverter-Defibrillator Magnets

Like pacemakers, magnet behavior in ICDs can be altered by programming. Most devices suspend tachyarrhythmia detection (and therefore therapy) when a magnet is appropriately placed to activate the reed switch. Some devices from Angeion, CPI, Pacesetter, and St. Jude Medical can be programmed to ignore magnet placement. Some Guidant/CPI ICDs have been programmed to ignore magnet placement due to a faulty magnet switch. *Anti-tachycardia therapy in some Guidant/CPI devices can be permanently disabled by magnet placement for 30 seconds.* In general, magnets will not affect anti-bradycardia pacing mode or rate. Interrogating the device and calling the manufacturer remain the most reliable methods for determining magnet response.

Preanesthetic Evaluation and Implanted Cardioverter-Defibrillator Reprogramming

All ICDs should have their anti-tachycardia therapy disabled before the induction of anesthesia and commencement of the procedure.[1] Guidelines from HRS-NASPE and the ASA Advisory suggest that every patient with an ICD have an in-office comprehensive evaluation every 1 to 4 months. Devices with Bi-V pacing must have a sufficiently short AV delay for sensed events to ensure that all ventricular activity is paced. Failure of ventricular pacing (either right or left) owing to native AV conduction or threshold issues has been associated with inappropriate antitachycardia therapy (i.e., shock).

Intraoperative or Procedure Management

At this time, no special monitoring (owing to the ICD) is required for the patient with an ICD. ECG monitoring and the ability to deliver external cardioversion or defibrillation must be present during the time of ICD disablement. Although many recommendations exist for defibrillator pad placement to protect the ICD, it must be remembered that the patient, not the ICD, is being treated.

Furthermore, no special anesthetic techniques have been advocated for the patient with an ICD. Most of these patients will have severely depressed systolic function, dilated ventricular cavities, and significant valvular regurgitation, and the choice of anesthetic technique should be dictated by the underlying physiologic derangements that are present. Conflicting data have been published regarding the choice of anesthetic agent(s) and changes to defibrillation threshold (DFT).

Anesthetic Considerations for Insertion of an Implanted Cardioverter-Defibrillator

Insertion of ICDs is mostly performed in the catheterization suite with only complicated cases referred to the operating room. The procedure requires defibrillation testing to ensure an acceptable margin of safety for the device. VT or ventricular fibrillation is induced by the introduction of premature beats timed to the vulnerable repolarization period. External adhesive pads are placed before the procedure and connected to an external cardioverter/defibrillator to provide "back-up" shocks should the device be ineffective. Monitored anesthesia care is typically chosen with a brief general anesthetic given for defibrillation testing. General anesthesia may be chosen for patients with severe concomitant diseases (e.g., chronic lung disease, sleep apnea) when control of the airway is desired. Simultaneous insertion of biventricular pacing systems with an ICD might necessitate a general anesthetic due to the length of the procedure and the often severe impairment of left ventricular function.

In addition to standard patient monitoring, continuous arterial blood pressure monitoring may be used even during monitored anesthesia care to rapidly assess for return of blood pressure after defibrillation testing. Repeated defibrillation testing is usually well tolerated without deterioration of cardiac function even in patients with left ventricular ejection fractions less than 35%. Nonetheless, means of pacing must be available should bradycardia develop after cardioversion/defibrillation. Often, however, restoration of circulatory function after defibrillation testing is accompanied by tachycardia and hypertension necessitating treatment with a short-acting β-blocker and/or vasoactive drugs.

Complications associated with ICD insertion include those related to insertion and those associated specifically with the device. Percutaneous insertion is typically via the subclavian vein, predisposing to pneumothorax. Cardiac injury including perforation is a remote possibility. Device-related complications include those associated with multiple shocks that may lead to myocardial injury or refractory hypotension.[19]

Postanesthesia Implanted Cardioverter-Defibrillator Evaluation

The ICD must be reinterrogated and reenabled. All events should be reviewed and counters should be cleared, because the next device evaluator might not receive information about the EMI experience of the patient and might make erroneous conclusions regarding the patient's arrhythmia events.[20]

SUMMARY

Preoperative

- Have any implanted pacemaker or defibrillator interrogated by a competent authority shortly before the procedure.
- Obtain a copy of this interrogation. Ensure that the device will pace the heart.
- Consider replacing any device near its elective replacement period in a patient scheduled to undergo either a major operation or surgery within 15 cm of the generator.
- Determine the patient's underlying rhythm, rate, and pacemaker dependency to determine the need for backup pacing support.
- If magnet use is planned, ensure that a magnet mode exists and verify its rate and pacing mode.
- Program rate responsiveness off, if present.
- Program rate enhancements off, if present.
- Consider increasing the pacing rate to optimize oxygen delivery to tissues for major operations.
- Disable antitachycardia therapy, if present.

Intraoperative

- Monitor cardiac rhythm/peripheral pulse with pulse oximeter (plethysmography) or arterial waveform.
- Disable the "artifact filter" on the ECG monitor.
- Avoid use of the monopolar electrosurgical unit (ESU).
- Use bipolar ESU if possible; if this is not possible, then pure cut (monopolar ESU) is better than "blend" or "coag."
- Place the ESU current return pad in such a way to prevent electricity from crossing the generator-heart circuit, even if the pad must be placed on the distal forearm and the wire covered with sterile drape.
- If the ESU causes ventricular oversensing and pacer quiescence, limit the period(s) of asystole.
- Temporary pacing might be needed, and consideration should be given to the possibility of pacemaker or defibrillator failure.

19

Postoperative

- Have the device interrogated by a competent authority postoperatively. Some rate enhancements can be reinitiated, and optimum heart rate and pacing parameters should be determined. The ICD patient must be monitored until the antitachycardia therapy is restored.

REFERENCES

1. Fleisher L, Beckman J, Brown K, et al: ACC/AHA 2007 guidelines on perioperative cardiovascular evaluation and care for noncardiac surgery. Circulation 116; 1971, 2007
2. American Society of Anesthesiology Practice Advisory for the Perioperative Management of Patients with Rhythm Management Devices: Pacemakers and implantable cardioverter-defibrillators. Anesthesiology 103:186, 2005
3. Rozner M: Pacemaker misinformation in the perioperative period: Programming around the problem. Anesth Analg 99:1582, 2004
4. Bernstein AD, Daubert JC, Fletcher RD, et al: The revised NASPE/BPEG generic code for antibradycardia, adaptive-rate, and multisite pacing. North American Society of Pacing and Electrophysiology/British Pacing and Electrophysiology Group. Pacing Clin Electrophysiol 25:260, 2002
5. Bristow MR, Saxon LA, Boehmer J, et al: Cardiac-resynchronization therapy with or without an implantable defibrillator in advanced chronic heart failure. N Engl J Med 350:2140, 2004
6. Rozner MA, Roberson JC, Nguyen AD: Unexpected high incidence of serious pacemaker problems detected by pre- and postoperative interrogations: A two-year experience. J Am Coll Cardiol 43:113A, 2004
7. Hauser R, Hayes D, Parsonnet V, et al: Feasibility and initial results of an Internet-based pacemaker and ICD pulse generator and lead registry. Pacing Clin Electrophysiol 24:82, 2001
8. Yildirim H, Adanair T, Atay A, et al: The effects of sevoflurane, isoflurane, and desflurane on QT interval of the ECG. Eur J Anaesthesiol 21:566, 2004
9. Pressly N: Review of MDR Reports reinforces concern about EMI. FDA User Facility Reporting No. 20. Published 1997. Available at: http://www.fda.gov/cdrh/fuse20.pdf. Accessed December 1, 2002
10. Rozner MA: MRI in the patient with a pacemaker: Caution is indicated. J Am Coll Cardiol. 2004
11. Trankina MF, White RD: Perioperative cardiac pacing using an atrioventricular pacing pulmonary artery catheter. J Cardiothorac Anesth 3:154, 1989
12. Gauss A, Hubner C, Meierhenrich R, et al: Perioperative transcutaneous pacemaker in patients with chronic bifascicular block or left bundle branch block and additional first-degree atrioventricular block. Acta Anaesthesiol Scand 43:731, 1999
13. Atlee JL III, Pattison CZ, Mathews EL, Hedman AG: Transesophageal atrial pacing for intraoperative sinus bradycardia or AV junctional rhythm: Feasibility as prophylaxis in 200 anesthetized adults and hemodynamic effects of treatment. J Cardiothorac Vasc Anesth 7:436, 1993
14. Niehaus M, de Sousa M, Klein G, et al: Chronic experiences with a single lead dual chamber implantable cardioverter defibrillator system. Pacing Clin Electrophysiol 26:1937, 2003
15. Moss AJ, Zareba W, Hall WJ, et al: Prophylactic implantation of a defibrillator in patients with myocardial infarction and reduced ejection fraction. N Engl J Med 346:877, 2002
16. Bardy GH, Lee KL, Mark DB, et al: Amiodarone or an implantable cardioverter-defibrillator for congestive heart failure. N Engl J Med 352:225, 2005
17. McClellan M, Tunis S: Medicare coverage of ICDs. N Engl J Med 352:222, 2005
18. Gras D, Leclercq C, Tang AS, et al: Cardiac resynchronization therapy in advanced heart failure: The multicenter InSync clinical study. Eur J Heart Fail 4:311, 2002
19. DiMarco JP: Implantable cardioverter-defibrillators. N Engl J Med 349:1836-1847, 2003
20. Goldberger Z, Lampert R: Implantable cardioverter-defibrillators: expanding implications and technologies. JAMA 295:809, 2006

IV

Chapter 20

Anesthesia for Heart, Lung, and Heart-Lung Transplantation

Joseph J. Quinlan, MD • Andrew W. Murray, MD • Alfonso Casta, MD

HEART TRANSPLANTATION

The history of heart transplantation spans almost a century. Canine heterotopic cardiac transplantation was first reported in 1905, but such efforts were doomed by ignorance of the workings of the immune system (Box 20-1). Further research in the late 1950s and early 1960s set the stage for the first human cardiac transplant by Barnard in 1966. However, there were few long-term survivors in this era, owing to continued deficiency in understanding and in modulating the human immune system, and the procedure fell into general disfavor. Continued research at selected centers (e.g., Stanford University) and lessons learned from renal transplantation led to greater understanding of the technical issues and immunology required, and by the early 1980s cardiac transplantation gained widespread acceptance as a realistic option for patients with end-stage cardiomyopathy.

Heart transplantation experienced explosive growth in the mid to late 1980s, but the annual number of heart transplants worldwide plateaued by the early 1990s at approximately 3500 per year. The factor limiting continued growth has been

BOX 20-1 *Heart Transplantation*

- Frequency of transplantation remains limited by donor supply.
- Pathophysiology before transplantation is primarily that of end-stage ventricular failure.
- Pathophysiology after transplantation reflects the effects of denervation.
- Allograft coronary vasculopathy is a frequent long-term complication.

a shortage of suitable donors. In 2004, there were approximately 3500 patients on the United Network for Organ Sharing cardiac transplant waiting list (includes all U.S. candidates), whereas only 2055 heart transplantations were performed in the United States during the 2003 calendar year. The median waiting time for a cardiac graft varies widely according to blood type (approximately 39 days for type AB recipients but up to 303 days for type O recipients). In aggregate, more than 48% of patients on the heart transplant list had spent more than 2 years waiting for a transplant.[1] The most frequent recipient indications for adult heart transplantation remain either idiopathic or ischemic cardiomyopathy. Other less common diagnoses include viral cardiomyopathy, systemic diseases such as amyloidosis, and complex congenital heart disease.

The 1-year survival after heart transplantation has been reported to be 79%, with a subsequent mortality rate of approximately 4% per year. There has been little change in the survival statistics over the past decade; the Organ Procurement and Transplant Network reports that the 1- and 3-year survivals after heart transplantation for those transplanted in the United States during the period 1999 through 2001 were approximately 85% and 77%, respectively. One-year survival after repeat heart transplantation more than 6 months after the original procedure is slightly lower (63%) but substantially worse if performed within 6 months of the original grafting (39%). Risk factors for increased mortality have been associated with recipient factors (prior transplantation, poor human leukocyte antigen [HLA] matching, ventilator dependence, age, and race), medical center factors (volume of heart transplants performed, ischemic time), and donor factors (race, gender, age). Early deaths are most frequently due to graft failure, whereas intermediate-term deaths are caused by acute rejection or infection. Late deaths after heart transplantation are most frequently due to allograft vasculopathy, post-transplant lymphoproliferative disease or other malignancy, and chronic rejection.

Recipient Selection

Potential candidates for heart transplantation generally undergo a multidisciplinary evaluation including a complete history and physical examination, routine hematology, chemistries (to assess renal and hepatic function), viral serology, electrocardiography, chest radiography, pulmonary function tests, and right- and left-sided heart catheterization. Ambulatory electrocardiography, echocardiography, and nuclear gated scans are performed if necessary. The goals of this evaluation are to confirm a diagnosis of end-stage heart disease that is not amenable to other therapies and that will likely lead to death within 1 to 2 years and to exclude extracardiac organ dysfunction that could lead to death soon after heart transplantation. Patients typically have stage D heart failure, New York Heart Association (NYHA) class IV symptoms, and a left ventricular ejection fraction (LVEF) of less than 20%. Although most centers eschew a strict age cutoff, the candidate should have a "physiologic" age younger than 60 years. Detecting pulmonary hypertension, and determining whether it is due to a fixed elevation of pulmonary vascular resistance (PVR), is crucial; early mortality due to graft failure is threefold higher in patients with elevated PVR (transpulmonary gradient > 15 mmHg or PVR > 150 dynes $\cdot$ sec $\cdot$ cm^{-5}). If elevated PVR is detected, a larger donor heart, a heterotopic heart transplant, or a heart-lung transplant may be more appropriate. Active infection and recent pulmonary thromboembolism with pulmonary infarction are additional contraindications to heart transplantation. The results of this extensive evaluation should be tabulated and available to the anesthesia team at all times, because heart transplantation is an emergency procedure.

Donor Selection and Graft Harvest

Once a brain-dead donor has been identified, the accepting transplant center must further evaluate the suitability of the allograft. Centers generally prefer donors to be previously free of cardiac illness and younger than 35 years of age, because the incidence of coronary artery disease markedly increases at older ages. However, the relative shortage of suitable cardiac donors has forced many transplant centers to consider older donors without risk factors and symptoms of coronary artery disease. If it is necessary and the services are available at the donor hospital, the heart can be further evaluated by echocardiography (for regional wall motion abnormalities) or coronary angiography to complement standard palpation of the coronaries in the operating room. The absence of sepsis, prolonged cardiac arrest, severe chest trauma, and a high inotrope requirement are also important. The donor is matched to the prospective recipient for ABO blood-type compatibility and size (within 20%, especially if the recipient has high PVR); a crossmatch is performed only if the recipient's preformed antibody screen is positive.

Donors can exhibit major hemodynamic and metabolic derangements that can adversely affect organ retrieval. The vast majority of brain-dead donors will be hemodynamically unstable.[2] Reasons for such instability include hypovolemia (secondary to diuretics or diabetes insipidus), myocardial injury (possibly a result of "catecholamine storm" during periods of increased intracranial pressure), and inadequate sympathetic tone due to brainstem infarction. Donors often also have abnormalities of neuroendocrine function such as low T_3 and T_4 levels. Donor volume status should be assiduously monitored, and inotropic and vasopressor therapy should be guided by data from invasive monitors.

Donor cardiectomy is performed through a median sternotomy and usually simultaneous with recovery of other organs such as lungs, kidneys, and liver. Just before cardiac harvesting, the donor is heparinized and an intravenous cannula is placed in the ascending aorta for administration of conventional cardioplegia. The superior vena cava (SVC) is ligated, and the inferior vena cava (IVC) is transected to decompress the heart, simultaneous with the administration of cold hyperkalemic cardioplegia into the aortic root. The aorta is cross-clamped when the heart ceases to eject. The heart is also topically cooled with ice-cold saline. After arrest has been achieved, the pulmonary veins are severed, the SVC is transected, the ascending aorta is divided just proximal to the innominate artery, and the pulmonary artery (PA) transected at its bifurcation. The heart is then prepared for transport by placing it in a sterile plastic bag that is placed in turn in another bag filled with ice-cold saline, all of which are carried in an ice chest. Of all the regimens tested, conventional cardioplegia has proved most effective in maintaining cardiac performance. The upper time limit for ex vivo storage of human hearts appears to be approximately 6 hours.

20

SURGICAL PROCEDURES

Orthotopic Heart Transplantation

Orthotopic heart transplantation is carried out via a median sternotomy, and the general approach is similar to that used for coronary revascularization or valve replacement. Patients will frequently have undergone a prior median sternotomy; repeat sternotomy is cautiously performed using an oscillating saw. The groin should be prepped and draped to provide a rapid route for cannulation for cardiopulmonary bypass (CPB) if necessary. After the pericardium is opened, the aorta is cannulated as distally as possible, and the IVC and SVC are individually cannulated via the high right atrium (RA). Manipulation of the heart before institution of CPB is limited if thrombus is detected in the heart with transesophageal echocardiography (TEE). After initiation of CPB and cross-clamping of the aorta, the heart is arrested and excised (Fig. 20-1). The aorta and PA are separated and divided just above the level of their respective valves, and the atria are transected at their grooves. A variant of this classic approach totally excises both atria, mandating bicaval anastomoses. This technique may reduce the incidence of atrial arrhythmias, better preserve atrial function by avoiding tricuspid regurgitation, and enhance cardiac output (CO) after transplantation.

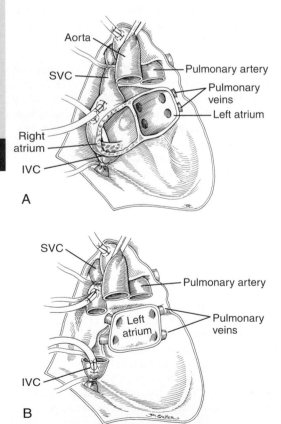

Figure 20-1 Mediastinum after excision of the heart but before allograft placement. Venous cannulas are present in the superior and inferior vena cavae, and the arterial cannula is present in the ascending aorta. **A,** Classic orthotopic technique. **B,** Bicaval anastomotic technique.

IV

The donor graft is then implanted with every effort to maintain a cold tissue temperature, beginning with the left atrial (LA) anastomosis. If the foramen ovale is patent, it is sutured closed. The donor RA is opened by incising it from the IVC to the base of the RA appendage (to preserve the donor sinoatrial node), and the RA anastomosis is constructed. Alternatively, if the bicaval technique is used, individual IVC and SVC anastomoses are sewn. The donor and recipient PAs are then brought together in an end-to-end manner, followed by the anastomosis of the donor to the recipient aorta. After removal of the aortic cross-clamp, the heart is de-aired via a vent in the ascending aorta. Just before weaning from CPB, one of the venous cannulas is withdrawn into the RA and the other removed. The patient is then weaned from CPB in the usual manner. After hemostasis is achieved, mediastinal tubes are placed for drainage, the pericardium is left open, and the wound is closed in the standard fashion.

Heterotopic Heart Transplantation

Although orthotopic placement of the cardiac graft is optimal for most patients, certain recipients are not candidates for the orthotopic operation, and instead the graft is placed in the right side of the chest and connected to the circulation in parallel with the recipient heart. The two primary indications for heterotopic placement are significant irreversible pulmonary hypertension and gross size mismatch between the donor and recipient. Heterotopic placement may avoid the development of acute right ventricular (RV) failure in the unconditioned donor heart in the presence of acutely elevated RV afterload.

Donor harvesting for heterotopic placement is performed in the previously described manner, except that the azygos vein is ligated and divided to increase the length of the donor SVC; the PA is extensively dissected to provide the longest possible main and right PA; and the donor IVC and right pulmonary veins are oversewn, with the left pulmonary veins incised to create a single large orifice. The operation is performed via a median sternotomy in the recipient, but the right pleura is entered and excised. The recipient SVC is cannulated via the RA appendage, and the IVC is cannulated via the lower RA. After arrest of the recipient heart, the LA anastomosis is constructed by incising the recipient LA near the right superior pulmonary vein and extending this incision inferiorly and then anastomosing the respective LA. The recipient RA-SVC is then incised and anastomosed to the donor RA-SVC, following which the donor aorta is joined to the recipient aorta in an end-to-side manner. Finally, the donor PA is anastomosed to the recipient main PA in an end-to-side manner if it is sufficiently long; otherwise, they are joined via an interposed vascular graft (Fig. 20-2).

Special Situations

Mechanical ventricular assist devices have been successfully used to "bridge" patients who would otherwise die of acute heart failure awaiting transplantation.[3] The technique of transplantation is virtually identical in such patients to that for ordinary orthotopic transplantation. However, repeat sternotomy is obligatory, and patients will often have been exposed to aprotinin during the assist device placement, increasing the probability of an anaphylactic response to the second aprotinin exposure. Although the incidence of anaphylaxis seems to be low, the team should be in a position to expeditiously initiate CPB before administering aprotinin in this setting. Placement of large-bore intravenous access is prudent because excessive hemorrhage can occur during the transplant procedure.

Rarely, patients will present for cardiac transplantation combined with transplantation of the liver. The cardiac allograft is usually implanted first to better enable the patient to survive potential hemodynamic instability associated with reperfusion of the hepatic

20

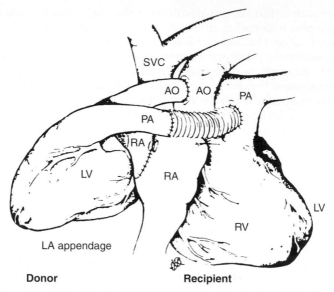

Figure 20-2 Placement of heterotopic graft in the right chest, with anastomoses to the corresponding native left and right atria, ascending aorta, and an interposition graft to the native pulmonary artery. LA = left atrial; LV = left ventricle; RA = right atrium; PA = pulmonary artery; AO = aorta; WVC = superior vena cava; RV = right ventricle. (From Cooper DKC, Lanza LP: Heart Transplantation: The Present Status of Orthotopic and Heterotopic Heart Transplantation. Lancaster, UK, MTP Press, 1984.)

allograft. Large-bore intravenous access is mandatory. A venous cannula can be left in the RA at the completion of the heart transplant procedure to serve as a return site for subsequent veno-veno bypass during liver transplantation.

Pathophysiology Before Transplantation

The pathophysiology of heart transplant candidates is predominantly end-stage cardiomyopathy. Such patients normally have both systolic dysfunction (characterized by decreased stroke volume and increased end-diastolic volume) and diastolic dysfunction, characterized by an elevated intracardiac diastolic pressure. As compensatory mechanisms to maintain CO fail, the elevated LV pressures lead to increases in pulmonary venous pressures and development of pulmonary vascular congestion and edema. A similar process occurs if RV failure also occurs. Autonomic sympathetic tone is increased in patients with heart failure, leading to generalized vasoconstriction as well as salt and water retention. Vasoconstriction and ventricular dilation combine to substantially increase myocardial wall tension. Over time, the high levels of catecholamines lead to a decrease in the sensitivity of the heart and vasculature to these agents via a decrease in receptor density (i.e., "down-regulation") and a decrease in myocardial norepinephrine stores.

Therapy for heart failure seeks to reverse or antagonize these processes. Almost all candidates will be maintained on diuretics; hypokalemia and hypomagnesemia secondary to urinary losses are likely, and the anesthesiologist must be alert to the possibility that a patient is hypovolemic from excessive diuresis. Another mainstay of therapy is vasodilators (e.g., nitrates, hydralazine, and angiotensin-converting enzyme inhibitors), which decrease the impedance to LV emptying and improve cardiac function and survival in patients with end-stage heart failure. Paradoxically, slow incremental β-blockade with agents such as carvedilol or metoprolol can also improve hemodynamics and exercise tolerance in some patients awaiting heart transplantation. Patients who are symptomatic despite these measures often require inotropic therapy. Digoxin is an effective but weak inotrope, and its use is limited by toxic side effects. Phosphodiesterase inhibitors such as amrinone, milrinone, and enoximone are efficacious, but chronic therapy is restricted by concerns about increased mortality in those receiving these agents. Therefore, inotrope-dependent patients are often treated with intravenous infusions of β-adrenergic agonists such as dopamine or dobutamine. Patients refractory to even these measures may be supported with intra-aortic balloon counterpulsation, but its use is fraught with significant vascular complications and essentially immobilizes the patient. Many patients with low CO are maintained on anticoagulants such as warfarin to prevent pulmonary or systemic embolization, especially if they have atrial fibrillation.

Pathophysiology after Transplantation

The physiology of patients after heart transplantation is of interest not only to anesthesiologists in cardiac transplant centers but also to the anesthesiology community at large because a substantial portion of these patients return for subsequent surgical procedures.

Cardiac denervation is an unavoidable consequence of heart transplantation. Many long-term studies indicate that reinnervation is absent or at best partial or incomplete in humans. Denervation does not significantly change baseline cardiac function, but it does substantially alter the cardiac response to demands for increased CO. Normally, increases in heart rate can rapidly increase CO, but this mechanism is not available to the transplanted heart. Heart rate increases only gradually with exercise, and this effect is mediated by circulating catecholamines. Increases in CO in response to exercise are instead mostly mediated via an increase in stroke volume. Therefore, maintenance of adequate preload in cardiac transplant recipients is crucial. Lack of parasympathetic innervation is probably responsible for the gradual decrease in heart rate after exercise seen in transplant recipients, rather than the usual sharp drop.

Denervation has important implications in the choice of pharmacologic agents used after cardiac transplantation. Drugs that act indirectly on the heart via either the sympathetic (ephedrine) or parasympathetic (atropine, pancuronium, edrophonium) nervous systems will generally be ineffective. Drugs with a mixture of direct and indirect effects will exhibit only their direct effects (leading to the absence of the normal increase in refractory period of the atrioventricular node with digoxin, tachycardia with norepinephrine infusion, and bradycardia with neostigmine). Thus, agents with direct cardiac effects (e.g., epinephrine or isoproterenol) are the drugs of choice for altering cardiac physiology after transplantation. However, the chronically high catecholamine levels found in cardiac transplant recipients may blunt the effect of α-adrenergic agents, as opposed to normal responses to β-adrenergic agents.[4]

Allograft coronary vasculopathy remains the greatest threat to long-term survival after heart transplantation. Allografts are prone to the accelerated development of an unusual form of coronary atherosclerosis that is characterized by circumferential, diffuse involvement of entire coronary arterial segments, as opposed to the conventional form of coronary atherosclerosis with focal plaques often found in eccentric positions in proximal coronary arteries. The pathophysiologic basis of this process remains elusive, but it is likely due to an immune cell-mediated activation of vascular endothelial cells to upregulate the production of smooth muscle cell growth

20

factors. More than half of all heart transplant recipients have evidence of concentric atherosclerosis 3 years after transplant, and more than 80% have this condition at 5 years.[5] Because afferent cardiac reinnervation is rare, a substantial portion of recipients with accelerated vasculopathy have silent ischemia. Noninvasive methods of detecting coronary atherosclerosis are insensitive for detecting allograft vasculopathy. Furthermore, coronary angiography often underestimates the severity of allograft atherosclerosis; other diagnostic regimens such as intravascular ultrasound and dobutamine stress echocardiography may detect morphologic abnormalities or functional ischemia, respectively, in the absence of angiographically significant lesions. Therefore, the anesthesiologist should assume that there is a substantial risk of coronary vasculopathy in any heart transplant recipient beyond the first 2 years, regardless of symptoms, the results of noninvasive testing, and even angiography.

Anesthetic Management
Preoperative Evaluation and Preparation

The preoperative period is often marked by severe time constraints due to the impending arrival of the donor heart. Nevertheless, a rapid history should screen for last oral intake, recent anticoagulant use, intercurrent deterioration of ventricular function, or change in anginal pattern; a physical examination should evaluate present volume status, and a laboratory review (if available) and a chest radiograph should detect the presence of renal, hepatic, or pulmonary dysfunction. Many hospitalized patients will be supported with inotropic infusions and/or an intra-aortic balloon pump, and the infusion rates and timing of the latter should be reviewed.

Equipment and drugs similar to those usually used for routine cases requiring CPB should be prepared. A β-agonist such as epinephrine should be readily available both in bolus form and as an infusion to rapidly treat ventricular failure; and an α-agonist such as phenylephrine or norepinephrine is useful to compensate for the vasodilatory effects of anesthetics, because even small decreases in preload and afterload can lead to catastrophic changes in CO and coronary perfusion in these patients.

Placement of invasive monitoring before induction will facilitate rapid and accurate response to hemodynamic events during induction. In addition to standard noninvasive monitoring, an arterial catheter and a PA catheter (with a long sterile sheath to allow partial removal during graft implantation) are placed after judicious use of sedation and local anesthetics. Placing the arterial catheter in a central site rather than the radial artery will avoid the discrepancy between radial and central arterial pressure often seen after CPB, but it may also be necessary to cannulate a femoral artery for arterial inflow for CPB if there has been a prior sternotomy. Floating the PA catheter into correct position may be difficult due to cardiac chamber dilation and severe tricuspid regurgitation. Large-bore intravenous access is mandatory, especially if a sternotomy has been previously performed, in which case external defibrillator/pacing patches may also be useful. The overall hemodynamic "picture" should be evaluated and optimized insofar as possible just before induction. If the hemodynamics seem tenuous, then starting or increasing an inotrope infusion may be advisable.

Induction

Most patients presenting for heart transplantation will not be in a fasting state and should be considered to have a "full stomach." Therefore, the induction technique should aim to rapidly achieve control of the airway to prevent aspiration while avoiding myocardial depression. A regimen combining a short-acting hypnotic with minimal myocardial depression (etomidate, 0.3 mg/kg), a moderate dose of narcotic to blunt the tachycardia response to laryngoscopy and intubation (fentanyl, 10 μg/kg), and succinylcholine (1.5 mg/kg) is popular; high-dose narcotic techniques with or without benzodiazepines have also been advocated. Vasodilation should be countered with an α-agonist. Anesthesia can be maintained with additional narcotic and sedatives (benzodiazepines or scopolamine).[6]

Intraoperative Management

After induction, the stomach can be decompressed with an orogastric tube and a TEE probe introduced while the bladder is catheterized. A complete TEE examination often reveals useful information not immediately available from other sources, such as the presence of cardiac thrombi, ventricular volume and contractility, and atherosclerosis of the ascending aorta and aortic arch. Cross-matched blood should be immediately available once surgery commences, especially if the patient has had a previous sternotomy; patients not previously exposed to cytomegalovirus should receive blood from donors who are likewise cytomegalovirus negative. Sternotomy and cannulation for CPB are performed as indicated earlier. The period before CPB is often uneventful, apart from arrhythmias and slow recovery of coronary perfusion due to manipulation of the heart during dissection and cannulation. The PA catheter should be withdrawn from the right side of the heart before completion of bicaval cannulation.

Once CPB is initiated, ventilation is discontinued and the absence of a thrill in the carotid arteries is documented. Most patients will have an excess of intravascular volume, and administration of a diuretic and/or the use of hemofiltration via the pump may be beneficial for increasing the hemoglobin concentration. A dose of glucocorticoid (methylprednisolone, 500 mg) is administered as the last anastomosis is being completed before release of the aortic cross-clamp to attenuate any hyperacute immune response. During the period of reperfusion an infusion of an inotrope is begun for both inotropy and chronotropy. TEE is used to monitor whether the cardiac chambers are adequately de-aired before weaning from CPB.

Weaning from bypass begins after ventilation is resumed and the cannula in the SVC is removed. The donor heart should be paced if bradycardia is present despite the inotropic infusion. Once the patient is separated from bypass, the PA catheter can be advanced into position. Patients with elevated PVR are at risk for acute RV failure and may benefit from a pulmonary vasodilator. Rarely, such patients require support with an RV assist device. TEE often provides additional useful information about right- and left-sided heart function and volume and documents normal flow dynamics through the anastomoses.

Protamine is then given to reverse heparin's effect after satisfactorily weaning from CPB. Continued coagulopathy despite adequate protamine is common after heart transplantation, especially if there has been a prior sternotomy. Treatment is similar to that used for other post-bypass coagulopathies: meticulous attention to surgical hemostasis, empirical administration of platelets, and subsequent addition of fresh frozen plasma and cryoprecipitate guided by subsequent coagulation studies. Antifibrinolytic infusions decrease blood loss, transfusion of red blood cells and clotting factors such as platelets, fresh frozen plasma, and cryoprecipitate, and blood donor exposures after heart transplant via repeat sternotomy. After adequate hemostasis is achieved, the wound is closed in standard fashion and the patient transported to the intensive care unit (ICU).

Postoperative Management and Complications

Management in the ICU after the conclusion of the procedure is essentially a continuation of the anesthetic management after CPB. The ECG, the arterial, central venous, and/or PA pressures, and the arterial oxygen saturation are monitored continuously.

20

Cardiac recipients will continue to require β-adrenergic infusions for chronotropy and inotropy for up to 3 to 4 days. Vasodilators may be necessary to control arterial hypertension and decrease impedance to LV ejection. Patients can be weaned from ventilatory support and extubated when the hemodynamics are stable and hemorrhage has ceased. The immunosuppressive regimen of choice (typically consisting of cyclosporine, azathioprine, and prednisone or of tacrolimus and prednisone) should be started after arrival in the ICU. Invasive monitoring can be withdrawn as the inotropic support is weaned, and mediastinal tubes are removed after drainage subsides (usually after 24 hours). Patients can usually be discharged from the ICU after 2 or 3 days.

Early complications after heart transplantation include acute and hyperacute rejection, cardiac failure, systemic and pulmonary hypertension, cardiac arrhythmias, renal failure, and infection. Hyperacute rejection is an extremely rare but devastating syndrome mediated by preformed recipient cytotoxic antibodies against donor heart antigens. The donor heart immediately becomes cyanotic from microvascular thrombosis and ultimately ceases to contract. This syndrome is lethal unless the patient can be supported mechanically until a suitable heart is found. Acute rejection is a constant threat in the early postoperative period and may present in many forms (e.g., low CO, arrhythmias). Acute rejection occurs most frequently during the initial 6 months after transplantation, so its presence is monitored by serial endomyocardial biopsies, with additional biopsies to evaluate any acute changes in clinical status. Detection of rejection mandates an aggressive increase in the level of immunosuppression, usually including pulses of glucocorticoid or a change from cyclosporine to tacrolimus. Low CO after transplantation may reflect a number of causes: hypovolemia, inadequate adrenergic stimulation, myocardial injury during harvesting, acute rejection, tamponade, or sepsis. Therapy should be guided by invasive monitoring, TEE, and endomyocardial biopsy. Systemic hypertension may be due to pain, so adequate analgesia should be obtained before treating blood pressure with a vasodilator. Because fixed pulmonary hypertension will have been excluded during the recipient evaluation, pulmonary hypertension after heart transplantation is usually transient and responsive to vasodilators such as prostaglandin E_1, nitrates, or hydralazine after either orthotopic or heterotopic placement.[7] Atrial and ventricular tachyarrhythmias are common after heart transplantation; once rejection has been ruled out as a cause, antiarrhythmics are used for conversion or control (except those acting via indirect mechanisms such as digoxin, or those with negative inotropic properties such as β-blockers and calcium channel blockers). Almost all recipients will require either β-adrenergic agonists or pacing to increase heart rate in the immediate perioperative period, but 10% to 25% of recipients will also require permanent pacing.[8] Renal function often improves immediately after transplantation, but immunosuppressives such as cyclosporine and tacrolimus may impair renal function. Finally, infection is a constant threat to immunosuppressed recipients. Bacterial pneumonia is frequent early in the postoperative period, with opportunistic viral and fungal infections becoming more common after the first several weeks.

LUNG TRANSPLANTATION

History and Epidemiology

Although the first human lung transplant was performed in 1963, surgical technical problems and inadequate preservation and immunosuppression regimens prevented widespread acceptance of this procedure until the mid 1980s (Box 20-2). Advances in these areas have since made lung transplantation a viable option for many patients

---

BOX 20-2   *Lung Transplantation*

- Broader donor criteria have decreased the time from listing to transplantation.
- Nitric oxide minimizes reperfusion injury.
- Donor lungs should be ventilated with a protective strategy (low inspired oxygen, low tidal volume/inspired pressure) after transplantation.

---

with end-stage lung disease. The frequency of both single- and double-lung transplants increased exponentially during the period up until 1993, with the sharpest growth in unilateral transplants. According to data collected by UNOS between 2000 and 2002, the annual frequency of lung transplantation remained stagnant, with the total number averaging in the vicinity of 1000. This is unchanged from the time between 1993 and 1995 when the numbers first leveled off. Further growth in lung transplantation is constrained by a shortage of donor organs, with demand for organs still vastly exceeding supply. It is estimated that in excess of a million individuals with end-stage lung disease are potential recipients of lung transplants.[9] Some had hoped that non–heart-beating donors would provide an alternative source of organs, but this has not been the case. The Organ Procurement and Transplantation Network currently registers approximately 4000 patients for lung transplantation. This number does not accurately reflect the number of organs required as some patients will require bilateral lung transplantation. Average time to transplant increased to as much as 451 days in 1999, but now about one fourth of patients receive a transplant within 251 days. Most of this improvement has been seen with recipients who are 50 years of age and older. One explanation for this may be increasing leniency in organ selection criteria. This seems to have not been associated with increasing mortality rates. Mortality for patients on the waiting list has also continued to decline, from a 1993 high of close to 250 per 1000 patient-years to approximately 140 in 2002. Although some of this improvement may be ascribed to better medical management of patients on the waiting list, it is also likely due to broadened criteria for acceptance for transplantation and subsequent inclusion of patients with less severe illness.

Increased experience with lung transplantation has been accompanied by a decrease in both operative and long-term mortality. For example, 30-day mortality for double-lung transplantation decreased from 44% in 1988 to 13.6% in 1991, whereas that for single-lung transplantation decreased from 22.7% to 12.6%.[10] As of the end of 1995, 3-year actuarial survival for recipients of both single- and double-lung transplants performed in the era 1992 to 1995 was approximately 60%, 10% better than for recipients transplanted in the previous 3-year interval. Even better survival data have been reported from centers with extensive experience with these procedures (1-year survival rates of 82% for double-lung recipients and 90% for single-lung recipients). Infection is the most frequent cause of death in the first year after transplant, but this is superceded in later years by bronchiolitis obliterans.

Some of the most challenging patients are those with cystic fibrosis. The 1-year survival of 79% and 5-year survival of 57% after lung transplantation have shown that despite the high incidence of poor nutrition and the almost ubiquitous colonization by multidrug-resistant organisms, these patients can still successfully undergo lung transplantation with acceptable outcome data.[11]

It is a sign of the maturity of lung transplantation procedures that survival data for repeat lung transplantation are also becoming available. A late 1991 survey of centers reported that actuarial survival after repeat transplantation was significantly worse than that of first-time recipients (e.g., 35% vs. greater than 75% at 1 year),[12] and

20

subsequent data have confirmed this observation. Infection and multiorgan failure before repeat transplant are associated with an almost uniformly fatal outcome.

Recipient Selection

Because donor lungs are scarce, it is important to select as recipients those most likely to benefit from lung transplantation. In general, candidates should be terminally ill with end-stage lung disease (NYHA class III or IV, with a life expectancy of approximately 2 years), be psychologically stable, and be devoid of serious medical illness (especially extrapulmonary infection) compromising other organ systems. Patients already requiring mechanical ventilation are poor candidates, although lung transplantation can be successful in such a setting. Other factors such as advanced age, previous thoracic surgery or deformity, and corticosteroid dependence may be regarded as relative contraindications by individual transplant centers. Hepatic disease due solely to right-sided heart dysfunction should not preclude candidacy.

Potential recipients undergo a multidisciplinary assessment of their suitability, including pulmonary spirometry, radiography (plain film and chest CT scan), and echocardiography or multiple gated image acquisition (MUGA) scan. Patients older than 40 years of age and those with pulmonary hypertension usually undergo left-sided heart catheterization to exclude significant coronary atherosclerosis or an intracardiac shunt. TEE may yield data (e.g., unanticipated atrial septal defect) that will alter subsequent surgical approach in approximately one fourth of patients with severe pulmonary hypertension. Candidates who are accepted are often placed on a physical conditioning regimen to reverse muscle atrophy and debilitation and to keep them within 20% of their ideal body weight. Because lung transplantation is an emergency procedure (limited by a lung preservation time of 6 to 8 hours), results of this comprehensive evaluation should be readily available to the anesthesia team at all times.

Donor Selection and Graft Harvest

The ongoing shortage of suitable donor organs has led to a liberalization of selection criteria. Prospective lung donors who were cigarette smokers are no longer rejected simply based on a pack-year history. CT has been used to assess the structural integrity of the lung, particularly in donors who have sustained traumatic chest injury. Lungs that have contusion limited to less than 30% of a single lobe can be considered adequate.[13] Greater use has also been made of organs from older but otherwise healthy donors (55 to 60 years old) especially when the ischemic period will be short. A clear chest radiograph, normal blood gas results, unremarkable findings on bronchoscopy and sputum stain, and direct intraoperative evaluation confirm satisfactory lung function. The lungs are matched to the recipient for ABO blood type and size (oversized lungs can result in severe atelectasis and compromise of venous return in the recipient, especially after double-lung transplantation). Donor serology and tracheal cultures guide subsequent antibacterial and antiviral therapy in the recipient.

Most lung grafts are recovered during a multivisceral donor harvest procedure. The heart is removed as described for heart transplantation, using inflow occlusion and cardioplegic arrest, with division of the IVC and SVC, the aorta, and the main PA. Immediately after cross-clamping, the pulmonary vasculature is flushed with ice-cold preservative solution, which often contains prostaglandin E_1. This is believed to promote pulmonary vasodilation, which aids homogeneous distribution of the preserving solution. Other additives that have been included are nitroglycerin and low-potassium 5% Dextran. The LA is divided so as to leave an adequate LA cuff for both the heart graft and lung graft(s) with the pulmonary veins. After explanation, the lung may also be flushed to clear all pulmonary veins of any clots. After the lung is inflated, the trachea (or bronchus for an isolated lung) is clamped, divided, and stapled closed. Inflating the lung has been shown to increase cold ischemia tolerance of the donor organ. The lung graft is removed, bagged, and immersed in ice-cold saline for transport.

Surgical Procedures

Because of the relative shortage of lung donors and the finding that recipients can gain significant exercise tolerance even with only one transplanted lung, single-lung transplantation is the procedure of choice for all lung transplant candidates, except when leaving one of the recipient's lungs in place would predispose to complications. For example, the presence of lung disease associated with chronic infection (cystic fibrosis and severe bronchiectasis) mandates double-lung transplantation to prevent the recipient lung from acting as a reservoir of infection and subsequently cross-contaminating the allograft. Patients with severe air trapping may require double-lung transplantation if uncontrollable ventilation-perfusion mismatching will be likely after transplantation. Lobar transplantation into children and young adults from living-related donors is discussed separately.

Single-Lung Transplant

The choice of which lung to transplant is usually based on multiple factors, including avoidance of a prior operative site, preference for removing the native lung with the worst ventilation-perfusion ratio, and donor lung availability. The recipient is positioned for a posterolateral thoracotomy, with the ipsilateral groin prepped and exposed in case CPB becomes necessary. With the lung deflated, a pneumonectomy is performed, with special care to preserve as long a PA segment as possible. After removal of the diseased native lung, the allograft is positioned in the chest with precautions to maintain its cold tissue temperature. The bronchial anastomosis is performed first. A "telescoping" anastomosis is used if there is significant discrepancy in size between the donor and the recipient. The object of the technique is to minimize the chance of dehiscence. Although it was once common to wrap bronchial anastomoses with omentum, wrapping produces no added benefit when a telescoping anastomosis is performed. The PA is anastomosed next, and finally the pericardium is opened and the allograft LA cuff containing the pulmonary venous orifices is anastomosed to the native LA. The pulmonary circuit is then flushed with blood and de-aired. The initial flush solution is usually cold (4°C) but is followed by a warm (37°C) flush. The warm flush is usually performed during final completion of the vascular anastomoses. The goal of the flushing is to achieve a controlled reperfusion. The contents of this solution are listed in Box 20-3. After glucocorticoid administration, the vascular clamps are removed, reperfusion is begun, and the lung reinflated with a series of ventilations to full functional residual capacity. After achieving adequate hemostasis and satisfactory blood gases, chest tubes are placed, the wound is closed, and the patient is transported to the ICU.

Double-Lung Transplant

Early attempts at double-lung transplantation using an en bloc technique via a median sternotomy were plagued by frequent postoperative airway dehiscence due to poor vascular supply of the tracheal anastomosis; by hemorrhage due to extensive mediastinal dissection (which also resulted in cardiac denervation); by the

BOX 20-3 *Warm Pulmonoplegia*

- Hematocrit 18% to 20%, leukocyte depleted
- L-Glutamate
- L-Aspartate
- Adenosine
- Lidocaine
- Nitroglycerin
- Verapamil
- Dextrose
- Insulin

requirement for complete CPB and cardioplegic arrest (to facilitate pulmonary arterial and venous anastomoses); and by poor access to the posterior mediastinum. The subsequent development of the bilateral sequential lung transplant technique via a "clamshell" thoracosternotomy (essentially two single-lung transplants performed in sequence) has avoided many of the problems inherent in the en bloc technique.[14] An alternative to using a clamshell incision in slender patients is an approach through two individual anterolateral thoracotomies. This results in a particularly pleasing cosmetic result in female patients because the scar falls in the breast crease. Use of CPB is optional, exposure of the posterior mediastinum is enhanced (improving hemostasis), and cardiac denervation can usually be avoided. Pleural scarring is usually extensive in patients with cystic fibrosis, and postoperative hemorrhage and coagulopathy are the rule if CPB is required.

Transplantation of both lungs is performed in the supine position. The groins are prepped and exposed in case CPB is required. If a clamshell incision is used, the arms are padded and suspended over the head on an ether screen. In the slender patient whose anteroposterior chest dimensions are normal, the arms may be tucked at the patient's sides. Recipient pneumonectomy and implantation of the donor lung are performed sequentially on both lungs in essentially the same manner as described above for a single-lung transplant. The native lung with the worst function should be transplanted first. In patients whose indication for transplantation is suppurative disease, the pleural cavity is pulse-lavaged with antibiotic-containing solution that has been tailored to that patient's antimicrobial sensitivity profile. In addition to this, the anesthesiologist irrigates the trachea and bronchi with diluted iodophore solution before the donor lung is brought onto the surgical field.

Pathophysiology before Transplantation

Patients with highly compliant lungs and obstruction of expiratory airflow cannot completely exhale the delivered tidal volume, resulting in positive intrapleural pressure throughout the respiratory cycle ("auto-PEEP" [positive end-expiratory pressure] or "intrinsic PEEP"), which decreases venous return and causes hypotension. The presence of auto-PEEP is highly negatively correlated with FEV_1 (percent predicted) and highly positively correlated with pulmonary flow resistance and resting hypercarbia. Hyperinflation is a frequent complication of single-lung ventilation during lung transplantation in patients with obstructive lung disease. Hyperinflation-induced hemodynamic instability can be diagnosed by turning off the ventilator for 30 seconds and opening the breathing circuit to the atmosphere. If the blood pressure returns to its baseline value, hyperinflation is the underlying cause. Hyperinflation

---

BOX 20-4   *Treatment of Intraoperative Right Ventricular Failure*

- Avoid large increases in intrathoracic pressure from:
  - Positive end-expiratory pressure (PEEP)
  - Large tidal volumes
  - Inadequate expiratory time
- Intravascular volume
  - Increase preload if pulmonary vascular resistance is normal.
  - Rely on inotropes (dobutamine) if pulmonary vascular resistance is increased.
- Maintain right ventricular coronary perfusion pressure with α-adrenergic agonists.
- Cautious administration of pulmonary vasodilators (avoid systemic and gas exchange effects)

  Prostaglandin E1 (0.05 to 0.15 µg/kg/min)

  Inhaled nitric oxide (20 to 40 ppm)

---

can be ameliorated with deliberate hypoventilation (decreasing both the tidal volume and/or rate).[15] Although this may result in profound hypercarbia, high carbon dioxide tensions are well tolerated in the absence of hypoxemia. PEEP may also decrease air trapping because it decreases expiratory resistance during controlled mechanical ventilation. However, the application of PEEP requires close monitoring, because if the level of extrinsic PEEP applied exceeds the level of auto-PEEP, further air trapping may result.

RV failure is frequently encountered in lung transplant recipients with pulmonary hypertension due to chronically elevated RV afterload. The response of the RV to a chronic increase in afterload is to hypertrophy, but eventually this adaptive response is insufficient. As a result, RV volume decreases and chamber dilation results. The following should be kept in mind when caring for patients with severe RV dysfunction (Box 20-4). First, increases in intrathoracic pressure may markedly increase PVR, leading to frank RV failure in patients with chronic RV dysfunction. Changes in RV function may occur immediately after adding PEEP, increasing tidal volume or decreasing expiratory time, and can have devastating consequences. In addition, although intravascular volume expansion in the presence of normal PVR increases CO, overzealous infusion in patients with elevated PVR increases RV end-diastolic pressure and RV wall stress, decreasing CO. Inotropes with vasodilating properties (such as dobutamine or milrinone) are often a better choice than volume for augmenting CO in the setting of elevated PVR. Furthermore, the RV has a higher metabolic demand yet a lower coronary perfusion pressure than normal. RV performance can be augmented by improving RV coronary perfusion pressure with α-adrenergic agents, provided these vasoconstrictors do not disproportionately elevate PVR. This can sometimes be a better choice than augmenting the perfusion pressure with β-adrenergic agents because the oxygen supply is increased without a large increase in oxygen demand. Finally, vasodilators such as nitroprusside or prostaglandin E_1 may be effective in decreasing PVR and improving RV dysfunction early in the disease process, when only mild to moderate pulmonary hypertension is present. However, they are of notably limited value in the presence of severe, end-stage pulmonary hypertension. Systemic vasodilation and exacerbation of shunting often limit their use. Inhaled nitric oxide has shown promise as a means of acutely decreasing PVR without altering systemic hemodynamics both during the explanation phase and after lung transplantation.[16] Nitric oxide decreases both PA pressure and intrapulmonary shunting. Further, the combination of inhaled nitric oxide and aerosolized prostacyclin had a synergistic effect, without causing deleterious effects on the systemic perfusion pressure. The use of nitric oxide with or without inhaled prostacyclin may be helpful in avoiding CPB in patients having lung transplantation.

20

Pathophysiology after Lung Transplantation

The implantation of the donor lung(s) causes marked alterations in recipient respiratory physiology. In single-lung recipients, the pattern of ventilation-perfusion matching depends on the original disease process. For example, with pulmonary fibrosis, blood flow and ventilation gradually divert to the transplanted lung, whereas in patients transplanted for diseases associated with pulmonary hypertension, blood flow is almost exclusively diverted to the transplanted lung, which still receives only half of the total ventilation. In such patients the native lung represents mostly dead-space ventilation. Transplantation results in obligatory sympathetic and parasympathetic denervation of the donor lung and therefore alters the physiologic responses of airway smooth muscle. Exaggerated bronchoconstrictive responses to the muscarinic agonist methacholine have been noted in some studies of denervated lung recipients. The mechanism of hyperresponsiveness may involve cholinergic synapses, inasmuch as they are the main mediators of bronchoconstriction. For example, electrical stimulation of transplanted bronchi (which activates cholinergic nerves) produces a hypercontractile response. This suggests either enhanced release of acetylcholine from cholinergic nerve endings due to an increased responsiveness of parasympathetic nerves or else loss of inhibitory innervation. Such effects are unlikely to be postsynaptic in origin because the number and affinity of muscarinic cholinergic receptors on transplanted human bronchi are similar to controls. Reinnervation during subsequent weeks to months has been demonstrated in several animal models, but there is no definitive evidence concerning reinnervation of transplanted human lungs. Mucociliary function is transiently severely impaired after lung transplantation and remains depressed for up to 1 year after the procedure. Thus, transplant recipients require particularly aggressive endotracheal suctioning to remove airway secretions.

Lung transplantation also profoundly alters the vascular system. The ischemia and reperfusion that are an obligatory part of the transplantation process damage endothelia. Cold ischemia alone decreases β-adrenergic cyclic adenosine monophosphate (cAMP)-mediated vascular relaxation by approximately 40%, and subsequent reperfusion produces even greater decreases in both cyclic guanosine monophosphate (cGMP)-mediated and β-adrenergic cAMP-mediated pulmonary vascular smooth muscle relaxation. Endothelial damage in the pulmonary allograft also results in "leaky" alveolar capillaries and the development of pulmonary edema. Pulmonary endothelial permeability is approximately three times greater in donor lungs than in healthy volunteers. Regulation of pulmonary vasomotor tone solely by circulating humoral factors is another side effect of denervation. Changes in either the levels of circulating mediators or in the responsiveness of the pulmonary vasculature to such mediators may result in dramatic effects on the pulmonary vasculature. An example of the former is the finding that the potent vasoconstrictor endothelin is present at markedly elevated levels (two to three times normal) immediately after transplantation and remains elevated for up to 1 week thereafter. Alterations in the response of denervated pulmonary vasculature to α_1-adrenergic agents and prostaglandin E_1, as well as a reduction in nitric oxide activity, have also been demonstrated in acutely denervated lung. Dysfunctional responses to mediators may be exaggerated if CPB is required. Pulmonary vascular resistance can be substantially decreased with the administration of inhaled nitric oxide after reperfusion. It remains unclear whether nitric oxide also ameliorates reperfusion injury. Several studies suggest that nitric oxide prevents or modulates reperfusion injury as measured by decreased lung water, lipid peroxidase activity, and neutrophil aggregation in the graft.[17] However, there are a number of studies that suggest that although nitric oxide has an effect on pulmonary hemodynamics, it does not ameliorate reperfusion injury.

Given these pathophysiologic derangements, it is not surprising that PVR increases in the transplanted lung. However, what the clinician observes in the lung transplant patient will depend on the severity of pulmonary vascular dysfunction present preoperatively. PA pressures decrease dramatically during lung transplantation in patients who had pulmonary hypertension before transplantation and remain so for weeks to months thereafter. Concomitant with the decrease in PA pressure, there is an immediate decrease in RV size after lung transplantation in those patients with preexisting pulmonary hypertension, as well as a return to a more normal geometry of the interventricular septum. Both of these effects are sustained over several weeks to months. Although echocardiographic indices of RV function (RV fractional area change) have not shown a consistent improvement in the immediate post-transplant period, several other studies have documented improvement in RV function during the first several months after lung transplantation. One striking finding was that persistent depression of RV function (defined as baseline RV fractional area change of less than 30% with failure to increase after transplant by at least 5% or by 20% of baseline) was statistically associated with death in the immediate perioperative period.

Anesthetic Management

Preoperative Evaluation and Preparation

Immediate pretransplant reevaluation pertinent to intraoperative management includes a history and physical examination to screen for intercurrent deterioration or additional abnormalities that affect anesthetic management. Particular attention should be given to recent physical status, especially when the transplant evaluation was performed more than 9 to 12 months previously. A decrease in the maximal level of physical activity from that at the time of initial evaluation can be a sign of progressive pulmonary disease or worsening RV function. Most patients are maintained on supplemental nasal oxygen, yet are mildly hypoxemic. Patients who are bedridden, or who must pause between phrases or words while speaking, possess little functional reserve and are likely to exhibit hemodynamic instability during induction. The time and nature of the last oral intake should be determined to aid in deciding the appropriate method of securing the airway. The physical examination should focus on evaluation of the airway for ease of laryngoscopy and intubation; the presence of any reversible pulmonary dysfunction such as bronchospasm; and signs of cardiac failure. New laboratory data are often not available before the beginning of anesthesia care, but special attention should be directed to evaluation of the chest radiograph for signs of pneumothorax, effusion, or hyperinflation because they may affect subsequent management.

Equipment necessary for this procedure is analogous to that used in any procedure where CPB and cardiac arrest are real possibilities. Special mandatory pieces of equipment include some method to isolate the ventilation to each lung. Although bronchial blockers have their advocates, double-lumen endobronchial tubes offer the advantages of easy switching of the ventilated lung, suctioning of the nonventilated lung, and facile independent lung ventilation postoperatively. A left-sided double-lumen endobronchial tube is suitable for virtually all lung transplant cases (even left lung transplants). Regardless of whether a bronchial blocker or double-lumen tube is used, a fiberoptic bronchoscope is absolutely required to rapidly and unambiguously verify correct tube positioning, evaluate bronchial anastomoses, and clear airway secretions. An adult-sized bronchoscope offers better field of vision and superior suctioning capability but can be used only with 41- or 39-Fr double-lumen tubes. A ventilator with low internal compliance is necessary to adequately ventilate the noncompliant lungs of recipients with restrictive lung disease or donor lungs with reperfusion injury. The added capability of the ventilator to deliver pressure-controlled ventilation is also important, especially for the patients who have pulmonary fibrotic disease or reperfusion injury. Single-lung recipients with highly compliant lungs may require independent lung ventilation with a second ventilator after transplantation. A PA catheter capable of estimating RV ejection fraction (RVEF) can be useful in diagnosing RV failure and its response to inotropes and vasodilators, as well as the response of the RV to clamping of the PA. However, RVEF catheters are not accurate in the presence of significant tricuspid regurgitation or when malpositioned. Continuous mixed venous oximetry is beneficial in evaluating tissue oxygen delivery in patients subject to sudden, severe cardiac decompensation in the course of the operation, as well as the responses to therapy. A rapid infusion system can be lifesaving in patients in whom major hemorrhage occurs due to anastomotic leaks, inadequate surgical ligation of mediastinal collateral vessels, chest wall adhesions, or coagulopathy after CPB.

Induction of Anesthesia

Patients presenting for lung transplantation frequently arrive in the operating room area without premedication. Indeed, many are admitted directly to the operating room from home. Due to the nature of the procedure planned, and many months on the transplant waiting list, these patients are often extremely anxious. Considering the risk of respiratory depression from sedatives in patients who are chronically hypoxic and/or hypercapnic, only the most judicious use of intravenous benzodiazepines or narcotics is warranted. Assiduous administration of adequate local anesthesia during placement of invasive monitoring will also considerably improve conditions for both the patient and anesthesiologist. The standard noninvasive monitoring typical of cardiovascular procedures (two electrocardiogram [ECG] leads including a precordial lead, blood pressure cuff, pulse oximetry, capnography, and temperature measurement) is used. Intravenous access sufficient to rapidly administer large volumes of fluid is required. Generally, two large-bore (16- or, preferably, 14-gauge catheters, or a 9-Fr introducer sheath) intravenous catheters are placed. Patients for bilateral sequential lung transplantation who will receive a "clamshell" thoracosternotomy should have intravenous catheters placed in the internal or external jugular veins, because peripherally placed intravenous catheters are often unreliable when the arms are bent at the elbow and suspended from the ether screen. An intra-arterial catheter is an absolute requirement for blood pressure monitoring and for obtaining specimens for arterial blood gases. Continuous monitoring via a fiberoptic electrode placed in the arterial catheter may occasionally be useful if this technology is available. The femoral artery should be avoided if possible because the groin may be needed as a site for cannulation for CPB. Although the radial or brachial artery may be used in single-lung transplantation patients, these sites are not optimal in those who will require CPB (e.g., en bloc double-lung transplants or patients with severe pulmonary hypertension) because the transduced pressure may inaccurately reflect central aortic pressure during and after CPB, as well as in patients undergoing a clamshell thoracosternotomy, because of the positioning of the arms. An axillary arterial catheter may be useful in the latter situations because it provides a more accurate measure of central aortic pressure and allows sampling blood closer to that perfusing the brain. This may be important if partial CPB with a femoral arterial cannula is used because differential perfusion of the upper and lower half of the body

IV

> ### BOX 20-5 *Key Principles of Anesthetic Induction for Lung Transplantation*
>
> - Secure the airway
>   - Intravenous rapid sequence induction versus gradual narcotic induction with continuous cricoid pressure
> - Avoid myocardial depression and increases in right ventricular afterload
> - Avoid lung hyperinflation

may result. A PA catheter is inserted via the internal or external jugular veins. A TEE probe is placed after the airway is secured. PA pressure monitoring is most useful in patients who have preexisting pulmonary hypertension, especially during induction and during initial one-lung ventilation and PA clamping. Position of the PA catheter can be verified by TEE to ensure that it is residing in the main PA.

If the procedure is planned without CPB, care should be taken to ensure that the patient would be kept at ideal physiologic temperature to minimize coagulopathy and increases in the Myo_2. This can be achieved with a warming blanket on the bed, on the patient's head and arms, and on the legs below the knees. A fluid warmer is also useful in this regard.

Three main principles should guide the formulation of a plan for induction: (1) protection of the airway; (2) avoidance of myocardial depression and increases in RV afterload in patients with RV dysfunction; and (3) avoidance and recognition of lung hyperinflation in patients with increased lung compliance and expiratory airflow obstruction (Box 20-5). All lung transplants are done on an emergency basis, and the majority of patients will have recently had oral intake and must be considered to have "full stomachs." Since aspiration during induction would be catastrophic, every measure must be taken to protect the airway. Patients with known or suspected abnormalities of airway anatomy should be intubated awake after topical anesthesia is applied to the airway. Although a conventional rapid-sequence intravenous induction with a short-acting hypnotic (e.g., etomidate 0.2 to 0.3 mg/kg), a small amount of narcotic (e.g., up to 10 µg/kg of fentanyl), and succinylcholine will usually be tolerated, patients with severe RV dysfunction may exhibit profound hemodynamic instability in response to this induction regimen. For such patients, a more gradual induction is recommended, with greater reliance on high doses of narcotics and ventilation with continuous application of cricoid pressure. Patients with bullous disease or fibrotic lungs requiring high inflation pressures may develop a pneumothorax during initiation of positive-pressure ventilation. Acute reductions in Sao_2 accompanied by difficulty in ventilating the lungs and refractory hypotension should generate strong suspicions that a tension pneumothorax has developed. RV function can be impaired during induction by drug-induced myocardial depression, by increases in afterload, or by ischemia secondary to acute RV dilation. Agents that act as myocardial depressants (e.g., thiopental) should be avoided in such patients. Increases in RV afterload can result from inadequate anesthesia, exacerbation of chronic hypoxemia and hypercarbia, and metabolic acidosis, as well as increases in intrathoracic pressure due to positive-pressure ventilation. Systemic hypotension is poorly tolerated because increased RV end-diastolic pressure will diminish net RV coronary perfusion pressure. In addition, chronic elevation of RV afterload increases the metabolic requirements of RV myocardium. Once the trachea is intubated and positive-pressure ventilation initiated, the avoidance of hyperinflation in patients with increased pulmonary compliance or bullous disease is crucial. Small tidal volumes and low respiratory rates and inspiratory/expiratory (I/E) ratios should be

---

BOX 20-6 *Management Principles for One-Lung Ventilation during Lung Transplantation*

- Tidal volume and respiratory rate
  - Maintain in patients with normal or decreased lung compliance (i.e., primary pulmonary hypertension, fibrosis)
  - Decrease both tidal volume and rate in patients with increased compliance (e.g., obstructive lung disease) to avoid hyperinflation ("permissive hypercapnia")
- Maintain oxygenation by
  - 100% Inspired oxygen
  - Applying continuous positive airway pressure (5 to 10 cm) to nonventilated lung
  - Adding positive end-expiratory pressure (5 to 10 cm) to ventilated lung
  - Intermittent lung re-inflation if necessary
  - Surgical ligation of the pulmonary artery of the nonventilated lung
- Be alert for development of pneumothorax on nonoperative side
  - Sharp drop in oxygen saturation, end-tidal carbon dioxide
  - Sharp rise in peak airway pressures
  - Increased risk with bullous lung disease
- Therapy
  - Relieve tension
  - Resume ventilation
  - Emergency cardiopulmonary bypass

---

used ("permissive hypercapnia"). If hemodynamic instability does occur with positive-pressure ventilation, the ventilator should be disconnected from the patient. If hyperinflation is the cause of hypotension, blood pressure will increase within 10 to 30 seconds of the onset of apnea. Ventilation can then be resumed at a tidal volume and/or rate compatible with hemodynamic stability.

Anesthesia can be maintained using a variety of techniques. A moderate dose of narcotic (5 to 15 μg/kg of fentanyl or the equivalent), combined with low doses of a potent inhalation anesthetic, offers the advantages of stable hemodynamics, a high inspired oxygen concentration, a rapidly titratable depth of anesthesia, and the possibility of extubation in the early postoperative period. Patients with severe RV dysfunction who cannot tolerate even low concentrations of inhalation anesthetics may require a pure narcotic technique. Nitrous oxide is generally not used, because of the requirement for a high inspired oxygen concentration throughout the procedure, and its possible deleterious effects if gaseous emboli or an occult pneumothorax is present.

Intraoperative Management

Institution of one-lung ventilation (OLV) occurs before hilar dissection and may compromise hemodynamics and/or gas exchange (Box 20-6). Patients with diminished lung compliance can often tolerate OLV with normal tidal volumes and little change in hemodynamics. In contrast, patients with increased lung compliance and airway obstruction will often exhibit marked hemodynamic instability, unless the tidal volume is decreased and the expiratory time is increased. The magnitude of hypoxemia generally peaks about 20 minutes after beginning OLV. Hypoxemia during OLV may be treated with continuous positive airway pressure (CPAP) applied to the nonventilated lung,[18] PEEP to the ventilated lung, or both. CPAP attempts to oxygenate the shunt fraction but may interfere with surgical exposure. PEEP attempts to minimize atelectasis in the ventilated lung but may concomitantly increase shunt through the nonventilated lung. Definitive treatment of shunt in the nonventilated

> **BOX 20-7** *Indications for Cardiopulmonary Bypass during Lung Transplantation*
>
> | | |
> |---|---|
> | Cardiac index | <2 L/min/m^2 |
> | S$\bar{v}o_2$ | <60% |
> | Mean arterial pressure | <50 to 60 mm Hg |
> | Sao$_2$ | <85% to 90% |
> | pH | <7.00 |

lung is provided by rapid isolation and clamping of the PA of the nonventilated lung. Pneumothorax on the nonoperative side may result during OLV if a large tidal volume is used.

PA clamping is usually well tolerated, except in the face of pulmonary hypertension with diminished RV reserve. If the degree of RV compromise is uncertain, a 5- to 10-minute trial of PA clamping is attempted, then the RV is evaluated by serial CO, RVEF measurements, and TEE. A significant decrease in CO may predict patients who will require extracorporeal support. Other indications for CPB in lung transplantation are listed in Box 20-7.

Patients with severe pulmonary hypertension (greater than two thirds of systemic pressure) will generally be placed on CPB before PA clamping. The intraoperative use of nitric oxide (20 to 40 ppm) may allow some procedures to proceed without the use of CPB.[19]

Lung transplantation can usually be performed without the aid of CPB; even during bilateral sequential lung transplantation, experienced teams use CPB for only about one fourth of patients. Although CPB may provide very stable hemodynamics, it is associated with an increased transfusion requirement. In addition, graft function (as reflected by alveolar-arterial oxygen gradient) may be compromised, endothelium-dependent cGMP- and β-adrenergic cAMP-mediated pulmonary vascular relaxation may be impaired to a greater degree, and a longer period of mechanical ventilation may be necessary. Several exceptional circumstances require CPB: the presence of severe pulmonary hypertension, because clamping of the PA will likely result in acute RV failure and "flooding" of the nonclamped lung; the repair of associated cardiac anomalies (e.g., patent foramen ovale, atrial or ventricular septal defects); treatment of severe hemodynamic or gas exchange instabilities; and living-related lobar transplantation. Hypercarbia is generally well tolerated and should not be considered a requirement for CPB per se. Thus, the frequency of CPB will depend on recipient population factors such as prevalence of end-stage pulmonary vascular disease and associated cardiac anomalies.

The use of femoral venous and arterial cannulas for CPB during lung transplantation may lead to poor venous drainage and/or "differential perfusion" of the lower and upper body. Moreover, native pulmonary blood flow continues and may act as an intrapulmonary shunt during CPB. In this case, the cerebral vessels receive this desaturated blood while the lower body is perfused with fully oxygenated blood from the CPB circuit. This effect is detectable by blood gas analysis of samples drawn from suitable arteries or appropriately located pulse oximeter probes. Treatment includes conventional measures to increase venous return and augment bypass flow or placing a venous cannula in the RA if this is feasible. The anesthesiologist should also maximize the inspired oxygen concentration and add PEEP to decrease intrapulmonary shunt. If all other measures fail, ventricular fibrillation can be induced using alternating current.

Extracorporeal membrane oxygenation (ECMO) has also been suggested as an alternative method of CPB during lung transplantation. It has been suggested that the use of ECMO with heparin-bonded circuits might improve the outcome of both single- and double-lung transplants by lessening the amount of pulmonary edema especially in those patients who need CPB due to hemodynamic instability or with primary pulmonary hypertension. An added benefit of this technique is also that it clears the operative field of bypass cannulas making left-sided transplant as unimpeded as right-sided transplant. There is no apparent increase in transfusion requirement. Another added benefit of using ECMO in situ is that reperfusion of the lungs can be more easily controlled since the CO transiting the newly transplanted lung can be precisely controlled. This is especially the case for patients with advanced pulmonary hypertension.[20]

If CPB is used, weaning from circulatory support occurs when the graft anastomoses are complete. Ventilation is resumed with a lung protection strategy. This technique in patients with decreased compliance related to acute respiratory distress syndrome had a 22% decrease in mortality when applying tidal volumes of 6 mL/kg and a plateau pressure less than 30 cm H_2O. Minimizing the inspired fraction of O_2 may help prevent generation of oxygen free-radicals and modulate reperfusion injury. Fio_2 can be decreased to the minimum necessary to maintain the Spo_2 at greater than 90%. Special attention should be directed to assessing and supporting RV function during this period, inasmuch as RV failure is the most frequent reason for failure to wean. Although the RV can often be seen in the surgical field, TEE is more valuable for visualizing this structure's functional properties at this juncture. Inotropic support with dobutamine or epinephrine as well as pulmonary vasodilation with nitroglycerin, nitroprusside, milrinone, or nitric oxide may be necessary if RV dysfunction is evident. Milrinone has the advantage of providing both inotropic and vasodilatory effects; however, its administration can be complicated by significant systemic hypotension necessitating the concomitant use of epinephrine or norepinephrine.

Coagulopathy after weaning from CPB is common. The severity of coagulopathy may be worse after double- than single-lung transplantation, probably due to the more extensive dissection, presence of collaterals and scarring, and the longer duration of CPB. Factors under the anesthesiologist's control include incomplete reversal of heparin's effects, which should be assayed by the activated coagulation time. Similarly, preexisting deliberate anticoagulation (e.g., due to warfarin) should be aggressively corrected with fresh frozen plasma. Because platelet dysfunction is common after CPB, empirical administration is justified if coagulopathy persists. The thrombotic and fibrinolytic systems are activated during lung transplantation, especially if CPB is used, and aprotinin can reduce this activation and perhaps reduce perioperative hemorrhage. The efficacy of ε-aminocaproic acid, tranexamic acid, and desmopressin (DDAVP) in this setting remains unknown.

Reperfusion without CPB is often accompanied by a mild to moderate decrease in systemic blood pressure and occasionally is complicated by severe hypotension. This is usually the result of profound systemic vasodilation. The etiology is unknown but may be due to ionic loads such as potassium or additives such as prostaglandin E_1 in preservation solutions or vasoactive substances generated during ischemia and reperfusion. This hypotension generally responds well to large doses of α-adrenergic agents and fortunately is short-lived. Agents of greatest use in this setting are norepinephrine and vasopressin. Ventilation is resumed with a lung protection strategy identical to that used when weaning from CPB.

Patients with preexisting increased lung compliance as found in chronic obstructive pulmonary disease can manifest great disparity in lung compliance after single-lung transplant. The donor lung usually exhibits normal to decreased compliance, depending on the presence of reperfusion injury. This will result in relative hyperinflation of the native lung and underinflation with loss of functional residual capacity in the donor lung. Hyperinflation of the native lung may cause hemodynamic instability due to mediastinal shift, especially if PEEP is applied. Therefore, patients exhibiting signs of hyperinflation during OLV, which improves with deliberate hypoventilation, should be treated with independent lung ventilation after reperfusion. To accomplish this, the patient's postoperative ventilator is brought to the operating room while the donor lung is being implanted. When all anastomoses are completed, the donor lung is ventilated with a normal tidal volume (8 to 10 mL/kg) and rate, with PEEP initially applied at 10 cm H_2O. These settings can be adjusted according to blood gases analysis. The vast majority of gas exchange will take place in the donor lung. The native lung is ventilated with a low tidal volume (2 to 3 mL/kg) and a low rate (2 to 4/min) without PEEP. The objective is to prevent this lung from overinflating or developing a large shunt. Carbon dioxide exchange occurs predominantly in the donor lung.

Although some degree of pulmonary edema is commonly detected by chest radiography postoperatively, it is uncommon to encounter severe pulmonary edema in the operating room immediately after reperfusion of the graft. However, when it does occur, postreperfusion pulmonary edema can be dramatic and life-threatening. Copious pink frothy secretions may require almost constant suctioning to maintain a patent airway and be accompanied by severe gas exchange and compliance abnormalities. Treatment includes high levels of PEEP using selective lung ventilation, diuresis, and volume restriction. Occasionally, patients may require support with ECMO for several days until reperfusion injury resolves; a high percentage of patients so treated ultimately survive.

Adequate analgesia is crucial for these patients to facilitate the earliest possible extubation, ambulation, and participation in spirometric exercises to enhance or preserve pulmonary function. Lumbar or thoracic epidural narcotic analgesia provides excellent analgesia while minimizing sedation. Epidural catheters can be placed prior to the procedure if time permits or after conclusion of the procedure. Placement of epidural catheters in cases where a high expectation exists for the necessity of CPB still remains a controversial topic. If CPB has been used or coagulopathy has developed, placement should be deferred until coagulation tests have normalized.

Postoperative Management and Complications

Routine postoperative management of the lung transplant recipient continues many of the monitoring modes and therapies begun in the operating room. Positive-pressure ventilation is continued for at least several hours; if differential lung ventilation was used intraoperatively, this is continued in the early postoperative period. Because the lung graft is prone to the development of pulmonary edema due to preservation/reperfusion and the loss of lymphatic drainage, fluid administration is minimized and diuresis encouraged when appropriate. When hemorrhage has ceased, the chest radiograph is clear, and the patient meets conventional extubation criteria, the endotracheal tube can be removed. Prophylactic antibacterial, antifungal, and antiviral therapy, as well as the immunosuppressive regimen of choice, is begun after arrival in the ICU.

Surgical technical complications are uncommon immediately after lung transplantation but may be associated with high morbidity. Pulmonary venous obstruction usually presents as acute, persistent pulmonary edema of the transplanted lung. Color-flow and Doppler TEE will show narrowed pulmonary venous orifices with turbulent, high-velocity flow and loss of the normal phasic waveform.

PA anastomotic obstruction should be suspected if PA pressures fail to decrease after reperfusion of the lung graft. If the right PA is obstructed, this is usually evident on a TEE examination in the same way as for pulmonary venous obstruction; it is usually much more difficult to adequately inspect the left PA anastomosis with TEE, although some centers have reported a high success rate. The diagnosis can be definitively made by measuring the pressure gradient across the anastomosis either by inserting needles on both sides of the anastomosis to transduce the respective pressures, or by advancing the PA catheter across it. However, care should be taken not to measure this gradient while the contralateral PA is clamped, because the shunting of the entire CO through one lung will exaggerate the gradient present. Angiography and perfusion scanning are also useful for making this diagnosis but are not immediately available in the operating room. Bronchial dehiscence or obstruction is extremely rare in the immediate perioperative period and can be evaluated by fiberoptic bronchoscopy.

Pneumothorax must be a constant concern for the anesthesiologist, especially involving the nonoperative side. Diagnosis of pneumothorax on the nonoperative side during a thoracotomy is extremely difficult. A sudden increase in inflation pressures with deterioration of gas exchange and possibly hypotension are characteristic. However, these same findings are possible with hyperinflation, mucus plugging, or malpositioning of the endobronchial tube. Transient cessation of ventilation and immediate fiberoptic bronchoscopy may rule out the former explanations, and the observation of an upward shift of the mediastinum in the surgical field may be observed in the presence of tension pneumothorax. If this diagnosis is strongly suspected, needle thoracostomy on the field may be lifesaving. Alternatively, the surgeon may be able to directly dissect across the mediastinum and decompress the nonoperative thorax, facilitating reinflation.

Tension pneumopericardium and postoperative hemothorax with complete ventilation-perfusion mismatch are other rare complications that have been reported after lung transplantation. Patients with pulmonary hypertension and RV hypertrophy may occasionally develop dynamic RV outflow obstruction when transplantation acutely decreases RV afterload; the diagnosis can be confirmed using TEE. Hyperacute rejection of a kind similar to that seen with heart transplantation has not been noted with lung transplantation.

The most common cause of death in the immediate perioperative period is graft dysfunction from reperfusion injury, which usually presents as hypoxemia, pulmonary infiltrates, poor lung compliance, pulmonary hypertension, and RV failure. If there are no technical reasons to account for pulmonary hypertension and RV failure, then graft dysfunction must be suspected. Unfortunately, few treatments will specifically ameliorate graft dysfunction, and therapy is largely supportive. Vasodilator therapy to directly decrease PVR and therefore RV afterload may improve hemodynamics and in some cases may improve gas exchange. Both prostaglandin E_1 and nitrates can reverse severe hypoxemia and pulmonary hypertension after lung transplantation, and the latter attenuate the increase in transcription of vasoconstrictor genes (such as for endothelin and platelet-derived growth factor) induced by hypoxia. Improvement in pulmonary hemodynamics and gas exchange in patients with graft dysfunction has also been reported with the administration of nitric oxide. Compared with historical control patients who developed graft dysfunction before the advent of nitric oxide, inhalation of nitric oxide decreased the duration of mechanical ventilation, frequency of airway complications, and mortality. Improved hemodynamics and gas exchange may reflect the ability of nitric oxide to compensate for the decrease in endothelium-derived relaxant factor activity after transplantation. If nitric oxide has been used

IV

to control pulmonary hypertension postoperatively it should be weaned gradually to avoid any rebound pulmonary vasoconstriction. Finally, extracorporeal membrane oxygenation may be employed to support the patient until there is adequate recovery of pulmonary function.

Rejection episodes are common and may occur as early as several days after transplantation. Rejection often presents as new infiltrates on chest radiograph in the setting of deteriorating gas exchange. Bronchoscopy with transbronchial biopsy helps to rule out other causes of deterioration and document acute changes consistent with rejection. Therapy for acute lung rejection consists of large pulses of corticosteroids such as methylprednisolone or changing the immunosuppressive agents (cyclosporine to tacrolimus or vice versa). Expired nitric oxide has been shown to be an indicator of chronic rejection in post–lung transplant patients. Measurements of expired nitric oxide have been shown to fall with the switch of cyclosporine to tacrolimus, reflecting a decrease in the inflammation in the pulmonary mucosa. Expired nitric oxide may be a useful tool to follow patients for the presence or change in chronic graft rejection.

One of the most serious complications of lung transplantation occurs late. Bronchiolitis obliterans is a syndrome characterized by alloimmune injury leading to obstruction of small airways with fibrous scar. Patients with bronchiolitis obliterans present with cough, progressive dyspnea, obstruction on flow spirometry, and interstitial infiltrates on chest radiograph. Therapy for this syndrome includes augmentation of immunosuppression, cytolytic agents (which have been used with varying degrees of success), or retransplantation in refractory cases.

Living-Related Lung Transplantation

The scarcity of suitable donor lungs has resulted in waiting times on transplant lists in excess of 2 years, during which as many as 30% of candidates succumb to their illness. Living-related lung transplantation programs have developed to address the needs of lung transplant candidates with acute deterioration expected to preclude survival. Successful grafting of a single lobe for children with bronchopulmonary dysplasia or Eisenmenger's syndrome, or two lobes for children and young adults with cystic fibrosis, has encouraged several centers to consider such procedures. The anesthetic management issues related to such undertakings have been reviewed.[21] Donor candidates will have undergone a rigorous evaluation to ensure that there are no contraindications to lobe donation and that the donation is not coerced. Donor lobectomy is performed via a standard posterolateral thoracotomy. Of special note to the anesthesiologist during such procedures is the requirement for OLV to optimize surgical exposure, the continuous infusion of prostaglandin E_1 to promote pulmonary vasodilation, and the administration of heparin and steroids just before lobe harvest. Anesthetic management of the recipient is identical to that for a standard lung transplant, except that the use of CPB is mandatory for bilateral lobar transplant.

HEART-LUNG TRANSPLANTATION

History and Epidemiology

The diminished frequency of heart-lung transplantation over the past decade reflects that it is being supplanted by lung transplantation. The number of heart-lung transplants worldwide peaked at 241 in 1989, and there has been a continual decline in subsequent years to approximately half that number. Approximately only 173

20

heart-lung transplant candidates were registered with UNOS as of early March 2005, less than 5% of the number on the lung transplant list. The most common recipient indications remain primary pulmonary hypertension, congenital heart disease (including Eisenmenger's syndrome), and cystic fibrosis.

One-year survival after heart-lung transplantation is 60%, significantly lower than that for isolated heart or lung transplantation. Mortality in subsequent years is approximately 4% per year, similar to that for heart transplantation. Risk factors for increased mortality after heart-lung transplant are recipient ventilator dependence, male recipient gender, and a donor age older than 40 years. Early deaths are most often due to graft failure or hemorrhage, whereas midterm and late deaths are primarily due to infection and bronchiolitis obliterans, respectively. Repeat heart-lung transplant is a rare procedure and likely to remain so because the 1-year survival after repeat heart-lung transplant is dismal (28%).

Recipient Selection

Candidates undergo an evaluation similar to that for lung transplant candidates. As more patients with pulmonary hypertension and cystic fibrosis are treated with isolated lung transplantation, it is likely that the indications for heart-lung transplantation will be limited to congenital heart disease with irreversible pulmonary hypertension that is not amenable to repair during simultaneous lung transplantation or diseases with both pulmonary hypertension and concomitant severe left ventricular dysfunction.

Donor Selection and Graft Harvest

Potential heart-lung donors must meet not only the criteria for heart donors but also those for lung donation, both described earlier in this chapter. Graft harvesting is carried out in a manner similar to that previously described for heart transplantation. After mobilization of the major vessels and trachea, cardiac arrest is induced with inflow occlusion and infusion of cold cardioplegia into the aortic root. After arrest, the pulmonary artery is flushed with a cold preservative solution often containing prostaglandin E_1. The ascending aorta, superior vena cava, and trachea are transected, and the heart-lung bloc is removed after it is dissected free of the esophagus. The trachea is clamped, and the graft is immersed in cold solution before being bagged for transport.

Surgical Procedures

The operation is generally performed through a median sternotomy, but a clamshell thoracosternotomy is also an acceptable approach. Both pleurae are incised. Any pulmonary adhesions are taken down before anticoagulation for bypass. Cannulae for CPB are placed in a manner similar to that for heart transplantation. After the aorta is cross-clamped, the heart is excised in a manner similar to that for orthotopic heart transplant. Each lung is then individually removed, including its pulmonary veins. The airways are divided at the level of the respective main bronchi for bibronchial anastomoses. For a tracheal anastomosis, the trachea is freed to the level of the carina without stripping its blood supply, and an anastomosis is constructed just above the level of the carina. The atrial anastomosis is performed in a manner similar to that for orthotopic heart transplantation, and finally the aorta is joined to the recipient aorta. After de-airing and reperfusion, the patient is weaned from CPB, hemostasis is achieved, and the wound is closed.

Pathophysiology before Transplantation

The pathophysiology of heart-lung transplant recipients combines the elements discussed earlier in this chapter. Patients usually have end-stage biventricular failure with severe pulmonary hypertension. The cardiac anatomy may be characterized by complex congenital malformations. If obstruction of pulmonary airflow is present, there is a danger of hyperinflation after application of positive-pressure ventilation.

Pathophysiology after Transplantation

Like isolated heart recipients, heart-lung transplant recipients' physiology is characterized by cardiac denervation; transient cardiac ischemic insult during graft harvest, transport, and implantation; and long-term susceptibility to accelerated allograft vasculopathy and rejection. As is the case for lung recipients, heart-lung recipients have denervated pulmonary vascular and airway smooth muscle responses, transient pulmonary ischemic insult, altered pulmonary lymphatic drainage, and impaired mucociliary clearance.

Anesthetic Management

The anesthetic management of heart-lung transplantation more closely resembles that of heart than lung transplantation, because the use of CPB is mandatory. After placement of invasive and noninvasive monitoring similar to that used for heart transplantation, anesthesia can be induced with any of the techniques previously described for heart and lung transplantation. Similar to lung transplantation, avoidance of myocardial depression as well as protection and control of the airway are paramount. Although a double-lumen endotracheal tube is not mandatory, it aids in exposure of the posterior mediastinum for hemostasis after weaning from CPB. Otherwise, anesthetic management before CPB is similar to that for heart transplantation.

A bolus of glucocorticoid (e.g., methylprednisolone, 500 mg) is given when the aortic cross-clamp is removed. After a period of reperfusion, an inotrope infusion is started, and the heart is inspected for adequate de-airing with TEE. Ventilation is resumed with normal tidal volume and rate and the addition of PEEP (5 to 10 cm) before weaning from CPB. After successful weaning from CPB, the pulmonary artery catheter can be advanced into the pulmonary artery again. Protamine is then administered to reverse heparin-induced anticoagulation. The inspired oxygen concentration can often be decreased to less toxic levels based on blood gas analysis.

Problems encountered after weaning from CPB are similar to those encountered after isolated heart or lung transplantation. Lung reperfusion injury and dysfunction may compromise gas exchange, so administration of crystalloid should be minimized. Occasionally, postreperfusion pulmonary edema may require support with high levels of PEEP and inspired oxygen in the operating room. Ventricular failure usually responds to an increase in β-adrenergic support. Unlike isolated heart or lung transplantation, frank right ventricular failure is uncommon immediately after heart-lung transplantation unless lung preservation was grossly inadequate. Coagulopathy is often present after heart-lung transplant and should be aggressively treated with additional protamine (if indicated), platelets, and fresh frozen plasma. Aprotinin can dramatically decrease hemorrhage after heart-lung transplant and reduce transfusion of red blood cells and platelets, and it is associated with a lower alveolar-arterial gradient for oxygen after transplantation.

20

Postoperative Management and Complications

The principles of the immediate postoperative care of heart-lung transplant recipients are a combination of those for isolated heart and lung recipients. Invasive and non-invasive monitoring done in the operating room is continued. Inotropic support is continued in a manner similar to that for heart transplantation. Ventilatory support is similar to that after lung transplantation; the lowest acceptable inspired oxygen concentration is used to avoid oxygen toxicity, and the patient is weaned from the ventilator after hemodynamics have been stable for several hours, hemorrhage has ceased, and satisfactory gas exchange is present. Diuresis is encouraged. Finally, the immunosuppressive regimen of choice is begun. Barring any complications, the patient can be discharged from the ICU after several days.

Infection is a more frequent and serious complication in heart-lung recipients than in isolated heart recipients. Bacterial and fungal infections are especially common in the first month after transplantation, with viral and other pathogens (*Pneumocystis carinii* and *Nocardia*) occurring in subsequent months.

Similar to isolated heart or lung transplants, rejection episodes are common early after heart-lung transplantation. Rejection may occur independently in either the heart or lung. Therapy is similar to that for rejection of isolated heart or lung grafts.

Heart grafts in heart-lung blocks are prone to accelerated coronary vasculopathy in a manner similar to those of isolated heart grafts. As with lung transplantation, a feared late complication of heart-lung transplantation is bronchiolitis obliterans. Clinical presentation is similar to that seen with lung transplant patients. Approximately one third of heart-lung recipients develop this process. Anecdotal reports indicate that most affected patients also have accelerated coronary vasculopathy.

SUMMARY

- The key factor limiting the number of cardiac transplants is a shortage of donors.
- The 1-year survival is 79%, with subsequent mortality of about 4% per year.
- Potential recipients have end-stage heart failure (stage D), New York Heart Association class IV symptoms, ejection fraction less than 20%, and a physiologic age younger than 60 years.
- Orthotopic heart transplantation is carried out via a median sternotomy, and the general approach is similar to that used for myocardial revascularization or valve replacement.
- Candidates for transplantation are frequently treated with diuretics, vasodilators, and β-blockers. Patients with end-stage disease may require inotropic drugs, intra-aortic balloon pump, or ventricular assist devices.
- After transplantation, the patient has a denervated heart, and heart rate increases only gradually with stress due to circulating catecholamines.
- Denervation means direct-acting cardiovascular drugs must be used to obtain a response, because indirect-acting drugs have a minimal or unpredictable response.
- Allograft-acquired coronary artery disease is the greatest threat to long-term survival of the patient after heart transplantation.
- Increased experience with lung transplantation has been accompanied by a decrease in both operative and long-term mortality.

IV

- Surgical complications are uncommon immediately after lung transplantation but may be associated with high mortality. Pneumothorax and infection are constant concerns. The most common cause of death in the perioperative period is graft dysfunction from reperfusion injury.

REFERENCES

1. Hunt SA: Taking heart: cardiac transplantation past, present, and future. N Engl J Med 355:231, 2006
2. Wood KE, Becker BN, McCartney JG, et al: Care of the potential organ donor. N Engl J Med 351:2730, 2004
3. Mehta SM, Aufiero TX, Pae WE: Combined Registry for the Clinical Use of Mechanical Ventricular Assist Pumps and the Total Artificial Heart in Conjunction with Heart Transplantation: Sixth official report. J Heart Lung Transplant 14:585, 1994
4. Borow KM, Neumann A, Arensman FW, et al: Cardiac and peripheral vascular responses to adrenoceptor stimulation and blockade after cardiac transplantation. J Am Coll Cardiol 14:1229, 1989
5. Gao SZ, Hunt SA, Schroeder JS, et al: Early development of accelerated graft coronary artery disease: Risk factors and course. J Am Coll Cardiol 28:673, 1996
6. Hensley FA, Martin DE, Larach DR, et al: Anesthetic management for cardiac transplantation in North America. J Cardiothorac Anesth 1:429, 1987
7. Villanueva FS, Murali S, Uretsky BF, et al: Resolution of severe pulmonary hypertension after heterotopic cardiac transplantation. J Am Coll Cardiol 14:1239, 1989
8. Jacquet L, Ziady G, Stein K, et al: Cardiac rhythm disturbances early after orthotopic heart transplantation: Prevalence and clinical importance of the observed abnormalities. J Am Coll Cardiol 16:832, 1990
9. Olson CM (ed): Diagnostic and therapeutic technology assessment: Lung transplantation. JAMA 269:931, 1993
10. Kaye MP: The Registry of the International Society for Heart and Lung Transplantation: Ninth official report. J Heart Lung Transplant 11:599, 1992
11. Quinlan JJ, Gasior TA, Firestone S, et al: Anesthesia for living-related (lobar) lung transplantation. J Cardiothorac Vasc Anesth 1996, 391:1996
12. Novick RJ, Kaye MP, Patterson GA, et al: Redo lung transplantation: A North American-European experience. J Heart Lung Transplant 12:5, 1993
13. Gilbert S, Dauber J, Hattler B, et al: Lung and heart-lung transplantation at the University of Pittsburgh 1982-2002. Clin Transplants 253, 2002
14. Kaiser LR, Pasque MK, Trulock EP, et al: Bilateral sequential lung transplantation: The procedure of choice for double-lung replacement. Ann Thorac Surg 52:438, 1991
15. Quinlan JJ, Buffington CW: Deliberate hypoventilation in a patient with air trapping during lung transplantation. Anesthesiology 78:1177, 1993
16. Adatia I, Lillehei C, Arnold JH, et al: Inhaled nitric oxide in the treatment of postoperative graft dysfunction after lung transplantation. Ann Thorac Surg 57:1311, 1994
17. Lang JD, Jr Leill W: Pro: Inhaled nitric oxide should be used routinely in patients undergoing lung transplantation. J Cardiothorac Vasc Anesth 15:7859, 2001
18. Triantafillow AN, Benumof JL, Lecamwasam HS: Physiology of the lateral decubitus position, the open chest, and one lung ventilation. In Kaplan JA, Slinger PD (ed), Thoracic Anesthesia, 3rd ed, Philadelphia, Churchill Livingstone, 2003, pp 71–94
19. Chetham P: Anesthesia for heart or single or double lung transplantation. J Card Surg 15:167, 2000
20. Pereszlenyi A, Lang G, Steltzer H, et al: Bilateral lung transplantation with intra- and postoperatively prolonged ECMO support in patients with pulmonary hypertension. Eur J Cardiothorac Surg 21:858, 2002
21. Veeken C, Palmer SM, Davis RD, Gricknik KP: Living-related lobar lung transplantation. J Cardiothorac Vasc Anesth 18:506, 2004

20

Chapter 21

New Approaches to the Surgical Treatment of End-Stage Heart Failure

Marc E. Stone, MD • Gregory W. Fischer, MD

According to the American Heart Association, there are approximately 6–7 million people in the United States with congestive heart failure (HF). Available statistics indicate that the incidence of HF in the population approaches 10 per 1000 after age 65, with 550,000 new cases each year. Heart failure (HF) is the leading cause of hospitalization in patients older than age 65, with a reported associated cost of $24 to $50 billion annually. On a global scale, HF reportedly affects 0.4% to 2.0% of the adult population.[1]

Despite great advances in the understanding of the pathophysiology of HF and the development of medications that can potentially attenuate the progression of that pathophysiology, morbidity and mortality from this disease remain very high. The incidence of hospitalization for HF rose by 70% during the 1990s, and patients with New York Heart Association (NYHA) class IV symptoms currently have a reported 1-year mortality rate of 30% to 50%. By comparison, the corresponding rates for

NYHA class I-II patients and class II-III patients are 5% and 10% to 15%, respectively. Thus, one of the major goals in the management of HF is the prevention of progression to advanced stages.

While many patients successfully achieve temporary relief of HF *symptoms* with medical management, the underlying pathophysiology inevitably progresses and pharmacologic interventions alone will eventually become inadequate in the vast majority. A variety of surgical procedures can be performed to improve cardiac function and potentially arrest (or even reverse) the progression to severe dysfunction, but until very recently, surgical intervention (short of transplantation or placement of a ventricular assist device) was considered contraindicated in patients with advanced HF. Surprisingly good outcomes with "corrective" interventions, however, have now resulted in patients presenting for surgical treatment of their HF on a regular basis.[2,3]

SURGICAL OPTIONS FOR HEART FAILURE

A growing number of surgical procedures exist (or have been developed) to relieve HF symptoms and arrest the progression of the disease through correction of abnormal myocardial depolarization, enhancement of myocardial blood supply, improvement in ventricular loading conditions, and restoration of more normal ventricular geometry. Box 21-1 provides a list of current surgical interventions for HF.

Cumulative worldwide experience with such interventions thus far suggests that these procedures not only relieve symptoms but may also attenuate or possibly arrest the progressive myocardial remodeling that accompanies chronic HF. In some cases, partial reversal of the adverse myocardial remodeling has been demonstrated and combination therapy (surgical intervention with targeted pharmacologic treatment) intended to enhance reverse remodeling is actively being investigated.[4]

Thus, interventions previously considered contraindicated by low ejection fraction (EF) are now being used precisely for that indication. It remains to be determined, however, which procedures will ultimately benefit which subpopulations of HF patients. Despite the common final pathway that leads to dilated pathophysiology seen in the majority of these patients, an individual's initial underlying etiology may again become an important consideration as these procedures are used earlier and earlier in the course of deterioration as a treatment intended to halt the progression of the disease.

21

BOX 21-1 *Surgical Options for the Management of Heart Failure*

- Cardiac resynchronization therapy with biventricular pacing
- Revascularization (coronary artery bypass grafting or percutaneous coronary artery stenting)
- Mitral valve repair or replacement
- Left ventricular reconstruction (e.g., with the Dor procedure or the Batista procedure)
- Dynamic cardiomyoplasty
- Extrinsic compression devices (e.g., the CorCap)
- Implantation of a left ventricular assist device (LVAD)
- Cardiac transplantation
- New therapies for congestive heart failure in various stages of development include transplantation of skeletal myoblasts and stem cells, "gene" therapy, and xenotransplantation.

REVASCULARIZATION

Coronary artery disease has become the most common etiology of HF. Of those patients currently listed for heart transplantation, 39% carry a primary diagnosis of ischemic heart disease.

Where viable myocardium and feasible targets exist, revascularization of chronically ischemic, hibernating myocardium can improve ventricular function, downgrade NYHA functional class, and improve prognosis. While the primary benefit of revascularization appears to be functional improvement of the LV, reducing ischemic substrate for arrhythmias and retarding adverse myocardial remodeling are important secondary benefits.

Despite an increased perioperative risk of morbidity and mortality in this population, the world's literature reports current survival between 57% and 75% at 5 years with in-hospital mortality between 1.7% and 11%. A recent review reported an 83.5% survival at 2 years after revascularization compared with only 57.2% survival in patients with congestive heart failure (CHF) who were not revascularized.[5] In general, morbidity and mortality tend to correlate inversely with EF and directly with NYHA functional class. Additional factors predisposing patients to higher morbidity and mortality include advanced age, female sex, hypertension, diabetes, and emergent operations. The decreases in morbidity and mortality after revascularization in this high-risk population in recent years are at least partially attributable to improvements in surgical technique and myocardial protection, but the concurrent performance of mitral valve repair and ventricular reshaping address the adverse ventricular loading conditions present and may also contribute to improved outcomes. The results of ongoing clinical trials evaluating combinations of surgical procedures (e.g., revascularization plus ventricular reshaping versus revascularization alone) are eagerly awaited.

The importance of determining the viability of myocardium in the area to be revascularized cannot be understated because the potential for recovery of function depends on residual contractile reserve, integrity of the sarcolemma, and metabolically preserved cellular function. Methods to detect viable myocardium include dobutamine echocardiography, single-photon emission computed tomography (SPECT), and positron-emission tomography (PET). While dobutamine stress echocardiography has often been shown to have the highest predictive accuracy, there are important limitations that need to be taken into account. Dobutamine stress echocardiography, for example, can have false-negative results if there is loss of contractile proteins in the presence of preserved function of the muscle fiber membrane.

CORRECTION OF MITRAL REGURGITATION

Mitral regurgitation (MR) may result from several different pathophysiologic states (e.g., leaflet prolapse, annular dilation, leaflet perforation), but the MR seen in patients with HF is most often functional, owing primarily to restriction of leaflet motion with subsequent limitation of leaflet coaptation because the papillary muscles are tethered by the dilated LV.

Historically, many physicians considered MR advantageous for the failing LV. It was believed that a low-pressure atrial "pop off" allowed the failing ventricle to protect itself from the high afterload of the systemic circulation and gave the illusion that the heart had a better overall contractile state than really existed. This misconception was "supported" by the fact that surgical replacement of the mitral valve was associated with a very high mortality rate in patients with depressed LV function. It is now

IV

known, however, that mitral valve replacement or repair can improve overall cardiac performance by eliminating the increased myocardial oxygen demand that accompanies the progressive pressure and volume overload due to MR.

Despite the slightly increased operative risk, the current literature supports mitral valve repair or replacement as beneficial to patients with severely depressed LV function, HF, and MR. In a recent series, Romano and Bolling reported operative mortality of 5% with 1- and 2-year survival rates of 80% and 70%, respectively.[6] Not only was long-term mortality reduced, but the increase in LV systolic function (on average by 10%) enabled a downgrading of NYHA class and resulted in an improved quality of life. It has been shown that 1-, 2-, and 5-year survival rates of 91%, 84%, and 77%, respectively, can be obtained in patients with LVEF less than 30%. In addition, the rate of re-hospitalization for HF was decreased during the period of follow-up compared with a cohort that did not receive a mitral repair. Thus, both medical and economic benefits may result from mitral valve repair in this population.

While the majority of end-stage HF patients will exhibit functional MR, there may be additional concurrent valvular pathology present in a given patient. An intraoperative transesophageal echocardiography (TEE) evaluation of the valvular anatomy, the mechanism of the MR, and direct surgical inspection will determine the feasibility of repair. It is generally believed that valve repair is preferable to valve replacement, because there are demonstrated hemodynamic advantages associated with preservation of the subvalvular apparatus[7] and long-term anticoagulation is not required.

LEFT VENTRICULAR RESHAPING

In 1996, Batista introduced the concept of surgically reshaping the dilated and failing LV of NYHA class IV patients to improve systolic performance. In the Batista procedure, resection of a wedge of normal myocardium from the LV apex to the base (laterally, between the papillary muscles) restored more normal ventricular geometry and decreased wall tension. Functional MR was also addressed during the Batista procedure by a valve replacement or repair. While many patients did benefit initially from this procedure (reduction of NYHA functional class to NYHA I in 57% and NYHA II in 33.3%), perioperative mortality was high (>20% in both Batista's own series and in the large Cleveland Clinic experience). Additionally, the experience of several centers was that many patients required rescue mechanical circulatory assistance after the procedure and many patients experienced a re-dilation of their LV, resulting in a return to NYHA class IV status. Thus, despite a short-lived period of initial enthusiasm in the 1990s, the Batista procedure has essentially been abandoned. The concept of ventricular reshaping, however, remains of interest.

The modified Dor procedure (endoventricular circular patch plasty) is successfully used to reshape the dilated, spherical LV of patients who have had an anterior wall myocardial infarction with resulting aneurysm and akinesis/dyskinesis. Essentially, a Dacron patch is placed within the LV cavity so as to exclude the large akinetic/dyskinetic area of the anterior wall. This restores LV geometry to a more normal elliptical shape and improves systolic function. When performed concurrently with coronary artery bypass grafting (CABG), significant early and late improvements in both NYHA functional class and EF have been demonstrated with an in-hospital mortality rate of 12%. A trial of 439 patients undergoing this procedure found an improved in-hospital mortality of 6.6% and an 18-month survival of 89.2%. In this series, CABG was performed concurrently in 89%, mitral valve repair in 22%, and mitral valve replacement in 4%.[8]

21

PROCEDURES TO ARREST THE DILATION OF THE FAILING VENTRICLE

The intent of extrinsic constraint is to arrest the progressive dilation of the failing ventricle. Decreasing the radius of the LV will reduce wall tension (Laplace's law), which will decrease myocardial oxygen demand. In addition, this may result in improved systolic and diastolic function, as well as subjective improvements in functional capacity. This type of ventricular reshaping can be accomplished with biological tissues and devices applied to the external surface of the heart.

Dynamic Cardiomyoplasty

Decades in development, this procedure was introduced into clinical practice in 1985 by Carpentier and Chachques. In dynamic cardiomyoplasty, an electrically stimulated flap of skeletal muscle (e.g., latissimus dorsi) was wrapped around the heart in an attempt to augment systolic function. Between 1985 and 1991, approximately 185 dynamic cardiomyoplasties were performed worldwide in 17 countries. Although subjective improvement was widely reported by patients who had undergone the procedure, objective measurements of significant functional improvement were inconsistent.

Acorn CorCap Cardiac Support Device

The CorCap Cardiac Support Device (Acorn Cardiovascular, Inc., Minneapolis, MN) is an investigational mesh fabric that is surgically wrapped around the heart in an attempt to prevent further dilation. This device has been shown in animal models to reduce wall stress, myocyte hypertrophy, and myocardial fibrosis. A global multicenter study by Oz and coworkers[9] showed promising results. There were significant reductions in LV end-diastolic dimensions, MR grade, and NYHA classification in patients 12 months after CorCap implantation. At the same time, a significant improvement was seen in LVEF and quality of life. Ongoing randomized clinical trials in Europe and the United States will further address the safety of implantation of the CorCap device and ultimate outcomes.

IV

CARDIAC RESYNCHRONIZATION THERAPY AND IMPLANTABLE CARDIOVERTER-DEFIBRILLATORS

The progression of disease resulting in advanced cardiac failure is typically accompanied by conduction defects and arrhythmias, and pacemakers and implantable cardioverter-defibrillators (ICDs) are commonly used in this population. In addition to the well-known defects in sinus or atrioventricular node function, intraventricular conduction defects delay the onset of RV or LV systole in 30% to 50% of patients with advanced HF.[10] This lack of coordination of LV and RV contractions further impairs CO and has been reported to increase the risk of death in this population.

Cardiac resynchronization therapy (CRT) entails biventricular pacing to optimize the timing of RV and LV contractions. The right atrium (RA) is paced by a lead in the RA, the RV by a lead in the RV, and the LV by a lead in a coronary vein (accessed via the coronary sinus). While CRT is more an interventional cardiology procedure than a surgical procedure per se, anesthesiologists are frequently asked to provide sedation (if not general anesthesia) for these sometimes lengthy implantation procedures.

Studies have shown that atrial-synchronized biventricular pacing (pacing the LV and RV in a carefully timed manner) can "resynchronize" RV and LV contraction, improving CO and overall hemodynamics. This enhances these patients' ability to exercise (which improves their NYHA functional class) and decreases the length and frequency of their hospitalizations, which improves their quality of life.[11]

Sudden death from ventricular fibrillation (VF) accounts for approximately 300,000 deaths annually in the United States. Patients with advanced HF experience VF with a frequency 6 to 9 times that of the general population, and VF causes 40% of all deaths in this population even in the absence of apparent disease progression based on symptoms. Thus, ICDs are commonly indicated for patients with advanced cardiac failure. An ICD is a device capable of arrhythmia detection and automatic defibrillation. ICDs successfully terminate VF in greater than 98% of episodes, and studies have demonstrated that an ICD increases survival and decreases the risk of sudden death in patients with ischemic cardiomyopathy and decreased LV function.[12]

The Comparison of Medical Therapy, Pacing, and Defibrillation in Heart Failure (COMPANION) trial studied 1500 patients at 128 U.S. centers. In this recently completed trial, compared with optimal pharmacologic therapy alone, CRT decreased the risk of the combined endpoint of death from or hospitalization for HF by 34%. The combination of CRT and ICD implantation reduced these risks by 40%. While many studies are ongoing, it is clear that CRT and ICDs significantly reduce morbidity and mortality in patients with advanced HF.

Pacemakers and ICDs are typically implanted in the electrophysiology suite by cardiologists using local anesthesia. Anesthesiologists are commonly asked to sedate or briefly induce anesthesia during these procedures so that proper functioning of the device(s) can be ascertained with patient amnesia during arrhythmia induction and therapy. Clinicians must consider all the same anesthetic issues and concerns when sedating/inducing one of these patients for device testing as one would for a surgical procedure in the operating room. Propofol or dexmedetomidine infusions are commonly used in small dosages; etomidate (0.05 to 0.1 mg/kg) is an alternative for patients with baseline hypotension. Many cardiologists use midazolam in this circumstance when an anesthesiologist cannot be present. Anesthesiologists may also choose a lighter plane of sedation if the risk of airway difficulty or gastric regurgitation is elevated.

21

VENTRICULAR ASSIST DEVICES

When cardiac failure is refractory to pharmacologic manipulations, mechanical circulatory assist devices are used as a temporary bridge-to-recovery, as a bridge-to-transplantation, or, in selected patients, as a final "destination therapy." While a thorough treatment of all mechanical circulatory assist devices is beyond the scope of this chapter, the following paragraphs introduce and briefly describe commonly used, currently available, U.S. Food and Drug Administration (FDA)–approved ventricular assist devices (VADs), as well as the next generation of miniaturized, totally implantable continuous-flow VADs, and the AbioCor total artificial heart (Abiomed, Danvers, MA).

Currently Available Ventricular Assist Devices: Indications and the Basic Strategy of Their Use

Mechanical circulatory assistance with a VAD has become common management of intractable cardiogenic shock that follows cardiac surgery, myocardial infarction (MI), or severe viral myocarditis, as well as in the patient with end-stage cardiomyopathy awaiting transplantation. All currently available VADs are pumps that collect blood returning to the heart and eject it downstream of the failing ventricle. Effectively, they take over the pumping function of the failing ventricle and can provide adequate systemic perfusion to prevent the devastating sequelae of cardiogenic shock (e.g., multisystem organ failure). With the potential exception of centrifugal pumps, currently approved VADs do not provide oxygenation or removal of waste from the blood—they simply act as pumps that can maintain perfusion of the body in the place of a failing ventricle.

While the VAD is acting to maintain the circulation, decompression of the failing ventricle will decrease ventricular wall tension and therefore myocardial oxygen demand. To decompress the failing ventricle, cannulas must be placed in the heart to divert blood to the pump, and all currently approved devices use essentially the same cannulation strategies within the heart and great vessels. For LV support, blood is drained from the LA or, more commonly, the LV apex and returned to the ascending aorta. For RV support, blood is drained from the RA or RV and returned to the main pulmonary artery. These cannulation strategies are common to all VADs currently approved for clinical use and are diagrammed in Figure 21-1.

Temporary Ventricular Assist Device Use: Bridge to Recovery

In patients in whom there has been an acute myocardial insult resulting in refractory cardiogenic shock but myocardial recovery *is* expected, a short-term VAD (e.g., the Abiomed BVS5000; Abiomed, Danvers, MA), an intermediate-term VAD (e.g., the Thoratec VAD system; Thoratec Laboratories, Pleasanton, CA, or the AB5000 ventricle; Abiomed, Danvers, MA), or standard centrifugal devices can support the circulation as a "bridge to recovery." The Abiomed BVS5000, the Thoratec, and the AB5000 ventricle are paracorporeal, pneumatically driven devices capable of providing pulsatile support for the LV (LVAD), the RV (RVAD), or both ventricles (BiVAD) as needed. With all these devices, the paracorporeal pump heads are connected to inflow and outflow cannulas anastomosed to the heart and great vessels. Table 21-1 summarizes the basic characteristics of these devices. The artificial blood contacting surfaces, unidirectional valves, and pulsatile nature of the pumping mechanism in these devices require that the patient be anticoagulated during support.

Regardless of the device used as a bridge-to-recovery, the patient may potentially be weaned from mechanical support as the ventricle recovers from the acute stunning it has sustained. Unfortunately, complications are frequent and recovery is not assured. In general, the best outcomes are obtained when rescue mechanical circulatory assistance is initiated as soon as the severity of the myocardial insult is recognized and truly appreciated. The best outcomes occur when:
- Support is commenced to correct marginal hemodynamics within 30 to 45 minutes of attempted pharmacologic treatment (with or without an intra-aortic balloon pump).
- The time between the first attempt to wean from CPB and biventricular support implant is less than 6 hours.

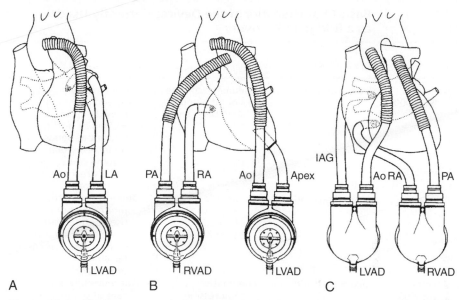

Ao   LA   PA   RA   Ao   Apex   Ao RA   PA

IAG

A   B   C

LVAD   RVAD   LVAD   LVAD   RVAD

Figure 21-1 The Thoratec ventricular assist device (VAD) and three cannulation approaches for univentricular left-sided heart support (**A**) and biventricular support (**B** and **C**). This figure illustrates the currently used cannulation strategies for all currently available ventricular assist devices. As described in the text, cannulas are placed in the heart and great vessels to divert blood returning to the failing side of the heart to the pump. The blood collected in the VAD blood chamber is then ejected into the arterial circulation immediately downstream of the failing ventricle. Ao = aorta; LA = left atrial appendage; PA = pulmonary artery; RA = right atrium; Apex = left ventricular apex; IAG = cannula inserted via the interatrial groove and directed toward the LA roof. (Reprinted with permission from Thoratec Corporation.)

- The biventricular support implant occurs as part of the initial operation.
- Due consideration is given to whether the patient requires univentricular or biventricular support.
- Hemostasis is ensured before leaving the operating room.

Poor outcomes occur when:

- Signs of other end organ failure are present.
- The patient is older than age 75 years.
- The patient is brought back to the operating room for implantation after a period of time.

Intermediate- to Long-Term Ventricular Assist Device Use: Bridge to Transplantation

In cases when no myocardial recovery is expected (e.g., end-stage cardiomyopathy) or when an acutely stunned LV fails to recover despite support with a short-term VAD, a long-term "implantable" LVAD (e.g., the Novacor LVAS; World Heart, Ottawa, Canada) is commonly used as a "bridge to transplantation." By providing effective CO in place of the failed native heart, this technology can stave off the end organ damage resulting from a rapidly deteriorating CO and allows severely decompensated transplant-eligible patients to potentially survive long enough to receive a

21

Table 21-1 Basic Characteristics of the Devices Currently Used as a Bridge to Recovery

Device	Fill Mechanism	Drive Mechanism	System Control and Output
Abiomed BVS5000	Gravity drainage	Pneumatic compression of blood chamber	Automatically adjusts rate of pumping to provide up to 5 L/min of outflow (output depends on intravascular volume status and downstream vascular resistances)
Thoratec	Vacuum assisted	Pneumatic compression of blood chamber	Depending on the mode of operation, user-defined settings determine the output (intravascular volume status is important)
Abiomed AB5000 ventricle	Vacuum assisted	Pneumatic compression of blood chamber	Automatically adjusts rate of pumping to provide up to 6 L/min of outflow (output depends on intravascular volume status and downstream vascular resistances)
Centrifugal pumps	Gravity drainage assisted by vortex	Centrifugal force drives blood	Output is dependent on user-defined speed of impeller rotation

IV

donor heart. An additional benefit of this application of VADs is an improved quality of life, often as an outpatient, while awaiting a new heart.

The Novacor (Fig. 21-2) and the HeartMate (World Heart, Inc., Oakland, CA) (Fig. 21-3) are the most commonly used bridge-to-transplantation devices for patients with advanced LV failure. Patients with biventricular failure are typically bridged with the Thoratec devices. While there are new and promising devices currently in clinical trials, the Thoratec is presently the only widely available mechanical circulatory support device capable of providing intermediate to long-term support of the native heart as a bridge-to-transplantation for patients who require biventricular support. According to the most recent voluntary Novacor, HeartMate, and Thoratec registries, more than 1700 patients have been implanted with the Novacor, more than 5600 with the HeartMate, and more than 2500 with the Thoratec worldwide. Of those implanted with the Thoratec for bridge to transplantation, 59% required biventricular assistance. Rates of successful bridging to transplantation with these devices are reportedly on the order of 51% to 78%.[13]

An implanted Novacor is shown in Figure 21-2, and a HeartMate is seen in Figure 21-3. As depicted, the pump heads of these devices are implanted in a surgically created pocket in the preperitoneal space. Inflow and outflow conduits are connected to the heart and great vessels as shown. Blood is drained to the

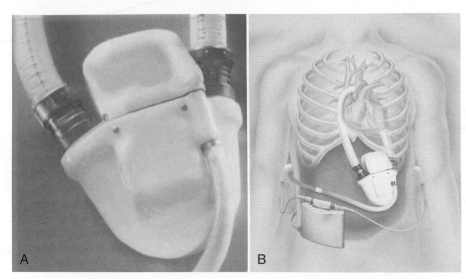

Figure 21-2 **A,** The Novacor LVAS. Inflow and outflow cannulas are at the *top,* and the drive line, which provides electrical power and system control, can be seen at the *bottom right.* **B,** The appearance of an implanted Novacor LVAS. Blood is drained from the LV apex to the pump and ejected into the ascending aorta. The pump head is completely implanted in the preperitoneal space of the abdomen. The current model requires that a cable from the device be tunneled through the abdominal wall to connect to the external system controller and power supply. (Reproduced with permission from WorldHeart, Inc.)

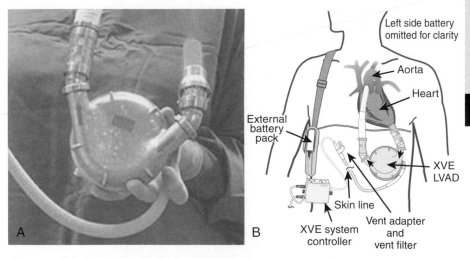

Figure 21-3 **A,** The HeartMate LVAS. The inflow and outflow cannulaes are at the *top,* and the drive line to bring power and system control is at the *bottom.* **B,** The appearance of an implanted HeartMate XVE LVAD. Blood is drained from the left ventricular apex to the pump and ejected into the ascending aorta. The pump head is completely implanted in the preperitoneal space of the abdomen. The current model requires that a cable from the device be tunneled through the abdominal wall to connect to the external system controller and power supply. (Reproduced with permission from Thoratec Laboratories, Inc.)

21

implanted pump head from the LV apex and is ejected in a pulsatile fashion into the ascending aorta. Adequate intravascular volume status is a critical factor in optimizing pump outputs.

Current versions of these devices require a percutaneous cable to connect the implanted pump heads to an external source of power and system control, potentially increasing the incidence of infection. Additional common complications of long-term VAD use include a high incidence of perioperative bleeding and subsequent potential for cerebral thromboembolism.

The Novacor requires formal anticoagulation with warfarin (target INR 2.5 to 3 times normal) because its blood chamber is composed of smooth polyurethane. In contrast, the blood chamber of the HeartMate has an antithrombogenic lining composed of sintered titanium microspheres that encourages the ingrowth and development of a neointima. For this reason, patients supported by a HeartMate do not require formal anticoagulation and are generally maintained only on aspirin (perhaps in combination with dipyridamole) depending on the preferences of the implanting center.

Permanent Ventricular Assist Device Use: Destination Therapy

A relatively new indication for long-term VAD use is "destination therapy." Destination therapy refers to the intentionally permanent implantation of an LVAD in a nontransplant eligible patient as a permanent management solution for end-stage cardiac failure. The availability of this indication is a great advance in the treatment of HF because while cardiac transplantation remains the ultimate intervention for advanced HF, the number of donor organs is severely limited in comparison with the number of those who would benefit, and the vast majority of patients with end-stage cardiac disease cannot realistically expect to be transplanted. Effectively, the intentionally permanent implantation of a mechanical assist device may be the best option available if the vast numbers of patients in the population with advanced HF are to survive.

Based on the encouraging results of the REMATCH trial,[14] the HeartMate LVAS was FDA-approved in 2002 for use as "destination therapy" in the United States. Briefly, REMATCH (Randomized Evaluation of Mechanical Assistance for the Treatment of Congestive Heart Failure) was conducted to determine if the HeartMate could be effective as an alternative therapy for patients with end-stage cardiac failure who are not eligible to receive a transplant. In addition to patient survival, the study collected data on the implanted patient's quality of life, the cost of the patient's care, and any adverse events that occurred during the treatment. In essence, the REMATCH study demonstrated that the use of a left-sided VAD was not only an effective tool to treat patients with advanced HF but also resulted in more than twice the survival rate and an improved quality of life in comparison to optimal medical management. This was especially the case if the patient was younger than 60 years. Summarized results of the REMATCH trial appear in Table 21-2.

Table 21-2 Summarized Results of the REMATCH Trial

	HeartMate	Medical Treatment
1-Year survival (patients <60 yr)	52% (74%)	25% (33%)
2-Year survival	23%	8%
Median survival	408 days	150 days

As of 2007, 512 patients have been sustained on the HeartMate devices for destination therapy in 67 centers. The longest duration of support is 2638 days (7.2 years), but the longest duration with a single pump is 3.5 years. Seventy seven patients have gone on to receive a heart transplant.

Complications of Currently Available Ventricular Assist Devices

Regardless of which short- or long-term device is in use, the major complications of VAD use include coagulopathic bleeding in the perioperative period, potential for thromboembolism during support, and infection. Sepsis is the leading cause of death. Additional complications of VAD use include RV failure while on isolated LV assistance (on the order of 30% due to the induced changes in RV geometry), potential device malfunction, and progressive multisystem organ failure despite VAD support.[15]

TOTAL ARTIFICIAL HEART

From the original pneumatically driven devices with their massive external control consoles to the totally implantable computer-controlled AbioCor Implantable Replacement Heart (Abiomed, Danvers, MA), the mechanical TAH has been the subject of intensive research and development for decades.

The Abiocor Implantable Replacement Heart (Fig. 21-4) represents a major advance in artificial heart technology because it is truly totally implantable; there are no percutaneous cables, conduits, or wires. The device is motor driven, so a source of compressed air to drive the pumping action is not required, allowing patients complete mobility. The device itself weighs approximately 2 pounds and is orthotopically implanted.

Transcutaneous energy transfer is used (in lieu of a percutaneous cable) to supply the motor-driven hydraulic pumping of the artificial ventricles with power

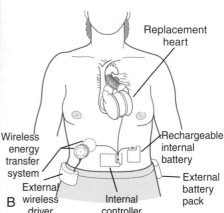

Figure 21-4   A, The AbioCor Implantable Replacement Heart. **B,** Orthotopic implantation of the AbioCor Implantable Replacement Heart. As discussed in the text, the native failed heart is removed, and the AbioCor is implanted orthotopically, anastomosed to cuffs of native atria and the great vessels. Transcutaneous energy transfer technology eliminates the need for percutaneous wires. Human clinical trials with this promising new device are ongoing. (For the latest information, visit www.abiomed.com. Reproduced with permission from Abiomed, Inc.)

and system control. Artificial unidirectional valves within the device mandate anticoagulation during support.

The Abiocor TAH was FDA-approved in 2006. The first and most successful implantation was performed by Gray and Dowling at the University of Louisville. Long-term survival of over 1 year has been achieved. It can now be used for inotropic dependent patients with end-stage HF requiring biventricular support who are transplant ineligible with less than 30 day expected survival without intervention.

NEW THERAPIES

Cellular Transplantation into the Myocardium

A novel approach to treating severe systolic dysfunction is the injection of harvested autologous skeletal muscle cells into the failing myocardium. This procedure can be performed either surgically at the end of a revascularization procedure or percutaneously in the catheterization laboratory.

The basic understanding of the remodeling process is that viable and contractile cardiomyocytes undergo apoptosis and become replaced by noncontractile tissue. This in turn leads to systolic and diastolic dysfunction. In an attempt to restore functionality, contractile cells are injected into this region. In clinical practice, myoblasts from the patient's quadriceps muscle have been used. Using the patient's own tissue has several advantages. First, the complications of pharmacologic immunosuppression are avoided. Second, there are no ethical problems in contrast to those frequently observed when fetal cells are used. Finally, the ease of harvest and processing makes this tissue ideal for this purpose.

Skeletal muscle cells, however, are histologically different from native cardiomyocytes. Adhesion molecules, which are found in native cardiomyocytes, are not found in skeletal myocytes. These adhesion molecules are important for adhesion to the extracellular matrix and for intercellular communication.

A frequently encountered occurrence in the phase I studies was the fact that many patients had episodes of ventricular tachycardia after the procedure. They were successfully treated with amiodarone or electric cardioversion. Phase II studies are now in progress in the United States and Europe. Many other cell types are now being experimentally injected into the myocardium or given intravenously in an attempt to regrow cardiac myocytes. These cells include adult bone marrow stem cells, embryonic stem cells, and cardiac progenitor cells found mainly in the atrium. They have been injected alone or with multiple growth factors such as granulocyte-macrophage colony-stimulating factor (GM-CSF), vasoactive endothelial growth factor (VEGF), and angiopoietin-1, which mobilize progenitor cells and induce new cell growth. The transplanted cells may morph into new cardiac muscle cells or they may improve cardiac function by boosting the growth of new blood vessels or releasing other growth factors that encourage cell proliferation and survival. Any of these effects could explain some of the early positive results seen to date.[16]

Gene Transfer in Cardiac Myocytes

Gene therapy has received much interest by the media during the past decade. Multiple research groups are trying to cure or at least alleviate symptoms brought on by HF through gene therapy. To change the genetic programming of a cell it is necessary to inoculate the cell with DNA. To achieve this goal, vectors are being used. Vectors commonly used range from plasmid DNA to different virus types (e.g., adenovirus, herpesvirus). The two cellular pathways that are being targeted are the sarcoplasmic reticulum and the β-adrenergic pathway. The targets of gene therapy are to increase β-adrenergic function, adenylyl cyclase, the V_2 vasopressin receptor, and sarcoplasmic reticulum Ca^{2+} ATPase (*SERCA2a*), while also decreasing phospholambam and β-adrenoreceptor kinase (*BARK 1*). All of these new therapies hold great promise and many trials are being done.[17]

ANESTHETIC CONSIDERATIONS IN THE PATIENT WITH SEVERELY IMPAIRED CARDIAC FUNCTION

Essential Considerations

Cardiac failure can be the common outcome of a variety of underlying causes, and patients may therefore present with widely varying clinical status. Some may appear quite compromised whereas others may appear surprisingly well compensated despite significant underlying pathophysiology. Regardless of what is planned surgically, achieving hemodynamic stability during the induction and maintenance of anesthesia requires a preoperative knowledge of the status of the coronary arteries (including prior bypass grafts or stents), the extent of any valvular regurgitation and/or stenosis that may be present, and whether there is significant pulmonary hypertension. Additionally, all patients with significant ventricular dysfunction require a thorough preoperative evaluation of the major organ systems (particularly the renal, hepatic, and central nervous systems) for impairment. The anesthetic plan can then take any existing organ dysfunction into consideration.

Preoperative Optimization

Patients with cardiac failure are medically optimized by pharmacologic manipulations of SVR (afterload reduction), β-blockade, and diuresis. Most medications should be continued throughout the perioperative period, but the decision as to whether to withhold angiotensin-converting enzyme inhibitors and diuretics should be made on an individual basis.

Patients with HF often require preinduction optimization of intravascular volume status, pharmacologic manipulations of inotropy and afterload, adjustments to pacemaker settings (where present), and, on occasion, elective placement of an intra-aortic balloon pump.

It is prudent to provide supplemental oxygen and monitor vital signs during the preoperative period. This is especially important if anxiolytic medications are given because this population will not tolerate sudden decreases in sympathetic tone, hypoxemia, or the potentially increased pulmonary vascular resistance that may accompany a respiratory acidosis if hypoventilation results from anxiolysis.

Intraoperative Considerations

Most procedures intended to improve cardiac function will require CPB, but the potential availability of bypass cannot be taken for granted because the function of even a severely depressed ventricle can still get worse, and it is well known that having to emergently institute CPB significantly increases morbidity and mortality. In

21

the prebypass period, further depression of cardiac function and significant increases in ventricular afterload must be avoided, which will increase myocardial oxygen demand and may cause ischemia. Preload, afterload, heart rate, and contractility must be continuously optimized for each patient at all times.

Where CPB will be used, it is generally prudent to consider employing an antifibrinolytic agent in an attempt to decrease bleeding in the postbypass period. In some patients, CPB may not be needed to insert an LVAD.

Anesthetic Agents and Technique

While the usual sedative and hypnotic agents may be tolerated in patients with mild cardiac failure, the failing heart is chronically compensated by a heightened adrenergic state, and removal of that sympathetic tone may lead to rapid decompensation with cardiovascular collapse during anesthetic induction. Patients with severely decreased ventricular function tend to decompensate quickly from physiologic and hemodynamic aberrations (e.g., hypercarbia, hypoxemia, hypotension, bradycardia/tachycardia, sudden alterations in volume status, and loss of sinus rhythm), and agents should be chosen and used in a manner likely to maintain hemodynamic stability. Additionally, agent selection should take into account any coexisting renal or hepatic insufficiency. Intravascular volume status needs to be carefully considered and continuously optimized for each individual patient. Inotropic and vasoactive agents, including ephedrine, phenylephrine, dopamine, epinephrine, milrinone, vasopressin, nitroglycerin, and nitroprusside should be available and judiciously used at the first sign of refractory hemodynamic instability.

Unfortunately, there can be no standard approach to these patients. Despite the perceived similarity of one patient with cardiac failure to another, each individual's underlying pathophysiology must be carefully considered and then anesthetic agents chosen that will best maintain the hemodynamic goals for that patient.

Traditionally, a technique based on high-dose opioid (e.g., total fentanyl dose 50 to 100 µg/kg, or total sufentanil dose 5 to 10 µg/kg) together with a neuromuscular blocking agent has been used for patients with severely depressed cardiac function. While such a technique will likely result in many hours of hemodynamic stability, potential disadvantages of this technique are that amnesia may not be adequate and the bradycardia and initial chest wall rigidity that typically accompany such an induction must be pharmacologically countered.

Etomidate (0.2 to 0.3 mg/kg IV) is usually the induction agent of choice in these patients because it causes neither a significant reduction in SVR nor a significant decrease in myocardial contractility. The decreases in vascular tone and myocardial contractility that accompany induction with propofol make this drug unsuitable for those with severely depressed cardiac function. Similarly, thiopental, with its propensity to cause myocardial depression and venodilation, with consequent decreases in CO, is not often used for these patients.

As a general rule, high doses of the potent inhalation agents are poorly tolerated in this population. While all of the inhalation agents (including nitrous oxide) are myocardial depressants to varying extents, enflurane and halothane are particularly potent in this regard and are generally avoided in patients with depressed ventricular function. Isoflurane, sevoflurane, and desflurane are more likely to be compatible with hemodynamic stability in the well-optimized patient, although isoflurane and desflurane must be used cautiously due to their particular tendency to decrease SVR. In comparison with the other currently available agents, sevoflurane appears to cause less myocardial depression and decrease in SVR. In addition to direct myocardial depression and vasodilation, the inhaled anesthetic agents may also affect myocardial automaticity, impulse conduction, and refractoriness, potentially resulting in reentry phenomena and arrhythmias.

Although its use in adults has decreased dramatically in recent years, ketamine remains an extremely useful agent in patients with severely decreased ventricular function. A ketamine induction (1 to 2.5 mg/kg IV or 2.5 to 5 mg/kg IM) followed by a maintenance infusion (50 to 100 µg/kg/min) will usually provide excellent hemodynamic stability while ensuring adequate analgesia and amnesia. Where feasible, midazolam is generally provided before giving ketamine in an attempt to lessen the potential post-emergence psychiatric side effects that may occur in some patients. Additional small doses (1 to 2 mg every 2 to 3 hours) or an infusion of midazolam (0.5 µg/kg/min) are often provided when a ketamine infusion is in use. For adults and older pediatric patients, a small intravenous dose of glycopyrrolate (e.g., 0.2 mg) is generally provided to act as an antisialagogue. Once on CPB, the ketamine infusion can be stopped, and moderate-to-high doses of narcotics administered.

Central venous access and pulmonary artery catheterization (PAC) are extremely useful (if not mandatory) in this patient population for several reasons. First, pharmacologic interventions are frequently necessary, and potent inotropic and vasoactive agents are preferably administered to the circulation through a central route. Second, the ability to follow and optimize trends of CO and other hemodynamic indices, as well as the ability to assess the efficacy of pharmacologic interventions to manipulate pulmonary vascular resistance, cannot be overlooked. Third, an extraordinarily useful monitor for evaluating the adequacy of oxygen delivery is measurement of mixed venous oxygen saturation.

Nowhere is TEE a more invaluable intraoperative tool than during surgical procedures intended to improve cardiac function, because the success of many of these procedures depends on specific information provided by the echocardiographer. For example, TEE visualization of the precise mechanism and location of mitral regurgitation often determines the feasibility of valve repair. TEE is used to assess the anatomy of the valve overall, as well as to specifically evaluate the leaflets for abnormal thickening, calcification, mobility, and points of coaptation with respect to the annular plane. Doppler analyses and color-flow mapping complement the two-dimensional evaluation and may provide additional information.

Transesophageal Echocardiography and Ventricular Assist Devices

The role of TEE where mechanical ventricular assist devices are concerned begins before placement of the device, with a TEE evaluation focused on detecting or ruling out specific anatomic pathologic processes that may prevent the device from functioning as intended, or lead to preventable complications, and often must be surgically addressed before starting support by the device.[18]

Pre-LVAD placement, TEE is used to detect specific anatomic pathologies that will[19]:
- Impair LVAD filling (e.g., mitral stenosis, severe tricuspid regurgitation, severe RV dysfunction)
- Decrease efficacy of LVAD ejection and LV decompression (e.g., aortic regurgitation)
- Cause complications once the LVAD is functioning (e.g., patent foramen ovale, atrial septal defect, intracardiac thrombus, ascending aortic atherosclerosis, mobile plaques)

During LVAD placement, TEE is used to:
- Ensure proper inflow cannula position in the center of the LV (pointing toward mitral valve)

21

- Ensure adequate de-airing of device before startup

Post-LVAD placement, TEE is used to:

- Ensure adequate LV decompression (but not complete obliteration of the LV cavity)
- Ensure RV function does not deteriorate
- Ensure tricuspid regurgitation does not worsen (or assess the need for a tricuspid valve annuloplasty)
- Reevaluate for patent foramen ovale (must be closed if detected)

Postoperative Considerations

By and large, improvements in ventricular function will not be immediately apparent in this population after the majority of surgical procedures described in this chapter. In fact, ventricular function is often worse after a major cardiotomy because there has often been some degree of myocardial stunning during CPB despite the best of myocardial protective techniques with modern cardioplegia. Generally, it will be necessary to optimize intravascular volume status and employ pharmacologic manipulations of afterload and contractility. Temporary pacing with epicardial wires placed during surgery is often used to optimize heart rate. In addition, meticulous management of electrolytes, coagulation status, and red blood cell mass is necessary.

One area that is often neglected in this population with sometimes tenuous hemodynamics is postoperative pain management. Patients with severely decreased ventricular function will not tolerate the stress response and tachycardia that accompany postoperative pain due to the increased myocardial oxygen demand (potentially leading to ischemia) and decreased diastolic filling time (potentially leading to decreased stroke volume). This combination is especially deleterious in patients with poor ventricular function and will exacerbate hemodynamic instability.

SUMMARY

- Congestive heart failure (HF) is a chronic progressive disease of epidemic proportion that costs billions of dollars annually.
- Current medical management alone is incapable of preventing the progression of HF to the advanced stages of the disease.
- Surgical options for the management of HF exist and are being increasingly used at an earlier stage in the course of the disease. Implantation of a mechanical circulatory assist device remains an attractive management option for advanced cardiac failure because the underlying problem is mechanical pump failure. Currently available pulsatile devices have been shown to be effective but have a high incidence of complications. The next generation of continuous-flow devices (currently in human clinical trials) promises increased device durability and fewer complications.
- Electrophysiologic maneuvers (e.g., biventricular pacing) can often improve cardiac output and decrease mortality in patients with advanced HF.
- New therapies (e.g., transplantation of skeletal myoblasts, stem cells, gene therapies) that can potentially reverse the adverse ventricular remodeling accompanying HF and improve ventricular function are under development and in various stages of human clinical trials but are years away from routine clinical applicability.

- The anesthetic management of patients presenting for "heart failure surgery" can be challenging due to the severely depressed cardiac function and the often debilitated state of the patient.
- Patients with end-stage HF often present with significant comorbidities that must be identified preoperatively.
- The intraoperative management of the patient with advanced HF requires a careful titration of anesthetic agents and continuous optimization of hemodynamics. Such optimization generally requires meticulous management of preload, afterload, heart rate, heart rhythm, and contractility, as well as judicious manipulation of systemic and pulmonary vascular resistances where necessary.
- Attention to postoperative pain management is critical in this population if exacerbations of hemodynamic instability are to be avoided.

REFERENCES

1. Neubauer S: The failing heart—an engine out of fuel. N Engl J Med 356:1140-1151, 2007
2. Vitali E, Colombo T, Fratto P, et al: Surgical therapy in advanced heart failure. Am J Cardiol 91(suppl):88F, 2003
3. Westaby S, Narula J: Preface: Surgical options in heart failure. Surg Clin North Am 84:15, 2004
4. Birks E, Tansley P, Hardy J, et al: Left ventricular assist device and drug therapy for the reversal of heart failure. N Engl J Med 355:1873, 2006.
5. Liao L, Cabell CH, Jollis JG, et al: Usefulness of myocardial viability or ischemia in predicting long-term survival for patients with severe left ventricular dysfunction undergoing revascularization. Am J Cardiol 93:1275, 2004
6. Romano MA, Bolling SF: Mitral valve repair as an alternative treatment for heart failure patients. Heart Fail Monit 4:7, 2003
7. Reese TB, Tribble CG, Ellman PI, et al: Mitral repair is superior to replacement when associated with coronary artery disease. Ann Surg 239:6715, 2004
8. Athanasuleas CL, Stanley AW, Jr Buckberg GD, et al: Surgical anterior ventricular endocardial restoration (SAVER) in the dilated remodeled ventricle after anterior myocardial infarction. RESTORE Group. Reconstructive Endoventricular Surgery, Returning Torsion Original Radius Elliptical Shape to the LV. J Am Coll Cardiol 37:1199, 2001
9. Oz MC, Konerzt WF, Kleber FX, et al: Global surgical experience with the acorn cardiac support device. J Thorac Cardiovasc Surg 126:983, 2003
10. Jarcho J: Resynchronizing ventricular contraction in heart failure. N Engl J Med 352:1594, 2005
11. Cleland J, Daubert J, Erdman E, et al: The effect of cardiac resynchronization on morbidity and mortality in heart failure. N Engl J Med 352:1539, 2005
12. Bardy E, Lee K, Mark D, et al: Amiodarone or an implanted cardioverter-defibrillator for congestive heart failure. N Engl J Med 352:225, 2005
13. Minami K, El-Banayosy A, Sezai A, et al: Morbidity and outcome after mechanical support using Thoratec, Novacor, and HeartMate for bridging to heart transplantation. Artif Organs 24:421, 2000
14. Rose EA, Gelijns AC, Moskowitz AJ, et al: Long-term use of a left ventricular assist device for end-stage heart failure. N Engl J Med 345:1435, 2001
15. Horton S, Khodaverdian R, Powers A, et al: Left ventricular assist device malfunction: A systemic approach to diagnosis. J Am Coll Cardiol 43:1574, 2004
16. Rosenstrauch D, Poglajen G, Zidar N, Gregoric I: Stem cell therapy for ischemic heart failure. Tex Heart Inst J 32:339, 2005
17. Chaudhri BB, del Monte F, Harding SE, et al: Gene transfer in cardiac myocytes. Surg Clin North Am: 84:141, 2004
18. Horton S, Khodaverdian R, Chatelain P, et al: Left ventricular assist device malfunction: An approach to diagnosis by echocardiography. J Am Coll Cardiol 45:1435, 2005
19. Mets B: Anesthesia for left ventricular assist device placement. J Cardiothorac Vasc Anesth 14:316, 2000

21

Section V
Extracorporeal Circulation

Chapter 22

Cardiopulmonary Bypass and the Anesthesiologist

Christina Mora-Mangano, MD • John L. Chow, MD • Max Kanevsky, MD

GOALS AND MECHANICS OF CARDIOPULMONARY BYPASS

The cardiopulmonary bypass (CPB) circuit is designed to perform four major functions: (1) oxygenation and carbon dioxide elimination, (2) circulation of blood, (3) systemic cooling and rewarming, and (4) diversion of blood from the heart to provide a bloodless surgical field. Typically, venous blood is drained by gravity from the right side of the heart into a reservoir that serves as a large mixing chamber for all blood return, additional fluids, and drugs. Because (in most instances) negative pressure is not employed, the amount of venous drainage is determined by the central venous pressure, the column height between the patient and reservoir, and resistance to flow in the venous circuitry.

Venous return may be decreased deliberately (as is done when restoring the patient's blood volume before coming off bypass) by application of a venous clamp. From the reservoir, blood is pumped to an oxygenator and heat exchanger unit before passing through an arterial filter and returning to the patient. Additional components

513

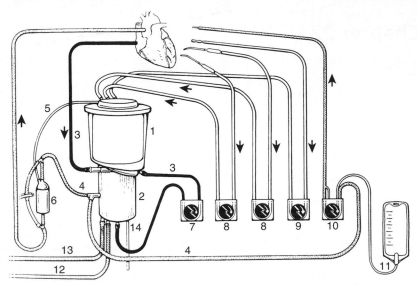

Figure 22-1 Components of the extracorporeal circuit: (1) integral cardiotomy reservoir; (2) membrane oxygenator bundle; (3) venous blood line; (4) arterial blood line; (5) arterial filter purge line; (6) arterial line filter; (7) venous blood pump (also called the arterial pump head; this pump forces venous blood through the membrane oxygenator and arterialized blood to the patient's aortic root); (8) cardiotomy suction pump; (9) ventricular vent pump; (10) cardioplegia pump; (11) crystalloid cardioplegia; (12) water inlet line; (13) water outlet line; and (14) gas inlet line. (From Davis RB, Kauffman JN, Cobbs TL, Mick SL: Cardiopulmonary Bypass. New York, Springer-Verlag, 1995, p 239.)

of the circuit generally include pumps and tubing for cardiotomy suction, venting, and cardioplegia delivery and recirculation, as well as in-line blood gas monitors, bubble detectors, pressure monitors, and blood sampling ports. A schematic representation of a typical bypass circuit is depicted in Figure 22-1.

The cannulation sites and type of CPB circuit used are dependent on the type of operation planned. Most cardiac procedures use full CPB, in which the blood is drained from the right side of the heart and returned to the systemic circulation through the aorta. The CPB circuit performs the function of heart and lungs. Aortoatriocaval cannulation is the preferred method of cannulation for CPB, although femoral arteriovenous cannulation may be the technique of choice for emergency access, repeat sternotomy, and other clinical settings in which aortic or atrial cannulation is not feasible. Procedures involving the thoracic aorta are often performed using partial bypass in which a portion of oxygenated blood is removed from the left side of the heart and returned to the femoral artery. Perfusion of the head and upper extremity vessels is performed by the beating heart, and distal perfusion is provided below the level of the cross-clamp by retrograde flow by the femoral artery. All blood passes through the pulmonary circulation, eliminating the need for an oxygenator.

PHYSIOLOGIC PARAMETERS OF CARDIOPULMONARY BYPASS

The primary objective of CPB is maintenance of systemic perfusion and respiration. Controversy arises with the question of whether systemic oxygenation and perfusion should be "optimal or maximal." Remarkably, after more than one-half century of CPB, there is continued disagreement regarding the fundamental management of extracorporeal circulation. Clinicians and investigators disagree on what are the best strategies for arterial blood pressure goals, pump flow, hematocrit, temperature, blood gas management, or mode of perfusion (pulsatile vs. nonpulsatile) (Box 22-1). Additional considerations of what is best relate to other goals of CPB: maintenance of homeostasis, facilitation of surgery, and avoidance of complications.[1]

Perfusion Pressure during Cardiopulmonary Bypass

Selection of perfusion pressure during CPB is based on balancing the demands of surgical access (bloodless field) with patient outcome (adequate oxygen delivery). Lower flow and pressure during CPB may optimize visualization, whereas higher flow and pressure may minimize patient complications. Determining the optimum perfusion pressure has been extremely challenging because no single study can adequately address all the complexities of CPB. Because of the brain's poor tolerance of ischemia, neurologic outcome has been the most common outcome studied in relation to perfusion pressure. The complicated relationship between neurologic outcome and perfusion pressure is likely related to two causes of adverse neurologic outcomes: hypoperfusion and embolism.

Between mean arterial pressures (MAP) of 50 and 150 mmHg, cerebral autoregulation maintains a relatively constant blood flow and oxygen delivery. During hypothermic CPB, the lower limit of cerebral autoregulation may be as low as 20 to 30 mmHg,[2] affording some additional protection against hypoperfusion. Increasing perfusion pressure to alleviate the risk of hypoperfusion may lead to greater embolic load and worse outcomes. Ultimately, the selection of perfusion pressure during CPB will need to be based on clinical outcome studies.

Subgroups at increased risk for adverse outcomes that may benefit from higher perfusion pressure during CPB include patients with severe atheromatous disease (cerebrovascular or aortic arch), advanced age, systemic hypertension, and diabetes. Increased cerebral dysfunction in the elderly may be a result of slower vasodilatation of cerebral resistance vessels during periods of rewarming and subsequent transient episodes of metabolism-flow mismatch with resultant ischemia. It is unknown what the effect of elevating perfusion pressure during rewarming would be on neurologic outcome. Hypertensive patients are generally accepted to have intact pressure-flow autoregulation, with a rightward shift in the cerebral autoregulation curve such that pressure-dependent flow patterns develop at higher perfusion pressures than in the normal population. In hypertensive patients the use of higher perfusion pressure during CPB is common practice. Patients with type 1 diabetes mellitus appear to have impaired metabolism-flow coupling during CPB. They also have some loss of pressure-flow autoregulation.

Once the CPB team has selected target perfusion pressures during CPB, a few technical issues emerge. Throughout this discussion perfusion pressure and MAP have been used almost interchangeably. In general, cerebral perfusion pressure is what is of most concern. Cerebral perfusion pressure is determined by the difference between MAP and the higher of central venous pressure and intracranial pressure. The latter values are usually less than 5 mmHg during CPB. However, in the presence of compromised cerebral venous drainage (malpositioned cannula, patient positioning), MAP will not accurately reflect cerebral perfusion pressure.

Measurement artifacts also play a role in perfusion pressure management. MAP may vary by as much as 20 mmHg over 30 seconds while pump flow is constant. The mechanism of this oscillation and its relation to outcome are unclear. A more common artifact is discordance between radial arterial and central arterial pressures during rewarming. This difference may be as great as 30% and is believed to occur from opening of arteriovenous shunts in the arm.

After acknowledging the technical issues of pressure monitoring, the CPB team is left to maintain the selected perfusion pressure. To achieve these perfusion pressure goals the team has two general options: alterations of pump flow or administration of vasoactive agents. Increasing pump flow may be used as a temporizing measure for hypotension if surgical demands allow it; however, this may come at the cost of dangerously reducing reservoir volume. Alternatively, phenylephrine and norepinephrine may be used to support perfusion pressure. In the case of hypertension, pump flow may be reduced, although this increases the potential for inadequate oxygen delivery; more commonly, a vasodilator, such as sodium nitroprusside or nitroglycerin, is employed. Isoflurane or another volatile anesthetic may be administered through the pump oxygenator, with careful attention paid to its use during weaning from CPB.

Nonpulsatile versus Pulsatile Perfusion

It remains uncertain whether pulsatile CPB improves outcome compared with standard, nonpulsatile CPB. Claims of advantages to pulsatile flow are effectively offset by conflicting studies of similar design.

The comparatively small size of the arterial inflow cannula can effectively filter out a large component of the pulsatile kinetic energy. Consequently, as achieved clinically, pulsatile flow may actually be quite similar energetically to nonpulsatile flow. This potentially unrecognized lack of difference in types of flow may partly explain the failure of pulsatile perfusion to alter hormone levels and clinical outcome.

Pump Flow during Bypass

Like perfusion pressure, pump flow during CPB represents a careful balance between the conflicting demands of surgical visualization and adequate oxygen delivery. Two theoretical approaches exist. The first is to maintain oxygen delivery during bypass at normal levels for a given core temperature. Although this may limit hypoperfusion, it does increase the delivered embolic load. The second approach is to use the lowest flows that do not result in end-organ injury. This approach offers the potential advantage of less embolic delivery as well as potential improved myocardial protection and surgical visualization.

During CPB, pump flow and pressure are related through overall arterial impedance, a product of hemodilution, temperature, and arterial cross-sectional area. This is important because the first two factors, hemodilution and temperature, are critical

V

determinants of pump flow requirements. Pump flows of 1.2 L/min/m^2 perfuse most of the microcirculation when the hematocrit is near 22% and hypothermic CPB is being employed. However, at lower hematocrits or periods of higher oxygen consumption these flows become inadequate.

Most perfusion teams also monitor mixed venous saturation, targeting levels of 70% or greater. Unfortunately, this level does not guarantee adequate perfusion of all tissue beds, because some (muscle, subcutaneous fat) may be functionally removed from circulation during CPB. Hypothermic venous saturation may overestimate end-organ reserves. Regional perfusion of various end-organs (brain, kidney, small intestine, pancreas, and muscle) has been quantified with a fluorescent microsphere technique.[3] Cerebral blood flow was unchanged at higher pump flows. Renal perfusion was maintained at flows of 1.9 and 1.6 L/min/m^2. Perfusion to the pancreas was constant at all flows, and small bowel perfusion varied linearly with pump flow. Muscle bed flows were decreased at all flows.

During CPB, most of the outcomes studied in relation to pump flow are those related to the organs at high risk for ischemic injury (i.e., kidney and brain). Much work has been applied to examining the relationship between renal dysfunction and pump flow. Preexisting renal disease is a consistent predictor of postoperative renal dysfunction, the incidence of which ranges between 3% and 5%. Renal function appears unaltered when pump flows greater than 1.6 L/min/m^2 are employed, but whether this management will affect outcomes in patients with preexisting renal dysfunction is less clear.

Bypass Temperature Management Strategy

Although hypothermic temperatures have been employed since the advent of extracorporeal circulation, the importance of reduced temperatures during bypass was challenged in the early 1990s.

Effects on Central Nervous System

The brain is arguably the organ most vulnerable to ischemic damage during CPB. Cerebral hypoperfusion and embolic phenomena are likely to occur in every patient undergoing bypass, resulting in ischemic events. It is believed that hypothermia provides protection from ischemic phenomena and resultant infarction by decreasing cerebral oxygen demands, maintaining energy (ATP, phosphocreatine) stores. Although the effect of reduced temperatures on metabolism is of importance, there is increasing evidence that the most important salutary effects of hypothermia on cerebral ischemia are not related to the reduction in metabolism but rather to the attenuation of the excitotoxic cascade.

Several groups of investigators have assessed the effect of normothermic temperatures during bypass on perioperative central nervous system events in cardiac surgery patients.[4] Mild hypothermia provides some magnitude of cerebral protection during CPB, whereas mildly hyperthermic temperatures (>37°C) exacerbate and amplify the ischemic injury associated with CPB.

Temperature Monitoring

Because the brain is vulnerable to hyperthermic temperatures, it is important to use the temperature-monitoring site most likely to reflect cerebral temperature. The most commonly used sites in cardiac surgery patients include esophageal, nasopharyngeal, tympanic, pulmonary arterial, rectal, urinary bladder, subcutaneous (or muscle), and cutaneous sites. Unfortunately, none of these monitoring locations

22

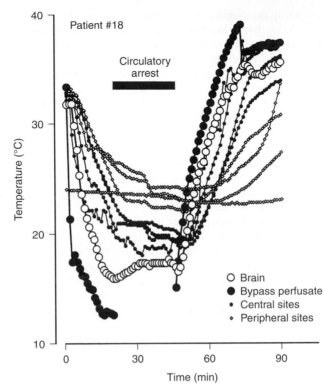

Figure 22-2 Graphic depiction of temperature-time relationship during cardiopulmonary bypass and deep hypothermic circulatory arrest. Temperatures are plotted every minute. Central sites are the nasopharynx, tympanic membrane, esophagus, and pulmonary artery. Peripheral sites are the bladder, rectum, axilla, and sole of the foot. The two slowest cooling central sites were tympanic membrane and esophagus. (From Stone JG, Young WL, Smith CR, et al: Do standard monitoring sites reflect true brain temperature when profound hypothermia is rapidly induced and reversed? Anesthesiology 82:344, 1995.)

has been demonstrated to reflect cerebral temperature reliably. With exposure of the brain, investigators have placed a thermocouple directly in the cerebral cortex. Brain temperature was compared with values obtained from sensors in eight locations.[5] Investigators found a poor concordance between cerebral temperature and values obtained at the other monitoring sites. Locations hypothesized to best reflect core temperature—tympanic membrane, esophagus, nasopharynx, pulmonary artery— sometimes overestimated cerebral temperature or underestimated brain tempera- ture. Because of the substantial variability noted in central temperature readings (Fig. 22-2) and lack of the concordance of central temperature measures in every patient, the investigators recommended the use of at least three measures of central or core temperature.

Acid-Base Strategy

The management of acid-base status during hypothermic CPB has been a long- standing source of debate. Understanding of the physiologic responses to hypo- thermia, and the influences of Pco_2 have led to shifts in clinical practice over the past decades. Two strategies exist for managing acid-base balance during periods of hypothermia: α-stat and pH-stat. The term α-stat was first proposed to describe the theory that acid-base regulation in vertebrate animals functioned during temperature fluctuation to maintain a constant ratio (α) of dissociated to undissociated forms of the imidazole ring on histidine. It is this protein charge state that is important in regulating pH-dependent cellular processes. Hypothermia increases the solubility of oxygen and carbon dioxide in the blood, leading to a decrease in Pco_2 and an increase in pH at lower temperatures. With α-stat blood gas management, the uncorrected (37°) pH is kept at 7.40 with the Pco_2 at 40 mmHg, creating a relative alkalosis at the patient's actual body temperature. This strategy is considered to be physiologic because the ionization state of histidine is unchanged over all temperature ranges and protein structure and function are preserved.

The pH-stat approach to acid-base balance maintains a pH of 7.40 and Pco_2 of 40 mmHg when corrected for body temperature, typically requiring the addition of CO_2 during hypothermic CPB. This method of blood gas management was generally favored until the mid 1980s because it was believed that the potent vasodilatory effects of CO_2 would provide increased cerebral blood flow and thereby minimize the risk of cerebral ischemia during CPB. It is now recognized that pH-stat management during hypothermia produces passive cerebral vasodilation, impairs autoregulatory responses to blood pressure changes and metabolic demands in the brain, and does not improve overall oxygen balance. In contrast, α-stat management preserves autoregulation and the relationship between cerebral blood flow and metabolism. Neither blood gas strategy has any significant effect on hypothermic cerebral metabolism. The increased CBF seen with pH-stat may also increase the risk of cerebral embolization or produce a steal phenomenon.[6]

Fluid Management

The choice of fluid for priming the extracorporeal circuit in CPB remains controversial. The idea of using nonblood prime was first introduced in 1959. This technique of hemodilution was found to be safe when combined with hypothermia to reduce oxygen consumption and demand. The use of nonblood primes and moderate hemodilution for CPB has become routine in most centers. A reduction in hematocrit from 40% to 20% allows cooling to 22°C without an increase in blood viscosity or required driving pressure. Hematocrit reduction may be achieved before bypass by means of acute normovolemic hemodilution in the hope of reinfusing the patient's own heparin-free blood, rather than allogeneic red blood cells, after CPB.

Several studies have investigated the differences between colloid and crystalloid priming solutions. In general, crystalloid solutions lead to decreased colloid osmotic pressure with a resultant increase in extracellular water retention, irrespective of the osmolarity of the pump prime. Albumin, unlike a pure crystalloid prime, can decrease the interaction of blood components with the bypass circuit by coating the fluid pathway surfaces. In their meta-analysis of 21 controlled trials enrolling 1346 patients, Russell and associates showed a notably smaller drop in on-bypass platelet counts in patients treated with albumin in the pump prime.[7]

Ultrafiltration during bypass can be used as a means of reducing excess water accumulation. Modified ultrafiltration describes the process of hemofiltration immediately after the cessation of bypass. This process results in a more consistent reduction in total body water with significant increases in hematocrit, myocardial contractility, cardiac index, and improved pulmonary compliance.

END-ORGAN EFFECTS OF CARDIOPULMONARY BYPASS

Myocardial Injury

Most coronary revascularization procedures are completed with the assistance of CPB. Although the completion of coronary anastomoses is facilitated by CPB (i.e., the surgeon can operate on a quiet, nonbeating heart), the heart is subjected to a series of events leading to ischemic myocardium during extracorporeal circulation. The operation, which is designed to preserve and improve myocardial function, is sometimes associated with myocardial damage (Box 22-2). The extent and incidence of this injury are dependent on the sensitivity and specificity of the diagnostic methods being used. However, most patients who undergo cardiac operations sustain some degree of myocardial injury. Although patients with normal ventricular function may tolerate these minor amounts of injury without detectable sequelae, those with impaired ventricular function preoperatively may not be able to tolerate the slightest injury. As the patient population for CPB continues to become older and have greater degrees of concomitant illness, understanding the physiology of and developing effective preventive strategies for myocardial injury during CPB are increasingly important. Because myocardial damage influences early and long-term results, the identification and control of factors associated with myocardial injury are critical to ensuring good outcomes. Although injury may be linked to anesthetic and surgical management, myocardial injury usually is thought to occur from inadequate myocardial protection during CPB.

Mechanisms

The underlying mechanism for most types of myocardial injuries during CPB is ischemia. Ischemia develops when oxygen demand outstrips its supply in the heart. This process involves a complex cascade of events that compromise high-energy phosphate and calcium homeostasis. Many reports confirm the role of high-energy phosphate depletion and intracellular calcium accumulation in the pathogenesis of myocardial damage during ischemia and subsequent reperfusion. Oxidative phosphorylation ceases when the tissue Po_2 falls below 5 to 10 mmHg. Then creatine phosphate (CP) and anaerobic production become the main sources of high-energy phosphate. These mechanisms are unfortunately limited. Creatine kinase (CK)–mediated transfer of high-energy phosphate from CP to adenosine diphosphate (ADP) provides an immediate source of energy; the amount of adenosine triphosphate (ATP) produced by transfer is limited initially by substrate availability and subsequently by lactate inhibition. Anaerobic production is inefficient and self-limiting because of accumulation of metabolites (i.e., lactate, pyruvate, and hydrogen ions) with inhibition of enzyme systems. As high-energy phosphate stores

---

BOX 22-2	*End Organs That Can Be Adversely Affected by Cardiopulmonary Bypass*

- Heart
- Brain
- Kidneys
- Gastrointestinal tract
- Endocrine system

become depleted, the cardiac cells are no longer able to maintain normal transport of calcium out of the cell. Energy-dependent mechanisms that lower intracellular ionized calcium concentration and terminate the contractile process fail because of a lack of high-energy phosphate. The cytosolic concentration of ionized calcium remains high, and energy use persists with the formation of rigor bonds between the contractile proteins. Continued energy use with calcium and proton-activated release of destructive lipoprotein lipase eventually leads to loss of cell integrity and function.

Certain specific events during CPB are associated with myocardial ischemia and injury (Table 22-1). These events lead to ischemia by increasing oxygen demands, decreasing oxygen supply, or a combination of both. When these factors are present together they potentiate myocardial damage. For example, the distended, fibrillating ventricle with a low perfusion pressure is particularly susceptible to damage.

Aortic Cross-Clamping

Aortic cross-clamping, potentially a major cause of myocardial injury during CPB, was a product of evolution. Initially, continuous aortic or direct coronary artery perfusion of the empty, beating heart was used to "protect" the myocardium during cardiac repairs. Ventricular fibrillation was frequently induced and maintained to "quiet" the heart and thereby improve exposure and prevent air embolism. Despite continuous perfusion, myocardial damage commonly occurred. Although myocardial protection improved with the addition of moderate cardiac hypothermia (28° to 32°C), operating conditions did not. Most surgeons found it difficult to perform precise repairs on the firm, bleeding, beating, or fibrillating heart. To improve exposure and minimize the complications associated with direct coronary cannulation for aortic valve replacement (AVR), myocardial ischemia was induced by aortic cross-clamping. However, the technique of normothermic or moderate hypothermic ischemic arrest is not without problems. First, the heart continues to beat for some time after application of the aortic cross-clamp, thereby compromising the anticipated improvement in operating conditions. Persistent electrical and mechanical activity during much of the ischemic period needlessly depletes high-energy phosphate and compromises post-repair ventricular performance. Second, few surgeons can complete a complex repair quickly enough to prevent significant myocardial damage in the unprotected heart. Third, the use of intermittent cross-clamping with periods of reperfusion does little to improve operating conditions or prevent necrosis. Reactive hyperemia after release of the aortic clamp continues to obscure the

22

Table 22-1	Factors Associated with Myocardial Injury during Cardiopulmonary Bypass
Abnormal perfusate composition	
Persistent ventricular fibrillation	
Inadequate myocardial perfusion	
Ventricular distention	
Ventricular collapse	
Coronary embolism	
Catecholamines	
Aortic cross-clamping	
Reperfusion	

operative field. Multiple short periods of reperfusion, particularly in the presence of VF, may potentiate rather than prevent ischemic damage. Defibrillation to improve reperfusion reintroduces the problem of systemic air embolism during open repairs.

Rapid cessation of electrical and mechanical activity immediately after aortic cross-clamping is desirable to potentiate surgical exposure and myocardial preservation. The extent of necrosis in unprotected myocardium is directly related to the duration of aortic cross-clamping. The ischemic time should be minimized. Variability among patients in terms of myocardial vulnerability makes it difficult to accurately predict safe periods of interval ischemia. Prolonged surgical time demands direct interventions to protect the myocardium. These focus along the lines of maximizing high-energy phosphate production while minimizing high-energy phosphate use and intracellular calcium accumulation during the ischemic period. Specific interventions include hypothermia, cardioplegia, β-adrenergic and calcium channel blockade, and adenosine-regulating compounds. Uninterrupted periods of ischemia provide the best operating conditions while minimizing the risk of reperfusion injury and air embolism.

Myocardial Protection

Myocardial protection strategies can be summarized with four basic concepts:

1. Myocardial protection begins with preparation of the heart before arrest.
2. Metabolic requirements should be reduced during the arrest interval.
3. A favorable metabolic milieu during arrest helps provide a margin of safety with reduced metabolism.
4. Reperfusion modification after an ischemic insult can minimize structural and functional damage to the myocardium.

The first concept includes phenomena under the direct control of the anesthesiologist. In the pre-bypass period, the heart should be prepared for ischemic arrest by optimizing myocardial metabolism and providing hemodynamic conditions that optimize myocardial oxygen supply-demand ratios.

Patients coming to cardiac surgery (especially in this era of same-day admissions) are frequently dehydrated and hypoglycemic. The anesthesiologist should rehydrate the patient and administer sufficient glucose to improve the heart's ability to tolerate ischemic arrest. Because the initiation of bypass is frequently accompanied by hypotension, the anesthesiologist should be prepared to administer vasoconstrictive drugs (e.g., phenylephrine) to maintain coronary perfusion pressure. Similarly, ventricular distention must be avoided (especially before fibrillatory arrest) because increases in left ventricular end-diastolic pressure decrease coronary perfusion pressures and greatly compromise subendocardial oxygen delivery. The anesthesiologist should monitor intraventricular volume with a transesophageal echocardiography (TEE) probe after the initiation of bypass. The surgeon can prevent ventricular distention by placing a hole in the left atrium, left ventricle, or pulmonary artery or by placing a vent in the left ventricle. Although negative pressure venting enhances the risk of intracavitary air entrapment, many surgeons prefer active venting to passive methods. Several pharmacologic interventions administered to patients or added to the cardioplegic solution may enhance myocardial protection. β-Receptor antagonists (e.g., propranolol, esmolol) provide myocardial protection by decreasing heart rate and myocardial metabolism. The heart rate should be maintained at less than 80 beats per minute in patients with ischemic heart disease in the pre-bypass period.

V

Brain Injury

The brain is highly susceptible to injury during CPB. Many clinicians believe that cerebral injuries after cardiac surgery are the most devastating adverse outcomes associated with CPB. A study of 2400 patients undergoing elective coronary artery bypass grafting (CABG) from 24 U.S. centers reported that 6.1% of patients suffer adverse postoperative gross neurologic or psychiatric central nervous system events. These patients remain in the intensive care unit and hospital for greater periods of time, and 1 in every 3 surviving patients does not return home but requires continued long-term care and rehabilitation.[8] (see chapter 23).

Renal Dysfunction

The effects of CPB on the renal system have significant health and economic impacts; however, despite intensive investigation into the pathogenesis and prevention of renal failure, there remains limited progress in the development of effective protective strategies in recent decades.[9] Because intravascular volume depletion and hypoperfusion can lead to exacerbation of renal ischemia and accentuate the risk for postoperative acute renal failure, avoidance of nephrotoxic agents and close attention to intravascular volume, blood pressure, and cardiac output (CO) are central in the effort to reduce the occurrence of acute renal failure after cardiac surgery.

Gastrointestinal Effects

The effects of CPB on the gastrointestinal system are complex and not fully elucidated. Although most patients undergoing cardiac surgery do not suffer adverse changes in gastrointestinal function, subclinical perturbations including transient elevations in hepatocellular enzymes and hyperamylasemia have been observed after CPB. Although the incidence of gastrointestinal complications after CPB is low (range, 0.3% to 3.7%), they are associated with significant morbidity and remarkably high mortality (range, 11% to 67%) compared with cardiac surgery patients without postoperative gastrointestinal compromise. The frequently reported adverse gastrointestinal outcomes include gastroesophagitis, upper and lower gastrointestinal hemorrhage, hyperbilirubinemia, hepatic and splenic ischemia, colitis, pancreatitis, cholecystitis, diverticulitis, mesenteric ischemia, as well as intestinal obstruction, infarction, and perforation.[10]

Although the pathophysiology of gastrointestinal complications after cardiac surgery is likely multifactorial, a unifying mechanism is splanchnic hypoperfusion. The gastrointestinal system is particularly vulnerable for ischemia due to the lack of autoregulation and to the preferential shunting of blood away from the gastrointestinal circulation during periods of hypotension. Hypothermia and nonpulsatile flow during CPB may be detrimental to mucosal perfusion. However, hypothermia has little effect on hepatic arterial blood flow and may actually increase portal flow. There is no significant difference in hepatic blood flow between pulsatile and nonpulsatile perfusion at high flow rates (2.4 L/min/m^2) during hypothermia. Perhaps more important to the development of inadequate gastrointestinal perfusion is the significant increase in total body oxygen consumption in the immediate hours after CPB. Visceral hypotension is the most significant factor in the development of gastrointestinal complications after cardiac surgery. Gut ischemia of sufficient duration impairs gastrointestinal tract barrier function. Studies evaluating gut permeability have shown that CPB is associated with an increase in mucosal permeability and systemic endotoxin concentration.

22

Endocrine and Inflammatory Responses

Endocrine Response

Cardiopulmonary bypass provokes a marked stress response, which has been quantified by measurements of hormones and vasoactive substances in plasma. Hypothermia, hemodilution, and nonpulsatile flow produce insulin, prostaglandin, and renin release during CPB and are potent stimuli for catecholamine release. Epinephrine levels increase throughout CPB with a ninefold increase that peaks during rewarming, after aortic cross-clamp release. Although striking, the magnitude of the catecholamine responses is comparable to that after syncope, myocardial infarction, strenuous exercise, or caffeine ingestion. It is likely that increased plasma catecholamine concentrations are in part due to decreased clearance. The heart and lungs, which serve as primary clearance organs for these substances, are partially or completely excluded from the circulation during much of CPB. Hypothermia slows all enzymatic processes responsible for metabolism.

Many other hormones increase during CPB. Vasopressin increases up to 20 times baseline levels during CPB. Some investigators suggest that vasopressin and angiotensin II are responsible for the elevations in SVR observed during CPB, and this may explain why vasopressin can be a useful drug to increase SVR on CPB in patients who are extremely vasodilated.[11]

Data from clinical and laboratory investigators now conclusively demonstrate the untoward affects of hyperglycemia in cardiac surgery. Aggressive control of perioperative glucose values represents the standard of care in cardiac surgery. Glucose values should be maintained at levels less than 200 mg/dL. Lower values (blood glucose 80 to 120 mg/dL) are likely superior to values of glucose more than 120 mg/dL. A protocol for management of glucose in cardiac surgery patients is outlined in Table 22-2.[12]

Immunologic Inflammatory Response

The physiologic insult of CPB results in a myriad of exaggerated, complex, and mostly pathologic immunologic events. The passage of blood through the extracorporeal circuit causes activation of complement, platelets, neutrophils, and proinflammatory kinins. At the conclusion of bypass, blood perturbed by the process of extracorporeal circulation reperfuses ischemic organs, exacerbating the local inflammatory responses in end organs, including the brain, kidney, heart, and lung. These phenomena result in whole-body inflammatory response and represent the collective effect of activation of the complement, fibrinolytic, kallikrein, and coagulation systems.

The complement system is formed by two interconnected cascades: the classical and the alternative pathways. The elements of the classical pathway are C1, C4, and C2, with subunits and fragments of these elements developing as the cascade progresses. The classical pathway is thought to be normally triggered by antigen-antibody complexes. The alternative pathway, bypassing C1, C4, and C2 to activate C3, is triggered by complex polysaccharides, lipopolysaccharides, IgA and IgD and by exposure of blood to foreign surfaces. The two pathways converge at C3 and lead to activation of the terminal components, C5 to C9. The fragments C3a and C5a are known anaphylatoxins.

With initiation of CPB, complement is thought to be activated through the alternative pathway. Exposure of blood to the CPB circuit initiates activation of the coagulation cascade by means of the Hageman factor (XII). Although the coagulation cascade is initiated, it is not completed because of the presence of heparin. Activated factor XII (XIIa) results in plasmin generation. Plasmin activates complement by

Table 22-2 Stanford University Adult Cardiac Anesthesia Continuous Insulin Infusion Protocol

Bolus and start infusion as follows:

Blood Glucose (mg/dL)	Insulin Bolus Units	Units/hr
<125	0	0
125 to 175	5	1
175 to 225	10	2
>225	15	3

Measure blood glucose values every 30 minutes intraoperatively!

Insulin Titration

Blood Glucose	Treatment
<75	Stop insulin; D5W and recheck in 30 min; when > 150, restart at 50% of previous rate.
75-100	Stop insulin; recheck in 30 min; restart at 50% of previous rate (unless < 0.25 U/hr).
101-125	If < 10% lower than last value, decrease by 0.5 U/hr. If > 10% lower than last value, decrease by 50%. If neither, continue current rate.
126-175	Continue current rate.
176-225	If lower than last value, continue current rate. If higher than last value, increase by 0.5 U/hr.
>225	If > 10% lower than last value, continue current rate. If < 10% lower or greater than last value increase by 1 U/hr. If > 225 and not decreased after three adjustments, double current rate.

22

C1 (classical pathway), cleaves C3 (alternative pathway), and cleaves factor XII, which activates the kallikrein-kinin systems. Complement activation can also occur through the classical pathway by heparin-protamine complexes. Complement activation leads to direct membrane injury by complement subunits, neutrophil activation, enhancement of phagocytosis due to interaction of complement components and phagocytic cells, and release of lysosomal enzymes. The complement fragments are stimulants that induce changes in neutrophil behavior, causing neutrophil activation and migration and the promotion of adhesive and secretory events. These phenomena contribute to the reperfusion injury observed in cardiac surgery patients. Activated neutrophils attach to the endothelium, causing translocation of P-selectin from intracellular vesicles to the cell membrane and platelet-activating factor (PAF) synthesis. Endothelial membrane-bound PAF leads to increased neutrophil adhesion and activation and neutrophil adhesion protein (CD11/CD18) expression. Ultimately, increases in adhesion molecule emission in the endothelium and other tissue cell types (e.g., myocytes, alveolar cells, glomerular or renal tubular epithelium) result in transmigration of neutrophils into the interstitial space and release of large amounts of free radicals. These phenomena are schematically presented in Figure 22-3.

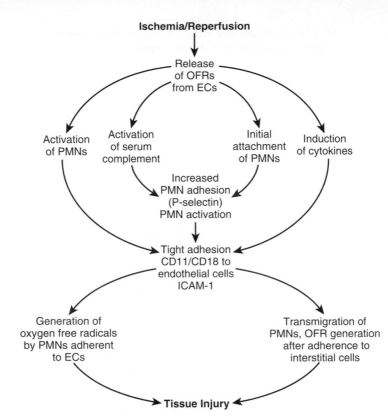

Figure 22-3 A schematic representation of the interactive components of the immune response that likely occurs during the postischemic inflammatory state after cardiopulmonary bypass. EC = endothelial cells; ICAM = intercellular adhesion molecules; OFR = oxygen free radicals; PMNs = polymorphonuclear leukocytes. (From Herskowitz A, Mangano DT: Inflammatory cascade: A final common pathway for perioperative injury? Anesthesiology 85:957, 1996.)

Although complement has been recognized as a significant factor in the development of the physiologic disturbances seen after cardiac surgery, endotoxins released into the bloodstream during CPB are also believed to play a significant role in the inflammatory cascade. Endotoxin binds to lipopolysaccharide-binding protein normally present in serum. This complex binds to specific receptors on macrophages with subsequent production of cytokines. The collective result of these cellular and humoral responses may be manifest by cardiovascular instability, pulmonary dysfunction, renal insufficiency, alterations in hemostasis, fever, and excess extravascular fluid retention.

Interventions aimed at reducing morbidity associated with the systemic inflammatory response seen after CPB may be directed at preventing or minimizing the activation of the various systems contributing to the response or at blocking the physiologic effects once activation occurs. Studies evaluating membrane versus bubble oxygenators have reported conflicting data regarding the degree of complement activation or clinical outcome.

Corticosteroids may play an important role in minimizing the inflammatory response by reducing complement activation, decreasing production of cytokines, and interfering with neutrophil adherence and migration. Most clinical trials have reported a beneficial effect on markers of inflammation (e.g., cytokine and

V

BOX 22-3 *Management before Cardiopulmonary Bypass*

- Anticoagulation
- Cannulation of the heart
- Careful monitoring
- Protection of the heart
- Preparation for cardiopulmonary bypass

---

complement levels, histamine release, leukocyte counts, endothelial activation). The use of aprotinin or other protease inhibitors has been shown to produce a dose-dependent reduction in complement activation, cytokine release, and neutrophil activation during cardiac surgery.

MANAGEMENT BEFORE BYPASS

An important objective of this phase is to prepare the patient for CPB (Box 22-3).[13] This phase invariably involves two key steps: anticoagulation and vascular cannulation. Heparin is still the anticoagulant clinically used for CPB. Dose, method of administration, and opinions as to what constitutes adequate anticoagulation vary. Heparin must be administered before cannulation for CPB, even if cannulation must be done emergently. Failure to do so is to risk thrombosis in the patient and extracorporeal circuit. After heparin has been administered, a period of 3 to 5 minutes is customarily allowed for systemic circulation and onset of effect. Various confirmatory tests of actual achievement of anticoagulation are performed if time permits.

Vascular Cannulation

The next major step in the pre-bypass phase is vascular cannulation. The goal of vascular cannulation is to provide access whereby the CPB pump may divert all systemic venous blood to the pump oxygenator at the lowest possible venous pressures and deliver oxygenated blood to the arterial circulation at pressure and flow sufficient to maintain systemic homeostasis.

Arterial Cannulation

Arterial cannulation is generally established before venous cannulation to allow volume resuscitation of the patient, should it be necessary. The ascending aorta is the preferred site for aortic cannulation because it is easily accessible, does not require an additional incision, accommodates a larger cannula to provide greater flow at a reduced pressure, and carries a lower risk of aortic dissection compared with other arterial cannulation sites (femoral or iliac arteries). Because hypertension increases the risk of aortic dissection during cannulation, the aortic pressure may be temporarily lowered (MAP < 80 mmHg during aortotomy and cannula insertion). Several potential complications are associated with aortic cannulation, including embolization of air or atheromatous debris, inadvertent cannulation of aortic arch vessels, aortic dissection, and other vessel wall injury.

Reviews and clinical reports emphasize the importance of embolization as the major mechanism of focal cerebral injury in cardiac surgery patients.[14] Intraoperative use of two-dimensional ultrasound to image the ascending aorta as a guide to selection of cross-clamping and cannulation sites is increasing. A femoral artery, rather than the ascending aorta, can be cannulated for systemic perfusion. Femoral

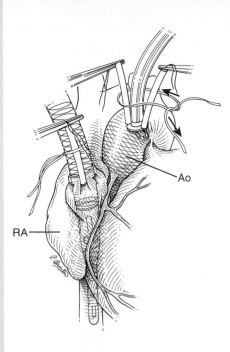

Figure 22-4 Aortic (Ao) and single, double-staged, right atrial (RA) cannulation. Notice the drainage holes of venous cannula in right atrium and inferior vena cava. (From Connolly MW: Cardiopulmonary Bypass. New York, Springer-Verlag, 1995, p 59.)

Ao

RA

cannulation is used when ascending aortic cannulation is considered relatively contraindicated, as in severe aortic atherosclerosis, aortic aneurysm or dissection, or known cystic medical necrosis. The anesthesiologist should seek evidence of cannula malposition by looking for unilateral blanching of the face, gently palpating carotid pulses, and checking for new unilateral diminution and by measuring blood pressure in both arms and checking for new asymmetries.

Venous Cannulation

Venous cannulation can be achieved using a single atrial cannula that is inserted into the right atrium and directed inferiorly (Fig. 22-4). Drainage holes are located in the inferior vena cava (IVC) and right atrium to drain blood returning from the lower extremities and the superior vena cava (SVC) and coronary sinus, respectively. This technique has the advantage of being simpler, faster and requiring only one incision; however, the quality of drainage can be easily compromised when the heart is lifted for surgical exposure. The bicaval cannulation technique, required in cases in which right atrial (RA) access is needed, involves cannulating the SVC and IVC (Fig. 22-5). Loops placed around the vessels can be tightened to divert all caval blood flow away from the heart. Blood returning to the right atrium from the coronary sinus will not be drained using this technique, so an additional vent or atriotomy is necessary.

During CPB, blood will continue to return to the left ventricle from a variety of sources, including the bronchial and thebesian veins, as well as blood that traverses the pulmonary circulation. Abnormal sources of venous blood include a persistent left SVC, systemic-to-pulmonary shunts, and aortic regurgitation. It is important to avoid left ventricular (LV) filling and distention during CPB to prevent myocardial rewarming and to minimize LV wall tension and limit myocardial oxygen demand. This can be accomplished with the use of a vent placed in the pulmonary artery, aortic root, or left ventricle, depending on the likely source of LV blood return.

Venous cannulas, using a two-stage or bicaval cannula, are large and can impair venous return from the IVC or SVC. Superior vena caval obstruction is detected by

V

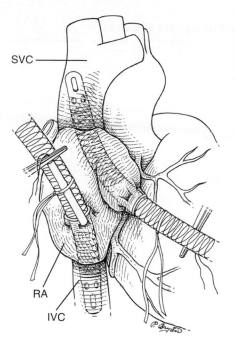

Figure 22-5   Position of two-vessel cannulation of right atrium (RA) with placement of drainage holes into superior vena cava (SVC) and inferior vena cava (IVC). The aortic cannula is not shown. (From Connolly MW: Cardiopulmonary Bypass. New York, Springer-Verlag, 1995, p 59.)

SVC

RA

IVC

venous engorgement of the head and neck, conjunctival edema, and elevated SVC pressure. Inferior vena caval obstruction is far more insidious, presenting only as decreased filling pressures because of lowered venous return.

Femoral venous cannulation is sometimes used to permit partial CPB without, or before, sternotomy or RA cannulation (e.g., repeat sternotomy, ascending aortic aneurysms). Because of their comparatively small size and placement in the distal IVC, femoral venous cannulas do not permit complete drainage of systemic venous blood and only partial CPB may be achieved. A long cannula with multiple fenestrations can be inserted through the femoral vein and passed to the level of the IVC-RA junction to enhance venous return.

Other Preparations

Once anticoagulation and cannulation are complete, CPB can be instituted. Because there is redundant pulmonary artery (PA) catheter length in the right ventricle, and the heart is manipulated during CPB, there is a tendency for distal migration of the PA catheter into pulmonary artery branches. This distal migration of the catheter increases the risks of "autowedging" and pulmonary artery perforation. During the pre-bypass phase it is advisable to withdraw the PA catheter 3 to 5 cm to decrease the likelihood of these untoward events. It is also advisable to check the integrity of all vascular access and monitoring devices. A PAC placed through an external jugular or subclavian vein can become kinked or occluded on full opening of the sternal retractor. If TEE is being used, the probe should be placed in the "freeze" mode and the tip of the scope placed in the neutral and unlocked position. Leaving the electronic scanning emitter on during hypothermic CPB adds heat to the posterior wall of the ventricle.

Before initiating CPB, the anesthesiologist should assess the depth of anesthesia and muscle relaxation. It is important to maintain paralysis to prevent patient movement that could result in dislodgment of bypass-circuit cannulae and prevent shivering

Table 22-3 Preparation for Bypass: Pre-bypass Checklist

1. Anticoagulation
   a. Heparin administered
   b. Desired level of anticoagulation achieved
2. Arterial cannulation
   a. Absence of bubbles in arterial line
   b. Evidence of dissection or malposition?
3. Venous cannulation
   a. Evidence of superior vena cava obstruction?
   b. Evidence of inferior vena cava obstruction?
4. Pulmonary artery catheter (if used) pulled back
5. Are all monitoring/access catheters functional?
6. Transesophageal echocardiograph (if used)
   a. In "freeze" mode
   b. Scope in neutral/unlocked position
7. Supplemental medications
   a. Neuromuscular blockers
   b. Anesthetics, analgesics, amnestics
8. Inspection of head and neck
   a. Color
   b. Symmetry
   c. Venous drainage
   d. Pupils

as hypothermia is induced (with the attendant increases in oxygen consumption). It is difficult to determine the depth of anesthesia during the various stages of CPB. Because blood pressure, heart rate, pupil diameter, and the autonomic nervous system are profoundly affected by extracorporeal circulation (e.g., the heart is asystolic; blood pressure is greatly influenced by circuit blood flow; sweating occurs with rewarming), these variables do not reliably reflect the anesthetic state. Although hypothermia decreases anesthetic requirements, it is necessary to provide analgesia, unconsciousness, and muscle relaxation during CPB. With the initiation of bypass and hemodilution, blood levels of anesthetics and muscle relaxants will acutely decrease. However, plasma protein concentrations also decrease, which increases the free-fraction and active drug concentrations. Every drug has a specific kinetic profile during CPB, and kinetics and pharmacodynamics during CPB will vary greatly among patients. Many clinicians administer additional muscle relaxants and opioids at the initiation of CPB. A vaporizer for potent inhalation drugs may be included in the bypass circuit. A final inspection of the head and neck for color, symmetry, adequacy of venous drainage (neck vein and conjunctiva engorgement), and pupil equality is reasonable to serve as a baseline for the anesthetic state. A summary of preparatory steps to be accomplished during the pre-bypass phase is given in Table 22-3.

INITIATION AND DISCONTINUATION OF BYPASS SUPPORT: AN OVERVIEW

Initiation of Cardiopulmonary Bypass

Uncomplicated Initiation

Once all preparatory steps have been taken, the perfusionist progressively increases delivery of oxygenated blood to the patient's arterial system, as systemic venous blood is diverted from the patient's right side of the heart, maintaining the pump's venous

Table 22-4   Checklist for Bypass Procedure

1. Assess arterial inflow
   a. Is arterial perfusate oxygenated?
   b. Is direction of arterial inflow appropriate?
   c. Evidence of arterial dissection?
   Patient's arterial pressure persistently low?
   Inflow line pressure high?
   Pump/oxygenator reservoir level falling?
   Evidence of atrial cannula malposition?
   Patient's arterial pressure persistently high or low?
   Unilateral facial swelling, discoloration?
2. Assess venous outflow
   a. Is blood draining to the pump/oxygenator's venous reservoir?
   Evidence of SVC obstruction?
   Facial venous engorgement or congestion, CVP elevated?
3. Is bypass complete?
   a. High CVP/low PA pressure?
   b. Impaired venous drainage?
   c. Low CVP/high PA pressure?
   d. Large bronchial venous blood flow?
   e. Aortic insufficiency?
   f. Arterial and PA pressure nonpulsatile?
   g. Desired pump flow established?
4. Discontinue drug and fluid administration
5. Discontinue ventilation and inhalation drugs to patient's lungs

CVP = central venous pressure; PA = pulmonary artery; SVC = superior vena cava.

reservoir volume. After full flow is achieved, all systemic venous blood is (ideally) draining from the patient to the pump reservoir. The central venous pressure (CVP) and pulmonary arterial pressure (PAP) should decrease to near zero (2 to 5 mmHg), whereas systemic flow, arterial pressure, and oxygenation are maintained at desired values. Table 22-4 outlines tasks to be completed within 5 minutes of initiating CPB.

Hypotension with Onset of Bypass

Systemic arterial hypotension (MAP = 30 to 40 mmHg) is relatively common on initiation of CPB. Much of this can be explained by the acute reduction of blood viscosity that results from hemodilution with nonblood priming solutions. MAP increases with initiation of hypothermia-induced vasoconstriction, along with levels of endogenous catecholamines and angiotensin. Treatment with α-agonists is *usually* not necessary. Of concern is the potential for myocardial and cerebral ischemia because hypothermia has not yet been achieved.

Until the aortic cross-clamp is applied, the coronary arteries are perfused with hemodiluted, nonpulsatile blood. If placement of the aortic cross-clamp is delayed, MAP should be maintained in the range of 60 to 80 mmHg to support myocardial perfusion, especially in the presence of known coronary stenosis or ventricular hypertrophy. This arterial pressure is likely adequate to maintain cerebral blood flow until hypothermia is induced.

Preparation for Separation

Before discontinuation of CPB, conditions that optimize cardiac and pulmonary function must be restored. To a great extent this is achieved by reversing the processes and techniques used to initiate and maintain CPB (Table 22-5).

Table 22-5 Preparation for Separation-from-Bypass Checklist

1. Air clearance maneuvers completed
2. Rewarming completed
   a. Nasopharyngeal temperature 36-37°C
   b. Rectal/bladder temperature ≥ 35°C, but ≤ 37°C
3. Address issue of adequacy of anesthesia and muscle relaxation
4. Obtain stable cardiac rate and rhythm (use pacing if necessary)
5. Pump flow and systemic arterial pressure
   a. Pump flow to maintain mixed venous saturation ≥ 70%
   b. Systemic pressure restored to normothermic levels
6. Metabolic parameters
   a. Arterial pH, Po_2, Pco_2 within normal limits
   b. Hct: 20%-25%
   c. K^+: 4.0-5.0 mEq/L
   d. Normal ionized calcium
7. Are all monitoring/access catheters functional?
   a. Transducers re-zeroed
   b. TEE (if used) out of freeze mode
8. Respiratory management
   a. Atelectasis cleared/lungs reexpanded
   b. Evidence of pneumothorax?
   c. Residual fluid in thoracic cavities drained
   d. Ventilation reinstituted
9. Intravenous fluids restarted
10. Inotropes/vasopressors/vasodilators prepared

Hct = hematocrit; TEE = transesophageal echocardiography.

Potential for Patient Awareness

It is not uncommon for patients to sweat during rewarming. This is almost certainly caused by perfusion of the hypothalamus (i.e., the thermoregulatory site) with blood that is warmer than the latter organ's set point (37°C). The brain is a high-flow organ and can be assumed to equilibrate fairly quickly (15 to 20 minutes) with cerebral perfusate temperature (i.e., nasopharyngeal temperature). A less likely but more disturbing possibility is that restoration of brain normothermia with decreased anesthetic concentration may result in inadequate depth of anesthesia and the potential for awareness. It is estimated that awareness occurs during cardiac surgery in 1% of patients.

Patient movement before discontinuation of CPB is extremely disruptive and may be genuinely life-threatening if it results in cannula dislodgment or disruption of the procedure. Additional muscle relaxant should be administered. If awareness is suspected, supplemental amnestics or anesthetics should be administered during rewarming. Because sweating stops almost immediately on discontinuation of bypass, continued sweating after emergence from CPB may be a sign of awareness. Neurologic monitors such as the Bispectral Index are being used by some clinicians to help judge the depth of anesthesia during and after weaning from CPB.[15]

Rewarming

When systemic hypothermia is used, body temperature is restored to normothermia by gradually increasing perfusate temperature with the heat exchanger. Time required for rewarming (i.e., heat transfer) varies with arterial perfusate temperature, patient temperature, and systemic flow. Excessive perfusate heating is not advisable for at least three key reasons: possible denaturation of plasma proteins, possible cerebral hyperthermia, and the fact that dissolved gas can condense into bubbles if the temperature gradient is too great. Because small increases (0.5°C) in cerebral temperature exacerbate ischemic injury in the brain, it is critical to perfuse the patient with blood temperatures at or below 37°C. Although this will increase the duration of rewarming, the risk of hyperthermic brain injury is greatly increased with hyperthermic blood temperatures. Many centers employ mild hypothermia (i.e., systemic temperature = 31° to 34°C) instead of moderate hypothermia (26° to 28°C), reducing the amount of heat transfer to achieve normothermia.

Rewarming may be enhanced by increasing pump flow, which thereby increases heat input. At levels of hypothermia routinely used (25° to 30°C), the patient behaves as if vasoconstricted (calculated SVR is relatively high). Increasing pump flow in this setting may result in unacceptable hypertension. There are two approaches to this problem: wait out the vasoconstriction or pharmacologically induce patient vasodilation. When rectal or bladder temperature approaches 30° to 32°C, patients appear to rapidly vasodilate. This is probably the result of decreasing blood viscosity or relaxation of cold-induced vasoconstriction with warming. Increasing pump flow at this point serves several purposes: increased heat transfer, support of systemic arterial pressure, and increased oxygen delivery in the presence of increasing oxygen consumption. Often, waiting for the patient to spontaneously "vasodilate" is sufficient; and with subsequent increased pump flows, rewarming will be adequate at separation from bypass support. Circumstances in which more aggressive rewarming may be needed include profound hypothermia with a large hypoperfused "heat sink" and late initiation of warming by accident or design.

Skeletal muscle and subcutaneous fat are relatively hypoperfused during CPB. These tissues cool slowly and are also slow to warm. Temperatures at high-flow regions (e.g., esophagus, nasopharynx) do not reflect the temperature of these tissues. Pharmacologic vasodilation allows an earlier increase in pump flow and delivery of warmed arterial blood to low-flow beds, making the rewarming process more uniform. Arteriolar vasodilators (e.g., sodium nitroprusside, hydralazine) are much more likely to be effective in this process than venodilators (e.g., nitroglycerin). Other aids to warming during or after CPB are heating blankets, warmed fluids, heated humidified gases, and increased room temperature. Sterile forced-air rewarming devices and servoregulated systems are also available.

Restoration of Systemic Arterial Pressure to Normothermic Value

After aortic cross-clamp release, the heart is again perfused through the native coronary arteries. Until the proximal anastomoses are made, myocardial perfusion may be compromised in the presence of a low MAP. Consequently, it is advisable to gradually increase MAP during rewarming to levels of 70 to 80 mmHg.

With discontinuation of CPB, a marked discrepancy often exists between blood pressure readings measured from the radial artery and the central aorta. Radial arterial catheters may underestimate central aortic systolic pressures by 10 to 40 mmHg. Discrepancies in MAP tend to be of a lesser magnitude (5 to 15 mmHg). Such a discrepancy is not present before CPB, nor is it present after CPB in all patients. Mechanisms are undefined, but evidence supports vasodilatory and arteriovenous shunting phenomena in the forearm and hand.

Removal of Intracardiac Air

At the end of the procedure, intracardiac air is present in virtually all cases that require opening the heart (i.e., valve repair or replacement, aneurysmectomy, septal defect repair, repair of congenital lesions). In such cases, it is important to remove as much air as possible before resumption of ejection. Surgical techniques differ. With

22

the aortic cross-clamp still applied, the surgeon or perfusionist can partially limit venous return and LV vent flow, causing the left atrium and left ventricle to fill with blood. Through a transventricular approach, the left ventricle then can be aspirated. The left atrium and left ventricle are ballotted to dislodge bubbles, and the cycle is repeated. The operating table can be rotated from side to side and the lungs ventilated to promote clearance of air from the pulmonary veins. Rather than transventricular aspiration, some surgeons vent air through the cardioplegia cannula or a needle vent in the ascending aorta. Before removal of the aortic cross-clamp, the patient is placed head down, so that bubbles will float away from the dependent carotid arteries. Some surgeons favor temporary manual carotid occlusion before cross-clamp removal, but safety and efficacy of this potentially dangerous maneuver are undocumented. A venting cannula is often left in the aorta at a location that should allow air pickup after resumption of ejection. The aortic cross-clamp can be temporarily reapplied for additional air-clearing maneuvers.

TEE has shown that routine air clearance techniques are not completely effective. Transcranial Doppler studies document a high incidence of intracranial gas emboli on release of the aortic cross-clamp or resumption of ejection. Three essential elements of air removal are mobilization of air by positive chamber filling, stretching of the atrial wall, and repeated chamber ballottement; removal of mobilized air by continuous ascending aortic venting; and proof of elimination by TEE.

Intracardiac air may be present in 10% to 30% of closed cardiac cases as well (e.g., CABG). During aortic cross-clamping, air may enter the aorta and left ventricle retrograde through native coronary arteries opened in the course of CABG surgery, particularly when suction is applied to vent the left side of the heart or aortic root. Efforts to expel air from the left ventricle and aortic root should be routine before unclamping the aorta. It is unclear to what extent gas emboli originating from the heart and aorta contribute to neurologic injury. However, microembolic load correlates with magnitude of cognitive dysfunction. Air ejected from the left ventricle can also travel to the coronary arteries, resulting in sudden and sometimes extreme myocardial ischemia and failure after separation from bypass.

Defibrillation

Before discontinuation of CPB, the heart must have an organized rhythm that is spontaneous or pacer induced. Ventricular fibrillation (VF), common after cross-clamp release and warming, will often spontaneously convert to some other rhythm. Prolonged VF is undesirable during rewarming for at least three reasons: (1) subendocardial perfusion is compromised in the presence of normothermic VF; (2) myocardial oxygen consumption is greater with VF compared with a beating heart at normothermia; and (3) if the left ventricle receives a large amount of blood (aortic insufficiency or bronchial return) in the absence of mechanical contraction, the left ventricle may distend. LV distention increases wall tension and further compromises subendocardial perfusion. On the other hand, early resumption of mechanical contraction may make some surgical procedures difficult (e.g., modification of distal anastomoses).

Defibrillation, when necessary, is accomplished with internal paddles at much lower energies than would be used for external cardioversion. In the adult, starting energies of 5 to 10 J are routine. Defibrillation is less effective when the heart has not fully rewarmed, and it is rarely successful if myocardial (perfusate) temperature is less than 30°C. Repeated attempts at defibrillation, particularly with escalating energy levels, can lead to myocardial injury. If defibrillation is not successful after two to four attempts, options include further warming, correction of blood gas and electrolyte abnormalities if present (high Po_2 and high normal serum potassium [K^+] seem favorable), increased MAP, and antiarrhythmic therapy. Bolus administration of 100 mg of lidocaine before the release of the cross-clamp significantly lowers the incidence of reperfusion ventricular fibrillation. Increasing coronary perfusion by increased MAP is believed to result in myocardial reperfusion and recovery of the energy state.

Restoration of Ventilation

Before discontinuation of CPB, the lungs must be reinflated. Positive pressure (20 to 40 cmH$_2$O) is repeatedly applied until all areas of atelectasis are visually reinflated. Attention is specifically directed at the left lower lobe, which seems more difficult to reexpand. Fluid that has collected in the thoracic cavities during CPB is removed by the surgeon; and if the pleural cavity has not been opened, evidence of pneumothorax is also sought. The tidal volume or ventilatory rate is increased 10% to 20% above pre-bypass values to compensate for increased Vd/Vt if present. Ventilation is resumed with 100% oxygen and subsequent adjustments in Fio$_2$ are made based on arterial blood gas analysis and pulse oximetry.

Correction of Metabolic Abnormalities and Arterial Oxygen Saturation

When rewarming is nearly complete and separation from CPB is anticipated to occur in 10 to 20 minutes, an arterial blood sample is taken and analyzed for acid-base status, Po$_2$, Pco$_2$, hemoglobin or hematocrit, potassium, glucose, and ionized calcium.

OXYGEN-CARRYING CAPACITY

Generally, a hematocrit of at least 20% to 25% is sought before discontinuation of bypass. The primary compensatory mechanism to ensure adequate systemic oxygen delivery in the presence of normovolemic anemia is increased CO. Increased CO results in an increased myocardial oxygen need, which is met by increased coronary oxygen delivery by coronary vasodilation. The lower limit of the hematocrit, below which increased CO can no longer support systemic oxygen needs, is reported to be 17% to 20% in dogs with *completely healthy hearts*. With increases in systemic Vo$_2$, such as occur with exercise, fever, or shivering, higher values of the hematocrit are required. Patients with good ventricular function and good coronary reserve (or good revascularization) might be expected to tolerate hematocrit values in the 20s. When ventricular function is impaired or revascularization is incomplete, hematocrit above 25% may aid in support of the systemic circulation and concomitantly lower myocardial oxygen requirements on discontinuation of bypass.

ARTERIAL PH

Considerable debate has centered on the extent to which acidemia affects myocardial performance and whether correction of arterial pH with sodium bicarbonate is advantageous or deleterious to the heart. Most clinical studies have found metabolic acidosis impairs contractility and alters responses to exogenous catecholamines. Hemodynamic deterioration is usually mild above pH 7.2 because of compensatory increases in sympathetic nervous system activity. Attenuation of sympathetic nervous system responses by β-blockade or ganglionic blockade increases the detrimental effect of acidosis. The ischemic or hypoxic myocardium has been found to be particularly vulnerable to detrimental effects of acidosis. Patients with poor contractile function or reduction of myocardial sympathetic responsiveness (e.g., chronic left ventricular failure), those treated with β-blockers, or those with myocardial ischemia are especially susceptible to the adverse effects of acidosis. For these reasons arterial pH is corrected to near-normal levels before discontinuation of CPB, using sodium bicarbonate. Concerns regarding carbon dioxide generation and acidification of the intracellular space can be obviated by slow administration and appropriate adjustment of ventilation, both of which are easily achieved during CPB.

22

ELECTROLYTES

Electrolytes most commonly of concern before discontinuation of CPB are potassium and calcium. Serum potassium concentration may be acutely low because of hemodilution with non–potassium-containing priming solutions or large-volume diuresis during CPB. More commonly, potassium concentration is elevated as a result of systemic uptake of potassium-containing cardioplegic solution; values exceeding 6 mEq/L are not uncommon. Other potential causes of hyperkalemia that must be considered are hemolysis, tissue ischemia or necrosis, and acidemia. Hypokalemia can be rapidly corrected during CPB with *relative* safety because the heart and systemic circulation are supported. Increments of 5 to 10 mEq of KCl over 1- to 2-minute intervals can be given directly into the oxygenator by the perfusionist, and potassium subsequently is rechecked. Depending on severity and urgency of correction, elevated potassium can be treated or reduced by any of several standard means: alkali therapy, diuresis, calcium administration, or insulin and glucose. Alternatively, hemofiltration can be used to lower serum potassium. While still on CPB, potassium-containing extracellular fluid is removed from the patient and replaced with fluid not containing potassium.

Ionized calcium is involved in the maintenance of normal excitation-contraction coupling and therefore in maintaining cardiac contractility and peripheral vascular tone. Low concentrations of ionized calcium lead to impaired cardiac contractility and lowered vascular tone. Concerns have been raised about the contribution of calcium administration to myocardial reperfusion injury and to the action of various inotropes. Some investigators argue in favor of measuring ionized calcium before discontinuation of CPB and to administer calcium in patients with low concentrations to optimize cardiac performance. Although they routinely measure ionized calcium before discontinuation of bypass, calcium salts are not routinely administered. When confronted with poor myocardial or peripheral vascular responsiveness to inotropes or vasopressors after bypass *in the presence of a low level of ionized calcium,* calcium salts should be administered to restore ionized calcium to normal (not elevated) levels in the hope of restoring responsiveness. The same strategy can be used for measuring and administering magnesium.

Other Final Preparations

Before separating from CPB, all monitoring and access catheters should be checked and calibrated. The zero-pressure calibration points of the pressure transducers are routinely checked. Not uncommonly, finger pulse oximeter probes do not have a good signal after CPB. In those cases, a nasal or ear probe is placed to obtain reliable oximetry. Intravenous infusions are restarted before separation from CPB, and their flow characteristics are assessed for evidence of obstruction or disconnection.

During warming and preparation for separation, an assessment should be made of the functional status of the heart and peripheral vasculature based on visual inspection, hemodynamic indices, and metabolic parameters. Based on this assessment, inotropes, vasodilators, and vasopressors thought likely to be necessary for successful separation from bypass should be prepared and readied for administration.

Separation from Bypass

After all preparatory steps are taken, CPB can be discontinued. Venous outflow to the pump or oxygenator is impeded by slowly clamping the venous line, and the patient's intravascular volume and ventricular loading conditions are restored by transfusion of perfusate through the aortic inflow line. When loading conditions are optimal, the aortic inflow line is clamped and the patient is separated from CPB.

V

BOX 22-4 *Perfusion Emergencies*

- Arterial cannula malposition
- Aortic dissection
- Massive air embolism
- Venous air lock
- Reversed cannulation

At this juncture it must be determined whether oxygenation, ventilation, and more commonly myocardial performance (systemic perfusion) are adequate. A discussion of these issues no longer involves CPB per se but, rather, applied cardiopulmonary physiology. Should separation fail for any reason, CPB can simply be reinstituted by unclamping the venous outflow and arterial inflow lines and restoring pump flow. This allows for support of systemic oxygenation and perfusion while steps are taken to diagnose and treat those problems that precluded successful separation.

PERFUSION EMERGENCIES

Accidents or mishaps occurring during CPB can quickly evolve into life-threatening emergencies (Box 22-4). Many of the necessary conditions of bypass (cardiac arrest, hypothermia, volume depletion) preclude the ability to resume normal cardiorespiratory function if an accident threatens the integrity of the extracorporeal circuit. Fortunately, major perfusion accidents occur infrequently and are rarely associated with permanent injury or death (Table 22-6). However, all members of the cardiac surgery team must be able to respond to perfusion emergencies to limit the likelihood of perfusion-related disasters.

Arterial Cannula Malposition

Ascending aortic cannulas can be malpositioned such that the outflow jet is directed primarily into the innominate artery, the left common carotid artery (rare), or the left subclavian artery (rare). In the first two circumstances, unilateral cerebral *hyperperfusion*, usually with systemic hypoperfusion, occurs, whereas flow directed to the subclavian artery results in global cerebral *hypoperfusion*. Despite the fact that not all combinations of arterial pressure monitoring site and cannula malposition produce systemic hypotension, it is commonly regarded as a cardinal sign of cannula malposition. For example, right arm blood pressure monitor and innominate artery cannulation, or left arm monitor and left subclavian artery cannulation may result in *high* arterial pressure on initiation of bypass. With other positioning and monitoring combinations, investigators report persistently low systemic arterial pressure (MAP = 25 to 35 mmHg), which is poorly responsive to increasing pump flow or vasoconstrictors. Over time (minutes), signs of systemic hypoperfusion (e.g., acidemia, oliguria) develop. Because a variable period of systemic hypotension with CPB initiation is nearly always seen with hemodilution, hypotension alone is not significant evidence to establish a diagnosis of arterial cannula malposition. On initiation of CPB and periodically thereafter, it is advisable to inspect the face for color change and edema, rhinorrhea, or otorrhea and to palpate the neck with onset of cooling for temperature asymmetry. EEG monitoring has been advocated as a method of detecting cannula malposition.

22

Table 22-6   Comparison of the Five Most Common Accidents from the Three Perfusion Surveys

Complication*	Stoney 1972-1977		Wheeldon 1974-1979		Kurusz 1982-1985	
	Incidents	PI/D	Incidents	PI/D	Incidents	PI/D
Air embolism	(2) 1.14	0.41	(2) 0.79	0.18	(6) 0.80	0.12
Coagulopathy	(1) 1.26	0.51	(6) 0.26	0.09	(8) 0.21	0.05
Electrical failure	(3) 0.67	0.01	(1) 1.00	0.06	(4) 0.84	0.003
Mechanical failure	(4) 0.38	0.02	(5) 0.27	0	(7) 0.30	0.007
Inadequate oxygenation	(5) 0.33	0.02	(3) 0.59	0	(3) 0.88	0.07
Hypoperfusion	—	—	(4) 0.30	0.18	(2) 0.96	0.15
Protamine reaction	—	—	—	—	(1) 2.80	0.22
Drug error	—	—	—	—	(5) 0.82	0.08

*The five most common complications for each study are listed as incidence per 1000 perfusions and the number of permanent injuries and mortalities as incidence per 1000 perfusions. The numbers in parentheses are the rank of each complication from most to least.

PI/D = permanent injury or death.

Data from Stoney WS, Alford WC Jr, Burrus GR, et al: Air embolism and other accidents using pump oxygenators. Ann Thorac Surg 29:336, 1980; Wheeldon DR: Can cardiopulmonary bypass be a safe procedure? In Longmore DB (ed): Towards Safer Cardiac Surgery. Lancaster, London, MTP, 1981, pp 427-446; and Kurusz M, Conti VR, Arens JF, et al: Perfusion accident survey. Proc Am Acad Cardiovasc Perf 7:57, 1986.

Two other arterial cannula malpositions are possible: abutment of the cannula tip against the aortic intima, which results in high line pressure, poor perfusion, or even acute dissection when bypass is initiated, and the cannula tip directed caudally toward the aortic valve. This may result in acute aortic insufficiency, with sudden left ventricular distention and systemic hypoperfusion on bypass. If the aortic inflow cannula is soft, aortic cross-clamping will occlude the arterial perfusion line, which can rupture the aortic inflow line. Suspicion of any cannula malposition must immediately be brought to the attention of the surgeon.

V

Aortic or Arterial Dissection

Signs of arterial dissection, often similar to those of cannula malposition, must also be sought continuously, especially on initiation of CPB. Dissection may originate at the cannulation site, aortic cross-clamp site, proximal vein graft anastomotic site, or partial occlusion (side-biting) clamp site. Dissections are due to intimal disruption, or more distally to fracture of atherosclerotic plaque. In either case, some systemic arterial blood flow becomes extraluminal, being forced into the arterial wall. The dissection propagates mostly in the direction of the systemic flow but not exclusively. Extraluminal blood compresses the luminal origins (take-offs) of major arterial branches such that vital organs (e.g., heart, brain, kidney, intestinal tract, spinal cord) may become ischemic. Because systemic perfusion may be low, and origins of the innominate and subclavian arteries may be compressed, probably the best sign of arterial dissection is persistently low systemic arterial pressure. Venous drainage to the pump decreases (blood is sequestered), and arterial inflow "line pressure" is usually inappropriately high. The surgeon may see the dissection if it involves the anterior or lateral ascending aorta (bluish discoloration), or both. It is possible the surgeon may *not* see any sign of dissection, because the dissection is out of view (e.g., posterior ascending aorta, aortic arch, descending aorta). Dissection can occur at any time before, during, or after CPB. As with cannula malposition, a suspicion of arterial dissection must be brought to the attention of the surgeon. The anesthesiologist must not assume that something is suddenly wrong with the arterial pressure transducer but should "think dissection."

After a dissection of the ascending aorta is diagnosed, immediate steps to minimize propagation must be taken. If it has occurred before CPB, the anesthesiologist should take steps to reduce MAP and the rate of rise of aortic pressure (dP/dt). If it occurs during CPB, pump flow and MAP are reduced to the lowest acceptable levels. Arterial perfusate is frequently cooled to profound levels (14° to 19°C) as rapidly as possible to decrease metabolic demand and protect vital organs. A different arterial cannulation site is prepared (e.g., the femoral artery is cannulated or the true aortic lumen is cannulated at a site more distal on the aortic arch). Arterial inflow is shifted to that new site in hopes that perfusing the true aortic lumen will reperfuse vital organs. The ascending aorta is cross-clamped just below the innominate artery, and cardioplegia is administered (into the coronary ostia or coronary sinus). The aorta is opened to expose the site of disruption, which is then resected and replaced. Reimplantation of the coronary arteries or aortic valve replacement, or both, may be necessary. The false lumina at both ends of the aorta are obliterated with Teflon buttresses, and the graft is inserted by end-to-end suture. With small dissections it is sometimes possible to avoid open repair by application of a partial occlusion clamp with plication of the dissection and exclusion of the intimal disruption. In some cases of arterial dissection during CPB, TEE has been found useful. Although provisional diagnoses were made on the basis of traditional signs, TEE allowed assessment of the origin and extent of dissection.[16] Diagnosis of arterial dissection has also been assisted by presence of EEG asymmetry.

Arterial dissections originating from femoral cannulation also necessitate reductions in arterial pressure, systemic flow, and temperature. If the operation is near completion, the heart may be transfused and CPB discontinued; otherwise, the aortic arch must be cannulated and adequate systemic perfusion restored to allow completion of the operation.

Massive Arterial Gas Embolus

Macroscopic gas embolus is a rare but disastrous CPB complication. Studies in 1980 reported incidences of recognized massive arterial gas embolism of 0.1% to 0.2%. The current incidence is probably lower because of the widespread use of reservoir level alarms and bubble detection devices. Between 20% and 30% of affected patients died immediately, with another 30% having transient or nondebilitating neurologic deficits, or both. Circumstances that most commonly contributed to these events were inattention to oxygenator blood level, reversal of left ventricular vent flow, or unexpected resumption of cardiac ejection in a previously opened heart.

The pathophysiology of cerebral gas embolism (macroscopic and microscopic) is not well understood. Tissue damage after gas embolization is initiated from simple mechanical blockage of blood vessels by bubbles. Although gas emboli may be absorbed or pass through the circulation within 1 to 5 minutes, the local reaction of platelets and proteins to the blood gas interface or endothelial damage is thought to potentiate microvascular stasis, prolonging cerebral ischemia to the point of infarction. Areas of marginal perfusion, such as arterial boundary zones, do not clear gas

22

emboli as rapidly as well-perfused zones, producing patterns of ischemia or infarction difficult to distinguish from those due to hypotension or particulate emboli.

Recommended treatment for massive arterial gas embolism includes immediate cessation of CPB with aspiration of as much gas as possible from the aorta and heart, assumption of steep Trendelenburg position, and clearance of air from the arterial perfusion line. After resumption of CPB, treatment continues with implementation or deepening of hypothermia (18° to 27°C) during completion of the operation, clearance of gas from the coronary circulation before emergence from CPB, and administration of glucocorticoids in an attempt to minimize cerebral edema. In many reports of patients suffering massive arterial gas embolus, seizures occurred postoperatively and were treated with anticonvulsants. Because seizures after ischemic insults are associated with poor outcomes, owing perhaps to hypermetabolic effects, prophylactic phenytoin seems reasonable. Hypotension has been shown to lengthen the residence time of cerebral air emboli and worsen the severity of resulting ischemia. Maintenance of moderate hypertension therefore is reasonable and clinically attainable to hasten clearance of emboli from the circulation and, hopefully, improve neurologic outcome.

Many clinicians have reported dramatic neurologic recovery when hyperbaric therapy is used for arterial gas embolism, even if delayed up to 26 hours after the event. Spontaneous recovery from air emboli has also been reported, and no prospective study of hyperbaric therapy in the cardiac surgery setting has been performed. Few institutions that do cardiac surgery have an appropriately equipped and staffed compression chamber to allow expeditious and safe initiation of hyperbaric therapy. Nonetheless, immediate transfer by air is often possible and should seriously be considered. It seems reasonable to expect that institutions that do cardiac surgery should have policies regarding catastrophic air embolism.

In 1980, Mills and Ochsner[17] suggested venoarterial perfusion as an alternative to hyperbaric therapy. Retrograde perfusion through the SVC cannula at 1.2 L/min at 20°C for 1 to 2 minutes was used in five of their eight patients with massive gas embolism. The goal was to flush air from the cerebral arterial circulation. None of the patients so treated had evidence of neurologic injury. Other reports using this technique have followed.

Venous Air Lock

Air entering the venous outflow line can result in complete cessation of flow to the venous reservoir, and this is called *air lock*. Loss of venous outflow necessitates immediate slowing, even cessation of pump flow, to prevent emptying the reservoir and subsequent delivery of air to the patient's arterial circulation. After an air lock is recognized, a search for the source of venous outflow line air must be undertaken (e.g., loose atrial purse string, atrial tear, open intravenous access) and repaired before reestablishing full bypass.

Reversed Cannulation

In this case, the venous outflow limb of the CPB circuit is incorrectly connected to the arterial inflow cannula and the arterial perfusion limb of the circuit is attached to the venous cannula. On initiation of CPB, blood is removed from the arterial circulation and returned to the venous circulation at high pressure. Arterial pressure is found to be extremely low by palpation and arterial pressure monitoring. Very low arterial pressures can also (more commonly) be due to dissection in the arterial tree. In the latter case, the perfusionist will rapidly lose volume, whereas with reversed cannulation, the perfusionist will have an immediate gross excess of volume. If high pump flow is established, venous or atrial rupture may occur. The CVP will be dramatically elevated, with evidence of facial venous engorgement.

Line pressure is the pressure in the arterial limb of the CPB circuit. Because arterial cannulas are much smaller than the aorta, there is always a pressure drop across the aortic cannula. Arterial inflow line pressure will always be considerably higher than systemic (patient) arterial pressure. The magnitude of the pressure drop depends on cannula size and systemic flow; small cannulas and higher flows result in greater gradients. The CPB pump must generate a pressure that overcomes this gradient to provide adequate systemic arterial pressure. For a typical adult (i.e., MAP of about 60 mmHg, systemic flow of about 2.4 L/min/m^2, and a 24-Fr aortic cannula), line pressure in an uncomplicated case usually ranges from 150 to 250 mmHg. The fittings on the arterial inflow line are plastic; the fittings and the line itself can rupture. Perfusionists typically do not want a line pressure in excess of 300 mmHg.

CPB must be discontinued and the cannula disconnected and inspected for air. If air is found in the arterial circulation, an air embolus protocol is initiated. Once arterial air is cleared, the circuit is correctly reconnected and CPB restarted. In adults, the venous outflow limb of the CPB circuit is a larger-diameter tubing than the arterial inflow tubing, precisely to eliminate reversed cannulation. This is why reversed cannulation is rare in adults, but it has happened. In pediatric cases, the arterial inflow and venous outflow limbs of the CPB circuit are close or equal in size.

SPECIAL PATIENT POPULATIONS

Care of the Gravid Patient during Bypass

Studies assessing the effects of cardiac surgery and CPB on obstetric physiology and fetal well-being are lacking. However, several reviews and many case reports describe individual experience in caring for the gravid patient and fetus during cardiac surgery and extracorporeal circulation. These surveys and anecdotal reports, along with an understanding of the well-documented physiology of pregnancy and the effects of cardiac therapeutics on fetal physiology, can serve as a basis for a rational approach to care for the pregnant patient and fetus during cardiac surgery.[18]

Maternal and Fetal Monitor Information

The pregnant patient undergoing cardiac surgery requires the usual monitors employed during cardiac surgery, as well as monitors that can assess fetal well-being. Monitors that help assess the adequacy of maternal cardiovascular performance and oxygen delivery to the fetus are of paramount importance. Little is known about the effects of cardiovascular drugs and other therapeutic measures on the pregnant cardiac patient undergoing CPB. Appropriate monitors permit the assessment of an individual therapy on maternal and fetal oxygen delivery.

Uterine activity should be monitored with a tocodynamometer applied to the maternal abdomen. This monitor transduces the tightening of the abdomen during uterine contractions. As is the case with other types of major surgeries, the tocodynamometer should not interfere with the conduct of cardiac surgery; if necessary, the monitor may be intermittently displaced by the operating surgeon. The use of an intra-amniotic catheter to monitor uterine activity and pressure may be inadvisable in a patient who will be fully heparinized. Intraoperative uterine contractions may have a deleterious effect on fetal oxygen delivery (by causing an increase in uterine venous pressure and decrease in uterine blood flow) and signal the onset of preterm labor. Use of the tocodynamometer is imperative, because it will provide

22

important information about the state of the uterus and allow intervention if necessary. Various reports have documented the common occurrence of uterine contractions during cardiac surgery and CPB. Uterine contractions may appear at any time during the perioperative period but occur most frequently immediately after the discontinuation of CPB and in the early ICU period. It is therefore important to leave the tocodynamometer in place after the completion of surgery. Although uterine contractions occur frequently in the perioperative course, they usually are effectively treated with magnesium sulfate, ritodrine, or ethanol infusions, and they do not result in preterm labor and fetal demise.

Fetal heart rate (FHR) monitors should be employed in all gravid patients after 16 weeks' gestation, because one of the primary perioperative goals is to avoid fetal loss. Use of an FHR monitor permits recognition of fetal distress and allows the clinician to institute measures to improve fetal oxygen delivery. The FHR monitor recognizes and records the FHR, FHR variability, and uterine contractions. A spinal electrode placed in the fetal scalp gives the most reliable fetal ECG and therefore the best FHR information. However, this method may be undesirable in the presence of maternal anticoagulation. External FHR monitoring, using ultrasound, phonocardiography, or external abdominal ECG, is less exact but preferable in this clinical setting.

The cardiac surgeon and perfusionist may not be familiar with uterine and FHR monitors; the anesthesiologist is accustomed to caring for these patients during labor and delivery and can assess uterine and FHR tracings. However, in some clinical circumstances, such as preoperative fetal distress, or anticipated need for emergency cesarean section during cardiac surgery, having a perinatologist or an obstetrician present during cardiac surgery may be desirable.

FHR is usually normal in the pre-bypass period but decreases precipitously with the initiation of CPB and remains below normal for the entire bypass period. There are many potential causes of this observed decrease in FHR. Persistent fetal bradycardia is a classic sign of acute fetal hypoxia. However, in the CPB setting, especially when hypothermia is employed, it is difficult to ascribe fetal bradycardia to hypoxia or to decreased fetal oxygen demand. Fetal tachycardia typically occurs after the discontinuation of bypass support. This tachycardia may represent a compensatory mechanism for the oxygen debt incurred during CPB. The FHR usually returns to normal by the end of the operative period.

Interventions optimizing maternal blood oxygen content, correcting any acid-base imbalance, and replenishing fetal glycogen stores may alleviate signs of fetal hypoxia. Some clinicians recommend an increase in CPB pump flow to improve fetal oxygen delivery.

Conducting the Bypass Procedure

The conditions of extracorporeal circulation—nonpulsatile blood flow, hypothermia, anemia, and requisite anticoagulation—will likely have a negative impact on fetal well-being during CPB. There are no studies that recommend a CPB management strategy in gravid patients. Recommendations are summarized (Table 22-7) for the management of bypass in pregnant patients.

BLOOD FLOW

Optimal CPB blood flow in the gravid patient is unknown. However, the increase in CO associated with pregnancy is well defined, and it might be argued that high blood flows during CPB are more physiologic in the gravid patient. It has been suggested that flow during CPB in the pregnant patient be maintained at a minimum of 3.0 L/min/m². A few reports demonstrate that increasing CPB circuit blood flow improves FHR, suggesting improvement in fetal oxygen delivery.

Table 22-7 Recommendations for the Conduct of Extracorporeal Circulation in the Gravid Patient

Variable	Recommended Value/ Characteristic	Rationale
Blood flow	3.0 L/min/m²	Cardiac index normally is increased during pregnancy.
Blood pressure (MAP)	60-70 mmHg	Uterine blood flow depends on maternal MAP.
Temperature	32-34°C	Mild hypothermia decreases fetal oxygen requirements and is less likely to cause fetal arrhythmia.
Oxygenator type	Membrane	Membrane oxygenators are associated with fewer embolic phenomena than bubblers.
Hematocrit	25%-27%	The quantity of oxygen carried in maternal blood (and therefore the oxygen available to the fetus) greatly depends on hemoglobin concentration.
Duration of perfusion	Minimized (?)	The duration of bypass is dictated by the complexity of the operative procedure.
Cardioplegia	?	
Pulsatile perfusion	?	

MAP = mean arterial pressure.

BLOOD PRESSURE

Under normal conditions, uterine blood flow is determined solely by maternal blood pressure, because the placental vasculature is maximally dilated. However, it is not known what factors determine uterine blood flow during the very abnormal condition of CPB. For example, catecholamine levels increase by several times during CPB; therefore, uterine vascular resistance may increase during extracorporeal circulation in response to increased levels of norepinephrine and epinephrine. However, regardless of the state of uterine vascular resistance during CPB, maternal blood pressure will be an important determinant of uterine blood flow and fetal oxygen delivery. Moderately high pressure (mean arterial pressure ≥ 65 mmHg) should be employed during perfusion in the gravid patient.

TEMPERATURE

There are theoretical advantages and disadvantages for normothermic and hypothermic CPB in the gravid patient. Hypothermia can cause fetal bradycardia and may lead to fetal ventricular arrhythmias resulting in fetal wastage. Rewarming after hypothermic bypass may precipitate uterine contractions and preterm labor. However, others reported the onset of uterine contractions at the time of discontinuation of bypass support in spite of normothermic perfusion. Uterine contractions also occur at various times in the post-bypass and postoperative periods. The association of uterine contractions with rewarming after hypothermic bypass is unclear.

Hypothermia may be protective to the fetus during extracorporeal circulation by decreasing fetal oxygen requirements. Perfusion temperatures of 25° to 37°C have been used in gravid patients undergoing CPB. There are no data that suggest hypothermia is harmful to the mother or fetus undergoing bypass. Normothermic CPB may increase the likelihood of untoward neurologic sequelae in the mother, an event that would be catastrophic in a woman with young children.

SUMMARY

- Cardiopulmonary bypass (CPB) provides extracorporeal maintenance of respiration and circulation at hypothermic and normothermic temperatures. CPB permits the surgeon to operate on a quiet, or nonbeating, heart at hypothermic temperatures, thus facilitating surgery in an ischemic environment.
- CPB is associated with a number of profound physiologic perturbations. The central nervous system, kidneys, gut, and heart are especially vulnerable to ischemic events associated with extracorporeal circulation.
- Controversy regarding the optimal management of blood flow, pressure, and temperature during CPB remains. Perfusion should be adequate to support ongoing oxygen requirements; mean arterial pressures of more than 70 mmHg may benefit patients with cerebral and/or diffuse arthrosclerosis. Arterial blood temperatures should never exceed 37.5°C.
- The initiation and termination of CPB are key phases of a cardiac surgery procedure, but the anesthesiologist must remain vigilant throughout the entire bypass.
- CPB is a complex system that is vulnerable to accidents. Careful and constant communication among the anesthesiologist, surgeon, perfusionist, and nurse is critical for patient safety.
- Minimally invasive cardiac surgery can be performed with port-access bypass circuits. This approach adds considerable complexity to the procedure and is not as popular as off-pump techniques for coronary artery bypass grafting.
- Bloodless cardiac surgery is possible, and numerous approaches including autotransfusion and hemodilution facilitate this goal.
- Total CPB can be tailored to produce deep hypothermic, circulatory arrest, or partial bypass. The special techniques require sophisticated monitoring and care.

REFERENCES

1. Edmunds LH: Cardiopulmonary bypass after 50 years. N Engl J Med 351:1603, 2004
2. Newman MF, Croughwell ND, White WD, et al: Effect of perfusion pressure on cerebral blood flow during normothermic cardiopulmonary bypass. Circulation 94:II353, 1996
3. Slater JM, Orszulak TA, Cook DJ: Distribution and hierarchy of regional blood flow during hypothermic cardiopulmonary bypass. Ann Thorac Surg 72:542, 2001
4. Mora CT, Henson MB, Weintraub WS, et al: The effect of temperature management during cardiopulmonary bypass on neurological and neuropsychological outcomes in coronary revascularization patients. J Thorac Cardiovasc Surg 112:514, 1996
5. Stone JG, Young WL, Smith CR, et al: Do standard monitoring sites reflect true brain temperature when profound hypothermia is rapidly induced and reversed? Anesthesiology 82:344, 1995
6. Kiziltan HT, Baltali M, Bilen A, et al: Comparison of alpha-stat and pH-stat cardiopulmonary bypass in relation to jugular venous oxygen saturation and cerebral glucose-oxygen utilization. Anesth Analg 96:644, 2003

7. Russell JA, Navickis RJ, Wilkes MM: Albumin versus crystalloid for pump priming in cardiac surgery: Meta-analysis of controlled trials. J Cardiothorac Vasc Anesth 18:429, 2004

8. Roach GW, Kanchuger M, Mora Mangano CT, et al: Adverse cerebral outcomes after coronary bypass surgery. N Engl J Med 335:1857, 1996

9. Mora Mangano CT, Diamondstone LS, Ramsay JG, et al: Renal dysfunction following myocardial revascularization: Risk factors, adverse outcomes and hospital resource utilization. Ann Intern Med 128:194, 1998

10. Perugini RA, Orr RK, Porter D, et al: Gastrointestinal complications following cardiac surgery: An analysis of 1477 cardiac surgery patients. Arch Surg 132:352, 1997

11. Holmes C, Landry D, Granton J: Vasopressin and the cardiovascular system. Crit Care 8:15, 2004

12. Ahmed Z, Lockhart CH, Weiner M, Klingensmith G: Advances in diabetic management: Implications for anesthesia. Anesth Analg 100:666, 2005

13. Jones RH: The year in cardiovascular surgery. J Am Coll Cardiol 45:1517, 2005

14. Wareing TH, Davila-Roman VG, Barzilai B, et al: Management of the severely atherosclerotic ascending aorta during cardiac operations: A strategy for detection and treatment. J Thorac Cardiovasc Surg 103:453, 1992

15. Liu E, Dhara S: Monitoring oxygenator expiratory isoflurane concentrations and the bispectral index to guide isoflurane requirements during cardiopulmonary bypass. J Cardiothorac Vasc Anesth 19:485, 2005

16. Troianos CA, Savino JS, Weiss RL: Transesophageal echocardiographic diagnosis of aortic dissection during cardiac surgery. Anesthesiology 75:149, 1991

17. Mills NL, Ochsner JL: Massive air embolism during cardiopulmonary bypass: Causes, prevention, and management. J Thorac Cardiovasc Surg 80:708, 1980

18. Pomini F, Mercogliano D, Cavalletti C, et al: Cardiopulmonary bypass in pregnancy. Ann Thorac Surg 61:259, 1996

22

Chapter 23

Organ Protection during Cardiopulmonary Bypass

Hilary P. Grocott, MD • Mark Stafford-Smith, MD

Modern cardiac surgery, heralded by the advent of cardiopulmonary bypass (CPB) more than 5 decades ago, continues to be challenged by the risk of organ dysfunction and the morbidity and mortality that accompanies it. Catastrophic organ system failure was common in the early days of CPB, but advances in perfusion, anesthesia, and surgical techniques have allowed most patients to undergo surgery without major morbidity or mortality. However, organ dysfunction ranging in severity from the most subtle to the most severe still occurs, manifesting most frequently in patients with decreased functional reserves or extensive comorbidities. With more than 1 million patients worldwide undergoing various cardiac operations annually, understanding organ dysfunction and developing perioperative organ protective strategies are of paramount importance.

A number of injurious common pathways may account for the organ dysfunction typically associated with cardiac surgery. CPB itself initiates a whole-body inflammatory response with the release of various injurious inflammatory mediators. Add to this the various preexisting patient comorbidities and the potential for organ ischemic injury due to embolization and hypoperfusion and it becomes clear why organ injury can occur. Most cardiac surgery, due to its very nature, causes some degree of myocardial injury. Other body systems can be affected by the perioperative insults associated with cardiac surgery (particularly CPB), including the kidneys, lungs, gastrointestinal tract, and central nervous system.

CENTRAL NERVOUS SYSTEM INJURY

Incidence and Significance of Injury

Central nervous system dysfunction after CPB represents deficits ranging from neurocognitive deficits, occurring in 25% to 80% of patients, to overt stroke, occurring in 1% to 5% of patients. The significant disparity between studies in the incidence of these adverse cerebral outcomes relates in part to their definition and to numerous methodologic differences in the determination of neurologic and neurocognitive outcome. Retrospective versus prospective assessments of neurologic deficits account for a significant portion of this inconsistency, as does the experience and expertise of the examiner. The timing of postoperative testing also affects determinations of outcome. For example, the rate of cognitive deficits is as high as 80% for patients at discharge, between 10% and 35% at 6 weeks or longer after coronary artery bypass grafting (CABG), and 10% to 15% more than a year after surgery. Higher rates of cognitive deficits recur 5 years after surgery, when as many as 43% of patients have documented deficits.

Although the incidence of this dysfunction varies greatly, the significance of these injuries cannot be overemphasized. Cerebral injury is a most disturbing outcome of cardiac surgery. To have a patient's heart successfully treated by the planned operation but discover that the patient no longer functions as well cognitively or is immobilized from a stroke can be devastating. There are enormous personal, family, and financial consequences of extending a patient's life with surgery, only to have the quality of the life significantly diminished. Mortality after CABG, although having reached relatively low levels in the past decade (approximately 1% overall), is increasingly attributable to cerebral injury.[1]

Risk Factors for Central Nervous System Injury

Successful strategies for perioperative cerebral and other organ protection begin with a thorough understanding of the risk factors, causes, and pathophysiology. Risk factors for central nervous system injury can be considered from several different perspectives. Most studies outlining risk factors take into account only stroke. Few describe risk factors for neurocognitive dysfunction. Although it is often assumed that their respective risk factors are similar, few studies have consistently reported the preoperative risks of cognitive loss after cardiac surgery. Factors such as a poor baseline (preoperative) cognitive state, years of education (i.e., more advanced education is protective), age, diabetes, and CPB time are frequently described.

Stroke is better characterized with respect to risk factors. Although studies differ somewhat as to all the risk factors, certain patient characteristics consistently correlate with an increased risk for cardiac surgery–associated neurologic injury. In a study of 2108 patients from 24 centers in a study conducted by the Multicenter Study of Perioperative Ischemia, incidence of adverse cerebral outcome after CABG surgery was determined and the risk factors analyzed.[2] Two types of adverse cerebral outcomes were defined. Type I included nonfatal

Table 23-1 Risk Factors for Adverse Cerebral Outcomes after Cardiac Surgery

Risk Factor	Type I Outcomes	Type II Outcomes
Proximal aortic atherosclerosis	4.52 [2.52 to 8.09]*	
History of neurologic disease	3.19 [1.65 to 6.15]	
Use of IABP	2.60 [1.21 to 5.58]	
Diabetes mellitus	2.59 [1.46 to 4.60]	
History of hypertension	2.31 [1.20 to 4.47]	
History of pulmonary disease	2.09 [1.14 to 3.85]	2.37 [1.34 to 4.18]
History of unstable angina	1.83 [1.03 to 3.27]	
Age (per additional decade)	1.75 [1.27 to 2.43]	2.20 [1.60 to 3.02]
Admission systolic BP > 180 mm Hg		3.47 [1.41 to 8.55]
History of excessive alcohol intake		2.64 [1.27 to 5.47]
History of CABG		2.18 [1.14 to 4.17]
Arrhythmia on day of surgery		1.97 [1.12 to 3.46]
Antihypertensive therapy		1.78 [1.02 to 3.10]

*Adjusted odds ratio [95% confidence intervals] for type I and type II cerebral outcomes associated with selected risk factors from the Multicenter Study of Perioperative Ischemia.

BP = blood pressure; CABG = coronary artery bypass graft surgery; IABP = intra-aortic balloon pump.

From Arrowsmith JE, Grocott HP, Reves JG, et al: Central nervous system complications of cardiac surgery. Br J Anaesth 84:378, 2000.

stroke, transient ischemic attack (TIA), stupor or coma at time of discharge, and death caused by stroke or hypoxic encephalopathy. Type II included new deterioration in intellectual function, confusion, agitation, disorientation, and memory deficit without evidence of focal injury. A total of 129 (6.1%) of the 2108 patients had an adverse cerebral outcome in the perioperative period. Type I outcomes occurred in 66 (3.1%) of 2108 patients, with type II outcomes occurring in 63 (3.0%) of 2108 patients. Stepwise logistic regression analysis identified eight independent predictors of type I outcomes and seven independent predictors of type II outcomes (Table 23-1).

Of all the factors in the Multicenter Study of Perioperative Ischemia analysis, age appears to be the most overwhelmingly robust predictor of stroke and of neurocognitive dysfunction after cardiac surgery. Age has a greater impact on neurologic outcome than it does on perioperative myocardial infarction or low cardiac output states after cardiac surgery (Fig. 23-1).

Atheromatous disease of the ascending, arch, and descending thoracic aorta has been consistently implicated as a risk factor for stroke in cardiac surgical patients. The increased use of transesophageal echocardiography (TEE) and epiaortic ultrasonography has added new dimensions to the detection of aortic atheromatous disease and the understanding of its relation to stroke risk. These imaging modalities have allowed the diagnosis of atheromatous disease to be made in a more sensitive and detailed manner, contributing greatly to the information regarding potential stroke risk. Studies have consistently reported higher stroke rates for patients with increasing atheromatous aortic involvement (particularly the ascending and arch segments). This relationship is outlined in Figure 23-2.

V

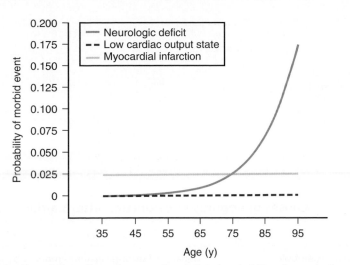

Figure 23-1 The relative effect of age on the predicted probability of neurologic and cardiac morbidity after cardiac surgery. (From Tuman KJ, McCarthy RJ, Najafi H, et al: Differential effects of advanced age on neurologic and cardiac risks of coronary artery operations. J Thorac Cardiovasc Surg 104:1510, 1992.)

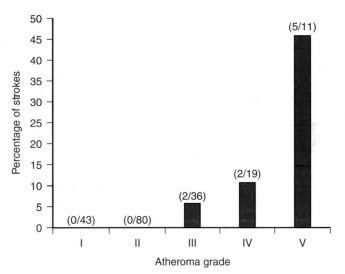

Figure 23-2 Stroke rate 1 week after cardiac surgery as a function of atheroma severity. Atheroma was graded by transesophageal echocardiography as follows: I, normal; II, intimal thickening; III, plaque < 5 mm thick; IV, plaque > 5 mm thick; V, any plaque with a mobile segment. (From Hartman GS, Yao FS, Bruefach M 3rd, et al: Severity of aortic atheromatous disease diagnosed by transesophageal echocardiography predicts stroke and other outcomes associated with coronary artery surgery: A prospective study. Anesth Analg 83:701, 1996.)

Cause of Perioperative Central Nervous System Injury

Because central nervous system dysfunction represents a wide range of injuries, differentiating the individual causes of these different types of injuries becomes somewhat difficult (Box 23-1). They are frequently grouped together and superficially

BOX 23-1   *Causes of Central Nervous System Complications after Cardiopulmonary Bypass*

- Cerebral emboli
- Global hypoperfusion
- Inflammation
- Cerebral edema
- Cerebral hyperthermia

Table 23-2   Causes of Cognitive Dysfunction after Cardiac Surgery

Cause	Possible Settings
Cerebral microemboli	Generated during cardiopulmonary bypass (CPB); mobilization of atheromatous material or entrainment of air from the operative field; gas injections into the venous reservoir of the CPB apparatus
Global cerebral hypoperfusion	Hypotension, occlusion by an atheromatous embolus leading to stroke
Inflammation (systemic and cerebral)	Injurious effects of CPB, such as blood interacting with the foreign surfaces of pump-oxygenator; upregulation of proinflammatory cyclooxygenase mRNA
Cerebral hyperthermia	Hypothermia during CPB; hyperthermia during and after cardiac surgery, such as aggressive rewarming
Cerebral edema	Edema from global cerebral hypoperfusion or from hyponatremia; increased cerebral venous pressure from cannula misplacement
Blood-brain barrier dysfunction	Diffuse cerebral inflammation; ischemia from cerebral microembolization or increased intracranial pressure
Pharmacologic influences	Anesthetic-related cognitive damage; necrosis of neonatal brains; proteomic changes
Genetic influences	Effects of single nucleotide polymorphisms on risk for Alzheimer's disease or for acute coronary syndromes and other thrombotic disorders

discussed as representing different severities on a continuum of similar injury. This likely misrepresents the different causes of these injuries. The following section addresses stroke and cognitive injury (Table 23-2).

Cerebral Embolization

Macroemboli (e.g., atheromatous plaque) and microemboli (i.e., gaseous and particulate) are generated during CPB, and many emboli find their way to the cerebral vasculature. Macroemboli are responsible for stroke, and microemboli are fundamental to the development of neurocognitive dysfunction. Sources for the microemboli are numerous and include those generated de novo from the interactions of blood within the CPB apparatus (e.g., platelet-fibrin aggregates) and those generated within the body by the production and mobilization of atheromatous material or entrainment of air from the operative field.[3]

Global Cerebral Hypoperfusion

The concept that global cerebral hypoperfusion during CPB may lead to neurologic and neurocognitive complications originates from the earliest days of cardiac surgery, when significant (in degree and time) systemic hypotension was a relatively common event. Although making intuitive sense (i.e., that hypotension would lead to global cerebral hypoperfusion), studies that have examined the relationship between mean arterial pressure (MAP) and cognitive decline after cardiac surgery have generally failed to show any significant relationship.

Temperature-Related Factors

During rewarming from hypothermic CPB there can be an overshoot in cerebral temperature due to aggressive rewarming generally aimed at decreasing time on CPB and overall operating room time. This cerebral hyperthermia may well be responsible for some of the injury that occurs in the brain.

Neuroprotective Strategies

Emboli Reduction

The aortic cannula may be very important to reduce cerebral emboli production. Placement of the cannula into an area of the aorta with a large atheroma burden may cause the direct generation of emboli from the "sandblasting" of atherosclerotic material in the aorta. The use of a distal aortic cannula, where the tip of the cannula lies beyond the origin of the cerebral vessels has also been found to reduce emboli load.

Blood that is returned from the surgical field though the use of the cardiotomy suction may significantly contribute to the particulate load in the CPB circuit and subsequently in the brain. The use of cell-salvage devices to process shed blood before returning it to the venous reservoir may minimize the amount of particulate- or lipid-laden material that contributes to embolization.

Management of Aortic Atherosclerosis

A combination of epiaortic scanning and atheroma avoidance techniques (with respect to cannulation, clamping, and vein graft anastomosis placement) have been used to attempt to reduce neurocognitive deficits.[4] The incidence of cognitive decline may be lower in patients who had an avoidance technique guided by epiaortic scanning compared with no epiaortic scanning. It is an area that requires more investigation. One of the difficulties in interpreting studies that have evaluated atheroma avoidance strategies is the absence of any form of blinding of the investigators. For the most part, a strategy is chosen based on the presence of known atheroma, and the results of these patients are compared with historical controls. Multiple techniques can be used to minimize atheromatous material liberated from the aortic wall from getting into the cerebral circulation. These range from optimizing placement of the aortic cannula in the aorta to an area relatively devoid of plaque to the use of specialized cannulas that reduce the sandblasting of the aortic wall. Alternative aortic cannulas and using different locations possess the ability to decrease embolization of atheromatous plaque. The avoidance of partial occlusion clamping for proximal vein graft anastomosis using a single-step automated anastomotic device and the use of alternatives to cross-clamping all possess the ability to mitigate injury due to embolization.

23

Acid-Base Management: α-Stat versus pH-Stat

Optimal acid-base management during CPB has long been debated. Theoretically, α-stat management maintains normal CBF autoregulation with the coupling of cerebral metabolism (CMR_{O_2}) to CBF, allowing adequate oxygen delivery while minimizing the potential for emboli. Although early studies were unable to document a difference in neurologic or neuropsychologic outcome between the two techniques, later studies showed reductions in cognitive performance when pH-stat management was used, particularly in cases with prolonged CPB times. pH-stat management (i.e., CO_2 is added to the fresh oxygenator gas flow) results in a higher CBF than is needed for the brain's metabolic requirements. This luxury perfusion risks excessive delivery of emboli to the brain. Except for congenital heart surgery, for which most outcome data support the use of pH-stat management due to its improvement in homogenous brain cooling before circulatory arrest, adult outcome data support the use of α-stat management.[5]

Mean Arterial Pressure Management during Cardiopulmonary Bypass

Although the data associating MAP with neurologic and neurocognitive outcome after CABG surgery are inconclusive, most data suggest that MAP during CPB is not a primary predictor of cognitive decline or stroke after cardiac surgery. However, with increasing age, MAP during CPB may play a role in improving cerebral collateral perfusion to regions embolized, improving neurologic and cognitive outcome.

Glucose Management

Hyperglycemia is a common occurrence during the course of cardiac surgery. Administration of cardioplegia containing glucose and stress response–induced alterations in insulin secretion and resistance increase the potential for significant hyperglycemia. Hyperglycemia has been repeatedly demonstrated to impair neurologic outcome after experimental focal and global cerebral ischemia. The explanation for this adverse effect likely relates to the effects that hyperglycemia have on anaerobic conversion of glucose to lactate, which ultimately cause intracellular acidosis and impair intracellular homeostasis and metabolism. A second injurious mechanism relates to an increase in the release of excitotoxic amino acids in response to hyperglycemia in the setting of cerebral ischemia. If hyperglycemia is injurious to the brain, the threshold for making injuries worse appears to be 180 to 200 mg/dL.

The appropriate type of perioperative serum glucose management and whether it adversely affects neurologic outcome in patients undergoing CPB remain unclear. The major difficulty in hyperglycemia treatment is the relative ineffectiveness of insulin therapy. Using excessive amounts of insulin during hypothermic periods may lead to rebound hypoglycemia after CPB. Chaney and associates[6] attempted to maintain normoglycemia during cardiac surgery with the use of an insulin protocol and came to the conclusion that even with aggressive insulin treatment, hyperglycemia is often resistant and may actually predispose to postoperative hypoglycemia. Attempting to mediate injury may actually predispose to additional injury.

Off-Pump Cardiac Surgery

Off-pump coronary artery bypass grafting (OPCAB) is frequently used for the operative treatment of coronary artery disease. Some preliminary data suggest less cognitive decline after OPCAB procedures, but most studies have not seen it eliminated altogether. The reasons for this are unclear but likely reflect on the complex pathophysiology involved. For example, if inflammatory processes play a role in initiating or propagating cerebral injury, OPCAB, with its continued use of sternotomy, heparin administration, and wide hemodynamic swings, all of which may contribute to a stress and inflammatory response, may be a significant reason why cognitive dysfunction is still seen. Ascending aortic manipulation, with its ensuing particulate embolization, is also still commonly used.

ACUTE RENAL INJURY

Despite the recognition, made more than 40 years ago, of acute renal injury as a serious complication of cardiac surgery, postoperative renal dysfunction persists today as an independent predictor of postoperative mortality. Even during procedures where there is no evidence of acute renal injury as reflected by a rise in serum creatinine, more subtle markers have demonstrated renal tubular injury. Patients with increasing degrees of acute renal injury after cardiac surgery require disproportionately more short- and long-term resources and have increasingly poorer outcome and greater costs.[7] The association of acute renal dysfunction with mortality and major morbidity may reflect its role as a marker of, rather than as a contributor to, the insult of cardiac surgery; however, there is compelling evidence that acute renal injury itself also contributes directly to adverse outcome. Accumulation of "uremic toxins" and release of inflammatory mediators from the injured kidney also appear to contribute significantly to remote organ dysfunction.

Incidence and Significance

Definitions and the incidence of renal injury vary, with approximately 8% to 15% of cardiac surgery patients sustaining a moderate renal injury (defined by a peak rise in the serum creatinine level of more than 1.0 mg/dL) and 1% to 5% requiring dialysis. Each type of cardiac surgical procedure has its own specific pattern of renal injury. As a result, surgical procedure type is an important variable when examining the incidence and severity of postoperative acute renal injury. For example, elevation of the serum creatinine level, a common marker of acute renal injury, typically peaks on the second day after CABG with CPB and, in most cases, returns to baseline by postoperative day 4 or 5.[8]

In-hospital mortality rates for CABG range from less than 1% for patients with subclinical renal injury to 20% for those with moderate renal injury, and rates exceed 60% when dialysis is required. Survivors of significant postoperative renal injury have higher in-hospital resource use. In addition to the direct relationship with renal injury of morbidity, mortality, and perioperative cost, intensive care unit stays are up to five to six times longer and overall hospital length of stay increases approximately three times. Patients with renal dysfunction are also more likely to be discharged to an extended-care facility, with its own associated costs. Accelerated long-term decline of renal function after cardiac surgery may lead to later end-stage renal disease.

Risk Factors for Surgery-Related Acute Renal Injury

Numerous studies have characterized risk factors for nephropathy after cardiac surgery (Table 23-3). Preoperative variables are most useful for renal risk stratification with intraoperative and postoperative issues contributing to overall clinical management decisions. Equivalent renal injury for a patient with preoperative renal

23

Table 23-3 Risk Factors for Renal Injury

Important Factors	Probably Not Important
Preoperative Factors	
Advanced age	Gender
Obesity	Renal artery stenosis
Preexisting renal insufficiency	
Diabetes	
Hyperglycemia	
Hypertension	
Ascending aortic atherosclerosis	
Peripheral vascular disease	
IABP	
COPD	
Loop diuretic therapy	
Corticosteroid therapy	
Nephrotoxins (radiocontrast dye, cyclosporin, aminoglycosides, cephalosporins, NSAIDs)	
Genetic variants	
Intraoperative Factors	
Aprotinin	Lysine analogs
Loop diuretic (increased risk)	Low-dose dopamine
Transfusion	Mannitol
Hyperglycemia	
Procedure type (CABG < valve < HCA)	
Emergency procedure	
Reoperation	
IABP	
CPB management	CPB management
Extended CPB duration	Hypothermia
Hemodilution	Blood pressure management
Postoperative Factors	
Low cardiac output	
Excessive inotrope use	
Prolonged ventilation	
Transfusion	
Sepsis	
CMV infection	

CABG = coronary artery bypass graft surgery; CPB = cardiopulmonary bypass; CMV = controlled mechanical ventilation; COPD = chronic obstructive pulmonary disease; HCA = hypothermic circulatory arrest; IABP = intra-aortic balloon pump; NSAIDs = nonsteroidal anti-inflammatory drugs.

V

dysfunction does result in a greater rise in serum creatinine due to the nonlinear relationship between reductions in glomerular filtration rate (GFR) and creatinine rise. Even small amounts of additional renal impairment may lead to dialysis for a surgical patient with severe renal disease at baseline.

Procedure-related risk factors include emergent and redo operations, valvular procedures, and operations requiring a period of circulatory arrest or extended durations of CPB. Infection and sepsis, atrial fibrillation, and indicators of low cardiac output states, including need for inotropic agents and insertion of an intra-aortic balloon pump (IABP) during surgery, also have been associated with renal impairment.

> **BOX 23-2** *Causes of Renal Injury during Cardiopulmonary Bypass*
>
> - Emboli
> - Renal ischemia
> - Reperfusion injury
> - Pigments, radiocontrast agents, aprotinin

Causes and Pathophysiology of Renal Injury

Ischemia-Reperfusion Injury

A long-standing assumption regarding the causes and pathophysiology of renal dysfunction after cardiac surgery is that hypoperfusion with resulting renal ischemia plays a central role (Box 23-2). This assumption is supported by an understanding of the precarious oxygen supply and demand physiology of the renal medulla, particularly during CPB, as well as the responsiveness of experimental acute renal injury to improved renal perfusion. However, clinically applied techniques directed at improving perfusion (e.g., including low-dose dopamine) and reducing oxygen consumption (e.g., loop diuretics) have been uniformly unsuccessful in cardiac surgical patients and in most other settings. Other risk factors supporting the ischemia-reperfusion hypothesis of acute renal injury and nephropathy after cardiac surgery include episodes of circulatory arrest and perioperative low cardiac output states and prolonged bypass duration.[9]

Drug-Related Nephropathy

Several agent-specific nephrotoxicities are relevant to cardiac surgery. Cephalosporin-related renal injury to the proximal renal tubule has been reported. Aminoglycoside antibiotics also have a potent nephrotoxic effect. Nonsteroidal anti-inflammatory drug nephrotoxicity is thought to be related to renal vasoconstriction from inhibition of locally synthesized endogenous renal vasodilator prostaglandins. Radiocontrast agents have also been shown to adversely effect renal function.

Concern continues regarding the use of antifibrinolytic agents during cardiac surgery. Benign proximal tubule effects of lysine analog agents cause "tubular proteinuria" in cardiac surgery patients; however, no change in the incidence of acute renal injury has been documented in longitudinal studies examining institutional rates of renal injury before and after periods of ε-aminocaproic acid use.[10] Aprotinin also interacts with the proximal renal tubule and is thought to saturate tubular transport mechanisms, resulting in tubular proteinuria. Aprotinin has been implicated in postoperative renal dysfunction after cardiac surgery.[11]

Pigment Nephropathy: Hemoglobinuria and Myoglobinuria

Severe intravascular hemolysis leading to release of hemoglobin in amounts sufficient to exceed the absorptive capacity of circulating haptoglobin and the normal renal metabolic reserve can lead to hemoglobinuria and acute renal injury. The deterioration in kidney function appears to be the result of a combination of renal vasoconstriction, direct cytotoxicity, and tubular obstruction by casts.

Although free hemoglobin is often seen in the urine during and after cardiac surgery, particularly after prolonged CPB, the significance of hemoglobinuria as a contributor to nephropathy after cardiac surgery is unknown. Myoglobinuria can occur

23

after femoral artery cannulation for CPB or IABP insertion if ipsilateral leg ischemia develops. Myoglobinuric acute renal failure has been reported after cardiac surgery with femoral artery cannulation, particularly in children. However, it is not clear that femoral artery cannulation is a concern for most patients.

Strategies for Renal Protection

Cardiopulmonary Bypass Management

Basic issues in the management of CPB that relate to the kidney involve the balance between oxygen supply and oxygen demand, particularly to the renal medulla. Perfusion pressure (i.e., MAP during CPB) and oxygen-carrying capacity (as related to hemodilution and transfusion) address the supply issues, with the use of hypothermia being directed at modulating renal oxygen demand.

Pharmacologic Intervention

DOPAMINE

Mesenteric dopamine-1 (D_1) receptor agonists increase renal blood flow, decrease renal vascular resistance, and enhance natriuresis and diuresis. Despite the absence of clinical evidence of renoprotection, this rationale has been used to justify the use of low-dose ("renal-dose") dopamine (<5 µg/kg/min) for decades. Despite the lack of benefit and accumulating concerns regarding the use of low-dose dopamine, continued use of this agent for renoprotection is prevalent.[12]

FENOLDOPAM

Fenoldopam mesylate, a benzazepine derivative, is a selective D_1-receptor agonist. Although first approved as an antihypertensive agent, fenoldopam has shown promise in the prevention of contrast-induced nephropathy. A recent meta-analysis by Landoni et al provides evidence that fenoldopam may confer significant benefits in preventing renal replacement therapy and reducing mortality in patients undergoing cardiovascular surgery.[13]

DIURETIC AGENTS

Diuretics increase urine generation by reducing reuptake of tubular contents. This can be achieved by numerous mechanisms, including inhibiting active mechanisms that lead to solute reuptake (e.g., loop diuretics), altering the osmotic gradient in the tubular contents to favor solute remaining in the tubule (e.g., mannitol), or hormonal influences that affect the balance of activities of the tubule to increase urine generation (e.g., atrial natriuretic peptide). The general renoprotective principle of diuretic agents is that increasing tubular solute flow through injured renal tubules will maintain tubular patency, avoiding some of the adverse consequences of tubular obstruction, including oliguria or anuria and possibly the need for dialysis.

MYOCARDIAL INJURY

From the earliest days of modern cardiac surgery, perioperative myocardial dysfunction, with its associated morbidity and mortality, has been reported. Evidence, including substantial subendocardial cellular necrosis, led to the conclusion that this injury resulted from an inadequate substrate supply to the metabolically active myocardium. Optimizing myocardial protection during cardiac surgery involves several compromises inherent in allowing surgery to be performed in a relatively immobile, bloodless field while preserving postoperative myocardial function. The fundamental tenets of this protection center on the judicious use of hypothermia along with the induction and maintenance of chemically induced electromechanical diastolic cardiac arrest. Despite continued efforts directed at myocardial protection, it is clear that myocardial injury, although reduced, still remains a problem, and with it, the representative phenotype of myocardial dysfunction.

Incidence and Significance of Myocardial Dysfunction after Cardiopulmonary Bypass

Unlike other organs at risk of damage during cardiac surgery, it is assumed, owing to the very nature of the target of the operation being performed, that all patients having cardiac surgery suffer some degree of myocardial injury. Although the injury can be subclinical, represented only by otherwise asymptomatic elevations in cardiac enzymes, it frequently manifests more overtly. The degree to which these enzymes are released by injured myocardium, frequently to levels sufficiently high to satisfy criteria for myocardial infarction, has been related to perioperative outcome after cardiac surgery. CK-MB values more than 10 times the upper limit of normal during the initial 48 hours after CABG were significantly associated with 6-month mortality ($P < .001$).[14]

Risk Factors for Myocardial Injury

With an increasingly sicker cohort of patients presenting for cardiac surgery,[15] many with acute ischemic syndromes (e.g., often with evolving myocardial infarction) or significant left ventricular dysfunction, the need has never been greater for optimizing myocardial protection to minimize the myocardial dysfunction consequent to aortic cross-clamping and cardioplegia. The continued increase in cardiac transplantation and other complex surgeries in the heart failure patient has served to fuel the search for better myocardial protection strategies.

Pathophysiology of Myocardial Injury

The metabolic consequences of oxygen deprivation become apparent within seconds of coronary artery occlusion. With the rapid depletion of high-energy phosphates, accumulation of lactate and intracellular acidosis in the myocytes soon follows, with the subsequent development of contractile dysfunction. When myocyte adenosine triphosphate levels decline to a critical level, the subsequent inability to maintain electrolyte gradients requiring active transport (e.g., Na^+, K^+, Ca^{2+}) leads to cellular edema, intracellular Ca^{2+} overload, and loss of membrane integrity.

Predictably with the release of the aortic cross-clamp and the restoration of blood flow, myocardial reperfusion occurs. With reperfusion the paradox, represented by the balance of substrate delivery restoration needed for normal metabolism that also can serve as the substrate for injurious free radical production, becomes a significant issue for consideration. Reperfusion causes a rapid increase in free radical production within minutes, and it plays a major role initiating myocardial stunning.

A potential additional mechanism for myocardial dysfunction specific to the setting of CPB relates to proposed acute alterations in β-adrenergic signal transduction.

Acute desensitization and downregulation of myocardial β-adrenergic receptors during CPB have been demonstrated after cardiac surgery. Although the role of the large elevations in circulating catecholamines seen with CPB on β-adrenergic malfunction is unclear, it has been proposed that an increased incidence of post-CPB low cardiac output states and reduced responsiveness to inotropic agents may, in part, be attributed to this effect.

Myocardial Protection during Cardiac Surgery: Cardioplegia

Optimizing the metabolic state of the myocardium is fundamental to preserving its integrity. The major effects of temperature and functional activity (i.e., contractile and electrical work) on the metabolic rate of myocardium have been extensively described.[16] With the institution of CPB, the emptying of the heart significantly reduces contractile work and myocardial oxygen consumption $M\dot{v}o_2$. Nullifying this cardiac work reduces the $M\dot{v}o_2$ by 30% to 60%. With subsequent reductions in temperature, the $M\dot{v}o_2$ further decreases, and with induction of cardiac arrest and hypothermia, 90% of the metabolic requirements of the heart can be reduced. Temperature reductions diminish metabolic rate for all electromechanical states (i.e., beating or fibrillating) of the myocardium.

Although cardiac surgery on the empty beating heart or under conditions of hypothermic fibrillation (both with the support of CPB) is sometimes performed, aortic cross-clamping with cardioplegic arrest remains the most prevalent method of myocardial preservation. Based on the principle of reducing metabolic requirements, the introduction of selective myocardial hypothermia and cardioplegia (i.e., diastolic arrest) marked a major clinical advance in myocardial protection. With the various additives in cardioplegia solutions (designed to optimize the myocardium during arrest and attenuate reperfusion injury) and the use of warm cardioplegia, the idea of delivering metabolic substrates (as opposed to solely reducing metabolic requirements) is also commonplace. Several effective approaches to chemical cardioplegia are employed. The clinical success of a cardioplegia strategy may be judged by its ability to achieve and maintain prompt continuous arrest in all regions of the myocardium, early return of function after cross-clamp removal, and minimal inotropic requirements for successful separation from CPB. Composition, temperature, and route of delivery constitute the fundamentals of cardioplegia-derived myocardial protection.

Composition of Cardioplegia Solutions

The composition of the various cardioplegia solutions used during cardiac surgery varies as much between institutions as it does between individual surgeons. In very general terms, cardioplegia can be classified into blood-containing and non–blood-containing (i.e., crystalloid) solutions. Table 23-4 outlines the various additives to cardioplegia solutions along with their corresponding rationale for use. Although all cardioplegia solutions contain higher than physiologic levels of potassium, solutions used for the induction of diastolic arrest contain the highest concentrations of potassium as opposed to solutions used for the maintenance of cardioplegia. In addition to adjustment of electrolytes, manipulation of buffers (e.g., bicarbonate, tromethamine), osmotic agents (e.g., glucose, mannitol, potassium), and metabolic substrates (e.g., glucose, glutamate, and aspartate) constitutes the most common variations in cardioplegia content.

Blood cardioplegia has the potential advantage of delivering sufficient oxygen to ischemic myocardium to sustain basal metabolism or even augment high-energy phosphate stores, as well as possessing free radical scavenging properties. The

Table 23-4	Strategies for the Reduction of Ischemic Injury with Cardioplegia	
Principle	**Mechanism**	**Component**
Reduce O_2 demand	Hypothermia	Blood, crystalloid, ice slush, lavage
	Perfusion	
	Topical/lavage	
	Asystole	KCl, adenosine(?), hyperpolarizing agents
Substrate supply and use	Oxygen	Blood, perfluorocarbons, crystalloid(?)
	Glucose	Blood, glucose, citrate-phosphate-dextrose
	Amino acids	Glutamate, aspartate
	Buffer acidosis	Hypothermia (Rosenthal factor), intermittent infusions
	Buffers	Blood, tromethamine, histidine, bicarbonate, phosphate
	Optimize metabolism	Warm induction (37°C), warm reperfusion
Reduce Ca^{2+} overload	Hypocalcemia	Citrate, Ca^{2+} channel blockers, K channel openers(?)
Reduce edema	Hyperosmolarity	Glucose, KCl, mannitol
	Moderate infusion pressure	50 mmHg

From Vinten-Johansen J, Thourani VH: Myocardial protection: An overview. J Extra Corpor Technol 32:38, 2000.

introduction of blood cardioplegia in the late 1970s followed recognition of the clinical utility of this technique.

Cardioplegia Temperature

The composition of cardioplegia solutions varies considerably; in contrast, myocardial temperature during cardioplegia is almost uniformly reduced to between 10°C and 15°C or less by the infusion of refrigerated cardioplegia and external topical cooling with ice slush. However, the introduction of warm cardioplegia has challenged this once universally considered necessity of hypothermia for successful myocardial protection. Although hypothermic cardioplegia is the most commonly used temperature, numerous investigations have examined tepid (27°C to 30°C) and warm (37°C to 38°C) temperature ranges for the administration of cardioplegia. Much of the work aimed at determining the optimum temperature of the cardioplegia solution centered on the fact that although hypothermia clearly offered some advantages to the myocardium in suppressing metabolism (particularly when intermittent cardioplegia was delivered), it may have some detrimental effects.

The deleterious effects of hypothermia include the increased risk of myocardial edema (through ion pump activity inhibition) and the impaired function of various membrane receptors on which some pharmacologic therapy depends (such as the various additives to the cardioplegia solutions). The other disadvantages of hypothermic cardioplegia, in addition to the production of the metabolic inhibition in the myocardium, are an increase in plasma viscosity and a decrease in red blood cell deformability. As a result, investigations aimed at using warmer cardioplegia temperatures have been explored.

23

BOX 23-3　*Uses for Retrograde Cardioplegia*

- Along with anterograde cardioplegia
- In the presence of aortic insufficiency
- For aortic valve surgery
- To perfuse severely diseased coronary arteries

Cardioplegia Delivery Routes

Retrograde cardioplegia, where a cardioplegia catheter is introduced into the coronary sinus, allows for almost continuous cardioplegia administration. Retrograde delivery is useful in settings where antegrade cardioplegia is problematic, such as with severe aortic insufficiency or during aortic root or aortic valve surgery (Box 23-3). It also allows the distribution of cardioplegia to areas of myocardium supplied by significantly stenosed coronary vessels. Retrograde cardioplegia has proved safe and effective for cardioplegia in patients with coronary artery disease and in those undergoing valve surgery. With the administration of retrograde cardioplegia, certain provisos should be considered. The acceptable perfusion pressure to limit perivascular edema and hemorrhage needs to be limited to less than 40 mmHg.[17]

GASTROINTESTINAL COMPLICATIONS

Incidence and Significance

Gastrointestinal complications after cardiac surgery, although occurring relatively infrequently (0.5% to 5.5%), portend a significantly increased incidence of overall adverse patient outcome. The variability in the reported incidence of gastrointestinal complications is partly a reflection of how they are defined and the variable patient and operative risk factors in the studied cohorts. Although the most commonly considered gastrointestinal complications include pancreatitis, gastrointestinal bleeding, cholecystitis, and bowel perforation or infarction, hyperbilirubinemia (total bilirubinemia > 3.0 mL/dL) has also been described as an important complication after cardiac surgery. In one of the largest prospective studies examining these complications after CPB, McSweeney and associates studied 2417 patients undergoing CABG (with or without concurrent intracardiac procedures) in a multicenter study in the United States. The overall incidence of gastrointestinal complications in this study was 5.5%, ranging from 3.7% for hyperbilirubinemia to 0.1% for major bowel perforation or infarction.[18]

In addition to their association with other morbid events, adverse gastrointestinal complications are significantly associated with increased mortality after cardiac surgery. The average mortality among subtypes of gastrointestinal complications in the study by McSweeney and associates was 19.6%, and in other reports the mortality rate ranges from 13% to 87%, with an overall average mortality of 33%. Even the seemingly insignificant complication of having an increased laboratory measurement of total bilirubin was associated with an odds ratio of death of 6.6 in the study of McSweeney and associates, compared with a death odds ratio of 8.4 for all adverse gastrointestinal outcomes combined. Apart from the significant effect on mortality, the occurrence of an adverse gastrointestinal outcome also significantly increases the incidence of perioperative myocardial infarction, renal failure, and stroke, as well as significantly prolonging intensive care unit and hospital length of stay.

Risk Factors

A long list of preoperative, intraoperative, and postoperative risk factors for gastrointestinal complications have been identified in a number of studies.[19] As many factors are associated with one another, it is only when these risk factors are examined in multivariable analyses that a more accurate understanding of what the most significant risk factors for visceral complications after cardiac surgery are. Preoperatively, age (>75 years), history of congestive heart failure, presence of hyperbilirubinemia (>1.2 mg/dL), combined cardiac procedures (e.g., CABG plus valve), repeat cardiac operation, preoperative ejection fraction less than 40%, preoperative elevations in partial thromboplastin time, emergency operations; intraoperatively, prolonged CPB, use of TEE, and blood transfusion; and postoperatively, requirements for prolonged inotropic vasopressor support, IABP use for the treatment of low cardiac output; and prolonged ventilatory support are all risk factors. These factors identify patients at high risk, and they lend some credence to the overall pathophysiology and suspected causes of these adverse events. If there is a common link between all these risks, it is that many of these factors would be associated with impairment in oxygen delivery to the splanchnic bed.

Pathophysiology and Etiology

Impairments in splanchnic perfusion commonly occur during even the normal conduct of cardiac surgery. When this is superimposed on an already depressed preoperative cardiac output or is associated with prolonged postoperative low cardiac output, the impairment in splanchnic blood flow is further perpetuated. The systemic inflammatory response to CPB itself can be initiated by splanchnic hypoperfusion by means of translocation of endotoxin from the gut into the circulation. De novo splanchnic hypoperfusion can be a result of the humoral vasoactive substances that are released by inflammation remote from the gut. Another etiologic factor for gastrointestinal complications directly related to splanchnic hypoperfusion is atheroembolism. Prolonged ventilator support is another etiologic factor for gastrointestinal complications. Several lines of investigation have described a relationship between prolonged ventilation and gastrointestinal adverse events; this likely results from a direct effect of positive-pressure ventilation impairing cardiac output and subsequently splanchnic perfusion.

23

Protecting the Gastrointestinal Tract during Cardiac Surgery

As with other aspects of organ protection, critical etiologic factors need to be addressed with specific targeted therapies (Box 23-4). Unfortunately, as with most other organ-protective strategies, the major limitation in making definitive recommendations is an overall lack of large, well-controlled, prospectively randomized studies to provide supportive data for any one particular technique.

Cardiopulmonary Bypass Management

Because CPB itself has been shown to impair splanchnic blood flow, modifications in how it is conducted may have some salutary effects on gastrointestinal tract integrity. Several studies have focused on the issue of the relative importance of pressure versus flow during CPB, demonstrating that it is likely more beneficial to maintain an adequate bypass flow rate than only maintaining pressure during bypass. The addition of significant vasoconstrictors to artificially maintain an adequate MAP in the presence of inadequate flow on CPB may lead to further compromise of splanchnic blood flow.

> **BOX 23-4** *Protecting the Gastrointestinal Tract during Cardiopulmonary Bypass*
>
> - Avoiding use of profound vasopressors
> - Maintaining a high perfusion flow
> - Reducing emboli-producing maneuvers

The optimal bypass temperature to protect the gut is also unknown. Just as aggressive rewarming can be injurious to the brain, there is some evidence that rewarming can cause increases in visceral metabolism, making any overshoot in temperature suspect by adversely altering the balance of gut oxygen consumption and delivery.

Drugs

A range of vasoactive drugs has been used to enhance splanchnic blood flow during CPB. It is likely that most of these drugs, such as the phosphodiesterase III inhibitors, dobutamine, and other inotropic agents, maintain or enhance splanchnic blood flow not because of a direct effect on the vasculature but by the inherent enhancement in cardiac output. An increasingly common drug in the setting of cardiac surgery is vasopressin. Although vasopressin can clearly augment systemic MAP, it does so at the cost of severe impairments to splanchnic blood flow. Although there are always trade-offs when choosing which vasoactive agent to use, if having a very low MAP is going to be detrimental to other organ systems, the choice to use vasopressin should at least be made with the knowledge that it can have an adverse effect on splanchnic blood flow.

Off-Pump Cardiac Surgery

There is little evidence that the use of off-pump cardiac surgery is in any way beneficial to the gastrointestinal tract. Three retrospective studies[20] have shown no differences in gastrointestinal complications. One reason for this lack of apparent difference between on-pump and off-pump cardiac surgery may again be related to the common denominator of splanchnic perfusion. OPCAB is fraught with hemodynamic compromise that may lead to prolonged periods of splanchnic hypoperfusion by itself or as a result of the concurrent administration of vasopressors to maintain normal hemodynamics during the frequent manipulations of the heart.

LUNG INJURY DURING CARDIAC SURGERY

Incidence and Significance

Pulmonary dysfunction was one of the earliest recognized complications of cardiac surgery employing CPB.[21] However, as improvements in operative technique and CPB perfusion technologies occurred, the overall frequency and severity of this complication decreased. Juxtaposed to the improvements in cardiac surgery, which led to an overall reduction in complications, is an evolving patient population that now comprises a higher-risk group with a higher degree of pulmonary comorbidities, increasing their risks of postoperative pulmonary dysfunction. With the advent of fast-track techniques, even minor degrees of pulmonary dysfunction have reemerged as significant contributors to patient morbidity and the potential need for extended postoperative ventilation. As with most postoperative organ dysfunction, there is a range of dysfunction severity. Arguably, some degree of pulmonary dysfunction occurs in most patients after cardiac surgery; however, it manifests clinically only when the degree of dysfunction is particularly severe or the pulmonary reserve is significantly impaired. As a result, even minor CPB-related pulmonary dysfunction can cause significant problems in some patients.

The full range of reported pulmonary complications includes simple atelectasis, pleural effusions, pneumonia, cardiogenic pulmonary edema, pulmonary embolism, and various degrees of acute lung injury ranging from the mild to the most severe (i.e., acute respiratory distress syndrome [ARDS]). Although the final common pathway in all these forms of pulmonary dysfunction complications is the occurrence of hypoxemia, these complications vary widely in their incidence, cause, and clinical significance.

Pathophysiology and Etiology

Studies have demonstrated bypass-induced changes in the mechanical properties (i.e., elastance or compliance and resistance) of the pulmonary apparatus (particularly the lung as opposed to the chest wall) and changes in pulmonary capillary permeability. Impairment in gas exchange has been demonstrated to be a result of atelectasis with concomitant overall loss of lung volume. Most research has focused on the development of increases in pulmonary vascular permeability (leading to various degrees of pulmonary edema) as the principal cause of the impaired gas exchange that occurs during cardiac surgery and results in a high alveolar-arteriolar gradient (A-a Do_2).

The cause of pulmonary dysfunction and ARDS after cardiac surgery is complex but largely revolves around the CPB-induced systemic inflammatory response with its associated increase in pulmonary endothelial permeability. A central etiologic theme is a significant upregulation in the inflammation induced because of the interaction between the blood and foreign surfaces of the heart-lung machine or the inflammation related to the consequences of splanchnic hypoperfusion with the subsequent translocation of significant amounts of endotoxin into the circulation. Endotoxin is proinflammatory, and it has direct effects on the pulmonary vasculature. Clinical studies have demonstrated an increase in circulating intracellular adhesion molecules after CPB in patients with development of acute lung injury. Pathologic examination of the lungs of patients manifesting ARDS has shown extensive injury to the tissue, including swelling and necrosis of endothelial cells and type I and II pneumocytes. Several studies have also identified transfusion of packed red blood cells (>4 units) as a risk factor for ARDS in the cardiac surgical patient.

Pulmonary Thromboembolism

Although not an injury to the lungs occurring as a direct result of CPB itself, deep vein thrombosis (DVT) and pulmonary embolism occur with regular frequency in the cardiac surgical population. The incidence of pulmonary embolism after cardiac surgery ranges from 0.3% to 9.5%, with a mortality rate approaching 20%. The incidence of pulmonary embolism appears to be lower after valve surgery compared with CABG, which may be due to the anticoagulation that is started soon after valve surgery.

The incidence of DVT is 17% to 46%, and most cases are asymptomatic. The higher incidences were reported from series that used lower extremity ultrasound to examine entire populations. DVT has been reported for the leg from which the saphenous vein grafts were harvested and for the contralateral leg.

BOX 23-5 *Strategies to Protect the Lungs*

- Reduced F_IO_2 during bypass
- Low postoperative tidal volume
- Corticosteroid avoidance
- Nitric oxide (?)

Pulmonary Protection

Ventilatory Strategies

Several studies have examined the use of continuous positive airway pressure (CPAP) during CPB as a means to minimize some of the changes in the A-a Do_2 gradient that occur after surgery. Overall, it is unlikely that CPAP plays any major role in preventing or treating the pulmonary dysfunction that occurs in the setting of cardiac surgery.

The inspired oxygen content of the gases that the lungs see during the period of apnea during CPB may have an effect on the A-a Do_2 gradient, probably because of the enhanced effect of higher F_IO_2 on the ability of atelectasis (so-called absorption atelectasis) on these gradients. With these findings in mind, it would be prudent to reduce the F_IO_2 to room air levels during CPB. Several simple therapies can be introduced before separation from CPB, including adequate tracheobronchial toilet and the delivery of several vital capacity breaths that may reduce the amount of atelectasis that has occurred during bypass (Box 23-5).

SUMMARY

- Understanding organ dysfunction produced by cardiopulmonary bypass (CPB) and organ protection strategies is important.
- Central nervous system injury from CPB ranges from neurocognitive deficits in 25% to 80% of patients to stroke in 1% to 5% of patients.
- Advanced age is the most important risk factor for stroke and neurocognitive dysfunction after CPB.
- Acute renal injury from CPB can contribute directly to poor outcomes.
- Drugs such as dopamine and diuretics do not prevent renal failure after CPB.
- Myocardial stunning represents injury caused by short periods of myocardial ischemia that can occur with CPB.
- Blood cardioplegia has the potential advantage of delivering oxygen to ischemic myocardium, whereas crystalloid cardioplegia does not carry much oxygen.
- Gastrointestinal complications after CPB include pancreatitis, gastrointestinal bleeding, bowel infarction, and cholecystitis.
- Pulmonary complications such as atelectasis and pleural effusions are common after cardiac surgery with CPB.
- Organ dysfunction cannot definitively be prevented with off-pump cardiac surgery.

REFERENCES

1. Newman MF, Grocott HP, Mathew JP, et al: Report of the substudy assessing the impact of neurocognitive function on quality of life 5 years after cardiac surgery. Stroke 32:2874, 2001
2. Arrowsmith JE, Grocott HP, Reves JG, et al: Central nervous system complications of cardiac surgery. Br J Anaesth 84:378, 2000

3. Djaiani G, Fedorko L, Borger M, et al: Mild to moderate atheromatous disease of the thoracic aorta and new ischemic brain lesions after conventional coronary artery bypass graft surgery. Stroke 35:e356, 2004
4. Bar-Yosef S, Anders M, Mackensen GB, et al: Aortic atheroma burden and cognitive dysfunction after coronary artery bypass graft surgery. Ann Thorac Surg 78:1556, 2004
5. Duebener LF, Hagino I, Sakamoto T, et al: Effects of pH management during deep hypothermic bypass on cerebral microcirculation: Alpha-stat versus pH-stat. Circulation 106(suppl 1):I103, 2002
6. Chaney MA, Nikolov MP, Blakeman BP, et al: Attempting to maintain normoglycemia during cardiopulmonary bypass with insulin may initiate postoperative hypoglycemia. Anesth Analg 89:1091, 1999
7. Stafford-Smith M, Phillips-Bute B, Reddan DN, et al: The association of postoperative peak and fractional change in serum creatinine with mortality after coronary bypass surgery. Anesthesiology 93:A240, 2000
8. Ostermann ME, Taube D, Morgan CJ, et al: Acute renal failure following cardiopulmonary bypass: A changing picture. Intensive Care Med 26:565, 2000
9. Sreeram GM, Grocott HP, White WD, et al: Transcranial Doppler emboli count predicts rise in creatinine after coronary artery bypass graft surgery. J Cardiothorac Vasc Anesth 18:548, 2004
10. Stafford-Smith M, Phillips-Bute B, Reddan DN, et al: The association of epsilon-aminocaproic acid with postoperative decrease in creatinine clearance in 1502 coronary bypass patients. Anesth Analg 91:1085, 2000
11. Mangano DT, Tudor JC, Dietzel C, et al: The risk associated with aprotinin in cardiac surgery. N Engl J Med 354:353, 2006
12. Bellomo R, Chapman M, Finfer S, et al: Low-dose dopamine in patients with early renal dysfunction: A placebo-controlled randomised trial. Australia and New Zealand Intensive Care Society (ANZICS) Clinical Trials Group. Lancet 356:2139, 2000
13. Landoni G, Biondi-Zoccai G, Marino G, et al: Fenoldopam reduces the need for renal replacement therapy and in-hospital death in cardiovascular surgery: A meta-analysis. J Cardiothorac Vasc Anesth 22:27, 2008
14. Chaitman BR: A review of the GUARDIAN trial results: Clinical implications and the significance of elevated perioperative CK-MB on 6-month survival. J Card Surg 18(suppl 1):13, 2003
15. Ferguson TB Jr, Hammill BG, Peterson ED, et al: A decade of change-risk profiles and outcomes for isolated coronary artery bypass grafting procedures. 1990-1999: A report from the STS National Database Committee and the Duke Clinical Research Institute. Society of Thoracic Surgeons. Ann Thorac Surg 73:480, 2002
16. Vinten-Johansen J, Thourani VH: Myocardial protection: An overview. J Extra Corpor Technol 32:38, 2000
17. Flack JE 3rd, Cook JR, May SJ, et al: Does cardioplegia type affect outcome and survival in patients with advanced left ventricular dysfunction? Results from the CABG Patch Trial. Circulation 102(suppl 3): III-84, 2000
18. McSweeney ME, Garwood S, Levin J, et al: Adverse gastrointestinal complications after cardiopulmonary bypass: Can outcome be predicted from preoperative risk factors? Anesth Analg 98:1610, 2004
19. Hessel EA 2nd: Abdominal organ injury after cardiac surgery. Semin Cardiothorac Vasc Anesth 8:243, 2004
20. Sanisoglu I, Guden M, Bayramoglu Z, et al: Does off-pump CABG reduce gastrointestinal complications? Ann Thorac Surg 77:619, 2004
21. Weissman C: Pulmonary complications after cardiac surgery. Semin Cardiothorac Vasc Anesth 8:185, 2004

23

Chapter 24

Transfusion Medicine and Coagulation Disorders

Bruce D. Spiess, MD • Jan Horrow, MD • Joel A. Kaplan, MD

Coagulation and bleeding assume particular importance when operations are performed on the heart using extracorporeal circulation. This chapter begins with a discussion of the depth and breadth of hemostasis relating to cardiac procedures, beginning with coagulation pathophysiology. The pharmacology of heparin and protamine is described next. This background is then applied to treatment of the bleeding patient.

OVERVIEW OF HEMOSTASIS

Proper hemostasis requires the participation of innumerable biological elements (Box 24-1). They can be divided into four topics to facilitate understanding: coagulation factors, platelet function, the endothelium, and fibrinolysis. The reader must realize this is for simplicity of learning and that in biology the activation creates many reactions and control mechanisms, all interacting simultaneously. The interaction of the platelets, endothelial cells, and proteins to either activate or deactivate coagulation is a highly buffered and controlled process. It is perhaps easiest to think of coagulation as a wave of biological activity occurring at the site of tissue injury (Fig. 24-1). Although there are subcomponents to coagulation itself the injury/control leading to hemostasis is a four-part event: initiation, acceleration, control, and lysis (recanalization/fibrinolysis). The initiation phase begins with tissue damage, which is really begun with endothelial cell destruction or dysfunction. This initiation

BOX 24-1 *Components of Hemostasis*

- Coagulation factor activation
- Platelet function
- Vascular endothelium
- Fibrinolysis and modulators of coagulation

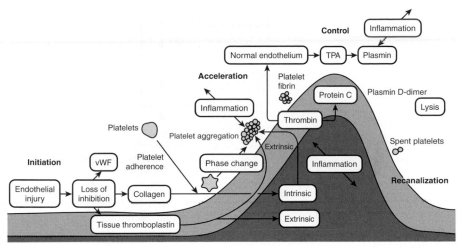

Figure 24-1 Coagulation is a sine wave of activity at the site of tissue injury. It goes through four stages: initiation, acceleration, control, and lysis/recanalization. (Redrawn with permission from Spiess BD: Coagulation function and monitoring. In Lichtor JL [ed]: Atlas of Clinical Anesthesia. Philadelphia, Current Medicine, 1996.)

phase leads to binding of platelets, as well as protein activations; both happen nearly simultaneously and each has feedbacks into the other. Platelets adhere and create an activation or acceleration phase that gathers many cells to the site of injury and creates a large number of biochemical protein cascade events. As the activation phase ramps up into an explosive set of reactions, counter-reactions are spun off, leading to control proteins damping the reactions. The surrounding normal endothelium exerts control over the reactions. Eventually the control reactions overpower the acceleration reactions and lysis comes into play.

The other key concept is that hemostasis is part of a larger body system—inflammation. Most of the protein reactions of coagulation control have importance in signaling inflammation and other healing mechanisms. It is no wonder that cardiopulmonary bypass (CPB) has such profound inflammatory effects when it is considered that each of the activated coagulation proteins and cell lines then feeds into upregulation of inflammation.

Protein Coagulation Activations

Coagulation Pathways

The coagulation factors participate in a series of activating and feedback inhibition reactions, ending with the formation of an insoluble clot. A *clot* is the total of platelet-to-platelet interactions leading to the formation of a platelet plug and then the

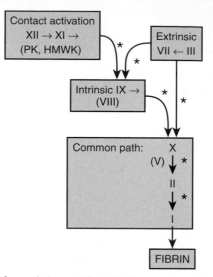

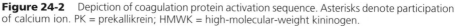

Figure 24-2   Depiction of coagulation protein activation sequence. Asterisks denote participation of calcium ion. PK = prekallikrein; HMWK = high-molecular-weight kininogen.

cross-linking of platelets to each other by way of the final insoluble fibrin that leads to a stable clot. Clotting is not simply the activation of proteins leading to more protein deposition.

With few exceptions, the coagulation factors are glycoproteins synthesized in the liver, which circulate as inactive molecules termed *zymogens*. Factor activation proceeds sequentially, with each factor serving as substrate in an enzymatic reaction catalyzed by the previous factor in the sequence. Hence, this has classically been called a "cascade" or "waterfall" sequence. Cleavage of a polypeptide fragment changes an inactive zymogen to an active enzyme. The active form is termed a *serine protease* because the active site for its protein-splitting activity is a serine amino acid residue. Many reactions require the presence of calcium ion (Ca^{2+}) and a phospholipid surface (platelet phosphatidylserine). The phospholipids occur most often either on the surface of an activated platelet or endothelial cell and occasionally on the surface of white cells. So anchored, their proximity to one another permits reaction rates profoundly accelerated (up to 300,000-fold) from those measured when the enzymes remain in solution. The factors form four interrelated arbitrary groups (Fig. 24-2): the contact activation and the intrinsic, extrinsic, and common pathways.

CONTACT ACTIVATION

Factor XII, high-molecular-weight kininogen (HMWK), prekallikrein (PK), and factor XI form the contact, or surface, activation group. Because factor XII autoactivates by undergoing a shape change in the presence of a negative charge, in vitro coagulation tests use glass, silica, kaolin, and other compounds with negative surface charge. One potential in vivo mechanism for factor XII activation is disruption of the endothelial cell layer, which exposes the underlying negatively charged collagen matrix. Activated platelets also provide negative charges on their membrane surfaces. HMWK anchors the other surface activation molecules, PK and factor XI, to damaged endothelium or activated platelets. Factor XIIa cleaves both factor XI, to form factor XIa, and PK, to form kallikrein.

INTRINSIC SYSTEM

Intrinsic activation forms factor XIa from the products of surface activation. Factor XIa splits factor IX to form factor IXa, with Ca^{2+} required for this process. Then factor IXa activates factor X with help from Ca^{2+}, a phospholipid surface (platelet), and a glycoprotein cofactor, factor VIIIa.

EXTRINSIC SYSTEM

Activation of factor X can proceed independently of factor XII by substances classically thought to be extrinsic to the vasculature. Any number of endothelial cell insults can lead to the production of tissue factor by the endothelial cell. At rest, the endothelial cell is very antithrombotic. However, with ischemia, reperfusion, sepsis, or cytokines, the endothelial cell will stimulate its production of intracellular NFκb and send messages for the production of messenger RNA for tissue factor production. This can happen quickly, and the resting endothelial cell can turn out large amounts of tissue factor. It is widely held today that the activation of tissue factor is what drives many of the abnormalities of coagulation after cardiac surgery, rather than contact activation.[1] Thromboplastin, also known as tissue factor, released from tissues into the vasculature, acts as a cofactor for initial activation of factor X by factor VII. Factors VII and X then activate one another with the help of platelet phospholipid and Ca^{2+}, thus rapidly generating factor Xa. Factor VIIa also activates factor IX, thus linking the extrinsic and intrinsic paths.

COMMON PATHWAY

Factor Xa splits prothrombin (factor II) to thrombin (factor IIa). The combination of factors Xa, Va, and Ca^{2+} is termed the *prothrombinase complex*. Factor Xa anchors to the membrane surface (of platelets) via Ca^{2+}. Factor Va, assembling next to it, initiates a rearrangement of the complex, vastly accelerating binding of the substrate, prothrombin. Most likely, the factor Xa formed from the previous reaction is channeled along the membrane to this next reaction step without detaching from the membrane.

Thrombin cleaves the fibrinogen molecule to form soluble fibrin monomer and polypeptide fragments termed *fibrinopeptides A* and *B*. Fibrin monomers associate to form a soluble fibrin matrix. Factor XIII, activated by thrombin, cross-links these fibrin strands to form an insoluble clot. Patients with lower levels of factor XIII have been found to have more bleeding after cardiac surgery.

VITAMIN K

Those factors that require calcium (II, VII, IX, X) depend on vitamin K to add between 9 and 12 γ-carboxyl groups to glutamic acid residues near their amino termini. Calcium tethers the negatively charged carboxyl groups to the phospholipid surface (platelets), thus facilitating molecular interactions. Some inhibitory proteins also depend on vitamin K (proteins C and S).

Modulators of the Coagulation Pathway

Thrombin, the most important coagulation modulator, exerts a pervasive influence throughout the coagulation factor pathways. It activates factors V, VIII, and XIII; cleaves fibrinogen to fibrin; stimulates platelet recruitment and chemotaxis of leukocytes and monocytes; releases tissue plasminogen activator (t-PA), prostacyclin, and nitric oxide from endothelial cells; releases interleukin-1 from macrophages; and with thrombomodulin, activates protein C, a substance that then inactivates factors Va and VIIIa. Note the negative feedback aspect of this last action. The latest thinking on coagulation function centers around the effects of thrombin. The platelets, tissue

24

factor, and contact activation all are interactive and are activated by a rent in the surface of the endothelium or through the loss of endothelial coagulation control. Platelets adhere to a site of injury and in turn are activated, leading to sequestration of other platelets. It is the interaction of all of those factors together that eventually creates a critical mass. Once enough platelets are interacting together, with their attached surface concomitant serine protease reactions, then a thrombin burst is created. Only when enough thrombin activation has been encountered in a critical time point, then a threshold is exceeded, and the reactions become massive and much larger than the sum of the whole. It is thought that the concentration and ability of platelets to react fully affect the ability to have a critical thrombin burst. CPB may affect the ability to get that full thrombin burst due to its effects on platelet number, platelet-to-platelet interactions, and the decreased amounts of protein substrates.

The many serine proteases that compose the coagulation pathways are balanced by serine protease inhibitors, termed *serpins.* This biological yin and yang leads to an excellent buffering capacity. It is only when the platelet-driven thrombin burst so overwhelms the body's localized anticoagulation or inhibitors that clot proceeds forward. Serpins include α_1-antitrypsin, α_2-macroglobulin, heparin cofactor II, α_2-antiplasmin, antithrombin (also termed antithrombin III), and others.

Antithrombin (ATIII) constitutes the most important inhibitor of blood coagulation. It binds to the active site (serine) of thrombin, thus inhibiting thrombin's action. It also inhibits, to a much lesser extent, the activity of factors XIIa, XIa, IXa, and Xa; kallikrein; and the fibrinolytic molecule plasmin. Thrombin bound to fibrin is protected from the action of antithrombin, thus explaining the poor efficacy of heparin in treating established thrombosis. ATIII is a relatively inactive zymogen. To be most effective antithrombin must bind to a unique pentasaccharide sequence contained on the wall of endothelial cells in the glycosaminoglycan surface known as heparan; the same active sequence is present in the drug heparin. An important note is that activated ATIII is active only against free thrombin. Most thrombin in its active form is either bound to glycoprotein-binding sites of platelets or in fibrin matrices. When blood is put into a test tube and clot begins to form (e.g., in an activated coagulation time [ACT]), 96% of thrombin production is yet to come. The vast majority of thrombin generation is on the surface of platelets and on clot-held fibrinogen. Platelets through their glycoprotein-binding sites and phospholipid folds protect activated thrombin from attack by ATIII. Therefore, the biological role of ATIII is to create an anticoagulant surface on endothelial cells. It is not present biologically to sit and wait for a dose of heparin before CPB.

Another serpin, *protein C,* degrades factors Va and VIIIa. Like other vitamin K–dependent factors, it requires Ca^{2+} to bind to phospholipid. Its cofactor, termed *protein S,* also exhibits vitamin K dependence. Genetic variants of protein C are less active and lead to increased risk for deep vein thrombosis and pulmonary embolism. When endothelial cells release thrombomodulin, thrombin then accelerates by 20,000-fold its activation of protein C. Activated protein C also promotes fibrinolysis.

Regulation of the extrinsic limb of the coagulation pathway occurs via tissue factor pathway inhibitor (TFPI), a glycosylated protein that associates with lipoproteins in plasma.[2] TFPI is not a serpin. It impairs the catalytic properties of the factor VIIa/tissue factor complex on factor X activation. Both vascular endothelium and platelets appear to produce TFPI. Heparin releases TFPI from endothelium, increasing TFPI plasma concentrations by as much as sixfold.[2]

von Willebrand factor (vWF), a massive molecule composed of disulfide-linked glycosylated peptides, associates with factor VIII in plasma, protecting it from proteolytic enzymes. It circulates in the plasma in its coiled inactive form. Disruption of the endothelium either allows for binding of vWF from the plasma or allows for

V

expression of vWF from tissue and from endothelial cells. Once bound, vWF uncoils to its full length and exposes a hitherto cryptic domain in the molecule. This A-1 domain has a very high affinity for platelet glycoproteins. Initially, vWF attaches to the GPIα platelet receptor, which slows platelet shear forces. This is not enough to bind the platelet, but it creates a membrane signal that allows for early shape change and expression of other glycoproteins, GPIb and GPIIb/IIIa. Then, secondary GPIb binding connects to other vWF nearby, binding the platelet and beginning the activation sequence. It bridges normal platelets to damaged subendothelium by attaching to the GPIb platelet receptor. An ensuing platelet shape change then releases thromboxane, β-thromboglobulin, and serotonin and exposes GPIIb/IIIa, which binds fibrinogen.

Platelet Function

Most clinicians think first of the coagulation proteins when considering hemostasis. Although no one element of the many that participate in hemostasis assumes dominance, platelets may be the most complex. Without platelets, there is no coagulation and no hemostasis. Without the proteins, there is hemostasis, but it lasts only 10 to 15 minutes as the platelet plug is inherently unstable and breaks apart under the shear stress of the vasculature. Platelets provide phospholipid for coagulation factor reactions; contain their own microskeletal system and coagulation factors; secrete active substances affecting themselves, other platelets, the endothelium, and other coagulation factors; and alter shape to expose membrane glycoproteins essential to hemostasis. Platelets have perhaps as many as 30 to 50 different types of cell receptors. The initial response to vascular injury is formation of a platelet plug. Good hemostatic response depends on proper functioning of platelet adhesion, activation, and aggregation (Fig. 24-3).

Platelet Adhesion

Capillary blood exhibits laminar flow, which maximizes the likelihood of interaction of platelets with the vessel wall. Red cells and white cells stream near the center of the vessels and marginate platelets. However, turbulence causes reactions in endothelium that leads to the secretion of vWF, adhesive molecules, and tissue factor. Shear stress is high as fast-moving platelets interact with the endothelium. When the vascular endothelium becomes denuded or injured, the platelet has the opportunity to contact vWF, which is bound to the exposed collagen of the subendothelium. A platelet membrane component, glycoprotein (GP)Ib, attaches to vWF, thus anchoring the platelet to the vessel wall. Independently, platelet membrane GPIa and GPIIa and IX may attach directly to exposed collagen, furthering the adhesion stage.

The integrin glycoproteins form diverse types of membrane receptors from combinations of 20 α and 8 β subunits. One such combination is GPIIb/IIIa, a platelet membrane component that initially participates in platelet adhesion. Platelet activation causes a conformational change in GPIIb/IIIa, which results in its aggregator activity.

Platelet adhesion begins rapidly—within 1 minute of endothelial injury—and completely covers exposed subendothelium within 20 minutes. It begins with decreased platelet velocity when GPIb/IX and vWF mediate adhesion, followed by platelet activation, GPIIb/IIIa conformational change, and then vWF binding and platelet arrest on the endothelium at these vWF ligand sites.[3]

Platelet Activation and Aggregation

Platelet activation results after contact with collagen, when adenosine diphosphate (ADP), thrombin, or thromboxane A_2 binds to membrane receptors, or from certain platelet-to-platelet interactions. Platelets then release the contents of their dense (δ)

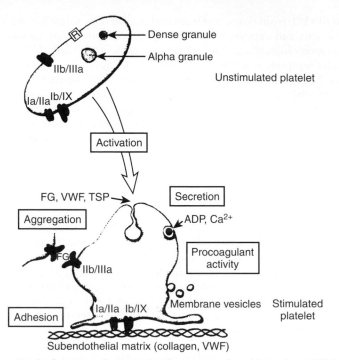

Figure 24-3   Platelet function in hemostasis. Glycoproteins Ib and IX and von Willebrand factor (vWF) mediate adhesion to the vessel wall. Glycoproteins IIb and IIIa and integrin molecules fibrinogen (FG) and thrombospondin (TSP) mediate platelet aggregation. (From George J, Shattil SJ: The clinical importance of acquired abnormalities of platelet function. N Engl J Med 324:27, 1991.)

granules and α granules. Dense granules contain serotonin, ADP, and Ca^{2+}; α granules contain platelet factor V (previously termed platelet factor 1), β-thromboglobulin, platelet factor 4, P-selectin, and various integrin proteins (vWF, fibrinogen, vitronectin, and fibronectin). Simultaneously, platelets employ their microskeletal system to change shape from a disk to a sphere, which changes platelet membrane GPIIb/IIIa exposure. Released ADP recruits additional platelets to the site of injury and stimulates platelet G protein, which in turn activates membrane phospholipase. This results in the formation of arachidonate, which platelet cyclooxygenase converts to thromboxane A_2. Other platelet agonists besides ADP and collagen include serotonin, a weak agonist, and thrombin and thromboxane A_2, both potent agonists. Thrombin is by far the most potent platelet agonist, and it can overcome all other platelet antagonists as well as inhibitors. In total, there are more than 70 agonists that can produce platelet activation and aggregation.

Agonists induce a shape change, increase platelet intracellular Ca^{2+} concentration, and stimulate platelet G protein. In addition, serotonin and thromboxane A_2 are potent vasoconstrictors. The presence of sufficient agonist material results in platelet aggregation. Aggregation occurs when the integrin proteins (mostly fibrinogen) released from α granules form molecular bridges between the GPIIb/IIIa receptors of adjacent platelets (the final common platelet pathway).

Prostaglandins and Aspirin

Endothelial cell cyclooxygenase synthesizes prostacyclin, which inhibits aggregation and dilates vessels. Platelet cyclooxygenase forms thromboxane A_2, a potent aggregating agent and vasoconstrictor. Aspirin irreversibly acetylates cyclooxygenase, rendering it inactive. Low doses of aspirin, 80 to 100 mg, easily overcome the finite amount of cyclooxygenase available in the nucleus-free platelets. However, endothelial cells can synthesize new cyclooxygenase. Thus, with low doses of aspirin, prostacyclin synthesis continues while thromboxane synthesis ceases, decreasing platelet activation and aggregation. High doses of aspirin inhibit the enzyme at both cyclooxygenase sites.

Reversible platelet aggregation is blocked by aspirin, as the platelet cyclooxygenase is inhibited. However, the more powerful agonists that yield the calcium release response can still aggregate and activate platelets, because cyclooxygenase is not required for those pathways.

Drug-Induced Platelet Abnormalities

Many other agents inhibit platelet function.[4] β-Lactam antibiotics coat the platelet membrane, whereas the cephalosporins are rather profound but short-term platelet inhibitors. Many cardiac surgeons may not realize that their standard drug regimen for antibiotics may be far more of a bleeding risk than aspirin. Hundreds of drugs can inhibit platelet function. Calcium channel blockers, nitrates, and β-blockers are ones commonly utilized in cardiac surgery. Nitrates are effective antiplatelet agents and that may be part of why they are of such benefit in angina, not just for their vaso-relaxing effect on large blood vessels. Nonsteroidal anti-inflammatory drugs (NSAIDs) reversibly inhibit both endothelial cell and platelet cyclooxygenase.

In addition to the partial inhibitory effects of aspirin and the other drugs just mentioned, new therapies have been developed that inhibit platelet function in a more specific manner. These drugs include platelet adhesion inhibitor agents, platelet-ADP-receptor antagonists, and GPIIb/IIIa receptor inhibitors (Table 24-1).

ADHESION INHIBITORS

Dipyridamole (Persantine) and cilostazol (Pletal) alter platelet adhesion by various mechanisms, including cyclic adenosine monophosphate (cAMP), phosphodiesterase III, and thromboxane A_2 inhibition. Dipyridamole has been used with warfarin in some patients with artificial valves and with aspirin in patients with peripheral vascular disease.

ADP RECEPTOR ANTAGONISTS

Clopidogrel (Plavix) and ticlopidine (Ticlid) are thienopyridine derivatives that inhibit the ADP receptor pathway to platelet activation. They have a slow onset of action because they must be converted to active drugs, and their potent effects last the lifetime of the platelets affected (5 to 10 days). Clopidogrel is the preferred drug because it has a better safety record than ticlopidine. It is administered orally once daily to inhibit platelet function and is quite effective in decreasing myocardial infarctions after percutaneous coronary interventions (PCIs). The combination of aspirin and clopidogrel has led to increased bleeding, but it is sometimes used in an effort to keep vessels and stents open. The thromboelastogram (TEG) with ADP added can be used to determine the degree of inhibition due to these drugs.

GPIIB/IIIA RECEPTOR INHIBITORS

These are the most potent (>90% platelet inhibition) and important platelet inhibitors because they act at the final common pathway of platelet aggregation with fibrinogen, no matter which agonist began the process. All of the drugs mentioned earlier work at earlier phases of activation of platelet function. These drugs are all administered by intravenous infusion, and they do not work orally. The GPIIb/IIIa inhibitors are often used in patients taking aspirin because they do not block thromboxane A_2 production.

24

Table 24-1 **Antiplatelet Therapy**

Drug Type	Composition	Mechanism	Indications	Route	Half-life	Metabolism
Aspirin	Acetylsalicylic acid	Irreversible COX inhibition	CAD, AMI, PVD, PCI, ACS	Oral	10 days	Liver, kidney
NSAIDs	Multiple	Reversible COX inhibition	Pain	Oral	2 days	Liver, kidney
Adhesion inhibitors (e.g., dipyridamole)	Multiple	Block adhesion to vessels	VHD, PVD	Oral	12 hr	Liver
ADP receptor antagonists (e.g., clopidogrel)	Thienopyridines	Irreversible inhibition of ADP binding	AMI, CVA, PVD, ACS, PCI	Oral	5 days	Liver
GPIIb/IIIa receptor inhibitors						
Abciximab (ReoPro)	Monoclonal antibody	Nonspecific—binds to other receptors	PCI, ACS	IV	12-18 hr	Plasma proteinase
Eptifibatide (Integrilin)	Peptide	Reversible—specific to GPIIb/IIIa	PCI, ACS	IV	2-4 hr	Kidney
Tirofiban (Aggrastat)	Nonpeptide-tyrosine derivative	Reversible—specific to GPIIb/IIIa	PCI, ACS	IV	2-4 hr	Kidney

COX = cyclooxygenase; CAD = coronary artery disease; AMI = acute myocardial infarction; PVD = peripheral vascular disease; PCI = percutaneous coronary intervention; ACS = acute coronary syndrome; VHD = valvular heart disease; CVA = cerebrovascular disease; IV = intravenous; ADP = adenosine diphosphate; GP = glycoprotein.

V

The dose of heparin is usually reduced when used with these drugs. Platelet activity can be monitored to determine the extent of blockade. Excessive bleeding requires allowing the short-acting drugs to wear off, while possibly administering platelets to patients receiving the long-acting drug abciximab. Most studies have found increased bleeding in patients receiving these drugs who required emergency CABG.

Vascular Endothelium

The cells that form the intima of vessels provide an excellent nonthrombogenic surface. Characteristics of this surface, which may account for its nonthrombogenicity, include negative charge; incorporation of heparan sulfate in the grid substance; the release of prostacyclin, nitric oxide, adenosine, and protease inhibitors by endothelial cells; binding and clearance of activated coagulation factors both directly, as occurs with thrombin, and indirectly, as evidenced by the action of thrombomodulin to inactivate factors Va and VIIIa via protein C; and stimulation of fibrinolysis.

Nitric oxide vasodilates blood vessels and inhibits platelets. Its mechanism involves activation of guanylate cyclase with eventual uptake of calcium into intracellular storage sites. Prostacyclin (PGI_2) possesses powerful vasodilator and antiplatelet properties. Endothelium-derived prostacyclin opposes the vasoconstrictor effects of platelet-produced thromboxane A_2. Prostacyclin also inhibits platelet aggregation, disaggregates clumped platelets, and, at high concentrations, inhibits platelet adhesion. Prostacyclin increases intracellular concentrations of cAMP, which inhibits aggregation. Thromboxane acts in an opposite manner. The mechanism of prostacyclin action is stimulation of adenylyl cyclase, leading to reduced intracellular calcium concentrations. Some vascular beds (e.g., lung) and atherosclerotic vessels secrete thromboxane, endothelins, and angiotensin, all vasoconstrictors, as well as prostacyclin. Activation of platelets releases endoperoxides and arachidonate. These substances, utilized by nearby damaged endothelial cells, provide substrate for prostacyclin production.

Fibrinolysis

Fibrin breakdown, a normal hematologic activity, is localized to the vicinity of a clot. It remodels formed clot and removes thrombus when endothelium heals. Like clot formation, clot breakdown may occur by intrinsic and extrinsic pathways. As with clot formation, the extrinsic pathway plays the dominant role in clot breakdown. Each pathway activates plasminogen, a serine protease synthesized by the liver, which circulates in zymogen form. Cleavage of plasminogen by the proper serine protease forms plasmin. Plasmin splits fibrinogen or fibrin at specific sites. Plasmin is the principal enzyme of fibrinolysis, just as thrombin is principal to clot formation. Plasma normally contains no circulating plasmin, because a scavenging protein, α_2-antiplasmin, quickly consumes any plasmin formed from localized fibrinolysis. Thus, localized fibrinolysis, not systemic fibrinogenolysis, accompanies normal hemostasis.

Extrinsic Fibrinolysis

Endothelial cells synthesize and release t-PA. Both t-PA and a related substance, urokinase plasminogen activator (u-PA), are serine proteases that split plasminogen to form plasmin. The activity of t-PA magnifies on binding to fibrin. In this manner also, plasmin formation remains localized to sites of clot formation. Epinephrine, bradykinin, thrombin, and factor Xa cause endothelium to release t-PA, as do venous occlusion and CPB.

24

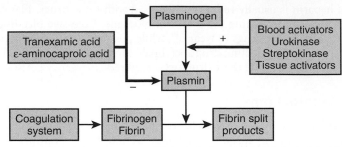

Figure 24-4 The fibrinolytic pathway. Antifibrinolytic drugs inhibit fibrinolysis by binding to both plasminogen and plasmin. Intrinsic blood activators (factor XIIa), extrinsic tissue activators (t-PA, u-PA), and exogenous activators (streptokinase, ASPAC) split plasminogen to form plasmin. (From Horrow JC, Hlavacek J, Strong MD, et al: Prophylactic tranexamic acid decreases bleeding after cardiac operations. J Thorac Cardiovasc Surg 99:70, 1990.)

Intrinsic Fibrinolysis

Factor XIIa, formed during the contact phase of coagulation, cleaves plasminogen to plasmin. The plasmin so formed then facilitates additional cleavage of plasminogen by factor XIIa, forming a positive feedback loop.

Exogenous Activators

Streptokinase (made by bacteria) and urokinase (found in human urine) both cleave plasminogen to plasmin, but do so with low fibrin affinity. Thus, systemic plasminemia and fibrinogenolysis as well as fibrinolysis ensue. Acetylated streptokinase plasminogen activator complex (ASPAC) provides an active site, which is not available until deacetylation occurs in blood. Its systemic lytic activity lies intermediate to those of t-PA and streptokinase. Recombinant t-PA (rt-PA; Alteplase) is a second-generation agent that is made by recombinant DNA technology and is relatively fibrin specific.

Clinical Applications

Figure 24-4 illustrates the fibrinolytic pathway, with activators and inhibitors. Streptokinase, ASPAC, and t-PA find application in the lysis of thrombi associated with myocardial infarction. These intravenous agents "dissolve" clots that form on atheromatous plaque. Clinically significant bleeding may result from administration of any of these exogenous activators or streptokinase.

Fibrinolysis also accompanies CPB. This undesirable breakdown of clot after surgery may contribute to postoperative hemorrhage and the need to administer allogeneic blood products. Regardless of how they are formed, the breakdown products of fibrin intercalate into sheets of normally forming fibrin monomers, thus preventing cross-linking. In this way, extensive fibrinolysis exerts an antihemostatic action.

HEPARIN

Pharmacology

Chemical Structure

The N-sulfated-D-glucosamine and L-iduronic acid residues of heparin alternate in copolymer fashion to form chains of varying length (Fig. 24-5). As a linear anionic polyelectrolyte, with the negative charges being supplied by sulfate groups, heparin demonstrates a wide spectrum of activity with enzymes, hormones, biogenic amines,

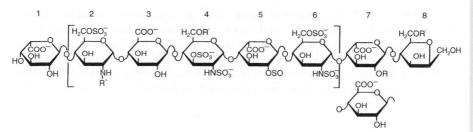

Figure 24-5 An octasaccharide fragment of heparin, a substituted alternating copolymer of iduronic acid and glucosamine. The leftmost sugar is iduronic acid. Note the numerous sulfate groups and the acetyl substitution on the second sugar. Variations in sugar substitutions and in chain length produce molecular heterogeneity. Brackets indicate the pentasaccharide sequence that binds to antithrombin. (From Rodén L: Highlights in the history of heparin. In Lane DA, Lindahl U [eds]: Heparin. Boca Raton, FL, CRC Press, 1989.)

and plasma proteins. A pentasaccharide segment binds to antithrombin. Heparin is a heterogeneous compound: the carbohydrates vary in both length and side chain composition, yielding a range of molecular weights from 5000 to 30,000, with most chains between 12,000 and 19,000. Today, the standard heparin is called unfractionated heparin (UFH).

Source and Biological Role

Heparin is found mostly in the lungs, intestines, and liver of mammals, with skin, lymph nodes, and thymus providing less plentiful sources. Abundance of heparin in tissues rich in mast cells suggests these as the source of the compound. Its presence in tissues with environmental contact suggests a biological role relating to immune function. Heparin may assist white blood cell movements in the interstitium after an immunologic response has been triggered.

Most commercial preparations of heparin now use pig intestine, 40,000 pounds of which yield 5 kg of heparin. Prevention of postoperative thrombosis constituted the initial clinical use of heparin in 1935.

Potency

Heparin potency is determined by comparing the test specimen against a known standard's ability to prolong coagulation. Current United States Pharmacopeia (USP) and British Pharmacopoeia (BP) assays use a PT-like method on pooled sheep's plasma obtained from slaughterhouses.

UFH dose should not be specified by weight (milligrams) because of the diversity of anticoagulant activity expected from so heterogeneous a compound. One USP unit of heparin activity is the quantity that prevents 1.0 mL of citrated sheep's plasma from clotting for 1 hour after addition of calcium. Units cannot be cross-compared among heparins of different sources, such as mucosal versus lung or low-molecular-weight heparin (LMWH) versus UFH or even lot to lot, because the assay used may or may not reflect actual differences in biological activity. None of these measures has anything to do with the effect of a unit on anticoagulation effect for human cardiac surgery.

Pharmacokinetics and Pharmacodynamics

The heterogeneity of UFH molecules produces variability in the relationship of dose administered to plasma level of drug. In addition, the relationship of plasma level to biological effect varies with the test system. A three-compartment model describes

24

heparin kinetics in healthy humans: rapid initial disappearance, saturable clearance observed in the lower dose range, and exponential first-order decay at higher doses. The rapid initial disappearance may arise from endothelial cell uptake. The reticuloendothelial system, with its endoglycosidases and endosulfatases, and uptake into monocytes, may represent the saturable phase of heparin kinetics. Finally, renal clearance via active tubular secretion of heparin, much of it desulfated, explains heparin's exponential clearance.

Male gender and cigarette smoking are associated with more rapid heparin clearance. The resistance of patients with deep vein thrombosis or pulmonary embolism to heparin therapy may be due to the release from thrombi of platelet factor 4 (PF4), a known heparin antagonist. Chronic renal failure prolongs elimination of high, but not low, heparin doses. Chronic liver disease does not change elimination.

Loading doses for CPB (200 to 400 units/kg) are substantially higher than those used to treat venous thrombosis (70 to 150 units/kg). Plasma heparin levels, determined fluorometrically, vary widely (2 to 4 units/mL) after doses of heparin administered to patients about to undergo CPB. The ACT response to these doses of heparin displays even greater dispersion. However, the clinical response to heparin administered to various patients is more consistent than suggested by in vitro measurements.

Actions and Interactions

Heparin exerts its anticoagulant activity via ATIII, one of the many circulating serine protein inhibitors (serpins), which counter the effects of circulating proteases. The major inhibitor of thrombin and factors IXa and Xa is ATIII; that of the contact activation factors XIIa and XIa is α_1-proteinase inhibitor; kallikrein inhibition arises mostly from C1 inhibitor. Antithrombin activity is greatly decreased at a site of vascular damage, underscoring its primary role as a scavenger for clotting enzymes that escape into the general circulation.

Antithrombin inhibits serine proteases even without heparin. The extent to which heparin accelerates antithrombin inhibition depends on the substrate enzyme: UFH accelerates the formation of the thrombin-antithrombin complex by 2000-fold but accelerates formation of the factor Xa-antithrombin complex by only 1200-fold. In contrast, LMWH fragments preferentially inhibit factor Xa. Enzyme inhibition proceeds by formation of a ternary complex consisting of heparin, antithrombin, and the proteinase to be inhibited (e.g., thrombin, factor Xa). For UFH, inhibition of thrombin occurs only on simultaneous binding to both antithrombin and thrombin. This condition requires a heparin fragment of at least 18 residues. A pentasaccharide sequence binds to antithrombin. LMWHs, consisting of chains 8 to 16 units long, preferentially inhibit factor Xa. In this case, the heparin fragment activates antithrombin, which then sequentially inactivates factor Xa; heparin and factor Xa do not directly interact (Fig. 24-6).

Several investigators have demonstrated continued formation of fibrinopeptides A and B, and prothrombin fragment F1.2 and thrombin-antithrombin complexes, despite clearly acceptable anticoagulation for CPB by many criteria. These substances indicate thrombin activity. The clinical significance of this ongoing thrombin activity has had limited study. The ACT must be more prolonged to prevent fibrin formation during cardiac surgery compared with during extracorporeal circulation without surgery, because surgery itself incites coagulation. UFH in conjunction with antithrombin appears to work in plasma only on free thrombin. When considering what is known today about thrombin burst and thrombin activity, heparin appears to be relatively inefficient, because there is not much free thrombin. Thrombin is held on the surface of activated platelets at various glycoprotein binding sites including the GPIIb/IIIa site. Most thrombin

V

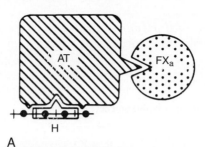

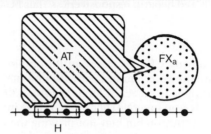

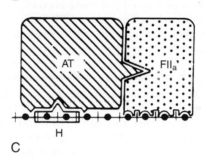

Figure 24-6   Antithrombin interaction (AT) with factor Xa may occur with either low-molecular-weight heparin (H) (**A**) or standard unfractionated heparin (**B**). Inhibition of thrombin (factor IIa), however, requires simultaneous binding of the heparin molecule to both antithrombin and thrombin (**C**). (From Holmer E, Soderberg K, Bergqvist D, Lindahl U: Heparin and its low-molecular-weight derivatives: Anticoagulant and antithrombotic properties. Haemostasis 16[suppl 2]:1, 1986.)

is fibrin bound, and heparin-antithrombin complexes do not bind at all to this thrombin unless the level of heparin is pushed far above what is used routinely for CPB. The idea behind using heparin for CPB is that by creating a large circulating concentration of activated antithrombin, whenever a thrombin molecule is produced, an available antithrombin molecule will be there to immediately bind to it before it can have any further activating effect. Clearly, that is unrealistic with the knowledge that thrombin exerts its main activity by binding to the surface of platelets.

Heparin Resistance

Patients receiving UFH infusions exhibit a much diminished ACT response to full anticoagulating doses of UFH for CPB (200 to 400 units/kg). With widespread use of heparin infusions to treat myocardial ischemia and infarction, heparin resistance or,

---

BOX 24-2 *Problems with Heparin as an Anticoagulant for Cardiopulmonary Bypass*

- Heparin resistance
- Heparin-induced thrombocytopenia
- Heparin rebound
- Heparin's heterogeneity and variable potency

---

more appropriately, "altered heparin responsiveness" has become more problematic during cardiac surgery (Box 24-2).[5]

Mechanism

Hemodilution accompanying CPB decreases antithrombin levels to about half of normal levels. There are, however, outlier patients who have profoundly low antithrombin levels. It is possible to see ATIII levels as low as 20% of normal, and these levels correspond to levels seen in septic shock and diffuse intravascular coagulation. However, supplemental antithrombin may not prolong the ACT, which means that the heparin available has been bound to sufficient or available antithrombin. The only way that the ACT would be prolonged is if there is excess heparin beyond available antithrombin. Reports of heparin resistance for CPB ascribe its occurrence variously to the use of autotransfusion, previous heparin therapy, infection, and ventricular aneurysm with thrombus.

The individual anticoagulant response to heparin varies tremendously. Some presumed cases of heparin resistance may represent nothing more than this normal variation. Regardless of cause, measurement of each individual's anticoagulant response to heparin therapy for CPB is warranted. Heparin resistance helps focus the debate regarding whether anticoagulation monitoring should measure heparin concentrations or heparin effect: the goal of anticoagulation is not to achieve heparin presence in plasma but to inhibit the action of thrombin on fibrinogen, platelets, and endothelial cells. Therefore, heparin effect is usually measured.

Treatment

Most commonly, additional heparin prolongs the ACT sufficiently for the conduct of CPB. Amounts up to 800 units/kg may be necessary to obtain an ACT of 400 to 480 seconds or longer. Whereas administration of fresh frozen plasma (FFP), which contains antithrombin, should correct antithrombin depletion and suitably prolong the ACT, such exposure to transfusion-borne infectious diseases should be avoided whenever possible. This modality is reserved for the rare refractory case. Rather than administer FFP, centers normally accepting only ACTs of 480 seconds or longer for CPB might consider accepting 400 seconds or less, or administering ATIII concentrate.

Antithrombin concentrate specifically addresses antithrombin deficiency. It is a solvent detergent-treated and heat-inactivated product providing greater protection against infectious disease transmission than that provided by FFP. The literature supports its success in treating heparin resistance during cardiac surgery. A multicenter study on the efficacy of using a recombinant human antithrombin (rhAT) in heparin-resistant patients undergoing CPB was published.[6] The patients received 75 units/kg of rhAT, which was effective in restoring heparin responsiveness in most patients. However, some patients still required FFP and the patients bled more than did a control group postoperatively.

V

> **BOX 24-3** *Considerations in Determining the Proper Dose of Protamine to Reverse Heparin*
>
> - The proper dose is very broad and difficult to know exactly.
> - The dose should be determined by a measurement of coagulation.
> - The dose should be administered over at least 10 minutes.

Heparin Rebound

Several hours after protamine neutralization for cardiac surgery, some patients develop clinical bleeding associated with prolongation of coagulation times. This phenomenon is often attributed to reappearance of circulating heparin. Theories accounting for "heparin rebound" include late release of heparin sequestered in tissues, delayed return of heparin to the circulation from the extracellular space via lymphatics, clearance of an unrecognized endogenous heparin antagonist, and more rapid clearance of protamine in relation to heparin. Studies demonstrating uptake of heparin into endothelial cells suggest that these cells may slowly release the drug into the circulation once plasma levels decline with protamine neutralization. It is doubtful how much heparin rebound contributes to actual bleeding. This phenomenon may be caused by TFPI release from the surface of endothelial cells or other causes of bleeding.

Treatment and Prevention

Although still debated by a few, most clinicians accept heparin rebound as a real phenomenon. However, clinical bleeding does not always accompany heparin rebound. When it does, administration of supplemental protamine will neutralize the remaining heparin (Box 24-3).

Heparin Effects other Than Anticoagulation

Unfractionated heparin was never biologically intended to circulate freely in plasma.[7] As such it has a number of underappreciated and untoward effects. All too often the effects of CPB have been asserted as causing a coagulopathy; however, the effect of heparin contributing to this has not been widely studied. That is because there has not been an alternative anticoagulant to compare with heparin until now. In the future, there may be better anticoagulants to use during cardiac surgery.

Heparin exerts its anticoagulant activity by activating a binding site on ATIII; and without antithrombin, heparin has no intrinsic anticoagulation effect. Antithrombin does have anticoagulant effects of its own, but its ability to bind to thrombin is increased 100- to 2000-fold by the presence of the pentasaccharide sequence of heparin. Less than one third of all mucopolysaccharides present in a dose of heparin contain the active pentasaccharide sequence. The other molecules may have a number of adverse properties.

UFH chelates calcium. When a large bolus dose of heparin is given, there is a slow and steady decline in blood pressure, probably due to decreased vascular resistance and decreased preload. Both arterial and venous vessels are dilated by the decrease in the calcium level. The heparin is given while patients are being prepared for CPB, and there are numerous mechanical events (i.e., catheters being inserted into the right atrium and vena cava and arrhythmias) that can be blamed for the hypotension, rather than the heparin itself.

24

Heparin is important for a number of angiogenesis and repair activities of tissue, and these effects may have something to do with its antineoplastic effect. Heparin also affects lipid, sodium and potassium, and acid-base metabolism. These effects are not usually seen acutely but come into play when patients have been on heparin infusions for days in the intensive care unit.

The immunologic effects of heparin are profound: 30% to 50% of cardiac surgery patients have heparin antibodies present in their blood by the time of hospital discharge. The clinical implications of these prevalent antibodies remain unknown.

Heparin-Induced Thrombocytopenia

Heparin normally binds to platelet membranes at GPIb and other sites and aggregates normal platelets by releasing ADP. A moderate, reversible, heparin-induced thrombocytopenia (HIT), now termed *type I,* has been known for half a century. The fact that heparin actually triggers an acute drop in platelet count should be considered a biological event, because heparin, even in trace amounts, triggers the expression of many different platelet glycoproteins. Some have termed this *activation* of platelets, but it is not total activation. Heparin's prolongation of the bleeding time is probably related to both activation of the platelets as well as heparin binding to the GPIb surface.

In contrast to these predictable effects of heparin, occasional patients develop progressive and severe thrombocytopenia ($<100,000/mm^3$), sometimes accompanied by a debilitating or fatal thrombosis. This syndrome is termed *type II heparin-induced thrombocytopenia* (HIT II). A platelet count in excess of $100,000/mm^3$ does not mean that HIT II is not present. A drop in platelet count in excess of 30% to 50% over several days in a patient who is receiving or who has just finished receiving heparin is probably HIT II.

Mechanism

These patients demonstrate a heparin-dependent antibody, usually IgG, although others are described, which aggregates platelets in the presence of heparin.[8] During heparin therapy, measured antibody titers remain low, owing to antibody binding to platelets. Titers rise after heparin therapy ceases; but paradoxically, antibody may be undetectable a few months later. Two other features are unexpected: first, the antibody does not aggregate platelets in the presence of excess heparin; and, second, not all reexposed patients develop thrombocytopenia.

The platelet surface contains complexes of heparin and PF4. Affected patients have antibody to this complex. Antibody binding activates platelets via their FcγII receptors and activates endothelium (Fig. 24-7). The activation of the platelet surface triggers a secondary thrombin release. Platelets can attach to each other creating what is known as a white clot syndrome. But if secondary thrombin generation is created through antibody activation of the platelets then a fibrin clot can be the result. In the absence of heparin, the heparin-PF4 antigen cannot form.

In the absence of an endothelial defect, the only responses to the antibody-antigen interaction are platelet consumption and thrombocytopenia. Atheroma rupture, endovascular interventions such as balloon angioplasty, vascular surgery, and other procedures that disrupt endothelium can provide a nidus for platelet adhesion and subsequent activation. PF4, released with platelet activation, binds to heparin locally, thus not only removing the inhibition of coagulation but also generating additional antigenic material (Fig. 24-8). Clumps of aggregated platelets thrombose vessels, resulting in organ and limb infarction. Amputation and/or death often occurs with established HIT with thrombosis (HITT). The presence of heparin-PF4 antibodies

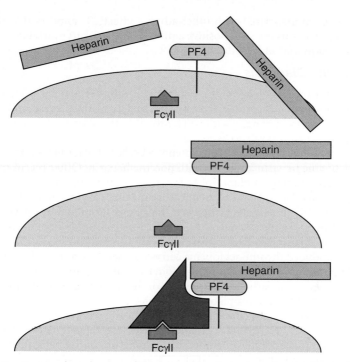

Figure 24-7 Presumed mechanism of the interaction among heparin, platelets, and antibody in heparin-induced thrombocytopenia. **Top,** Platelet factor 4 (PF4) released from platelet granules is bound to the platelet surface. **Middle,** Heparin and PF4 complexes form. **Bottom,** The antibody binds to the PF4-heparin complex and activates platelet FcγII receptors.

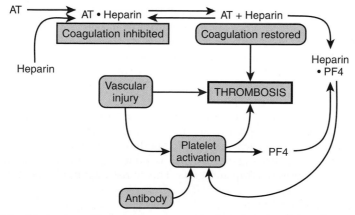

Figure 24-8 Mechanism of thrombosis accompanying heparin-induced thrombocytopenia. Normally, heparin and antithrombin (AT) form a complex that inhibits coagulation. Platelet factor 4 (PF4), released from platelets upon activation, binds heparin and drives the dissociation reaction of the antithrombin-heparin complex to the right, restoring coagulation locally. Restored coagulation mechanisms and activated platelets form thrombus in the presence of vascular injury. (Adapted from Parmet JL, Horrow JC: Hematologic diseases. In Benumof J [ed]: Anesthesia and Uncommon Diseases, 3rd ed. Philadelphia, WB Saunders, 1997.)

24

has recently been associated with other adverse effects. It appears that if a patient undergoes cardiac surgery with positive antibodies, the risk of mortality and/or myocardial infarction may at least double.

Incidence and Diagnosis

Estimates of the true incidence of this syndrome are confounded by different diagnostic thresholds for platelet count, varying efforts to detect other causes, and incomplete reports. After 7 days of therapy with UFH, probably 1% of patients develop HIT; after 14 days of therapy the prevalence is 3%. Using a platelet count of 100,000/mm^3, multiple reports comprising more than 1200 patients revealed an overall incidence of HIT of 5.5% with bovine heparin and 1.0% with porcine heparin. Other recent research has found the preoperative incidence of ELISA-positive patients to be between 6.5% to 10%. This means that antibodies are present and that may not mean that thrombocytopenia is occurring. Of great interest is that many more patients develop positive tests for ELISA antibodies by days 7 to 30 after cardiac surgery. Somewhere between 25% and 50% of patients develop these antibodies.

Heparin-induced thrombocytopenia can occur not only during therapeutic heparin administration but also with low prophylactic doses, although the incidence is dose related. Even heparin flush solution or heparin-bonded intravascular catheters can incite HIT. Cases of platelet-to-platelet adhesion creating a "white clot" in otherwise normal patients have been observed in the oxygenator and the reservoir of CPB machines. The fact that such events have been reported even when all other tests appeared normal signals the unpredictable nature of the heparin-PF4 antibody as well as the biological activity of UFH.

Although HIT usually begins 3 to 15 days (median, 10 days) after heparin infusions commence, it can occur within hours in a patient previously exposed to heparin. Platelet count steadily decreases to a nadir between 20,000 and 150,000/mm^3. Absolute thrombocytopenia is not necessary; only a significant decrease in platelet count matters, as witnessed by patients with thrombocytosis who develop thrombosis with normal platelet counts after prolonged exposure to heparin. Occasionally, thrombocytopenia resolves spontaneously despite continuation of heparin infusion.

Clinical diagnosis of HIT requires a new decrease in platelet count during heparin infusion. Laboratory confirmation is obtained from several available tests. In the serotonin release assay, patient plasma, donor platelets, and heparin are combined. The donor platelets contain radiolabeled serotonin, which is released when donor platelets are activated by the antigen-antibody complex. Measurement of serotonin release during platelet aggregation at both low and high heparin concentrations provides excellent sensitivity and specificity.

A second assay measures more traditional markers of platelet degranulation in a mixture of heparin, patient plasma, and donor platelets. The most specific test is an enzyme-linked immunosorbent assay for antibodies to the heparin-PF4 complex.

Measurement of platelet-associated IgG is poorly specific for HIT, because of numerous other causes of antiplatelet IgG. This test should not be used in the diagnosis of HIT.

Heparin-Induced Thrombocytopenia with Thrombosis

The incidence of HITT is 1.7% with bovine heparin and 0.3% with porcine heparin; thus, thrombosis accompanies more than one in five cases of HIT. It is clear that the longer patients are on heparin the more likely it is that they will develop antibody; and with the knowledge that today close to 50% of cardiac patients develop antibodies, it is possible that a significant number of long-term or early mortalities might be due to undiagnosed HITT. In several studies in the catheterization laboratory, it has been shown that if HITT antibodies are present before the performance of angioplasty, the mortality and combined morbidity are greatly increased, perhaps double or more. One study has been carried out in almost 500 patients undergoing CABG surgery looking for the presence of antibodies and outcome. The incidence of antibody-positive patients was approximately 15%, and their length of stay in the hospital and mortality were more than doubled. Occasional rare situations in which the CPB circuit suddenly clots or when there is early graft thrombosis or whole-body clotting may all be variants of HITT, but none of these cases can be readily studied because they are so rare. If such an occurrence does happen, HITT should be in the differential diagnosis. The occurrence of thrombosis at first seems paradoxical. However, HITT has as its hallmark a huge thrombin burst that can occur all over the body. With such massive thrombin generation the triggering of thrombosis is natural. Thrombosis may then activate the fibrinolytic system to produce a picture of consumptive coagulopathy.

From 15% to 30% of patients who develop HIT with thrombosis will develop severe neurologic complications, require amputation of a limb, or die. Lower limb ischemia constitutes the most frequent presentation. Venous clots occur probably as frequently as arterial ones but are not detected as often. Unfortunately, no test predicts the thrombosis component of HIT; thrombosis should be anticipated in the presence of vascular injury, such as puncture sites for catheterization.

Treatment and Prevention

In the absence of surgery, bleeding from thrombocytopenia with HIT is rare. In contrast to other drug-induced thrombocytopenias, in which severe thrombocytopenia commonly occurs, more moderate platelet count nadirs characterize HIT. Platelet transfusions are not indicated and may incite or worsen thrombosis. Heparin infusions must be discontinued, and an alternative anticoagulant should be instituted. LMWHs can be tested in the laboratory using serotonin release before patient administration. Although thrombosis may be treated with fibrinolytic therapy, surgery is often indicated. No heparin should be given for vascular surgery. Monitoring catheters should be purged of heparin flush, and heparin-bonded catheters should not be placed. Antiplatelet agents, such as aspirin, ticlopidine, or dipyridamole, which block adhesion and activation and, thus, PF4 release, provide ancillary help.

The patient presenting for cardiac surgery who has sustained HIT in the past presents a therapeutic dilemma. Antibodies may have regressed; if so, a negative serotonin release assay using the heparin planned for surgery will predict that transient exposure during surgery will be harmless. However, no heparin should be given at catheterization or in flush solutions after surgery.

Patients with HIT who require urgent surgery may receive heparin once platelet activation has been blocked with aspirin and dipyridamole or, in the past, the prostacyclin analog iloprost. Unfortunately, iloprost is no longer available. The problem with this strategy is obtaining sufficient blockade of platelet activity.

Another alternative, delaying surgery to wait for antibodies to regress, may fail because of the variable offset of antibody presence and the unpredictable nature of platelet response to heparin rechallenge. Plasmapheresis may successfully eliminate antibodies and allow benign heparin administration. Finally, methods of instituting anticoagulation without heparin may be chosen.

585

Table 24-2 **Therapeutic Options for Anticoagulation for Bypass in Patients with Heparin-Induced Thrombocytopenia***

1. Ancrod
2. Low-molecular-weight heparin or heparinoid (test first!)
3. Alternative thrombin inhibitor (hirudin, bivalirudin, argatroban)
4. Use a single dose of heparin, promptly neutralize with protamine, *and*
   a. Delay surgery so antibodies can regress; *or*
   b. Employ plasmapheresis to decrease antibody levels; *or*
   c. Inhibit platelets with iloprost, aspirin and dipyridamole (Persantine), abciximab, or RGD blockers

In all cases
1. No heparin in flush solutions
2. No heparin-bonded catheters
3. No heparin lock intravenous ports

*No agent is indicated for anticoagulation in CPB at this time.

BOX 24-4 *Potential Replacements as an Anticoagulant for Cardiopulmonary Bypass*

- Ancrod
- Low-molecular-weight heparins
- Factor Xa inhibitors
- Bivalirudin or other direct thrombin inhibitors
- Platelet receptor inhibitors

LMWH heparin, as an alternative to UFH, has been used for urgent surgery. While LMWHs can also induce thrombocytopenia, by displaying different antigenic determinants, they may prove acceptable alternatives for patients who develop HIT from UFH. Table 24-2 summarizes the therapeutic options available for urgent cardiac surgery in patients with HIT.

New Modes of Anticoagulation

The hemostatic goal during CPB is complete inhibition of the coagulation system. Unfortunately, even large doses of heparin do not provide this, as evidenced by formation of fibrinopeptides during surgery. Despite being far from the ideal anticoagulant, heparin still performs better than its alternatives. Current substitutes for heparin include ancrod, a proteinase obtained from snake venom that destroys fibrinogen; heparin fragments, which provide less thrombin inhibition than the parent, unfractionated molecule; direct factor Xa inhibitors; and direct thrombin inhibitors (Box 24-4).

Ancrod

Ancrod abnormally cleaves fibrinogen, resulting in its rapid clearance by the reticuloendothelial system. Thrombin, thus, has no substrate on which to act. Proper patient preparation for CPB (plasma fibrinogen, 0.4 to 0.8 g/L) requires more than 12 hours. Replenishment of fibrinogen via hepatic synthesis is slow; cryoprecipitate and/or FFP administration will speed restoration of coagulation. Patients anticoagulated in this fashion bleed more and require more cryoprecipitate and FFP compared with heparin-anticoagulated patients. Ancrod is not commercially available in the United States.

Direct Thrombin Inhibitors

Hirudin, a single-chain polypeptide containing 65 amino acids with a molecular weight of 7000 and produced by the medicinal leech *Hirudo medicinalis,* binds directly to thrombin without need of a cofactor or enzyme, inhibiting all the proteolytic functions of thrombin. This inhibition includes actions on fibrinogen; factors V, VIII, and XIII; and platelets.

Modifications of hirudin include hirugen, a synthetic peptide containing residues 53-64 of the native hirudin, and hirulog, formed by attaching the amino acid sequence d-phe-pro-arg-pro-(gly) to the amino-terminal end of hirugen. Hirugen inhibits thrombin's action on fibrinogen, but not on factor V. Hirulog has full inhibitory properties but is slowly cleaved by thrombin itself to a hirugen-like molecule.

Hirudin depends on renal excretion; renal failure prolongs its elimination half-life of 0.6 to 2.0 hours. Although there are no known direct neutralizing agents for these drugs, administration of prothrombin complex may partially restore coagulation by enhancing thrombin generation. Clinical trials of hirudin compounds have yielded mixed results. It has been used for patients with HITT but the longer half-life of approximately 90 minutes means that many of these patients bleed after cardiac surgery. Hirudin is highly antigenic and will lead to immune complexes being created to itself in about 40% of patients. If it is used a second time, the overall incidence of anaphylaxis may be as high as 10% of all patients who have received it before.

New direct thrombin inhibitors are now available (Fig. 24-9).[9] These include argatroban and bivalirudin. Argatroban is a derivative of arginine and is a relatively small molecule. It binds at the active cleavage site of thrombin and stops thrombin's action on serine proteases. It is completely hepatically cleared and has a half-life of 45 to 55 minutes with prolongation when liver function is depressed or liver blood flow is decreased. There is no reversal agent for argatroban. It has been approved by the U.S. Food and Drug Administration (FDA) for anticoagulation in the face of HITT, but there has not been, to date, a large-scale prospective randomized trial for cardiac surgery or any type of comparison to heparin/protamine. Some case reports do exist of successful usage of argatroban in HITT patients with acceptable amounts of postoperative bleeding. It has been more commonly utilized in the ICU for patients with hypercoagulable syndromes and HITT.

Bivalirudin is a synthetic peptide based on the structure of hirudin (previously called hirulog). Pharmacologists have taken the active amino acids at either end of the hirudin molecule and biosynthesized them. One active site competitively binds to the fibrinogen-binding site of thrombin, and the other 20-amino-acid sequence binds to the active serine cleavage site of thrombin. The two sequences of amino acids are connected together by a tetraglycine spacer. This fully manufactured molecule is highly specific for thrombin and has the unique property that it binds to both clot-bound and free thrombin. Heparin binds only to free plasma thrombin. Bivalirudin has a shorter half-life than argatroban and hirudin; the half-life is approximately 20 to 25 minutes. Like the other direct thrombin inhibitors, it also has no reversal agent analogous to protamine. So when it is used, it must wear off. Bivalirudin undergoes destruction by the molecule to which it binds and deactivates, thrombin; it spontaneously is destroyed by thrombin (proteolytic cleavage). The more thrombin activation that is present (i.e., the less bivalirudin that is present), the shorter is the half-life. Only about 20% of the molecular activity is eliminated by renal clearance. In mild to moderate renal failure, the effect on bivalirudin clearance is fairly small.

24

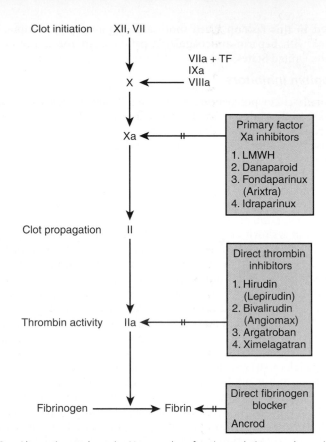

Clot initiation   XII, VII

VIIa + TF
IXa
X ← VIIIa

Xa ←—‖—

Primary factor
Xa inhibitors

1. LMWH
2. Danaparoid
3. Fondaparinux
   (Arixtra)
4. Idraparinux

Clot propagation   II

Direct thrombin
inhibitors

1. Hirudin
   (Lepirudin)
2. Bivalirudin
   (Angiomax)
3. Argatroban
4. Ximelagatran

Thrombin activity   IIa ←—‖—

Fibrinogen ——→ Fibrin ←—‖—

Direct fibrinogen
blocker

Ancrod

Figure 24-9   Alternatives to heparin. New modes of anticoagulation are shown in the boxes on the right side of the figure where they inhibit either factor Xa, thrombin, or fibrinogen. LMWH = low-molecular-weight heparin.

V

Several clinical trials of bivalirudin for cardiology procedures or cardiac surgery have been completed and published. Other ongoing and pivotal trials aiming for FDA approval are under way comparing bivalirudin to heparin/protamine for both on- and off-pump CABG cases as well as for patients with HITT. Bivalirudin has been FDA approved as a primary anticoagulant for angioplasty. In trials comparing bivalirudin to either heparin/protamine alone or heparin plus the use of a IIb/IIIa inhibitor, bivalirudin was found to have at least equal or better safety and less bleeding than either of the other therapies. When compared with heparin/protamine alone in PCI, bivalirudin was found to be superior, not just in bleeding, but also in terms of morbidity and mortality (as a combined endpoint). In a trial of 100 off-pump CABG patients randomized to receive either bivalirudin or heparin/protamine, bleeding and outcome were equal between the groups.[10] These patients underwent recatheterization at 3 months, and it was found that the bivalirudin patients had overall better flow down their grafts than did the patients who had received heparin/protamine. A phase I/II safety trial of bivalirudin in 30 on-pump CABG patients has also shown good safety, but no comparison was carried out to look at advantages against heparin/protamine. At this time, considerable research is ongoing and whether bivalirudin will prove superior to heparin/protamine for routine CABG is yet to be seen.[11] When used, the doses for CPB have been a 0.75-mg/kg bolus followed by an infusion at 1.75 mg/kg/hr titrated to the ACT (target, 2.5 times baseline). The CPB system is also primed with 50 mg, and no stasis can be allowed in the CPB circuit due to metabolism of bivalirudin during CPB. The infusion is stopped 15 to 30 minutes before CPB is discontinued, and patients bleed for up to 4 to 6 hours. In off-pump coronary artery bypass grafting similar doses to ACT targets of 350 to 450 seconds have been used.

In the face of HITT syndrome, case reports continue to show effectiveness and utility of bivalirudin. This is an off-label use of the drug because it has not been FDA approved.

PROTAMINE

Pharmacology

Protamine neutralizes heparin-induced anticoagulation. It is a nitrogenous alkaline substance from sperm heads of salmon. Composed of nearly two-thirds arginine, protamines contain many positive charges. Their biological role is to associate with the negatively charged phosphate groups of nucleic acids.

Neutralization of heparin-induced anticoagulation is the primary use of protamine. Formation of complexes with the sulfate groups of heparin forms the basis for this "antidote" effect. Protamine neutralizes the antithrombin effect of heparin far better than its anti–factor Xa effect. This distinction may arise from the need for thrombin, but not factor Xa, to remain complexed to heparin for antithrombin to exert its inhibitory effect. Because porcine mucosal heparin has more potent anti–factor Xa activity than bovine lung heparin, today's available heparin may prove to be more difficult to neutralize with protamine. Protamine's poor efficacy in neutralizing anti–factor Xa activity limits the utility of LMWH compounds as anticoagulants for CPB.

In the presence of circulating heparin, protamine forms large complexes with heparin. Excess protamine creates larger complexes. The reticuloendothelial system may then dispose of these particles by endocytosis. Although this action has not been proved, macrophages in the lung may constitute the site for elimination of these complexes, because intravenous administration of protamine permits formation of heparin/protamine complexes in the pulmonary circulation first. Proteolytic degradation of the protamine complexed to heparin conceivably results in free heparin. Protamine degradation in vivo proceeds by the action of circulating proteases, among them carboxypeptidase N, an enzyme that also clears anaphylatoxins and kinin pathway products. The time course of protamine disappearance from plasma in patients remains poorly investigated.

The recommended dose of protamine to neutralize heparin varies widely. This variability has been accounted for by differences in timing, temperature, and other environmental factors; choices for coagulation tests and outcome variables; and speculation and unproven assumptions. Protamine titration tests at the conclusion of CPB can determine the amount of heparin remaining in the patient. With automated versions of this test and simple assumptions regarding the volume of distribution of heparin, the amount needed to neutralize the heparin detected in the patient's vasculature can easily be calculated.

An alternative scheme splits a calculated dose of protamine of 1 mg/100 units into two separate doses: an initial dose (75% of the total) after CPB, with the remainder after reinfusion of blood from the bypass circuit. This scheme prevented increased plasma heparin levels and prolongation of the activated partial thromboplastin time (aPTT), compared with a control group. The ACT remained unchanged, perhaps a reflection of its insensitivity to small amounts of circulating heparin.

Adverse Reactions

The potential for a deleterious response to protamine administration raises serious questions and difficult choices in clinical care before, during, and after cardiac operations.

Rapid Administration

PERIPHERAL CARDIOVASCULAR CHANGES

Systemic hypotension from protamine occurs with rapid injection.[12] Decreased systemic vascular resistance (SVR) accompanies the systemic hypotension, whereas venous return and cardiac filling pressures decrease.

What constitutes slow administration? A neutralizing dose given over 5 minutes or longer will rarely engender cardiovascular changes. Systemic hypotension from rapid injection in humans has been ascribed to pharmacologic displacement of histamine from mast cells by the highly alkaline protamine, similar to the mechanism by which curare, morphine, and alkaline antibiotics (e.g., vancomycin and clindamycin) cause hypotension.

EFFECTS ON CARDIAC INOTROPY

Cardiac output (CO) predictably decreases after rapid administration when preload is allowed to decrease. Initial reports indicated a myocardial depressant effect. Patients with established ventricular compromise might suffer further degradation of contractile performance upon exposure to unbound protamine.

Platelet Reactions

The most underappreciated reaction to protamine is thrombocytopenia. When protamine is administered, it binds heparin wherever it comes into contact with it. It may find heparin attached to the surface of platelets and then coat the surface of the platelets with heparin/protamine complexes. It is also possible that heparin and protamine could form cross-links between platelets because the protamine is polycationic and can bind a number of heparin molecules. The end result is a decrease in platelet count within 10 to 15 minutes of administration of protamine. The usual is roughly a 10% drop in platelet count, but it can be larger, when normalization of coagulation is expected. It appears that the platelets are sequestered by the reticuloendothelium and particularly the pulmonary vasculature. It is unclear if those patients with the largest drop in platelets develop the worst bleeding or if they are at the highest risk of pulmonary vasoconstriction and pulmonary hypertension secondary to thromboxane release. The sequestered platelets come back into the circulation over the next few hours, and by 1 to 4 hours the platelet count returns toward normal.

Anaphylactoid Reaction

ALLERGY, ANAPHYLAXIS, AND ADVERSE RESPONSES

Not all adverse responses to protamine are allergic reactions. Hypersensitivity allergic reactions involve release of vasoactive mediators resulting from antigen-antibody interaction. The broader term *anaphylactoid reaction* includes not only severe immediate hypersensitivity allergy, termed *anaphylaxis*, but also other life-threatening idiosyncratic responses of nonimmunologic origin.[13]

DIABETES MELLITUS

Patients receiving protamine-containing insulin develop antibodies to protamine. Between 38% and 91% of these patients demonstrate an antiprotamine IgG; far fewer patients develop an antiprotamine IgE. Do these antibodies cause adverse responses to protamine administration? Few patients with diabetes actually develop hemodynamic compromise from protamine.

PRIOR EXPOSURE TO PROTAMINE

Previous protamine exposure may occur at catheterization, at prior vascular surgery, or at dialysis. Multiple exposures at intervals of about 2 weeks maximize the chance of an allergic response.

A single intravenous exposure to protamine will engender an IgG or IgE antibody response in 28% of patients. Nevertheless, many thousands of patients each year receive protamine at both catheterization and then later at surgery without sequelae. They offer evidence of the safety of this sequence and the rarity of intravenous exposure to protamine generating clinically significant antibodies.

FISH ALLERGY

Salmon is a vertebrate, or true fish (also known as "fin" fish), as opposed to shellfish, which are invertebrates. Patients allergic to fin fish can respond to protamine with anaphylaxis. No data link shellfish and protamine allergies.

VASECTOMY

Within 1 year of vasectomy, 22% of men develop cytotoxic (IgG) antibody to human protamine, which may cross-react with salmon protamine due to similarity among protamines. These autoantibodies exist in weak titers, however. Prospective studies demonstrate that patients with prior vasectomy receive protamine during cardiac surgery without adverse response.

Pulmonary Vasoconstriction

Several years after pulmonary artery catheters achieved common usage and case reports sensitized clinicians to adverse responses to protamine, Lowenstein and associates reported a series of cases in which protamine caused systemic hypotension, decreased left atrial pressure, elevated rather than decreased pulmonary artery pressure, and right ventricular distention and failure.[14] Unlike in anaphylaxis, plasma histamine levels do not change during this idiosyncratic, catastrophic pulmonary vasoconstriction, thus justifying a separate classification for this unusual response. The duration of pulmonary hypertension may vary substantially from brief episodes to those requiring reinstitution of CPB.

Animal models of type III protamine responses demonstrate that heparin must precede the protamine, that heparin/protamine complexes activate the complement pathway, and that blockade of complement activation attenuates pulmonary damage. Furthermore, leukocytes respond to complement activation by forming free radicals, which stimulate the arachidonate pathway. Blockade of this pathway mitigates the pulmonary response, whereas antihistamines do not. Figure 24-10 summarizes the speculative mechanisms of various adverse responses to protamine.

Theoretically, slow administration should limit type III reactions, because large heparin/protamine complexes would less likely form. Slow dilute infusion (see later) has decreased this adverse response to protamine.

On detection of sudden pulmonary hypertension and systemic hypotension, protamine infusion should cease, as should administration of any cardiovascular depressant. Administration of a heparin bolus should be considered in an attempt to reduce heparin/protamine complex size. Excess heparin would theoretically attract protamine away from large complexes to yield a larger number of smaller size particles. If hemodynamics have not deteriorated sufficiently to warrant immediate reinstitution of CPB, 70 units/kg of heparin should be tried first, then 300 units/kg

24

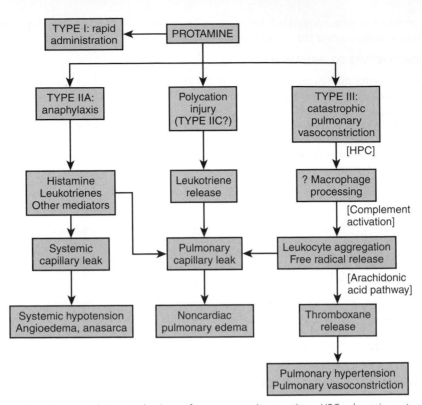

Figure 24-10 Speculative mechanisms of some protamine reactions. HPC = heparin-protamine complex. (From Horrow JC: Heparin reversal of protamine toxicity: Have we come full circle? J Cardiothorac Vasc Anesth 4:539, 1990.)

if that fails. Inotropic support should be selected so as not to worsen the pulmonary hypertension; isoproterenol (0.1 to 0.2 μg/kg bolus followed by 0.1 to 0.3 μg/kg/min) or milrinone appear best suited for this purpose. Milder cases may revert without intervention, merely by halting protamine administration, a highly desirable outcome insofar as the treatments outlined above all extract a price, whether it be arrhythmias from inotropes or bleeding from heparin. Rechallenge with protamine should be avoided.

Guidelines for Clinical Use

The most important principle in avoiding adverse responses to protamine is to administer the drug slowly. Dilution aids this goal by limiting the impact of an undetected rapid administration. A neutralizing dose (3 mg/kg, or 21 mL on average of a 10-mg/mL solution) can be added to 50 mL of clear fluid; then the diluted drug can be administered into a central vein by infusion over 10 to 15 minutes. It is important to provide a carrier flow when administering by peripheral vein, so that the long tubing does not slowly fill with drug rather than the drug enter the patient. Additional doses of undiluted protamine are given from small syringes (5 mL) at a maximum rate of 20 mg/min to adults. Proper choice of materials (small syringes, small drop administration sets, and use of diluent) helps protect against too-rapid drug delivery.

Slow administration should decrease the likelihood of a type I and a type III adverse response. However, anaphylactic response (type IIA) may occur at any delivery rate.

Alternatives to Protamine

This section discusses techniques for neutralizing heparin other than administration of protamine.

Hexadimethrine

This synthetic polycation is 1.1 to 2.0 times more potent than protamine. Hexadimethrine (Polybrene) engenders the same biological responses as protamine when administered rapidly: systemic hypotension, decreased SVR, and rapid disappearance from plasma. Pulmonary hypertension occurs after hexadimethrine neutralization of UFH. Patients allergic to protamine have received hexadimethrine without adverse effects. After reports of renal toxicity, hexadimethrine was withdrawn from clinical use in the United States. Animal studies confirm glomerular injury from hexadimethrine.

Heparinase

The enzyme heparinase, bonded to an exit filter of an experimental bypass circuit and interposed at the conclusion of CPB, decreased blood heparin levels within two passes. Current filters achieve 90% heparin removal with a single pass.

Systemic administration of the enzyme heparinase I, produced by *Flavobacterium*, results in a return of the ACT to normal in an ex vivo model, animal models of CPB, and human volunteers. Initial investigation in patients undergoing elective coronary artery bypass grafting operations confirms the utility of heparinase in neutralizing heparin-induced anticoagulation.[15]

Because the enzyme remains in the vasculature for some time after administration (the half-life is 12 minutes in healthy subjects), should an immediate need arise to reinstitute CPB, patients would require not only repeat doses of heparin, but also an infusion of heparin to counter the lingering effects of the enzyme.

BLEEDING PATIENT

After cardiac surgery, some patients bleed excessively. Chest tube drainage of more than 10 mL/kg in the first hour after operation or a total of more than 20 mL/kg over the first 3 hours after operation for patients weighing more than 10 kg is considered significant. Also, any sudden increase of 300 mL/hr or more after minimal initial drainage in an adult usually indicates anatomic disruption warranting surgical intervention.

The TEG has been extensively tested both alone and in conjunction with a number of other tests including prothrombin time (PT), platelet count, and fibrinogen. The TEG has been shown to have the best predictive accuracy for postoperative bleeding.[16] Using an algorithm based on the TEG and other tests, blood product utilization was cut considerably. Chest tube bleeding was not different, but the TEG did predict which patients might bleed abnormally. Work with TEG monitoring has shown that it can detect both hypocoagulable states as well as hypercoagulable states. New additives to the testing make it sensitive to the ADP receptor platelet antagonists as well as the GPIIb/IIIa inhibitors.

Insult of Cardiopulmonary Bypass

More so than patient factors, CPB itself acts to impair hemostasis. Bypass activates fibrinolysis, impairs platelets, and affects coagulation factors. Hypothermia, employed in most centers during CPB, adversely affects hemostasis as well.

24

Fibrinolysis

Numerous investigations support the notion that CPB activates the fibrinolytic pathway. Despite clinically adequate doses and blood concentrations of heparin, coagulation pathway activity persists. Formation of prothrombin and fibrinopeptide fragments and thrombin/antithrombin complexes document continued thrombin activity in this setting. The site of thrombin activity probably resides in the extracorporeal circuit, which contains a large surface of thrombogenic material. Thrombin activation results in fibrinolytic activity. Activation of fibrinolysis may be localized to those external sites of fibrin formation. Plasminogen activator concentrations rise during CPB, whereas levels of its inhibitor PAI-1 remain unchanged. This scenario is consistent with activation of fibrinolysis during CPB. Neither of the labels "primary" or "secondary" applies to the fibrinolysis peculiar to bypass.

Previous generations of oxygenators may have engendered systemic fibrinogenolysis more easily due to their more thrombogenic designs. In these (now more uncommon) instances of fibrinolysis, the TEG may demonstrate clot lysis. Even when fibrinolysis remains limited to the sites of extravascular fibrin formation, the fibrin degradation products so formed might impair hemostasis. In many cases, the mild fibrinolytic state engendered during CPB resolves spontaneously with little clinical impact.

Platelet Dysfunction

Thrombocytopenia occurs during CPB as a result of hemodilution, heparin, hypothermia-induced splenic sequestration of platelets, and platelet destruction from the blood-gas and blood-tissue interfaces created by cardiotomy suction, filters, and bubble oxygenators. Platelet count rarely dips below 50,000/mm^3, however.

Not only does the number of platelets decrease during CPB, but remaining platelets become impaired by partial activation. Fibrinogen and fibrin, which adhere to artificial surfaces of the extracorporeal circuit, form a nidus for platelet adhesion and aggregation. A reduced content of platelet α granules constitutes the evidence for partial activation. Nearly one third of circulating platelets undergo α-granule release during CPB. Bypass also depletes platelet glycoprotein receptors Ib and IIb/IIIa. These platelets cannot respond fully when subsequent hemostatic stimuli call for release of granule contents. Use of frequent cardiotomy suction and bubble oxygenators aggravates the extent of platelet activation.

Activation of the fibrinolytic system may contribute to platelet dysfunction. Local formation of plasmin affects platelet membrane receptors. Antifibrinolytic medications preserve platelet function and prevent some platelet abnormalities that occur during bypass.

Clotting Factors

Denaturation of plasma proteins, including the coagulation factors, occurs at blood-air interfaces. Liberal use of cardiotomy suction and prolonged use of oxygenators potentially impair coagulation by decreasing coagulation factor availability. Hemodilution also decreases factor concentrations. However, rarely do coagulation factor levels fall below the thresholds for adequate formation of fibrin in adult surgery.

Hypothermia

Hypothermia potentially affects hemostasis in many ways. First, the splanchnic circulation responds to hypothermia with sequestration of platelets. After warming, the accompanying thrombocytopenia reverses over 1 hour. Second, transient platelet

V

> **BOX 24-5** *Useful Drugs to Reduce Bleeding during Cardiac Surgery*
>
> - Aprotinin
> - Tranexamic acid or ε-aminocaproic acid
> - Recombinant factor VIIa
> - Desmopressin

dysfunction occurs, evidenced by a platelet shape change, increased adhesiveness, inhibition of ADP-induced aggregation, and decreased synthesis of both thromboxane and prostacyclin. Third, a specific heparin-like inhibitor of factor Xa becomes more active. Protamine cannot neutralize this factor, which might be heparan.

Fourth, hypothermia slows the enzymatic cleavage on which activation of coagulation factors depends. Many biological phenomena display a 7% attenuation of activity for each decrease of 1°C in temperature. While coagulation factor structure remains unaltered, formation of fibrin may be sluggish when the patient is cold. Fifth, hypothermia accentuates fibrinolysis. The fibrin degradation products so formed then impair subsequent fibrin polymerization. Cold-induced injury of vascular endothelium can release thromboplastin, which then incites fibrin formation and activates fibrinolysis.

Prevention of Bleeding

The possible transmission of serious viral illness during transfusion of blood products and impairment of immune function generate concern among clinicians and patients. Many techniques attempt to limit viral exposure, including donation of autologous blood or directed blood, blood scavenging during and after surgery, and efforts to limit perioperative hemorrhage.

Pharmacologic Factors

HEPARIN AND PROTAMINE

The prudent clinician's admonition to administer no drug to excess applies well to this pair of essential drugs. Too little heparin invites active fibrin formation during CPB with consumption of clotting factors and platelets and excessive activation of the fibrinolytic system. Too much heparin risks postoperative heparin rebound. With too little protamine, the remaining unneutralized heparin impairs hemostasis by its anticoagulant action. Doses of protamine excessive enough to overwhelm the endogenous proteases may exert an anticoagulant effect, as well as invite polycation-induced lung injury and pulmonary vasoconstriction. The optimal approach utilizes coagulation testing to estimate the appropriate heparin and protamine doses and confirms both adequate anticoagulation and its neutralization.

Desmopressin

This analog of vasopressin provides more potent and longer lasting antidiuretic activity than vasopressin, with little vasoconstriction (Box 24-5). Like the parent compound and like epinephrine and insulin, desmopressin releases coagulation system mediators from vascular endothelium. Factor VIII coagulant activity increases 2- to 20-fold and is maximal 30 to 90 minutes after injection. Factor XII levels also increase. In response to desmopressin, endothelium releases the larger multimers of vWF, as well as t-PA and prostacyclin. Nevertheless, the overall effect of desmopressin is procoagulant, perhaps because of the impact of factor VIII and vWF.

24

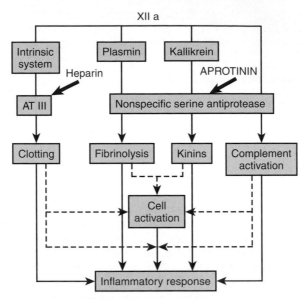

XII a

Intrinsic system

Plasmin

Kallikrein

Heparin

APROTININ

AT III

Nonspecific serine antiprotease

Clotting

Fibrinolysis

Kinins

Complement activation

Cell activation

Inflammatory response

Figure 24-11 Actions of aprotinin on the contact coagulation system, fibrinolytic pathway, and complement activation. (From Royston D: The serine antiprotease aprotinin [Trasylol]: A novel approach to reducing postoperative bleeding. Blood Coag Fibrin 1:55, 1990.)

The optimal dose of desmopressin is 0.3 µg/kg. Intravenous, subcutaneous, and intranasal routes are all acceptable. After plasma redistribution with an 8-minute half-life, metabolism in liver and kidney and urinary excretion yield a plasma half-life of 2.5 to 4 hours. Levels of factor VIII persist in plasma long after desmopressin excretion due to the release of vWF. Rapid intravenous administration decreases systemic blood pressure and SVR, possibly by prostacyclin release or stimulation of extrarenal vasopressin V_2 receptors. The drug's antidiuretic action poses no problem in the absence of excessive free water administration.

SYNTHETIC ANTIFIBRINOLYTICS

Effective fibrinolysis inhibition requires an intravenous loading dose of 10 mg/kg for tranexamic acid followed by 1 mg/kg/hr or 50 mg/kg of ε-aminocaproic acid followed by infusions of 25 mg/kg/hr. Infusion rates require downward adjustment when serum creatinine is elevated.

Several investigations, using prophylactic antifibrinolytics, document a savings in blood loss, as well as in blood transfused in a general population of cardiac surgery patients. By commencing administration of tranexamic acid before CPB, chest tube drainage in the first 12 hours after operation decreased by 30% and the likelihood of receiving banked blood within 5 days of operation decreased from 41% to 22%. Prophylactic antifibrinolytics may spare platelet function by inhibiting the deleterious effects of plasmin. Administration of very large doses of antifibrinolytics appears to offer no greater savings. Cardiac surgery patients undergoing repeat operation may benefit particularly from prophylactic antifibrinolytic administration.[17]

APROTININ

Bovine lung provides the source of this 58-residue polypeptide serine protease inhibitor. Aprotinin inhibits a host of proteases, including trypsin, plasmin, kallikrein, and factor XIIa activation of complement (Fig. 24-11). The adult intravenous dose for

V

surgical hemostasis is 2 million kallikrein inhibitor units (KIU) for both patient and bypass pump, followed by 600,000 KIU/hr. The elimination half-life of aprotinin, 7 hours, is considerably longer than that of the synthetic antifibrinolytics; after 6 days, aprotinin continues to be excreted in the urine.

Royston and coworkers documented more than a fourfold reduction in blood loss during repeat cardiac surgery. Subsequent studies using high-dose aprotinin confirmed conservation of blood products and a reduction in bleeding, ranging from 29% to 50%. Studies clearly demonstrate decreased fibrinolysis in aprotinin-treated patient groups; preservation of platelet GPIb, or blockade of a plasmin-mediated platelet defect may also explain the hemostatic mechanism of aprotinin.

High-dose aprotinin alone prolongs the celite ACT. Most investigators simply avoid the celite ACT and use kaolin ACT. The kaolin ACT adsorbs about 98% of aprotinin and any intrinsic antithrombin effect that aprotinin has is therefore mitigated. It is recommended to use the kaolin ACT and keep the length of ACT time the same as if aprotinin was not being used. An animal protein, aprotinin can cause anaphylaxis, although this is uncommon (<1 in 1000). Aprotinin costs significantly more than equivalent doses of synthetic antifibrinolytic drugs. The discussion and argument about cost effectiveness of aprotinin versus other antifibrinolytics has continued for more than 10 years. The major concerns today with aprotinin are its adverse effects on renal function and overall cardiovascular outcome; These concerns led to its removal from the market in 2007.[18]

Determine the Cause

The complexity of human hemostasis, augmented by unexpected behavior of coagulation tests, can lead to confusion in the diagnosis of bleeding after cardiac surgery. *Anatomic sources* of bleeding frequently present once systemic blood pressure achieves sufficient magnitude. Some clinicians prefer to identify these sources before chest closure with a provocative test (i.e., allowing brief periods of hypertension). Generous chest tube drainage early after operation suggests an anatomic source. Retained mediastinal clot may engender a consumptive coagulopathy. A widened mediastinum on chest radiograph suggests the need for surgical drainage.

Nonsurgical causes of bleeding (platelets, coagulation factors, and fibrinolysis) usually manifest as a generalized ooze. Inspection of vascular access puncture sites aids in this diagnosis. Bleeding from other areas not manipulated during surgery (stomach, bladder) may also occur.

Coagulation tests aid diagnosis. Because the PT and aPTT are usually prolonged by several seconds after CPB, only values more than 1.5 times control suggest factor deficiency. Elevation of the ACT should first suggest unneutralized heparin, then factor deficiency.

A decreased platelet count, usually denoting hemodilution or consumption, requires correction with exogenous platelets in any bleeding patient. However, bleeding patients with insufficient functional platelets may demonstrate normal platelet counts early after operation. For this reason, clinicians have sought rapid diagnostic tests of platelet function and attempted correlation with bleeding after CPB.

Low plasma fibrinogen occurs from excessive hemodilution or factor consumption and is corrected with cryoprecipitate or FFP. The thrombin time is useful here. Most clinical laboratories can perform this test with rapid turnaround. A prolonged thrombin time denotes unneutralized heparin, insufficient fibrinogen, or high concentrations of fibrin degradation products. Finally, direct measurement of fibrin degradation products denotes fibrinolytic activity. In the absence of a cause for a consumptive coagulopathy, antifibrinolytic therapy may be useful.

24

Table 24-3	A Treatment Plan for Excessive Bleeding after Cardiac Surgery	

Action	Amount	Indication
Rule out surgical cause	—	No oozing at puncture sites; chest radiograph
More protamine	0.5 to 1 mg/kg	ACT > 150 s or aPTT > 1.5 times control
Warm the patient	—	"Core" temperature < 35°C
Apply PEEP*	5 to 10 cm H_2O	—
Desmopressin	0.3 µg/kg IV	Prolonged bleeding time
Aminocaproic acid	50 mg/kg, then 25 mg/kg/hr	Elevated D-dimer or teardrop-shaped TEG tracing
Tranexamic acid	10 mg/kg, then 1 mg/kg/hr	Elevated D-dimer or teardrop-shaped TEG tracing
Platelet transfusion	1 U/10 kg	Platelet count < 100,000/mm³
Fresh frozen plasma	15 mL/kg	PT or aPTT > 1.5 times control
Cryoprecipitate	1 U/4 kg	Fibrinogen < 1 g/L or 100 mg/dL

*Positive end-expiratory pressure (PEEP) is contraindicated in hypovolemia.
ACT = activated coagulation time; PT = prothrombin time; aPTT = activated partial thromboplastin time; TEG = thromboelastographic.

Table 24-3 lists a treatment plan for excessive bleeding after cardiac surgery. Interventions appear not in order of likelihood but rather by priority of consideration. Thus, surgical causes should be ruled out before seizing on the diagnosis of a consumptive coagulopathy. The priority will also vary among institutions, depending on the availability and cost of resources. This table provides a simple algorithm for treating postoperative bleeding. More complete schemes present a daunting level of complexity that deter implementation (Fig. 24-12).

Adjunctive Therapy

WARMING

Bleeding patients with core or intermediate zone temperatures below 35°C will benefit from warming efforts, both passive (warm ambient temperature, adequate body coverings, low ventilator fresh gas flows, airway heat and humidity exchangers) and active (heated humidifiers, warmed intravenous fluids, forced air convective warming blankets). All too often, in the effort to maintain intravascular volume, intensive care unit personnel administer liters of room-temperature (≤20°C) or refrigerated (0° to 4°C) fluids, which render patients hypothermic.

POSITIVE END-EXPIRATORY PRESSURE

One popular method to limit bleeding after cardiac surgery is application of positive end-expiratory pressure (PEEP) (5 to 10 cm H_2O). A tamponade effect in the mediastinum may explain this salutary effect.

BLOOD PRESSURE

Maintenance of systemic blood pressure in the low-normal range promotes tissue perfusion while limiting leakage around suture lines. Adequate depth of anesthesia during surgery and sufficient postoperative analgesia and sedation should be verified before initiating vasodilator therapy.

V

Management of the Bleeding Cardiac Surgical Patient

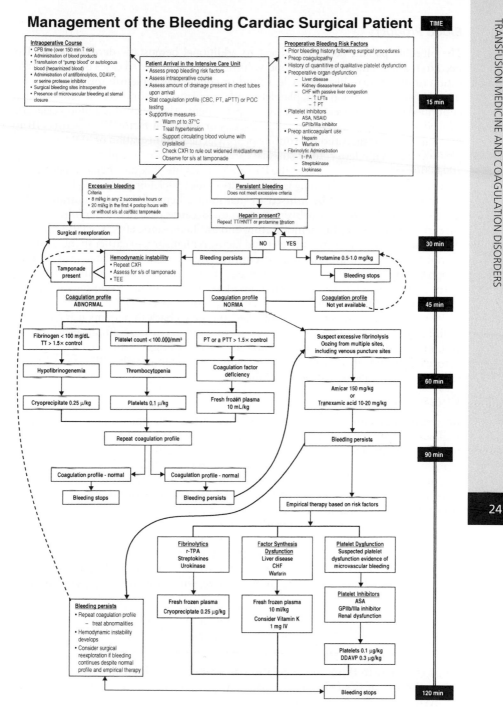

Figure 24-12 Algorithm for treating excessive bleeding. (From Milas B, Johes D, Gorman R: Management of bleeding and coagulopathy after heart surgery. Semin Thorac Cardiovasc Surg 12:326, 2000.)

Blood Products

The bleeding patient becomes subject to additional hemostatic derangements. The need to maintain intravascular blood volume arises in nearly all cases before identification of the cause of bleeding. Clear fluid or colloid will replenish intravascular volume. However, red blood cells, platelets, and coagulation factors become diluted when continued bleeding is treated with such replacement. Also, packed red blood cells and banked whole blood do not provide platelets or sufficient factor V or factor VIII to maintain hemostasis. Although routine prophylactic administration of FFP or platelets plays no role in modern cardiac surgical care, demonstration of a platelet count below 100,000/mm^3 or prolongation of the PT or aPTT despite adequate heparin neutralization *in a patient actively bleeding* is an indication for platelet or plasma replacement.

Banked blood should be infused to maintain a hemoglobin concentration that allows appropriate oxygen delivery to tissues. Because patients undergoing cardiac surgery also experience the hemodiluting and antihemostatic effects of CPB, the prudent clinician will commence platelet and factor replenishment earlier in the course of hemorrhage while awaiting laboratory confirmation. Each unit of platelet concentrate supplies about 10^{11} platelets, which increases the platelet count by about 20,000/mm^3 in the adult. Enough plasma accompanies platelet concentrates to supply the equivalent of 1.0 to 1.5 units of plasma for each 6 units of platelets.

Shed mediastinal blood can be collected and given back to patients using a closed drainage system. The drainage fluid, often collected in citrate, contains little fibrinogen. Presence of tissue and other debris in this fluid suggests the need for filtration before reinfusion. Shed mediastinal fluid supplies red blood cells without risk of viral transmission via allogeneic blood products.

Drugs

Recombinant factor VIIa (rFVIIa NovoSeven) has been approved for use in hemophiliacs who are resistant to factor VIII concentrates. When rFVIIa is administered, it binds to tissue factor and activates factor X leading to thrombin and fibrin formation. These then activate platelets. Thrombin generation and clotting take place on the surface of platelets and at sites of injury.[19,20] Numerous reports have been published of the off-label use of this "rescue agent" to stop bleeding in surgical patients, including cardiac surgical patients after CPB.

In hemophiliacs, the recommended dose is 90 µg/kg. However, reports in cardiac surgical patients have suggested doses of 30 µg/kg, while continuing ongoing component therapy and monitoring the PT/international normalized ratio. The half-life is about 2 hours and the dose may have to be repeated if bleeding continues. Most of the anecdotal reports have been positive, with a marked decrease in bleeding taking place.

SUMMARY

- It is easiest to think of coagulation as a wave of biological activity occurring at the site of tissue injury consisting of initiation, acceleration, control, and lysis.
- Hemostasis is part of a larger body system—inflammation. The protein reactions in coagulation have important roles in signaling inflammation.
- Thrombin is the most important coagulation modulator, interacting with multiple coagulation factors, platelets, tissue plasminogen activator, prostacyclin, nitric oxide, and various white blood cells.

V

- The serine proteases that compose the coagulation pathway are balanced by serine protease inhibitors, termed *serpins*. Antithrombin is the most important inhibitor of blood coagulation.
- Platelets are the most complex part of the coagulation process, and antiplatelet drugs are important therapeutic agents.
- Heparin requires antithrombin to anticoagulate blood and is not an ideal anticoagulant for cardiopulmonary bypass. Newer anticoagulants are actively being sought to replace heparin.
- Protamine can have many adverse effects. Ideally, a new anticoagulant will not require reversal with a toxic substance like protamine.
- Antifibrinolytic drugs are often given during cardiac surgery; these drugs include ε-aminocaproic acid and tranexamic acid.
- Recombinant factor VIIa is the latest drug to be studied as a "rescue agent" to stop bleeding during cardiac surgery. It appears to be very effective but has not yet been studied adequately.
- Every effort should be made to avoid transfusion of banked blood products during routine cardiac surgery. In fact, bloodless surgery is a reality in many cases.

REFERENCES

1. Edmunds Jr. LH: Blood-surface interactions during cardiopulmonary bypass. J Card Surg 8:404, 1993
2. Fischer R, Kuppe H, Koster A: Impact of heparin management on release of tissue factor pathway inhibitor during cardiopulmonary bypass. Anesthesiology 100:1040, 2004
3. Savage B, Saldivar E, Ruggeri ZM: Initiation of platelet adhesion by arrest onto fibrinogen or translocation on von Willebrand factor. Cell 84:289, 1996
4. Lange RA, Hillis LD: Antiplatelet therapy for ischemic heart disease. N Engl J Med 350:277, 2004
5. Koster A, Fischer T, Grunendel M, et al: Management of heparin: Resistance and cardiopulmonary bypass: The effect of 5 different anticoagulation strategies on hemostatic activation. J Cardiothorac Vasc Anesth 18:131, 2004
6. Avidan M, Levy J, Scholz J, et al: A phase III, double blind, placebo-controlled, multicenter study on the efficacy of recombinant human antithrombin in heparin-resistant patients scheduled to undergo cardiac surgery necessitating cardiopulmonary bypass. Anesthesiology 102:276, 2005
7. Day JRS, Landis RC, Taylor KM: Heparin is more than just an anticoagulant. J Cardiothorac Vasc Anesth 18:93, 2004
8. Godal HC: Heparin-induced thrombocytopenia. In Lane DA, Lindahl U (eds): Heparin, Boca Raton, FL, CRC Press, 1989, p 533
9. Dinisio M, Middeldorp S, Buller H: Direct thrombin inhibitors. N Engl J Med 353:1028, 2005
10. Merry AF, Raudkivi P, White HD, et al: Anticoagulation with bivalirudin (a direct thrombin inhibitor) vs heparin: A randomized trial in OPCAB graft surgery. Ann Thorac Surg 77:925, 2004
11. Koster A, Spiess BD, Chew DP, et al: Effectiveness of bivalirudin as a replacement for heparin during cardiopulmonary bypass in patients undergoing coronary artery bypass grafting. Am J Cardiology 93:356, 2004
12. Welsby I, Newman M, Phillips-Bute B, et al: Hemodynamic changes after protamine administration. Anesthesiology 102:308, 2005
13. Horrow JC: Protamine allergy. J Cardiothorac Vasc Anesth 2:225, 1988
14. Kirklin JK: Prospects for understanding and eliminating deleterious effects of cardiopulmonary bypass. Ann Thorac Surg 51:529, 1991
15. Michelsen LG, Kikura M, Levy JH, et al: Heparinase I (Neutralase) reversal of systemic anticoagulation. Anesthesiology 85:339, 1996
16. Cammerer U, Dietrich W, Rampf T, et al: The predictive value of modified computerized thromboelastography and platelet function analysis for postoperative blood loss in routine cardiac surgery. Anesth Analg 96:51, 2003
17. Shore-Lesserson L, Reich DL, Vela-Cantos F, et al: Tranexamic acid reduces transfusions and mediastinal drainage in repeat cardiac surgery. Anesth Analg 83:18, 1996
18. Smith PK, Shah AS: The role of aprotinin in a blood-conservation program. J Cardiothoracic Vasc Anesth 18(suppl):S24, 2004
19. Roberts H, Monroe D, Hoffman M: Safety profile of recombinant factor VIIa Semin Hematol 41(suppl 1):101, 2004
20. Tanaka K, Waly A, Cooper W, Levy J: Treatment of excessive bleeding in Jehovah's Witness patients after cardiac surgery with recombinant factor VIIa. Anesthesiology 98:1513, 2003

24

Chapter 25

Discontinuing Cardiopulmonary Bypass

Jack S. Shanewise, MD • Roberta Hines, MD • Joel A. Kaplan, MD

Cardiopulmonary bypass (CPB) has been used since the 1950s to facilitate surgery on the heart and great vessels, and even with the increased interest in off-pump coronary artery bypass grafting (CABG) CPB remains a critical part of most cardiac operations. Managing patients with CPB remains one of the defining characteristics of cardiac surgery and cardiac anesthesiology. Discontinuing CPB is a necessary part of every operation involving extracorporeal circulation. Through this process, the support of the circulation by the bypass pump and oxygenator is transferred back to the patient's heart and lungs. In this chapter we review important considerations involved with discontinuing CPB and present an approach to managing this critical component of a cardiac operation, which may be routine and easy or extremely complex and difficult. The key to success in discontinuing CPB is proper preparation. The period during and immediately after weaning from CPB is usually very busy for the anesthesiologist, and having to do things that could have been accomplished earlier in the operation is not helpful. The preparations for bringing a patient off CPB may be organized into several parts: general preparations, preparing the lungs, preparing the heart, and final preparations.

GENERAL PREPARATIONS

Temperature

Because at least moderate hypothermia is used during CPB in most cardiac surgery cases, it is important that the patient is sufficiently rewarmed before attempting to wean from CPB (Table 25-1). Initiation of rewarming is a good time to consider whether additional drugs need to be given to keep the patient anesthetized. Anesthetic vaporizers need to be off for 10 to 20 minutes before coming off CPB to clear the agent from the patient if so desired. Monitoring the temperature of a highly perfused tissue such as the nasopharynx is useful to help prevent overheating the brain during rewarming, but these temperatures may rise more rapidly than others, such as bladder, rectum, or axilla temperatures, leading to inadequate rewarming and temperature dropoff after CPB as the heat continues to distribute throughout the body. Different institutions have various protocols for rewarming, but the important point is to warm gradually, avoiding hyperthermia of the central nervous system while getting enough heat into the patient to prevent significant dropoff after CPB.[1] After CPB, there is a tendency for the patient to lose heat, and measures to keep the patient warm such as fluid warmers, a circuit heater-humidifier, and forced-air warmers should be set up and turned on before weaning from CPB. The temperature of the operating room may need to be increased as well; this is probably an effective measure to keep a patient warm after CPB, but it may make the scrubbed and gowned personnel uncomfortable.

Laboratory Results

Arterial blood gas analysis should be obtained before weaning from CPB and any abnormalities corrected. Severe metabolic acidosis depresses the myocardium and should be treated with sodium bicarbonate or tromethamine (Tham). The optimal hematocrit for weaning from CPB is controversial and probably varies from patient to patient.[2] It makes sense that sicker patients with lower cardiovascular reserve may benefit from a higher hematocrit, but the risks and adverse consequences of transfusion need to be considered as well. Suffice it to say that the hematocrit should be measured and optimized before weaning from CPB. The serum potassium level should be measured before weaning from CPB and may be high due to cardioplegia or low, especially in patients receiving loop diuretics. Hyperkalemia may make establishing an effective cardiac rhythm difficult and can be treated with sodium bicarbonate, calcium chloride, or insulin, but the levels usually decrease quickly after cardioplegia has been stopped. Low serum potassium levels should probably be corrected before coming off CPB, especially if arrhythmias

25

Table 25-1	General Preparations for Discontinuing Cardiopulmonary Bypass	
Temperature	**Laboratory Results**
Adequately rewarm before weaning from CPB	Correct metabolic acidosis
Avoid overheating the brain	Optimize hematocrit
Start measures to keep patient warm after CPB	Normalize K^+
Use fluid warmer, forced air warmer	Consider giving Mg^{2+} or checking Mg^{2+} level
Warm operating room	Check Ca^{2+} level and correct deficiencies

Table 25-2 Preparing the Lungs for Discontinuing Cardiopulmonary Bypass

1. Suction trachea and endotracheal tube, if needed.
2. Inflate lungs gently by hand.
3. Ventilate with 100% oxygen.
4. Treat bronchospasm with bronchodilators.
5. Check for pneumothorax and pleural fluid.
6. Consider need for positive end-expiratory pressure, intensive care unit ventilator, and nitric oxide.

are present. Administration of magnesium to patients on CPB decreases postoperative arrhythmias and may improve cardiac function, and many centers routinely give all CPB patients magnesium sulfate. Theoretical disadvantages include aggravation of vasodilation and inhibition of platelet function.[3,4] If magnesium is not given routinely, the level should be checked before weaning from CPB and deficiencies corrected. The ionized calcium level should be measured, and significant deficiencies corrected before discontinuing CPB. Many centers give all patients a bolus of calcium chloride just before coming off CPB because it transiently increases contractility and systemic vascular resistance. However, it has been argued that this practice is to be avoided because calcium may interfere with catecholamine action and aggravate reperfusion injury.

PREPARING THE LUNGS

As the patient is weaned from CPB and the patient's heart starts to support the circulation, the lungs again become the site of gas exchange, delivering oxygen and eliminating carbon dioxide. Before weaning from CPB, the lung function must be restored (Table 25-2). The lungs are reinflated by hand gently and gradually, with sighs using up to 30 cmH$_2$O pressure, and then mechanically ventilated with 100% oxygen. Care should be taken not to allow the left lung to injure an in situ internal mammary artery graft as the lung is reinflated. The compliance of the lungs can be judged by their feel with hand ventilation, with stiff lungs suggesting more difficulty with oxygenation or ventilation after CPB. If visible, both lungs should be inspected for residual atelectasis, and they should be rising and falling with each breath. Ventilation alarms and monitors should be activated. If prolonged expiration or wheezing is detected, bronchodilators should be given. The surgeon should inspect both pleural spaces for pneumothorax, which should be treated with chest tubes. Any fluid present in the pleural spaces should be removed before attempting to wean the patient from CPB.

PREPARING THE HEART

Preparing the heart to resume its function pumping blood involves optimizing the five hemodynamic parameters that can be controlled: rhythm, rate, contractility, afterload, and preload (Table 25-3).

Rhythm

There must be an organized, effective, and stable cardiac rhythm before attempting to wean from CPB. This can occur spontaneously after removal of the aortic cross-clamp, but the heart may resume electrical activity with ventricular fibrillation.

Table 25-3	Preparing the Heart for Discontinuing Cardiopulmonary Bypass
Parameter	**Preparation**
Rhythm	Normal sinus rhythm is ideal.
	Defibrillate if necessary when temperature > 30°C.
	Consider antiarrhythmic drugs if ventricular fibrillation persists more than a few minutes.
	Try synchronized cardioversion for atrial fibrillation or flutter.
	Look at the heart to diagnose atrial rhythm.
	Try atrial pacing if AV conduction exists.
	Try AV pacing for heart block.
Heart rate	Rate should be between 75 and 95 beats per minute in most cases.
	Treat slow rates with electrical pacing.
	Treat underlying causes of fast heart rates.
	Heart rate may decrease as the heart fills.
	Control fast supraventricular rates with drugs and then pace as needed.
	Always have pacing available during heart surgery.
Contractility	Inotropic support is more likely needed with depressed cardiac function before CPB, advanced age, long bypass or clamp time, poor preservation, or incomplete revascularization.
	Look for the vigorous "snap" of a heartbeat with good contractility.
	If depressed contractility is likely, begin inotropic drugs before weaning from CPB.
	Severely impaired function may require mechanical support.
Afterload	Systemic vascular resistance is a major component of afterload.
	Keep MAP between 60 and 80 mmHg at full CPB flow.
	Consider a vasoconstrictor if the MAP is low and a vasodilator if the MAP is high.
Preload	End-diastolic volume is the best measure of preload and can be seen with TEE.
	Filling pressures provide a less direct measure of preload.
	Consider baseline filling pressures.
	Assess RV volume and function with direct inspection.
	Assess LV volume and function with TEE.
	Cardiac distention may cause MR and TR.

AV = atrioventricular; CPB = cardiopulmonary bypass; LV = left ventricular; MAP = mean arterial pressure; MR = mitral regurgitation; RV = right ventricular; TEE = transesophageal echocardiography; TR, tricuspid regurgitation.

25

If the blood temperature is greater than 30°C, the heart may be defibrillated with internal paddles applied directly to the heart using 10 to 20 J. Defibrillation at lower temperatures may be unsuccessful because extreme hypothermia can cause ventricular fibrillation. If ventricular fibrillation persists or recurs repeatedly, antiarrhythmic drugs such as lidocaine or amiodarone may be administered to help achieve a stable rhythm. It is not unusual for the rhythm to remain unstable for several minutes immediately after cross-clamp removal, but persistent or recurrent ventricular fibrillation should prompt concern about impaired coronary blood flow. Because it provides an atrial contribution to ventricular filling and a normal, synchronized contraction of the ventricles, normal sinus rhythm is the ideal cardiac rhythm for weaning from CPB. Atrial flutter or fibrillation, even if present before CPB, can often be converted to normal sinus rhythm with synchronized cardioversion, especially if antiarrhythmic drugs are administered. It is often helpful to look directly at the heart when there is any question about the cardiac rhythm. Atrial contraction, flutter, and fibrillation are easily seen on CPB. Ventricular arrhythmias should be treated by correcting underlying causes such as potassium or magnesium deficits and, if necessary, with antiarrhythmic drugs such as amiodarone. If asystole or complete heart block occurs after cross-clamp removal, electrical pacing with temporary epicardial pacing wires may be needed to achieve an effective rhythm before weaning from CPB. If atrioventricular conduction is present, atrial pacing should be attempted because, as with normal sinus rhythm, it provides atrial augmentation to filling and synchronized ventricular contraction. Atrioventricular sequential pacing is used when there is heart block, which is frequently present for 30 to 60 minutes as the myocardium recovers after cross-clamp removal. Ventricular pacing remains the only option if no organized atrial rhythm is present, but this sacrifices the atrial "kick" to ventricular filling and the more efficient synchronized ventricular contraction of the normal conduction system.

Rate

In most situations for adult patients, the heart rate (HR) should be between 75 and 95 beats per minute for weaning from CPB. Lower rates may theoretically be desirable for hearts with residual ischemia or incomplete revascularization. Higher HRs may be needed for hearts with limited stroke volume, such as after ventricular aneurysmectomy. Slow HRs are best treated with electrical pacing, but β-agonist or vagolytic drugs also may be used to increase the HR. Tachycardia before weaning from CPB is more worrisome and difficult to deal with, and treatable causes such as inadequate anesthesia, hypercarbia, and ischemia should be identified and corrected. The HR often decreases as the heart is filled in the weaning process, and electrical pacing should always be immediately available during cardiac surgery. Supraventricular tachycardias should be electrically cardioverted if possible, but drugs such as β-antagonists or calcium channel antagonists may be needed to control the ventricular rate if they persist, most typically occurring in patients with chronic atrial fibrillation. If drug therapy lowers the rate too much, pacing may be used.

Contractility

The contractile state of the myocardium should be considered before attempting to wean from CPB. The likelihood of decreased contractility requiring inotropic support after CPB is greater with preexisting ventricular impairment (e.g., low ejection fraction, high left ventricular end-diastolic pressure [LVEDP] preoperatively or before CPB), advanced age, long CPB time, long aortic cross-clamp time, inadequate myocardial preservation, and incomplete revascularization. A heart with good contractility often has a vigorous snap with contraction that can be seen while on CPB, in contrast to the weak contractions of a heart with impaired contractility, but it may be difficult to assess global ventricular function while the heart is empty and on CPB. If significant depression of contractility is likely, inotropic support can be started before attempting to wean the patient from CPB. If depressed myocardial contractility becomes evident during weaning, the safest approach is to prevent cardiac distention by resuming CPB, resting the heart for 10 to 20 minutes while inotropic therapy with a catecholamine or phosphodiesterase inhibitor drug is started. Extreme depression of contractile function of the myocardium may require mechanical support with an intra-aortic balloon pump (IABP) or ventricular assist device (VAD).

Afterload

An important component of afterload in patients is the systemic vascular resistance (SVR). While on CPB at full flow, usually about 2.2 L/min/m², mean arterial pressure (MAP) is directly related to SVR and indicates whether the SVR is appropriate, too high, or too low. Low SVR after CPB can cause inadequate systemic arterial perfusion pressure, and high SVR can significantly impair cardiac performance, especially in patients with poor ventricular function. SVR is usually within a reasonable range when the arterial pressure is between 60 and 80 mmHg at full pump flow. If below that range, infusion of a vasopressor may be needed to increase SVR before attempting to wean from CPB. If the MAP is high while on CPB, vasodilator therapy may be needed.

Preload

In the intact heart, the best measure of preload is end-diastolic volume. Less direct clinical measures of preload include left atrial pressure (LAP), pulmonary artery occlusion pressure (PAOP), and pulmonary artery diastolic pressure, but there may be a poor relationship between end-diastolic pressure and volume during cardiac surgery. Transesophageal echocardiography (TEE) is a useful tool for weaning from CPB because it provides direct visualization of the end-diastolic volume and contractility of the left ventricle.[5] The process of weaning a patient from CPB involves increasing the preload (i.e., filling the heart from its empty state on CPB) until an appropriate end-diastolic volume is achieved. When preparing to discontinue CPB, some thought should be given to the appropriate range of preload for the particular patient. The filling pressures before CPB may indicate what they need to be after CPB; a heart with high filling pressures before CPB may require high filling pressures after CPB to achieve an adequate preload.

FINAL PREPARATIONS

The final preparations before discontinuing CPB include leveling the operating table, re-zeroing the pressure transducers, ensuring the proper function of all monitoring devices, confirming that the patient is receiving only intended drug infusions, ensuring the immediate availability of resuscitation drugs and appropriate fluid volume, and verifying that the lungs are being ventilated with 100% oxygen (Table 25-4).

Table 25-4	Final Preparations for Discontinuing Cardiopulmonary Bypass	
Anesthesiologist's Preparations	**Surgeon's Preparations**
Level operating table	Remove macroscopic collections of air from the heart
Re-zero transducers	Control major sites of bleeding
Activate monitors	CABG lying nicely without kinks
Check drug infusions	Cardiac vents off or removed
Have resuscitation drugs and fluid volume on hand	Clamps off the heart and great vessels
Reestablish TEE/PA catheter monitoring	Tourniquets around caval cannulas loose

CABG = coronary artery bypass graft; TEE = transesophageal echocardiography; PA = pulmonary artery.

The surgeon must confirm that he or she has completed the necessary preparations in the surgical field before discontinuing CPB. Macroscopic collections of air in the heart should be evacuated before starting to wean from CPB. These are most easily detected with TEE, which can also be helpful in monitoring and directing the de-airing process. Major sites of bleeding should be controlled, cardiac vent suction should be off, all clamps on the heart and great vessels should be removed, coronary artery bypass grafts should be checked for kinks and bleeding, and tourniquets around the caval cannulas should be loosened or removed before starting to wean a patient from CPB.

ROUTINE WEANING FROM CARDIOPULMONARY BYPASS

There should be close and clear communication among the perfusionist, the surgeon, and the anesthesiologist while weaning a patient from CPB, and the surgeon or the anesthesiologist should be in charge of the process. The anesthesiologist should be positioned at the head of the table, able to readily see the CPB pump and perfusionist, the heart and the surgeon, and the anesthesia monitor display. If present, the TEE display should also be easily in view. Weaning a patient from CPB is accomplished by diverting blood back into the patient's heart by occluding the venous drainage to the CPB pump. The arterial pump flow is decreased simultaneously as the pump reservoir volume empties into the patient and the heart's contribution to systemic flow increases. This can be accomplished most abruptly by simply clamping the venous return cannula and transfusing blood from the pump until the heart fills and the preload appears to be adequate. Some patients will tolerate this method of discontinuing CPB, but many will not, and a more gradual transfer from the pump to the heart is usually desirable. The worse the function of the heart, the slower the transition from full CPB to off CPB needs to be.

Before beginning to wean the patient from CPB, the perfusionist should communicate to the physicians involved three important parameters: the current flow rate of the pump, the volume in the pump reservoir, and the oxygen saturation of venous blood returning to the pump from the patient. The current flow rate of the pump indicates the stage of weaning as it is decreased. Weaning is just beginning at full flow, is well under way when down to 2 or 3 L/min in adults, and is almost finished at less than 2 L/min. The reservoir volume indicates how much blood is available for transfusion to fill the heart and lungs as CPB is discontinued. If the volume is low, less than 400 to 500 mL in adults, more fluid may need to be added to the reservoir before weaning from CPB. The oxygen saturation of the venous return $(S\overline{v}o_2)$ gives an indication of the adequacy of peripheral perfusion during CPB. If the $S\overline{v}o_2$ is greater than 60%, oxygen delivery during CPB is adequate; if it is less than 50%, oxygen delivery is inadequate, and measures to improve delivery (e.g., increase pump flow or hematocrit) or decrease consumption (e.g., give more anesthetic agents or neuromuscular blocking drugs) need to be taken before coming off CPB. An $S\overline{v}o_2$ between 50% and 60% is marginal and must be followed closely. As the patient is weaned from CPB, a rising $S\overline{v}o_2$ suggests that the net flow to the body is increasing and that the heart and lungs will support the circulation; a falling $S\overline{v}o_2$ indicates that tissue perfusion is decreasing and that further intervention to improve cardiac performance will be needed before coming off CPB.

The actual process of weaning from CPB begins with partially occluding the venous return cannula with a clamp. This may be done in the field by the surgeon or at the pump by the perfusionist. This causes blood to flow into the right ventricle. As the right ventricle fills and begins to pump blood through the lungs, the left side

V

of the heart will begin to fill. When this occurs, the left ventricle will begin to eject, and the arterial waveform will become pulsatile. Next, the perfusionist will gradually decrease the pump flow rate. As more of the venous return goes through the heart and less to the pump reservoir, it becomes necessary to gradually decrease the pump flow to avoid emptying the pump reservoir. One approach to weaning from CPB is to bring the filling pressure being monitored (e.g., central venous pressure [CVP], PAOP, LAP) to a specific, predetermined level somewhat lower than may be necessary and then assess the hemodynamics. Volume (preload) of the heart may also be judged by direct observation of its size or with TEE. Further filling is done in small increments (50 to 100 mL) while closely monitoring the preload until the hemodynamics appear satisfactory as judged by the arterial pressure, the appearance of the heart, and the trend of the $S\bar{v}o_2$. It is typically easy to see the right-sided heart volume and function directly in the surgical field and the left side of the heart with TEE, and combining the two observations is a useful approach for weaning from CPB. Overfilling and distention of the heart should be avoided because it may stretch the myofibrils beyond the most efficient length and dilate the annuli of the mitral and tricuspid valves, rendering them incompetent, which is easily detected with TEE. If the patient has two venous cannulae, the smaller of the two may be removed when the pump flow is one half of the full flow rate to improve movement of blood from the great veins into the right atrium. When the pump flow has been decreased to 1 L/min or less in an adult and the hemodynamics are satisfactory, the venous cannula may be completely clamped and the pump flow turned off. At this point, the patient is "off bypass."

This is a critical juncture in the operation. The anesthesiologist should pause a moment to make a brief scan of the patient and monitors to confirm that the lungs are being ventilated with oxygen, the hemodynamic status is acceptable and stable, the electrocardiogram shows no new signs of ischemia, the heart does not appear to be distending, and the drug infusions are functioning as desired. Further fine-tuning of the preload is accomplished by transfusing 50- to 100-mL boluses from the pump reservoir through the arterial cannula and observing the effect on hemodynamics. If there is acute failure of the circulation as evidenced by unstable rhythm, falling arterial and rising filling pressures, or visible distention of the heart, the patient is put back on CPB by unclamping the venous return cannula and turning on the arterial pump flow. Once back on CPB, an assessment of the cause of failure to wean is made and appropriate interventions undertaken before attempting to wean again. When the hemodynamics appear to be stable and adequate, the surgeon may remove the venous cannula from the heart.

The next step in discontinuing CPB is to transfuse as much as possible of the blood remaining in the pump reservoir into the patient before removal of the arterial cannula. This is usually easier and quicker than transfusing through the intravenous infusions after decannulation. The blood in the venous cannula and tubing (usually about 500 mL) may be drained into the reservoir for transfusion. The patient's venous capacitance can be increased by raising the head of the bed (i.e., reverse Trendelenburg position) or giving nitroglycerin, being more cautious with these maneuvers in patients with impaired cardiac function. Filling the vascular space with the head up and while infusing nitroglycerin increases the ability to cope with volume loss after decannulation by allowing rapid augmentation of the central vascular volume by leveling the bed and decreasing the nitroglycerin infusion rate.

After discontinuing CPB, the anticoagulation by heparin is reversed with protamine. Depending on institutional preference, protamine may be administered before or after removal of the arterial cannula. Giving it before removal allows for continued

25

transfusion from the pump and easier return to CPB if there is a severe protamine reaction. Giving protamine after removal of the arterial cannula probably decreases the risk of thrombus formation and systemic embolization. After the infusion of protamine is started, pump suction return to the reservoir should be stopped to keep protamine out of the pump circuit in case subsequent return to CPB becomes necessary. Protamine should be given slowly through a peripheral intravenous catheter over 7 to 15 minutes while watching for systemic hypotension and pulmonary hypertension, which may indicate that an untoward (allergic) reaction to protamine is occurring.[6] Technically flawed coronary artery bypass grafts may thrombose after protamine administration, causing acute ischemia and mimicking a protamine reaction.

When transfusion of the pump reservoir blood is completed, a thorough assessment of the patient's condition should be made before removing the arterial cannula, because after this is done returning to CPB becomes much more difficult. The cardiac rhythm should be stable. Cardiac function is assessed by evaluating pressures, cardiac output, and TEE. Hemodynamics should be satisfactory and stable. Adequate oxygenation and ventilation should be confirmed by arterial blood gas analysis or pulse oximetry and capnography. Bleeding from the heart should be at a manageable level before removal of the arterial cannula. The perfusionist should not have to transfuse significant amounts of blood through the arterial cannula before removing it, because it may be difficult to keep up with the blood loss through intravenous infusions alone. Bleeding sites behind the heart may have to be repaired on CPB if the patient cannot tolerate lifting the heart to expose the problem area. At the time of arterial decannulation, the systolic pressure should be between 85 and 105 mmHg to minimize the risk of dissection or tearing of the aorta. The head of the bed may be raised, or small boluses of a short-acting vasodilator (e.g., nitroglycerin, nitroprusside) may be given to lower the systemic blood pressure as necessary. Tight control of the arterial blood pressure may be needed for a few minutes until the cannulation site is secure.

When the arterial cannula has been removed, the heparin effects are reversed with protamine, and the hemodynamic status remains stable, the routine process of discontinuing CPB is complete. However, in patients with poor ventricular function after CPB, multiple drugs or even mechanical assist devices may be required throughout the rest of the operation and continued in the intensive care unit.

PHARMACOLOGIC MANAGEMENT OF VENTRICULAR DYSFUNCTION

Perioperative ventricular dysfunction is usually a transient state of contractile impairment that may require temporary support with positive inotropic agents. In a subset of patients, contractility may be significantly depressed such that combination therapy with positive inotropes and vasodilator agents is needed to effectively improve cardiac output and tissue perfusion. The use of mechanical assist devices is reserved for conditions of overt or evolving cardiogenic shock.

Severe ventricular dysfunction, specifically the low cardiac output syndrome (LCOS), occurring after CPB and cardiac surgery differs from chronic congestive heart failure (CHF) (Box 25-1). Patients emerging from CPB have hemodilution, moderate hypocalcemia, hypomagnesemia, and altered potassium levels. Depending on temperature and depth of anesthesia, these individuals may demonstrate low, normal, or high SVR. Increasing age, female sex, decreased LV ejection fraction, and increased duration of CPB are associated with a greater likelihood that inotropic support will be needed after CABG surgery (Table 25-5).

> ### BOX 25-1   *Risk Factors for the Low Cardiac Output Syndrome after Cardiopulmonary Bypass*
>
> - Preoperative ventricular dysfunction
> - Myocardial ischemia
> - Poor myocardial preservation
> - Reperfusion injury
> - Inadequate cardiac surgical repair or revascularization

Table 25-5   Patient Characteristics Associated with the Use of Inotropic Drug Support

Variable	No Inotropic Drug Support* (n=58)	Inotropic Drug Support* (n=70)	P
Age (yr)	57±8	62±8	.005
Sex			
Female (%)	10	26	.027
Male (%)	90	74	
Collateral circulation (%)	64	73	.271
WMA (%)	78	84	.334
Patients demonstrating cardiac enlargement (%)	7	21	.021
Baseline LVEDP (mm Hg)	14±7	16±6	.044
Postcontrast LVEDP (mm Hg)	21±8	24±7	.054
Change in LVEDP (mm Hg)	7±6	7±7	.534
EF (%)	61±11	54±13	.002
PT (min)	106±30	125±37	.004
IT (min)	42±15	50±19	.009

*All values except for sex, collateral circulation, WMA, and patients demonstrating cardiac enlargement are expressed as mean±SD.

WMA = wall motion abnormalities identified during preoperative radiographic-contrast ventriculography; LVEDP = left ventricular end-diastolic pressure; EF = preoperative ejection fraction calculated from end-diastolic and end-systolic measurements from radiograph-contrast ventriculography; PT = total duration of cardiopulmonary bypass (pump time); IT = duration of aortic cross-clamping (ischemic time).

From Royster RL, Butterworth JF, Prough DS, et al: Preoperative and intraoperative predictors of inotropic support and long-term outcome in patients having coronary bypass grafting. Anesth Analg 72:729, 1991.

Contractile dysfunction during or after cardiac surgery can result from preexisting impairment in contractility or be a new-onset condition. Abnormal contraction, especially in the setting of coronary artery disease (CAD), usually is caused by myocardial injury resulting in ischemia or infarction. The magnitude of contractile dysfunction corresponds to the extent and duration of injury. Brief periods of myocardial oxygen deprivation (<10 minutes) produce regional contractile dysfunction, which can be rapidly reversed by reperfusion. Extension of the ischemia to 15 to 20 minutes is also associated with restoration of cardiac function with reperfusion; however, this process is very slow and can take hours to days. This condition of postischemic reversible myocardial dysfunction in the presence of normal flow is referred to as *myocardial stunning*. Irreversible cell injury will occur with longer periods of ischemia, producing a myocardial infarction characterized by release of intracellular enzymes, disruption of cell membranes, influx of calcium, persistent contractile dysfunction, and eventual cellular swelling and necrosis.

Table 25-6 Management of Cardiac Dysfunction

Physiologic Variable	Management
Heart rate and rhythm	Maintain normal sinus rhythm, avoid tachycardia; for tachycardia or bradycardia, consider pacing or chronotropic agents (atropine, isoproterenol, epinephrine), correct acid-base disturbances and electrolytes, and review current medications.
Preload	Reduce increased preload with diuretics or venodilators (nitroglycerin or sodium nitroprusside); monitor CVP, PCWP, and SV; obtain echocardiogram to rule out ischemia, valvular lesions, tamponade, and intracardiac shunts; consider using inotropes, IABP, or both.
Afterload	Avoid increased afterload (increased wall tension); use vasodilators (sodium nitroprusside); avoid hypotension; maintain coronary perfusion pressure; consider IABP, inotropes devoid of α_1-adrenergic effects (dobutamine or milrinone), or both IABP and inotropes.
Contractility	Assess hemodynamics, rule out ischemia/infarction, assess rate/rhythm, preload, and afterload; use inotropes; if uncertain, obtain echocardiogram to assess cardiac function. Consider combination therapy with inotropes and vasodilators and/or assist devices (IABP/LVAD/RVAD).
Oxygen delivery	Increase Fio$_2$ and CO; check ABGs and chest radiograph; mechanical ventilation if indicated; correct acid-base disturbances.

Fio$_2$ = inspired oxygen concentration; ABGs = arterial blood gas; CO = cardiac output; CVP = central venous pressure; IABP = intra-aortic balloon pump; PCWP = pulmonary capillary wedge pressure; SV = stroke volume.

In addition to the previously described factors, right ventricular (RV) dysfunction and failure are potential sources of morbidity and mortality after cardiac surgery. Numerous factors may predispose patients to the development of perioperative RV dysfunction, including CAD, RV hypertrophy, previous cardiac surgery, and operative considerations such as inadequate revascularization or hypothermic protection. Technical and operative difficulties are associated with various cardiac surgical procedures (e.g., right ventriculotomy), RV trauma, rhythm and conduction abnormalities, injury to the right ventricle during cessation of CPB, or protamine reaction.

The following discussion provides an overview of the pharmacologic approach to management of perioperative ventricular dysfunction in the setting of cardiac surgery. Management goals are described in Table 25-6. These are extensions of the routine preparations made for discontinuing CPB shown in Table 25-3.

Sympathomimetic Amines

Sympathomimetic drugs (i.e., catecholamines) are pharmacologic agents capable of providing inotropic and vasoactive effects (Box 25-2). Catecholamines exert positive inotropic action by stimulation of the β_1-receptor. The predominant hemodynamic effect of a specific catecholamine depends on the degree to which the various α-, β-, and dopaminergic receptors are stimulated (Tables 25-7 and 25-8).

The physiologic effect of an adrenergic agent is determined by the sum of its actions on α-, β-, and dopaminergic receptors. The effectiveness of any adrenergic agent will be influenced by the availability and responsiveness of adrenergic receptors.

BOX 25-2   *Pharmacologic Approaches to Ventricular Dysfunction*

- Inotropic drugs
- Phosphodiesterase inhibitors
- Vasodilators
- Vasopressors
- Metabolic supplements

Table 25-7   Sympathomimetics

Drug	Dosage		Site of Action		Mechanism of Action
	Intravenous	Infusion	α	β	
Methoxamine	2-10 mg	—	++++		Direct
Phenylephrine	50-500 μg	10 mg/500 mL 20 μg/mL 10-50 μg/min	++++	±	Direct
Norepinephrine	—	8 mg/500 mL 16 μg/mL 2-16 μg/min	++++	+++	Direct
Metaraminol	100 μg	20-200 mg/500 mL 40-400 μg/mL 40-500 μg/min	++++	+	Direct and indirect
Epinephrine	2-16 μg	4 mg/500 mL 8 μg/mL 2-10 μg/min	+++	+++	Direct
Ephedrine	5-25 mg	—	+	++	Direct and Indirect
Dopamine	—	400 mg/500 mL 800 μg/mL 2-30 μg/kg/min	++	+++	Direct and indirect
Dobutamine	—	250 mg/500 mL 500 μg/mL 2-20 μg/kg/min	+	++++	Direct
Dopexamine	—	0.5-4.0 μg/kg/min		++	Direct
Isoproterenol	1-4 μg	2 mg/500 mL 4 μg/mL 1-5μg/min		++++	Direct

25

Chronically elevated levels of plasma catecholamines (e.g., chronic CHF and long CPB time) cause downregulation of the number and sensitivity of β-receptors. Maintenance of normal acid-base status, normothermia, and electrolytes also improve the responsiveness to adrenergic-receptor stimulation.

The selection of a drug to treat ventricular dysfunction is influenced by pathophysiologic abnormalities as well as by the physician's preference. If LV performance is decreased primarily as a result of diminished contractility, the drug chosen should increase contractility. Although β-agonists improve contractility and tissue perfusion, their effects may increase myocardial oxygen consumption (MVo_2) and reduce coronary perfusion pressure (CPP). However, if the factor most responsible for decreased cardiac function is hypotension with concomitantly reduced CPP, use of an α-adrenergic agonist can increase blood pressure and improve diastolic coronary perfusion.

Catecholamines are also effective for treating primary RV contractile dysfunction, with all of the $β_1$-adrenergic agonists augmenting RV contractility,

Table 25-8 Hemodynamic Effects of Catecholamines and Phosphodiesterase Inhibitors

Drug	CO	dp/dt	HR	SVR	PVR	PCWP	MVo₂
Dobutamine 2-12 µg/kg/min*	⇑⇑⇑⇑	⇑	⇑⇑⇑	⇓	⇓	⇓ or ⇔	⇑
Dopamine							
0-3 µg/kg/min	⇑	⇑	⇑	⇓	⇓	⇑	⇑
3-8 µg/kg/min	⇑⇑⇑	⇑	⇑	⇓	⇓	⇑	⇑
>8 µg/kg/min	⇑⇑⇑	⇑	⇑⇑⇑	⇑	⇔ (⇑)	⇑ or ⇔	⇑⇑⇑
Isoproterenol 0.5-10 µg/kg/min	⇑⇑⇑	⇑⇑⇑	⇑⇑⇑	⇓⇓⇓	⇓	⇓	⇑⇑⇑
Epinephrine 0.01-0.4 µg/kg/min	⇑⇑⇑	⇑	⇑	⇑ (⇓)	(⇑)	⇑ or ⇔	⇑⇑⇑
Norepinephrine 0.01-0.3 µg/kg/min	⇑	⇑	⇔ (⇑⇓)	⇑⇑⇑	⇔	⇔	⇑
PDE inhibitors†	⇑⇑⇑	⇑	⇑	⇓⇓⇓	⇓⇓	⇓⇓	⇓

*The indicated doses represent the most common dose ranges. For the individual patient, a deviation from these recommended doses might be indicated.

†PDE inhibitors are usually given as a loading dose followed by a continuous infusion: amrinone: 0.5-1.5 mg/kg loading dose, 10-30 µg/kg/min continuous infusion; milrinone: 50 µg/kg loading dose, 0.375-0.75 µg/kg/min continuous infusion.

CO = cardiac output; dp/dt = myocardial contractility; HR = heart rate; SVR = systemic vascular resistance; PVR = pulmonary vascular resistance; PCWP = pulmonary capillary wedge pressure; MVo₂ = myocardial oxygen consumption; PDE inhibitors = phosphodiesterase inhibitors.

Modified from Lehmann A, Boldt J: New pharmacologic approaches for the perioperative treatment of ischemic cardiogenic shock. J Cardiothorac Vasc Anesth 19:97-108, 2005.

Studies have documented the efficacy of epinephrine, norepinephrine, dobutamine, isoproterenol, dopamine, and phosphodiesterase-III (PDE-III) inhibitors in managing RV contractile dysfunction. When decreased RV contractility is combined with increased afterload, agents that exert vasodilator and positive inotropic effects should be used, including epinephrine, isoproterenol, dobutamine, and the PDE-III inhibitors.

Epinephrine

Epinephrine stimulates α- and β-adrenergic receptors in a dose-dependent fashion. It is frequently the inotrope of choice after CPB (Box 25-3). Doses of 10, 20, and 40 ng/kg/min increased stroke volume by 2%, 12%, and 22%, respectively, and increased cardiac index (CI) by 0.1, 0.7, and 1.2 L/min/m². The HR also increased, but by no more than 10 beats per minute at any dose. Epinephrine is frequently used after cardiac surgery to support the function of the "stunned" reperfused heart. During emergence from CPB, Butterworth and colleagues showed epinephrine (30 ng/kg/min) increased CI and stroke volume by 14% without increasing HR.[7] In cardiac surgical patients, epinephrine infusion (0.01 to 0.4 µg/kg/min) effectively increases cardiac output, minimally increases HR, and has acceptable side effects.

Dobutamine

Dobutamine is a synthetic catecholamine that generally produces dose-dependent increases in cardiac output and reductions in diastolic filling pressures. The effects of epinephrine (30 ng/kg/min) were compared with those of dobutamine (5 µg/kg/min) in 52 patients recovering from CABG surgery.[7] Both drugs significantly and similarly

V

> **BOX 25-3** *Inotropic Drugs*
>
> - Epinephrine
> - Norepinephrine
> - Dopamine
> - Dobutamine
> - Isoproterenol

---

increased stroke volume index, but epinephrine increased the HR by only 2 beats per minute whereas dobutamine increased the HR by 16 beats per minute.

In addition to increasing contractility, dobutamine may have favorable metabolic effects on ischemic myocardium. Intravenous and intracoronary injections of dobutamine increase coronary blood flow in animal studies. In paced cardiac surgical patients, dopamine increased oxygen demand without increasing oxygen supply whereas dobutamine increased myocardial oxygen uptake and coronary blood flow. However, because increases in HR are a major determinant of $M\dot{V}O_2$, these favorable effects of dobutamine could be lost if dobutamine induces tachycardia. During dobutamine stress-echocardiography, segmental wall motion abnormalities suggestive of myocardial ischemia can occur as a result of tachycardia and increases in $M\dot{V}O_2$.[8]

Dopamine

Dopamine is an endogenous catecholamine and an immediate precursor of norepinephrine and epinephrine. Its actions are mediated by stimulation of adrenergic receptors and specific postjunctional dopaminergic receptors (D_1-receptors) in the renal, mesenteric, and coronary arterial beds. In low doses (0.5 to 3.0 µg/kg/min), dopamine predominantly stimulates the dopaminergic receptors; at doses ranging from 3 to 7 µg/kg/min, it activates most adrenergic receptors in a nonselective fashion; and at higher doses (>10 µg/kg/min), dopamine behaves as a vasoconstrictor. The dose-dependent effects of dopamine are not very specific and can be influenced by multiple factors, such as receptor regulation, concomitant drug use, and interindividual and intraindividual variability.

Dopamine is unique in comparison with other endogenous catecholamines because of its effects on the kidneys. It has been shown to increase renal artery blood flow by 20% to 40% by causing direct vasodilation of the afferent arteries and indirect vasoconstriction of the efferent arteries. This results in an increase in glomerular filtration rate and in oxygen delivery to the juxtamedullary nephrons.

Despite favorable effects, dopamine has several undesirable features that may limit its use. Its propensity to raise HR and cause tachyarrhythmias can result in demand-related myocardial ischemia. After cardiac surgery, dopamine causes more frequent and less predictable degrees of tachycardia than dobutamine or epinephrine at doses that produce comparable improvement in contractile function.

Norepinephrine

Norepinephrine is used primarily to treat vasodilated patients after CPB. The α-adrenergic agonists benefit certain patients with circulatory failure refractory to inotropic and fluid therapy. Phenylephrine, norepinephrine, or vasopressin may be used to restore MAP in patients with a low SVR after CPB (i.e., vasoplegia syndrome).[9] When RV dysfunction primarily is a result of decreased CPP, vasoconstrictors can be used to optimize RV performance.

25

Isoproterenol

Isoproterenol is a potent, nonselective β-adrenergic agonist, devoid of α-adrenergic agonist activity. Isoproterenol dilates skeletal, renal, and mesenteric vascular beds and decreases diastolic blood pressure. The potent chronotropic action of isoproterenol, combined with its propensity to decrease CPP, limits its usefulness in patients with CAD. Applications include treatment of bradycardia (especially after orthotopic heart transplantation), pulmonary hypertension, and heart failure after congenital cardiac surgery. Isoproterenol remains the inotrope of choice for stimulation of cardiac pacemaker cells in the management of acute bradyarrhythmias or atrioventricular heart block. It reduces refractoriness to conduction and increases automaticity in myocardial tissues. The tachycardia seen with isoproterenol is a result of direct effects of the drug on the sinoatrial and atrioventricular nodes and reflex effects caused by peripheral vasodilation. It is routinely used in the setting of cardiac transplantation for increasing automaticity and inotropy and for its vasodilatory effect on the pulmonary arteries.

Phosphodiesterase Inhibitors

The PDE-III inhibitors amrinone (inamrinone) and milrinone increase cyclic adenosine monophosphate, calcium flux, and calcium sensitivity of contractile proteins. These drugs have a similar mode of action because they are noncatecholamine and nonadrenergic agents. They do not rely on β-receptor stimulation for their positive inotropic activity. As a result, the effectiveness of the PDE-III inhibitors is not altered by previous β-blockade nor is it reduced in patients who may experience β-receptor downregulation. In addition to their positive inotropic effects, these agents produce systemic and pulmonary vasodilation. As a result of this combination of hemodynamic effects (i.e., positive inotropic support and vasodilation), the term *inodilator* has been used to describe these drugs (Box 25-4).

Because these agents exert their hemodynamic effects by a nonadrenergic mechanism of action, when used in combination with β-agonists they have an additive effect on myocardial performance. Investigators have demonstrated the clinical application of combination therapy using PDE-III inhibitors and dopamine, phenylephrine, epinephrine, and nitroglycerin.[10]

A second-generation PDE-III inhibitor, milrinone has a similar hemodynamic profile to amrinone; however, its positive inotropic action is 15 to 30 times that of amrinone. Thrombocytopenia has been a potential clinical concern with the administration of PDE-III inhibitors, particularly amrinone. However, no significant reduction in platelet count occurred after 48 hours of milrinone infusion in cardiac surgical patients. Intravenous milrinone has been studied extensively and demonstrates a favorable short-term effect in CHF and ventricular dysfunction after CPB.[11]

V

BOX 25-4 *Inodilator Drugs*
• Inamrinone
• Milrinone
• Dobutamine
• Epinephrine plus nitroprusside ("epipride")

Milrinone, like other PDE-III inhibitors, appears to increase cardiac output without increasing overall MV_{O_2}. Data also suggest that milrinone may improve myocardial diastolic relaxation (i.e., positive "lusitropic" effect) and augment coronary perfusion. The proposed mechanism for this effect on diastolic performance is that by decreasing LV wall tension, ventricular filling is enhanced and myocardial blood flow and oxygen delivery are optimized.

The ability of short-term administration of milrinone to augment ventricular performance in patients undergoing cardiac surgery was shown in the results from the European Milrinone Multicentre Trial Group.[12] In this prospective study, intravenous milrinone was studied in patients after CPB. All patients received a bolus infusion of milrinone at 50 µg/kg over 10 minutes, followed by a maintenance infusion of 0.375, 0.5, or 0.75 µg/kg/min for 12 hours. Significant increases in stroke volume and CI were observed. In addition, significant decreases in pulmonary capillary wedge pressure (PCWP), CVP, PAP, MAP, and SVR were seen. Eighteen patients (14%) had arrhythmias; most occurred in the group receiving 0.75 µg/kg/min. Two arrhythmic events were deemed serious; both were bouts of rapid atrial fibrillation occurring with the higher dose.

After CPB, a loading dose of milrinone at 50 µg/kg, followed by a continuous infusion of 0.5 µg/kg/min, resulted in a significant increase in cardiac output. Butterworth and colleagues[13] also studied the pharmacokinetics and pharmacodynamics of milrinone in adult patients undergoing cardiac surgery; milrinone (25, 50, or 75 µg/kg) was given if the CI was less than 3.0 L/min/m² after separation from CPB. All three doses of milrinone significantly increased CI. The 50- and 75-µg/kg doses produced significantly greater increases in CI than the 25-µg/kg dose. The 75-µg/kg dose produced increases in CI comparable with the 50-µg/kg dose, but it was associated with more hypotension, despite administration of intravenous fluid, blood, and a phenylephrine infusion. The initial redistribution half-lives were 4.6, 4.3, and 6.9 minutes, and the terminal elimination half-lives were 63, 82, and 99 minutes for the 25-, 50-, and 75-µg/kg doses, respectively. The results of these investigations suggest that for optimizing hemodynamic performance (while minimizing any potential for arrhythmias), the middle dose range (i.e., loading dose of 50 µg/kg) of milrinone may be most efficacious with a continuous infusion of 0.5 µg/kg/min, leading to a plasma concentration of more than 100 mg/mL. In patients with poor LV function, the loading dose should be given during CPB to avoid a decrease in MAP and to minimize the need for other inotropes on discontinuing CPB.

Vasodilators

The indications for using vasodilators such as nitroglycerin or nitroprusside in cardiac surgery include management of perioperative systemic or pulmonary hypertension, myocardial ischemia, and ventricular dysfunction complicated by excessive pressure or volume overload (Box 25-5). In most conditions, nitroglycerin or nitroprusside may be used. Both share common features such as rapid onset, ultra-short half-lives (several minutes), and easy titratability. Nevertheless, there are important pharmacologic differences between nitroglycerin and nitroprusside. In the setting of ischemia, nitroglycerin is preferred because it selectively vasodilates coronary arteries without producing a coronary "steal." Likewise, in the management of ventricular volume overload or RV pressure overload, nitroglycerin may offer some advantage over nitroprusside. It has a predominant influence on the venous bed such that preload can be reduced without significantly compromising systemic arterial pressure. The benefits of nitroglycerin are improvement in stroke volume, reduction in wall tension and MV_{O_2}, increased perfusion to the subendocardium as a result of a lower

25

LVEDP, and maintenance of CPP. Nitroprusside is a more potent arterial vasodilator and may potentiate myocardial ischemia due to a coronary steal phenomenon or a reduction in coronary perfusion pressure. Its greater potency, however, makes nitroprusside the vasodilator of choice for management of perioperative hypertensive disorders and for afterload reduction during or after surgery for regurgitant valvular lesions.

Additional uses of vasodilators include management of RV dysfunction. Sodium nitroprusside can augment cardiac output by decreasing RV afterload and PVR. Similarly, nitroglycerin has been shown to decrease PVR, transpulmonary pressure, and mean PAP and to increase cardiac output in patients with elevated PVR resulting from mitral valve disease. Although nitroglycerin and nitroprusside decrease the impedance to RV ejection and increase the RV ejection fraction by reducing afterload, they are nonspecific pulmonary vasodilators. As a result, new studies have focused on the ability of agents such as prostaglandins (particularly prostaglandin E_1), nitric oxide, and the PDE-III inhibitors to more specifically decrease PVR.

Despite proven benefits of vasodilator therapy in the management of CHF, they can be difficult drugs to use in treatment of perioperative ventricular dysfunction. This is most evident in cases of the LCOS when impaired pump function is complicated by inadequate perfusion pressure. In these situations, multidrug therapy with vasoactive and cardioactive agents is warranted (i.e., nitroglycerin or nitroprusside plus epinephrine or milrinone and norepinephrine). Combination therapy enables greater selectivity of effect. The unwanted side effects of one drug can be avoided while supplementing the desired effects with another agent.[14] To maximize the desired effects of any particular combination of agents, frequent assessment of cardiac performance with a pulmonary artery catheter and TEE is needed. This allows the Starling curve and the pressure-volume loops to be visualized as they are shifted up and to the left with therapy.

Additional Pharmacologic Therapy

Following the steps outlined in Tables 25-3 and 25-6, most patients can be weaned off of CPB. However, a small percentage will be difficult to safely remove from CPB because of their chronic end-stage CHF or an acute insult during cardiac surgery producing cardiogenic shock. These patients will probably require mechanical circulatory support. However, while instituting these further steps, some clinicians try additional pharmacologic therapy.

Controversial Older Treatments

Some studies suggest that a reduction in plasma thyroid hormone concentration may be the cause of decreased myocardial function after CPB. Some patients exhibit signs of hypothyroidism, including decreases in HR, CI, and myocardial and systemic

Table 25-9 Emerging Drugs for Heart Failure and Cardiogenic Shock

Drug*	CO	PCWP	AP	HR	Arrhyth.	Onset	Offset	Diur.	Shock
Toborinone	⇑⇑⇑	⇓⇓⇓	⇑ or ⇓	⇔	⇑⇑⇑⇑	Short	Moderate	⇔	No
L-Simendan	⇑⇑⇑	⇓	⇓	⇑	⇔	Short	Very long	⇔	Yes
Tezosentan	⇑⇑⇑	⇓	⇓	⇔	⇔	Short	Short	⇔	No
Nesiritide	⇑	⇓⇓⇓	⇓	⇔	⇔	Short	Long	⇑⇑⇑	No
L-NAME	⇓	⇑⇑⇑	⇑⇑⇑⇑	(⇓)	?	Short	Moderate	⇑	Yes

*Positive inotropic drugs: toborinone: phosphodiesterase inhibitor. l-Simendan: levosimendan, calcium sensitizer. Vasodilating drugs: tezosentan: endothelin antagonist. Nesiritide: natriuretic peptide. Vasoconstricting drug: L-NAME: N^G-nitro-l-arginine-methyl ester, inhibitor of nitric oxide synthase.

CO = cardiac output; PCWP = pulmonary capillary wedge pressure; AP = arterial pressure; HR = heart rate; Arrhyth. = arrhythmogenic potential; Diur. = diuresis; Shock = cardiogenic shock; No = not yet used in patients with cardiogenic shock; Yes = already used in patients with cardiogenic shock.

Modified from Lehman A, Boldt J: New pharmacologic approaches for the perioperative treatment of ischemic cardiogenic shock. J Cardiothorac Vasc Anesth 19:97, 2005.

oxygen consumption and increases in arteriovenous oxygen difference and SVR. Multiple investigators have documented declines in the circulating triiodothyronine (T_3) concentration during and after CPB, and the most dramatic decreases in T_3 are seen at the end of CPB and during the first few hours after CPB. The reduced thyroid hormone concentrations after CPB may exacerbate myocardial stunning and the LCOS encountered in the post-CPB period. Thyroid hormone in the form of an intravenous T_3 infusion (2 µg/hr to a total dose of 0.5 µg/kg) has been used during cardiac surgery. This therapy has resulted in increases in the MAP and HR and reductions in LAP and CVP in patients who initially could not be weaned from CPB. Some of these patients have been successfully weaned from CPB and have required lower doses of dobutamine and other cardiac drug support after treatment with thyroid hormone.

The administration of glucose-insulin-potassium or just glucose and insulin has been found to be useful for metabolic support of the heart after CPB. The trauma of cardiac surgery produces insulin resistance, which restricts the availability of carbohydrates to the heart. The increased level of catecholamines during CPB may also put further strain on the energy metabolism of the heart, whereas insulin may improve this situation.[15] The administration of high-dose insulin has been compared with dopamine in patients undergoing CABG surgery. The infusion of dopamine (7 µg/kg/min) alone induced metabolic changes unfavorable to the myocardium, whereas dopamine plus insulin increased carbohydrate use with cessation of cardiac uptake of free fatty acids.

New Treatments for Heart Failure and Cardiogenic Shock

Levosimendan is a new positive inotropic drug belonging to the class of calcium sensitizers. The drug stabilizes the calcium-induced conformational change in cardiac troponin C and prolongs the effective cross-bridging time. In contrast to other positive inotropic drugs, levosimendan does not increase intracellular calcium. The drug has vasodilating and anti-ischemic properties produced by opening K^+-ATP channels[16] (Table 25-9).

Levosimendan is recommended by the European Society of Cardiology for treatment of acute worsening of heart failure and for acute heart failure after myocardial infarction.[17] It has also been found to enhance contractile function of stunned myocardium in patients with acute coronary syndromes. It is available clinically in Europe and is undergoing evaluation in the United States. The use of levosimendan has been reported in cardiac surgical patients with high perioperative risk, compromised LV function, difficulties in weaning from CPB, and severe RV failure after mitral valve replacement. The doses used were 12 µg/kg as a 10-minute loading dose, followed by an infusion of 0.1 µg/kg/min. It has been used preoperatively, during emergence from CPB, and in the postoperative period for up to 28 days. The potential for levosimendan to produce increased contractility, decreased resistance, minimal metabolic cost, and no arrhythmias makes it a potentially useful addition to the treatments for patients with LCOS or RV failure.

Nesiritide is a recombinant human brain–type natriuretic peptide with vasodilatory and diuretic effects. In patients with heart failure, intravenous nesiritide acts as a vasodilator and reduces preload; SVR is decreased, and CI subsequently increases. The drug has no positive inotropic effects. Compared with nitroglycerin and dobutamine, nesiritide had a greater effect on decreasing preload than nitroglycerin, and it did not cause as many arrhythmias as dobutamine. Its ultimate role in the treatment of acute heart failure is uncertain, but it may augment the vasodilators or diuretics.

Numerous other drugs are being studied for their uses in patients with acute decompensated heart failure and cardiogenic shock. These drugs include positive inotropic agents such as toborinone (a PDE-III inhibitor), vasodilators such as tezosentan (a specific and potent dual endothelin-receptor antagonist), and vasopressors such as L-NAME (a nitric oxide inhibitor) (see Table 25-9). These various drugs may prove useful for certain types of cardiovascular problems in the future.

INTRA-AORTIC BALLOON PUMP COUNTERPULSATION

The IABP is a device that is designed to augment myocardial perfusion by increasing coronary blood flow during diastole and unloading the left ventricle during systole. This is accomplished by mass displacement of a volume of blood (usually 30 to 50 mL) by alternately inflating and deflating a balloon positioned in the proximal segment of the descending aorta. The gas used for this purpose is carbon dioxide (because of its great solubility in blood) or helium (because of its inertial properties and rapid diffusion coefficients). Inflation and deflation are synchronized to the cardiac cycle by the electronics of the balloon console producing counterpulsations. The results of effective use of the IABP are often quite dramatic. Improvements in cardiac output, ejection fraction, coronary blood flow, and MAP are frequently seen, as well as decreases in aortic and ventricular systolic pressures, LVEDP, PCWP, LAP, HR, frequency of premature ventricular contractions, and suppression of atrial arrhythmias.

Indications and Contraindications

Since its introduction, the indications for the IABP have grown (Table 25-10). The most common use of the IABP is for treatment of cardiogenic shock. This may occur after CPB or after cardiac surgery in patients with shock preoperatively with acute postinfarction ventricular septal defects or mitral regurgitation, those who require stabilization before surgery, or patients who decompensate hemodynamically during cardiac catheterization. Patients with myocardial ischemia refractory to coronary vasodilation and afterload reduction are stabilized with an IABP before cardiac catheterization, and some patients with severe CAD will prophylactically

Table 25-10	**Intra-Aortic Balloon Pump Counterpulsation Indications and Contraindications**

Indications	Contraindications

1. Cardiogenic shock
   a. Myocardial infarction
   b. Myocarditis
   c. Cardiomyopathy
2. Failure to separate from CPB
3. Stabilization of preoperative patient
   a. Ventricular septal defect
   b. Mitral regurgitation
4. Stabilization of noncardiac surgical preoperative patient
5. Procedural support during coronary angiography
6. Bridge to transplantation
	1. Aortic valvular insufficiency
	2. Aortic disease
	   a. Aortic dissection
	   b. Aortic aneurysm
	3. Severe peripheral vascular disease
	4. Severe noncardiac systemic disease
	5. Massive trauma
	6. Patients with "do not resuscitate" instructions

have an IABP inserted before undergoing CABG or off-pump coronary artery bypass surgery.[18]

Contraindications to IABP use are relatively few. The presence of severe aortic regurgitation or aortic dissection is listed as an absolute contraindication for the IABP, although successful reports of its use in patients with aortic insufficiency or acute trauma to the descending thoracic aorta have appeared.

Insertion Techniques

In the initial development of the IABP, insertion was by surgical access to the femoral vessels. In the late 1970s, refinements in IABP design allowed the development of percutaneous insertion techniques. Now the technique most commonly used, percutaneous IABP insertion is rapidly performed with commercially available kits.

The femoral vessel with the greater pulse is sought by careful palpation. The length of the balloon to be inserted is estimated by laying the balloon tip on the patient's chest at Louis' angle and appropriately marking the distal point corresponding to the femoral artery. Care must be taken when removing the balloon from its package to follow the manufacturer's procedures exactly so as not to cause perforation of the balloon before insertion. Available balloons come wrapped and need only be appropriately deflated before removal from the package. The femoral artery is entered with the supplied needle, a J-tipped guidewire is inserted to the level of the aortic arch, and the needle is removed. The arterial puncture site is enlarged with the successive placement of an 8-Fr dilator and then a 10.5- or 12-Fr dilator and sheath combination (Fig. 25-1). In the adult-sized (30- to 50-mL) balloons, only the dilator needs to be removed, leaving the sheath and guidewire in the artery. The balloon is threaded over the guidewire into the central aorta and into the previously estimated correct position in the proximal segment of the descending aorta. The sheath is gently pulled back to connect with the leakproof cuff on the balloon hub, ideally so that the entire sheath is out of the arterial lumen to minimize risk of ischemic complications to the distal extremity. Alternatively, the sheath may be stripped off the balloon shaft much like a peel-away pacemaker lead introducer, thereby entirely removing the sheath from the insertion site. At least one manufacturer offers a "sheathless" balloon for insertion.

25

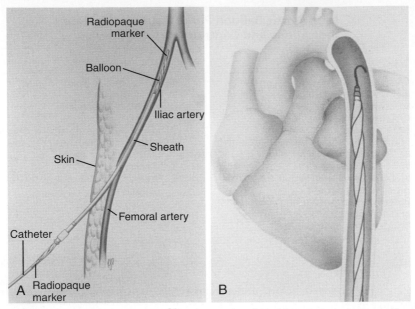

Figure 25-1 Diagram of intra-aortic balloon pump (IABP) insertion. **A,** Cannulation and insertion of the balloon through the femoral artery. Notice the tightly wrapped balloon as it traverses the sheath. A guidewire is not visible in this drawing. **B,** Correct positioning of balloon in the proximal descending aorta. The J-tipped guidewire is seen exiting from the balloon's central lumen. (**A,** Courtesy of Datascope Corporation; **B,** Courtesy of Kontron, Inc.)

If fluoroscopy is available during the procedure, correct placement is verified before fixing the balloon securely to the skin. Position may also be checked by radiography or echocardiography after insertion. If an indwelling left radial arterial catheter is functioning at the time of insertion, a reasonable estimate of position may be made by watching balloon-mediated alteration of the arterial pulse waveform (Fig. 25-2). After appropriate positioning and timing of the balloon, 1:1 counterpulsation may be initiated. The entire external balloon assembly should be covered in sterile dressings.

Removal of a percutaneously inserted IABP may be by the open (surgical removal) or closed technique. If a closed technique is chosen, the artery should be allowed to bleed for several seconds while pressure is maintained on the distal artery after balloon removal to flush any accumulated clot from the central lumen. This maneuver helps prevent distal embolization of clot. Pressure is then applied for 20 to 30 minutes on the puncture site for hemostasis. If surgical removal is chosen, embolectomy catheters may be passed antegrade and retrograde before suture closure of the artery.

Alternate routes of IABP insertion exist. The balloon may be placed surgically through the femoral artery. This is now performed without the use of an end-to-side vascular conduit, although this placement still requires a second surgical procedure for removal. In patients in whom extreme peripheral vascular disease exists or in pediatric patients in whom the peripheral vasculature is too small, the ascending aorta or aortic arch may be entered for balloon insertion. These approaches necessitate median sternotomy for insertion and usually require reexploration for removal. Other routes of access include the abdominal aorta and the subclavian, axillary, and iliac arteries. The iliac approach may be especially useful for pediatric cases.

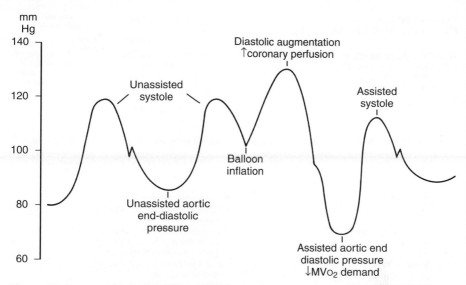

Figure 25-2 Arterial waveforms seen during intra-aortic balloon pump (IABP) assist. The first two waveforms are unassisted, and the last is assisted. Notice the decreased end-systolic and end-diastolic pressures and augmented diastolic pressures caused by IABP augmentation and the (correct) point at which balloon inflation occurs. These are waveforms generated by a correctly positioned and timed balloon. (Courtesy of Datascope Corporation.)

Timing and Weaning

There are a number of different manufacturers of IABP systems commercially available. The basic console design includes electrocardiographic and arterial blood pressure waveform monitoring and printing, balloon volume monitoring, triggering selection switches, adjustments for inflation and deflation timing, battery backup power sources, and gas reservoir. Some of these systems have become quite sophisticated, with advanced computer microprocessor circuits allowing triggering based on pacemaker signals or detection of and compensation for aberrant rhythms such as atrial fibrillation. Portable models exist for transportation of patients by ground, helicopter, or air ambulances.

For optimal effect of the IABP, inflation and deflation need to be correctly timed to the cardiac cycle. Although a number of variables, including positioning of the balloon within the aorta, balloon volume, and the patient's cardiac rhythm, can affect the performance of the IABP, basic principles regarding the function of the balloon must be followed. Balloon inflation should be timed to coincide with aortic valve closure, or aortic insufficiency and LV strain will result. Similarly, late inflation will result in a diminished perfusion pressure to the coronary arteries. Early deflation will cause inappropriate loss of afterload reduction, and late deflation will increase LV work by causing increased afterload, if only transiently. These errors and correct timing diagrams are illustrated in Figures 25-2 and 25-3.

As the patient's cardiac performance improves, the IABP support must be removed in stages rather than abruptly. Judicious application and dosing of vasodilator and inotropic medications can assist this procedure. The balloon augmentation may be reduced in steps from 1:1 counterpulsation to 1:2 and then to 1:4, with appropriate intervals at each stage to assess hemodynamic and neurologic stability, cardiac output, and mixed venous oxygen saturation changes. After appropriate observation at 1:4 or 1:8 counterpulsation, balloon assistance can be safely discontinued, and the device can be removed by one of the methods discussed. If percutaneous removal is

Premature deflation of the IAB during the diastolic phase

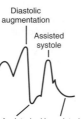

Waveform characteristics:
- Deflation of IAB is seen as a sharp drop following diastolic augmentation
- Suboptimal diastolic augmentation
- Assisted aortic end-diastolic pressure may be equal to or greater than the unassisted aortic end-diastolic pressure
- Assisted systolic pressure may rise

Physiologic effects:
- Suboptimal coronary perfusion
- Potential for retrograde coronary and carotid blood flow
- Angina may occur as a result of retrograde coronary blood flow
- Suboptimal afterload reduction
- Increased MVO_2 demand

A

Deflation of the IAB late in diastolic phase as aortic valve is beginning to open

Waveform characteristics:
- Assisted aortic end-diastolic pressure may be equal to the unassisted aortic end-diastolic pressure
- Rate of rise of assisted systole is prolonged
- Diastolic augmentation may appear widened

Physiologic effects:
- Afterload reduction is essentially absent
- Increased MVO_2 consumption due to the left ventricle ejecting against a greater resistance and a prolonged isovolumetric contraction phase
- IAB may impede left ventricular ejection and increase the afterload

B

Inflation of the IAB before aortic valve closure

Waveform characteristics:
- Inflation of IAB before dicrotic notch.
- Diastolic augmentation encroaches onto systole (may be unable to distinguish)

Physiologic effects:
- Potential premature closure of aortic valve
- Potential increased in LVEDV and LVEDP or PCWP
- Increased left ventricular wall stress or afterload
- Aortic regurgitation
- Increased MVO_2 demand

C

Inflation of the IAB markedly after closure of the aortic valve

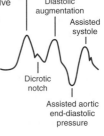

Waveform characteristics:
- Inflation of the IAB after the dicrotic notch.
- Absence of sharp V
- Suboptimal diastolic augmentation

Physiologic effects:
- Suboptimal coronary artery perfusion

D

Figure 25-3 Alterations in arterial waveform tracings caused by errors in timing of intra-aortic balloon pump (IABP). **A,** The balloon was deflated too early. **B,** The balloon was deflated too late. **C,** The balloon was inflated too early. **D,** The balloon was inflated too late. (Courtesy of Datascope Corporation.)

chosen, an appropriate interval for reversal of anticoagulation (if employed) before removal of the balloon should be allowed.

Complications

Several complications have been associated with IABP use (Table 25-11). The most frequently seen complications are vascular injuries, balloon malfunction, and infection.[19,20]

Table 25-11	**Intra-Aortic Balloon Pump Counterpulsation Complications**	
Vascular	**Miscellaneous**	**Balloon**
Arterial injury (perforation, dissection)	Hemolysis	Perforation (before insertion)
Aortic perforation	Thrombocytopenia	Tear (during insertion)
Aortic dissection	Infection	Incorrect positioning
Femoral artery thrombosis	Claudication (after removal)	Gas embolization
Peripheral embolization	Hemorrhage	Inadvertent removal
Femoral vein cannulation	Paraplegia	
Pseudoaneurysm of femoral vessels	Entrapment	
Lower extremity ischemia	Spinal cord necrosis	
Compartment syndrome	Left internal mammary artery occlusion	
Visceral ischemia		

SUMMARY

- The key to success in weaning from cardiopulmonary bypass (CPB) is proper preparation.
- After rewarming the patient, correcting any abnormal blood gases, and inflating the lungs, be sure to turn on the ventilator!
- To prepare the heart for discontinuing CPB, optimize the cardiac rhythm, heart rate, myocardial contractility, preload, and afterload.
- The worse the heart's condition, the more gradually CPB should be weaned. If hemodynamic values are not adequate, immediately return to CPB. Assess the problem, and choose an appropriate pharmacologic intervention before trying to terminate CPB again.
- Perioperative ventricular dysfunction usually is caused by myocardial stunning and is a temporary state of contractile dysfunction that should respond to positive inotropic drugs.
- In addition to left ventricular dysfunction, right ventricular failure is a possible source of morbidity and mortality after cardiac surgery.
- Epinephrine is frequently the inotropic drug of choice when terminating CPB because of its mixed α- and β-adrenergic stimulation.
- Milrinone is an excellent inodilator drug that can be used alone or combined with other drugs such as epinephrine for discontinuing CPB in patients with poor ventricular function.
- In patients with high preloads, vasodilators such as nitroglycerin or nitroprusside may markedly improve ventricular function.
- Intra-aortic balloon pump counterpulsation increases coronary blood flow during diastole and unloads the left ventricle during systole. These effects can help in weaning patients with poor left ventricular function and severe myocardial ischemia.

REFERENCES

1. Grigore AM, Grocott HP, Mathew JP, et al: Neurologic Outcome Research Group of the Duke Heart Center. The rewarming rate and increased peak temperature alter neurocognitive outcome after cardiac surgery. Anesth Analg 94:4, 2002
2. Spiess BD: Blood transfusion for cardiopulmonary bypass: The need to answer a basic question. J Cardiothorac Vasc Anesth 16:535, 2002

3. Boyd WC, Thomas SJ: Pro: Magnesium should be administered to all coronary artery bypass graft surgery patients undergoing cardiopulmonary bypass. J Cardiothorac Vasc Anesth 14:339, 2000

4. Grigore AM, Mathew JP: Con: Magnesium should not be administered to all coronary artery bypass graft surgery patients undergoing cardiopulmonary bypass. J Cardiothorac Vasc Anesth 14:344, 2000

5. Cheung AT, Savino JS, Weiss SJ, et al: Echocardiographic and hemodynamic indexes of left ventricular preload in patients with normal and abnormal ventricular function. Anesthesiology 81:376, 1994

6. Park KW: Protamine and protamine reactions. Int Anesthesiol Clin 42:135, 2004

7. Butterworth JF 4th, Prielipp RC, Royster RL, et al: Dobutamine increases heart rate more than epinephrine in patients recovering from aortocoronary bypass surgery. J Cardiothorac Vasc Anesth 6:535, 1992

8. Kertai MD, Poldermans D: The utility of dobutamine stress echocardiography for perioperative and long-term cardiac risk assessment. J Cardiothorac Vasc Anesth 19:520, 2005

9. Kristof AS, Magder S: Low systemic vascular resistance state in patients undergoing cardiopulmonary bypass. Crit Care Med 27:1121, 1999

10. Royster RL, Butterworth JF 4th, Prielipp RC, et al: Combined inotropic effects of amrinone and epinephrine after cardiopulmonary bypass in humans. Anesth Analg 77:662, 1993

11. Levy JH, Bailey JM, Deeb JM: Intravenous milrinone in cardiac surgery. Ann Thorac Surg 73:325, 2002

12. Feneck RO: Intravenous milrinone following cardiac surgery: I. Effects of bolus infusion followed by variable dose maintenance infusion. The European Milrinone Multicentre Trial Group. J Cardiothorac Vasc Anesth 6:554, 1992

13. Butterworth JF 4th, Hines RL, Royster RL, James RL: A pharmacokinetic and pharmacodynamic evaluation of milrinone in adults undergoing cardiac surgery. Anesth Analg 81:783, 1995

14. Felker JM: Inotropic therapy for heart failure: An evidence-based approach. Am Heart J 142:393, 2001

15. Wallin M, Barr G, Owall A, et al: The influence of glucose-insulin-potassium on GH/IGF-1/IGFBP-1 axis during elective coronary artery bypass surgery. J Cardiothorac Vasc Anesth 17:470, 2003

16. Lehmann A, Boldt J: New pharmacologic approaches for the perioperative treatment of ischemic cardiogenic shock. J Cardiothorac Vasc Anesth 19:97, 2005

17. Remme W, Swedberg K, and the Task Force for the Diagnosis and Treatment of Heart Failure, European Society of Cardiology: Guidelines for the diagnosis and treatment of chronic heart failure, Eur Heart J 22:1527, 2001

18. Stone G, Ohman E, Miller M, et al: Contemporary utilization and outcomes of intra-aortic balloon counterpulsation in acute myocardial infarction: The Benchmark Registry. J Am Coll Cardiol 41:1940, 2003

19. Craver J, Murrah C: Elective intra-aortic balloon counterpulsation for high-risk off-pump coronary artery bypass operations. Ann Thorac Surg 71:1220, 2001

20. Ferguson J, Cohen M, Freedan R, et al: The current practice of intra-aortic balloon counterpulsation: Results from the Benchmark Registry. J Am Coll Cardiol 38:1456, 2001

V

Section VI
Postoperative Care

Chapter 26

Postoperative Cardiac Recovery and Outcomes

Davy C.H. Cheng, MD • Daniel Bainbridge, MD

Care of the cardiac surgical patient has become increasingly specialized and patient care has become more complicated. Not only are clinical outcomes important, reflected in mortality and morbidity statistics, but the costs associated with delivering patient care are also playing an increasingly greater role in determining clinical practice.

Cardiac anesthesia itself has fundamentally shifted from a high-dose narcotic technique to a balanced approach using moderate-dose narcotics, shorter-acting muscle relaxants, and volatile anesthetics. This has primarily been driven by a realization that high-dose narcotics delay extubation and recovery after surgery. This new paradigm has also led to renewed interest in perioperative pain management involving multimodal techniques that facilitate rapid tracheal extubation such as regional blocks, intrathecal morphine, and supplementary nonsteroidal anti-inflammatory drugs (NSAIDs). In addition to changes in anesthetic practice, the type of patients presenting for cardiac surgery is changing. Patients are now older and have more associated comorbidities (stroke, myocardial infarction [MI], renal failure). Treatment options for coronary artery disease have expanded, ranging from medical therapy only to percutaneous interventions and surgery. Surgical options, however, have also expanded and include conventional coronary artery bypass grafting (CABG), off-pump coronary artery bypass grafting (OPCAB), minimally direct invasive coronary artery bypass grafting (MIDCAB), and robotically assisted coronary artery bypass grafting (RACAB) techniques. Change has also taken place in the recovery of cardiac patients. Whereas cardiac surgical procedures used to be associated with a high mortality and long intensive care unit (ICU) stays, today's moderate doses of narcotics allow for rapid ventilator

---

---

weaning and discharge from the ICU within 24 hours. This has prompted a shift from the classic model of recovering patients in the traditional ICU manner, with weaning protocols and intensive observation, to management more in keeping with the recovery room practice of early extubation and rapid discharge. This, in turn, has shifted the care of cardiac patients to more specialized postcardiac surgical recovery units.

Finally, clinical outcomes have driven change in the management of cardiac patients and are increasingly the focus of research. Intraoperative management now exists within the continuum of preoperative assessment and postoperative care. The outcomes of a patient within the hospital setting are only one small aspect of success. Long-term mortality, morbidity, and quality-of-life indicators are becoming the gold standard in determining benefit or harm interventions.

FAST TRACK CARDIAC SURGERY CARE

Anesthetic Techniques

There have been few trials comparing inhalation agents for fast track cardiac anesthesia (FTCA). Several studies have examined the effectiveness of propofol versus inhalation agents, most demonstrated reductions in myocardial enzyme release (CK-MB, troponin I) and preservation of myocardial function in patients receiving inhalation agents.[1] Although this endpoint is a surrogate for myocardial damage and does not show improved outcome per se, CK-MB release after CABG may be associated with poor outcome (Box 26-1).

The choice of muscle relaxant in FTCA is important to reduce the incidence of muscle weakness in the cardiac recovery area (CRA), which may delay tracheal extubation. Randomized trials have compared rocuronium (0.5 to 1 mg/kg) versus pancuronium (0.1 mg/kg) and found significant differences in residual paralysis in the ICU, and statistically significant delays were found in the time to extubation in the pancuronium group.[2] None of the trials used reversal agents, so the use of pancuronium appears acceptable as long as neostigmine or edrophonium is administered to patients with residual neuromuscular weakness.

There have been several trials examining the use of different short-acting narcotic agents during FTCA. In these trials, fentanyl, remifentanil, and sufentanil were all found to be efficacious for early tracheal extubation. The anesthetic drugs and their suggested dosages are given in Table 26-1.

Evidence Supporting Fast Track Cardiac Recovery

There are several randomized trials and a meta-analysis of randomized trials that have addressed the question of safety of FTCA.[3] None of the trials was able to demonstrate differences in outcomes between the fast track group and the conventional anesthesia group, but meta-analysis of the randomized trials demonstrated a reduction in the

Table 26-1   Suggested Dosages for Fast Track Cardiac Anesthesia

Induction

Narcotic
  Fentanyl, 5 to 10 μg/kg
  Sufentanil, 1 to 3 μg/kg
  Remifentanil, infusions of 0.5 μg/kg/min to 1.0 μg/kg/min
Muscle relaxant
  Rocuronium, 0.5 to 1 mg/kg
  Vecuronium, 1 to 1.5 mg/kg
Hypnotic
  Midazolam, 0.05 to 0.1 mg/kg
  Propofol, 0.5 to 1.5 mg/kg

Maintenance

Narcotic
  Fentanyl, 1 to 5 μg/kg
  Sufentanil, 1 to 1.5 μg/kg
  Remifentanil, infusions of 0.5 μg/kg/min to 1.0 μg/kg/min
Hypnotic
  Inhalational 0.5 to 1 MAC
  Propofol, 50 to 100 μg/kg/min

Transfer to Cardiac Recovery Area

Narcotic
  Morphine, 0.1 to 0.2 mg/kg
Hypnotic
  Propofol, 25 to 75 μg/kg/min

MAC=minimal alveolar concentration.
From Mollhoff T, Herregods L, Moerman A, et al: Comparative efficacy and safety of remifentanil and fentanyl in "fast track" coronary artery bypass graft surgery: A randomized, double-blind study. Br J Anaesth 87: 718, 2001; Engoren M, Luther G, Fenn-Buderer N: A comparison of fentanyl, sufentanil, and remifentanil for fast-track cardiac anesthesia. Anesth Analg 93: 859, 2001; and Cheng DC, Newman MF, Duke P, et al: The efficacy and resource utilization of remifentanil and fentanyl in fast-tract coronary artery bypass graft surgery: A prospective randomized, double-blinded controlled, multi-center trial. Anesth Analg 92:1094, 2001.

duration of intubation by 8 hours (Fig. 26-1) and the ICU length of stay by 5 hours in favor of the fast track group. However, the length of hospital stay was not statistically different.

One concern with FTCA is the potential for an increase in the incidence of adverse events, notably awareness. Awareness in patients undergoing FTCA was systematically investigated and the reported incidence of explicit intraoperative awareness was 0.3%. This is comparable to the reported incidence during conventional cardiac surgery. This suggests that FTCA does not increase the incidence of awareness compared with conventional cardiac surgery.

FTCA appears safe in comparison to conventional high-dose narcotic anesthesia. It reduces the duration of ventilation and ICU length of stay considerably without increasing the incidence of awareness or other adverse events. It also appears effective at reducing costs and resource utilization. As such, it is the standard of care in many cardiac centers. The usual practice at many institutions is to treat all patients as fast track candidates with the goal of allowing early tracheal extubation for every patient. However, if complications occur that would prevent early tracheal extubation, then the management strategy is modified accordingly. It has been demonstrated that the risk factors for delayed tracheal extubation (>10 hours) are increased age, female gender, postoperative use of intra-aortic balloon pump (IABP), inotropes, bleeding,

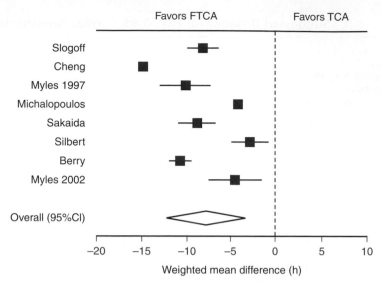

Figure 26-1 Forrest plot showing the weighted mean difference in extubation times. The overall effect was an 8.1-hour reduction in extubation times. FTCA=fast track cardiac anesthesia; TCA=traditional cardiac anesthesia.

and atrial arrhythmia. The risk factors for prolonged ICU length of stay (>48 hours) are those of delayed tracheal extubation plus preoperative MI and postoperative renal insufficiency. Care should be taken to avoid excess bleeding (antifibrinolytics) and to treat arrhythmias either prophylactically or on occurrence (β-blockers, amiodarone).

Postcardiac Surgical Recovery Models

The failure of many randomized FTCA trials to show reductions in resource utilization likely stems from the traditional ICU models used by these centers during the study period. Even when trials were combined in a meta-analysis, the ICU length of stay was reduced only by 5 hours despite patients being extubated a mean of 8 hours earlier.[3] Typically, patients who are extubated within the first 24 hours of ICU admission are transferred to the ward on postoperative day 1 in the morning or early afternoon. This allows the following daytime cardiac cases to have available ICU beds but prevents patient transfers during night-time hours. Two models have been proposed to deal with this issue: the parallel model and the integrated model. In the parallel model, patients are admitted directly to a CRA, where they are monitored with 1:1 nursing care until tracheal extubation. Following this, the level of care is reduced to reflect reduced nursing requirements with ratios of 1:2 or 1:3. Any patients requiring overnight ventilation are transferred to the ICU for continuation of care. The primary drawback with the parallel model is the physical separation of the CRA and ICU, which leads to two separate units and thus does not eliminate the requirement to transfer patients. The integrated model overcomes these limitations because all patients are admitted to the same physical area, but postoperative management such as nursing-to-patient ratio is variable based on patient requirements. Because nursing care accounts for 45% to 50% of ICU costs, reducing the nursing requirements where possible creates the greatest saving. Other cost savings from reductions in arterial blood gases measurement, use of sedative drugs, and ventilator maintenance are small. The goal is a postoperative unit that allows variable levels of monitoring

> **BOX 26-2** *Initial Management of the Fast Track Cardiac Anesthesia Patient*
>
> - Normothermia
> - Hemoglobin > 7.0 g/dL
> - $Paco_2$ of 35 to 45 mm Hg
> - Sao_2 > 95%
> - Mean blood pressure of 50 to 70 mm Hg
> - Potassium level of 3.5 to 5.0 mEq/L
> - Blood glucose < 200 mg/dL

and care based on patient need. Furthermore, FTCA has been demonstrated to be a safe and cost-effective practice that decreases resource utilization after patient discharge from the index hospitalization up to 1-year follow-up.[4]

INITIAL MANAGEMENT OF FAST TRACK CARDIAC ANESTHESIA PATIENTS: THE FIRST 24 HOURS

On arrival in the CRA, initial management of cardiac patients consists of ensuring an efficient transfer of care from operating room staff to CRA staff while at the same time maintaining stable patient vital signs. The anesthesiologist should relay important clinical parameters to the CRA team. To accomplish this, many centers have devised hand-off sheets to aid in the transfer of care. The patient's temperature should be recorded, and, if it is low, active rewarming measures should be initiated with the goal of rewarming the patient to 36.5°C. Shivering may be treated with low intravenous doses of meperidine (12.5 to 25 mg). Hyperthermia, however, is common within the first 24 hours after cardiac surgery and may be associated with an increase in neurocognitive dysfunction, possibly as a result of hyperthermia exacerbating cardiopulmonary bypass (CPB)–induced neurologic injury (Box 26-2).

Ventilation Management: Admission to Tracheal Extubation

Ventilatory requirements should be managed with the goal of early tracheal extubation (Table 26-2). Arterial blood gas samples are initially drawn within 30 minutes after admission and then repeated as necessary. Patients should be awake and cooperative, hemodynamically stable, and have no active bleeding with coagulopathy. Respiratory strength should be assessed by hand grip or head lift to ensure complete reversal of neuromuscular blockade. The patient's temperature should be above 36°C, preferably normothermic. When these conditions are met and arterial blood gas results are within the normal range, tracheal extubation may take place. Blood for arterial blood gas analysis should be drawn about 30 minutes after tracheal extubation to ensure adequate ventilation with maintenance of Pao_2 and $Paco_2$. Inability to extubate patients as a result of respiratory failure, hemodynamic instability, or large amounts of mediastinal drainage will necessitate more complex weaning strategies. Some patients may arrive after extubation in the operating room. Careful attention should be paid to these patients. The patient's respiratory rate should be monitored every 5 minutes during the first several hours. A blood sample should be drawn on admission and 30 minutes later to ensure the patient is not retaining carbon dioxide.

26

Table 26-2 Ventilation Management Goals during the Initial Trial of Weaning from Extubation

Initial ventilation parameters
    A/C at 10 to 12 beats per minute
    Tidal volume 8 to 10 mL/kg
    PEEP 5 cm H_2O
Maintain arterial blood gases
    pH 7.35 to 7.45
    Pa_{CO_2} 35 to 45
    $Pa_{O_2} > 90$
    Saturations $> 95\%$
Extubation criteria
    Arterial blood gases as above
    Awake and alert
    Hemodynamically stable
    No active bleeding (<400 mL/2 hr)
    Temperature $> 36°C$
    Return of muscle strength (>5 seconds, head lift/strong hand grip)

A/C = assist-controlled ventilation; PEEP = positive end-expiratory pressure.

If the patient's respirations become compromised, ventilatory support should be provided. Simple measures such as reminders to breathe may be effective in the narcotized/anesthetized patient. Low intravenous doses of naloxone (0.04 mg) may also be beneficial. Trials of continuous positive airway pressure (CPAP) or bilevel positive airway pressure (BiPAP) may provide enough support to allow adequate ventilation. Reintubation should be avoided because it may delay recovery; however, it may become necessary if the just-mentioned measures fail, resulting in hypoxemia, hypercarbia, and a declining level of consciousness.

Regulation of Hemoglobin Level

Anemia is common during and after cardiac surgery as a result of both dilutional changes and bleeding. While a hemoglobin transfusion threshold of 10 g/dL was once common, increasing evidence suggests that a threshold of 7 g/dL is reasonably safe. However, in the post-CPB period, patients with incomplete revascularization or with poor target vessels may require a higher transfusion threshold. As a result, blood transfusions should be individualized for each patient but should certainly be used to maintain a minimal hemoglobin level of 7 g/dL.

Management of Bleeding

Chest tube drainage should be checked every 15 minutes after ICU admission to assess a patient's coagulation status. Because blood loss is commonly divided into two types, surgical or medical, determining the cause of bleeding is often difficult. When bleeding exceeds 400 mL/hr during the first hour, 200 mL/hr for each of the first 2 hours, or 100 mL/hr over the first 4 hours, returning to the operating room for chest reexploration should be considered. The clinical situation must be individualized for each patient, however, and in the presence of a known coagulopathy, more liberal blood loss before chest reexploration may be acceptable. There are numerous medical causes for bleeding after cardiac surgery. Platelet dysfunction after cardiac surgery is common. Residual heparinization is common after cardiac surgery and frequently occurs

> **BOX 26-3** *Management of the Bleeding Patient*
>
> - Review activated coagulation time, prothrombin time, international normalized ratio, platelet count.
> - Give protamine if due to excess heparin (reinfusion of pump blood).
> - Treat medical cause: platelets, fresh frozen plasma, cryoprecipitate if secondary to decreased fibrinogen.
> - Treat surgical cause: reexploration.

when either heparinized pump blood is transfused after CPB or insufficient protamine is administered. Fibrinolysis is also very common after CPB, predominantly caused by a host of activated inflammatory and coagulation pathways. Coagulation factors may decrease from activation at air-blood interfaces or from dilution with the CPB pump priming solution. Hypothermia may also aggravate the coagulation cascade and lead to further bleeding. Conventional coagulation tests are helpful to identify the coagulation abnormality contributing to the bleeding. Common laboratory testing includes activated partial thromboplastin time, international normalized ratio, platelet count, fibrinogen level, and D-dimers. Unfortunately, with most conventional measures 20 to 40 minutes lapse before results are available (Box 26-3). The use of point-of-care testing such as thromboelastography has been demonstrated to reduce transfusion requirements without increasing blood loss and is commonly used, especially following difficult cardiac cases.

Electrolyte Management

Hypokalemia is common after cardiac surgery, especially if diuretics were given intraoperatively. Hypokalemia contributes to increased automaticity and may lead to ventricular arrhythmias, ventricular tachycardia, or ventricular fibrillation. Treatment consists of potassium infusions (20 mEq of potassium in 50 mL of D_5W infused over 1 hour) until the potassium exceeds 3.5 mEq/mL. In patients with frequent premature ventricular contractions caused by increased automaticity, a potassium level of 5.0 mEq/mL may be desirable. Hypomagnesemia contributes to ventricular preexcitation and may contribute to atrial fibrillation. Management consists of intermittent boluses of magnesium—1 to 2 g over 15 minutes. Hypocalcemia is also frequent during cardiac surgery and may reduce cardiac contractility. Intermittent boluses of calcium chloride or calcium gluconate (1 g) may be required (Table 26-3).

Glucose Management

Diabetes is a common comorbidity (up to 30%) and is a known risk factor for adverse outcome in patients presenting for cardiac surgery. Hyperglycemia itself is common during CPB. The risk factors for hyperglycemia include diabetes, administration of corticosteroids before CPB, volume of glucose-containing solutions administered, and use of epinephrine infusions. Poor perioperative glucose control is associated with increases in mortality and morbidity, including an increased risk of infection and a prolonged duration of ventilation.[5] In a large prospective, randomized, controlled trial of tight glucose control (blood glucose levels of 4.1 to 6.5 mmol/L) during postoperative ICU stay, reductions in mortality were shown by the authors compared with more liberal glucose control (blood glucose levels of 12 mmol/L). This trial enrolled both diabetic and nondiabetic hyperglycemic patients who underwent cardiothoracic surgery and demonstrates that tight management

Table 26-3 Common Electrolyte Abnormalities and Possible Treatment Options

Hypokalemia ($K^+ < 3.5$ mmol/L)
    SSx: muscle weakness, ST-segment depression, "u" wave, T wave flat, ventricular preexcitation
    Rx: IV KCl at 10 to 20 mEq/hr via central catheter
Hyperkalemia ($K^+ > 5.2$ mmol/L)
    SSx: muscle weakness, peaked T wave, loss of P wave, prolonged PR/QRS
    Rx: $CaCl_2$ 1 g, insulin/glucose, HCO_3^-, diuretics, hyperventilation, dialysis
Hypocalcemia (ionized $Ca^{2+} < 1.1$ mmol/L)
    SSx: hypotension, heart failure, prolonged QT interval
    Rx: $CaCl_2$ or Ca gluconate
Hypercalcemia (ionized $Ca^{2+} > 1.3$ mmol/L)
    SSx: altered mental state, coma, ileus
    Rx: dialysis, diuretics, mithramycin, calcitonin
Hypermagnesemia ($Mg^{2+} > 0.7$ mmol/L)
    SSx: weakness, absent reflexes
    Rx: stop Mg infusion, diuresis
Hypomagnesemia ($Mg^{2+} < 0.5$ mmol/L)
    SSx: arrhythmia, prolonged PR and QT intervals
    Rx: Mg infusion 1 to 2 g

SSx = signs and symptoms, Rx = treatment.

of glucose is beneficial in the CRA. Given all the associated risks of hyperglycemia, attempts should be made to maintain euglycemia throughout the perioperative setting in all patients presenting for surgery.

Pain Control

Pain control after cardiac surgery has become a concern as narcotic doses have been reduced to facilitate fast track protocols. Intravenous morphine is still the mainstay of treatment for post–cardiac surgery patients. The most common approach is patient-demanded, nurse-delivered intravenous morphine, and this treatment remains popular because of 1:1 to 1:2 nursing typically provided during cardiac recovery. However, with a change to more flexible nurse coverage and, therefore, higher nurse-to-patient ratios, patient-controlled analgesia (PCA) morphine is becoming increasingly popular (Table 26-4).

Medications for Risk Reduction after Coronary Artery Bypass Graft Surgery

CABG surgery itself reduces the risk of mortality and angina recurrence, but several medical management issues may help maintain the long-term benefit after CABG surgery. Specifically, the use of aspirin, β-blockers, and lipid-lowering agents has been demonstrated to prolong survival and/or reduce graft restenosis (Box 26-4).

Aspirin

Several studies have demonstrated the efficacy of aspirin use on graft patency and reductions in MI and mortality after CABG surgery.[6] A large observational study showed a reduction in mortality of nearly 3% and a reduction in MI rate of 48% with the early use of aspirin postoperatively (within 48 hours). Dosages of aspirin have ranged from 100 mg daily to 325 mg three times a day orally. Both ticlopidine and

Table 26-4　Pain Management Options after Cardiac Surgery

Patient-Controlled Analgesia
May be of benefit in a step-down unit
Reduced 24-hour morphine consumption demonstrated in two of seven randomized trials

Intrathecal Morphine
Doses studied: 500 μg to 4 mg
May be of benefit to reduce intravenous use of morphine
May be of benefit in reducing Visual Analog Scale pain scores
*Potential for respiratory depression
Ideal dosing not ascertained; range from 250 to 400 μg

Thoracic Epidurals
Common dosages from literature
　Ropivacaine 1% with 5 μg/mL fentanyl at 3 to 5 mL/hr
　Bupivacaine 0.5% with 25 μg/mL morphine at 3 to 10 mL/hr
　Bupivacaine 0.5% to 0.75% at 2 to 5 mL/hr
Reduced pain scores
Shorter duration of intubation
*Risk of epidural hematoma difficult to quantify

Nonsteroidal Anti-inflammatory Drugs
Common dosages from literature
　Indomethacin, 50 mg to 100 mg PR twice daily
　Diclofenac, 50 to 75 mg PO/PR every 8 hours
　Ketorolac, 10 to 30 mg IM/IV every 8 hours
Reduces narcotic utilization
Many different drugs studied; difficult to determine superiority of a given agent

*May increase serious adverse events (one trial using cyclooxygenase-2–specific inhibitors)

BOX 26-4　*Medications for Risk Reduction after Coronary Artery Bypass Graft Surgery*

- Aspirin: all patients after coronary artery bypass grafting
- Clopidogrel: patients who have contraindication to aspirin (may have superior efficacy compared with aspirin)
- β-Blockers: especially with perioperative myocardial infarction
- Lipid-lowering agents

26

clopidogrel may be suitable alternatives in patients who are allergic to aspirin. Clopidogrel, through reductions in all-cause mortality, stroke, and MI, may be superior to aspirin in patients who return with recurrent ischemic events after cardiac surgery.[7] Ticlopidine, however, should be used with caution because it may cause neutropenia (necessitating white blood cell counts to be monitored during initial use). Clopidogrel has a lower incidence of adverse reactions compared with ticlopidine and is therefore preferred as a second-line agent when aspirin is contraindicated.

Anticoagulation for Valve Surgery

Anticoagulation should be started in the early postoperative period for patients who have undergone valve replacement with either a mechanical or bioprosthesis and should also be considered when atrial fibrillation complicates the postoperative course. The recommended prophylactic regimens for patients with both mechanical and bioprosthetic heart valves are shown in Table 26-5.

Table 26-5 Suggested Antithrombotic Therapy for Heart Valve Prophylaxis

	Drug	Class
1. First 3 months after valve replacement	Warfarin, INR 2.5 to 3.5	I
2. Three months or longer after valve replacement		
A. Mechanical valve		
AVR and no risk factor*		
Bileaflet valve or Medtronic Hall valve	Warfarin, INR 2 to 3	I
Other disk valves or Starr-Edwards valve	Warfarin, INR 2.5 to 3.5	I
AVR + risk factor*	Warfarin, INR 2.5 to 3.5	I
MVR	Warfarin, INR 2.5 to 3.5	I
B. Bioprosthesis		
AVR and no risk factor*	Aspirin, 80 to 100 mg/d	I
AVR and risk factor*	Warfarin, INR 2 to 3	I
MVR and no risk factor*	Aspirin, 80 to 100 mg/d	I
MVR and risk factor*	Warfarin, INR 2.5 to 3.5	I
3. Addition of aspirin, 80 to 100 mg once daily if not on aspirin		IIa
4. Warfarin, INR 3.5 to 4.5 in high-risk patients when aspirin cannot be used		IIa
5. Warfarin, INR 2.0 to 3.0 in patients with Starr-Edwards AVR and no risk factor		IIb
6. Mechanical valve, no warfarin therapy		III
7. Mechanical valve, aspirin therapy only		III
8. Bioprosthesis, no warfarin and no aspirin therapy		III

*Risk factors: atrial fibrillation, left ventricular dysfunction, previous thromboembolism.
AVR = aortic valve replacement, MVR = mitral valve replacement.
Modified from Task Force on Practice Guidelines (Committee on Management of Patients with Valvular Heart Disease): ACC/AHA guidelines for the management of patients with valvular heart disease. A report of the American College of Cardiology/American Heart Association. J Am Coll Cardiol 32:1486-1588, 1998.

VI

MANAGEMENT OF COMPLICATIONS

Complications are frequent after cardiac surgery. Although many are short-lived, some complications, such as stroke, are long-term catastrophic events that seriously affect a patient's functional status.[8] The incidence and predisposing risk factors are well studied for many of the complications (Table 26-6). Many of these complications have specific management issues, which may improve recovery after surgery (Box 26-5).

Delirium

Delirium is defined generally as an acute transient neurologic condition with impairment of cognitive function, attention abnormalities, and altered psychomotor activity. It often includes a disorder with the sleep-wake cycle. It is fairly common after cardiac surgery with a prevalence of 8% to 15%.[9] Risk factors associated with delirium include age, previous history of stroke, duration of surgery, duration of aortic cross-clamp, atrial fibrillation, and blood transfusion. Interestingly, delirium is self-limited and does not adversely affect patient outcome or

Table 26-6   Common Complications after Cardiac Surgery

Complication	Incidence	Risk Factors
Stroke	2% to 4%	Age Previous stroke/transient ischemic attack Peripheral vascular disease Diabetes Unstable angina
Delirium	8% to 15%	Age Previous stroke Duration of surgery Duration of aortic cross-clamp Atrial fibrillation Blood transfusion
Atrial fibrillation	Up to 35%	Age Male gender Previous atrial fibrillation Mitral valve surgery Previous congestive heart failure
Renal failure	1%	Low postoperative cardiac output Repeat cardiac surgery Valve surgery Age Diabetes

---

BOX 26-5   *Treatment of Complications after Coronary Artery Bypass Surgery*

Stroke

- Supportive treatment
- Avoid potential aggravating factors such as hyperglycemia, hyperthermia, and severe anemia

Delirium

- Usually self-limited
- Requires close observation
- May require sedatives (midazolam, lorazepam)

Atrial Fibrillation

- Rate control: calcium channel blockers, β-blockers, digoxin
- Rhythm control: amiodarone, sotalol, procainamide
- Thromboembolic prophylaxis: for atrial fibrillation > 48 hours

Left Ventricular Dysfunction

- Volume
- Inotropes: epinephrine, milrinone, norepinephrine
- Mechanical support: intra-aortic balloon pump

Renal Failure

- Remove the causative agent (nonsteroidal anti-inflammatory drugs, antibiotics)
- Hemodynamic support if necessary
- Supportive care

26

hospital length of stay. Treatment is supportive, involving close observation of patients, and sedatives (midazolam, diazepam) or antipsychotics (haloperidol) as required.

Atrial Fibrillation

Atrial fibrillation after cardiac surgery is common and occurs in up to 35% of patients. While the cause is not completely understood, it is associated with an increase in mortality, stroke, and prolonged hospital stay. Known risk factors include age, male gender, previous episode, mitral valve surgery, and a history of congestive heart failure.[10] Prevention and treatment of atrial fibrillation can be achieved effectively with amiodarone, sotalol, magnesium, or β-blockers. Biatrial pacing may also be effective prophylaxis. Management of atrial fibrillation consists of rate control with conversion to sinus rhythm or anticoagulation. Several studies conducted to determine which strategy was superior were unable to find a difference between treatment strategies (AFFIRM and RACE trials).[11,12]

Rate control may be achieved with a β-blocker or a calcium channel blocker. Digoxin may also be effective, but it is difficult to achieve therapeutic levels quickly. An observational review of the AFFIRM trial suggests that β-blockers are superior to either calcium channel blockers or digoxin for rate control in AF. Conversion to sinus rhythm in the stable patient may be achieved with amiodarone, sotalol, or procainamide. Amiodarone is more commonly used in acute management of postoperative atrial fibrillation (150 to 300 mg IV) than other antiarrhythmics, particularly in patients with compromised ventricular function, because it causes little cardiac depression. Finally, persistent atrial fibrillation over 48 to 72 hours requires thromboembolic prophylaxis. Warfarin is recommended for patients at high risk of thromboembolic complications (previous stroke, congestive heart failure, diabetes mellitus, age), with an INR between 2 and 3 considered therapeutic.

Left Ventricular Dysfunction

Patients who have an unstable intraoperative course should have pulmonary artery filling pressures correlated to TEE findings and the results then passed to the recovery unit to allow for optimal initial management in the recovery unit. If the patient remains unstable in the ICU, then TEE can be used and cardiac function reassessed. When hypovolemia is thought to be the underlying cause of hypotension/low cardiac output, then colloids are initially used to optimize filling, because third spacing of fluids is common after CPB. The intravascular hypovolemia is best treated with the use of small intermittent boluses of colloid with continuous reassessment of central venous pressure, pulmonary artery pressure, wedge pressure, systemic pressures, or left ventricular end-diastolic area.[13]

If ventricular dysfunction is the main cause of hypotension/low cardiac output state, then inotropes and vasopressors should be added. Epinephrine (0.02 to 0.04 μg/kg/min) or dopamine (3 to 5 μg/kg/min) is commonly used to support patients coming off CPB and is usually continued into the ICU. If systolic pressure remains low, then the epinephrine infusion is usually increased to allow for greater α-receptor action (vasoconstriction). For patients with a low cardiac output or poor myocardial function on TEE, milrinone is commonly used (with or without a full loading dose). When volume and medical strategies are insufficient, especially in the presence of ischemic heart disease, mechanical support is used. IABPs are used in approximately 3% of cardiac surgical patients.[14]

POSTOPERATIVE RISK AND OUTCOME

One question that every patient asks and every anesthesiologist answers concerns the risks from this operation and the recovery course. Although seemingly a straightforward question, it gets to the heart of current medical practice, namely, assessing risk, weighing potential treatment options, determining best evidence for each patient, and then prescribing a course of treatment with the ultimate goal of providing the best possible care. It is important to know risk factors associated with cardiac surgery and to review treatment options for patients with specific reference to outcomes. This should all be placed within the context of cost and resource utilization, especially as medicine increasingly involves economic realities.[15-18]

SUMMARY

- Cardiac anesthesia has fundamentally shifted from a high-dose narcotic technique to a balanced approach using moderate-dose narcotics, shorter-acting muscle relaxants, and volatile anesthetics.
- This new paradigm has also led to renewed interest in perioperative pain management involving multimodal techniques that facilitate rapid tracheal extubation such as regional blocks, intrathecal morphine, and supplementary nonsteroidal anti-inflammatory drugs.
- This has prompted a shift from the classic model of recovery for patients in the traditional intensive care unit manner, with weaning protocols and intensive observation, to management more in keeping with the recovery room practice of early extubation and rapid discharge, which has shifted the care of cardiac patients to more specialized postcardiac surgical recovery units.
- Fast track cardiac anesthesia appears to be safe in comparison to conventional high-dose narcotic anesthesia, but if complications occur that would prevent early tracheal extubation, then the management strategy should be modified accordingly.
- The goal of a postcardiac surgery recovery model is a postoperative unit that allows variable levels of monitoring and care based on patient needs.
- The initial management in the postoperative care of fast track cardiac surgical patients consists of ensuring an efficient transfer of care from operating room staff to cardiac recovery area staff while at the same time maintaining stable patient vital signs.
- It is important to know risk factors associated with cardiac surgery and to review treatment options for patients with specific reference to outcomes, all placed within the context of cost and resource utilization, especially as medicine increasingly involves economic realities.
- There are many risk assessment models for cardiac surgery, but one primary drawback of scoring systems is the geographic variability that occurs among institutions, especially ones that are geographically and/or politically distinct and may not have the same risk factors for their cardiac surgery programs.

26

REFERENCES

1. De Hert SG, Cromheecke S, ten Broecke PW, et al: Effects of propofol, desflurane, and sevoflurane on recovery of myocardial function after coronary surgery in elderly high-risk patients. Anesthesiology 99:314, 2003
2. Murphy GS, Szokol JW, Marymont JH, et al: Recovery of neuromuscular function after cardiac surgery: pancuronium versus rocuronium. Anesth Analg 96:1301, 2003

3. Myles PS, Daly DJ, Djaiani G, et al: A systematic review of the safety and effectiveness of fast-track cardiac anesthesia. Anesthesiology 99:982, 2003

4. Cheng DC, Wall C, Djaiani G, et al: Randomized assessment of resource use in fast-track cardiac surgery 1 year after hospital discharge. Anesthesiology 98:651, 2003

5. Goldberg PA, Sakharova OV, Barrett PW, et al: Improving glycemic control in the cardiothoracic intensive care unit: Clinical experience in two hospital settings. J Cardiothorac Vasc Anesth 18:690, 2004

6. Mangano DT: Aspirin and mortality from coronary bypass surgery. N Engl J Med 347:1309, 2002

7. Bhatt DL, Chew DP, Hirsch AT, et al: Superiority of clopidogrel versus aspirin in patients with prior cardiac surgery. Circulation 103:363, 2001

8. Lahtinen J, Biancari F, Salmela E, et al: Postoperative atrial fibrillation is a major cause of stroke after on-pump coronary artery bypass surgery. Ann Thorac Surg 77:1241, 2004

9. Bucerius J, Gummert JF, Borger MA, et al: Predictors of delirium after cardiac surgery delirium: Effect of beating-heart (off-pump) surgery. J Thorac Cardiovasc Surg 127:57, 2004

10. Mathew JP, Fontes ML, Tudor IC, et al: A multicenter risk index for atrial fibrillation after cardiac surgery. JAMA 291:1720, 2004

11. Hagens VE, Ranchor AV, Van Sonderen E, et al: Effect of rate or rhythm control on quality of life in persistent atrial fibrillation. Results from the Rate Control Versus Electrical Cardioversion (RACE) Study. J Am Coll Cardiol 43:241, 2004

12. Olshansky B, Rosenfeld LE, Warner AL, et al: The Atrial Fibrillation Follow-up Investigation of Rhythm Management (AFFIRM) study: Approaches to control rate in atrial fibrillation. J Am Coll Cardiol 43:1201, 2004

13. Swenson JD, Bull D, Stringham J: Subjective assessment of left ventricular preload using transesophageal echocardiography: Corresponding pulmonary artery occlusion pressures. J Cardiothorac Vasc Anesth 15:580, 2001

14. Marra C, De Santo LS, Amarelli C, et al: Coronary artery bypass grafting in patients with severe left ventricular dysfunction: A prospective randomized study on the timing of perioperative intraaortic balloon pump support. Int J Artif Organs 25:141, 2002

15. Legrand VM, Serruys PW, Unger F, et al: Three-year outcome after coronary stenting versus bypass surgery for the treatment of multivessel disease. Circulation 109:1114, 2004

16. Khan NE, De Souza A, Mister R, et al: A randomized comparison of off-pump and on-pump multivessel coronary artery bypass surgery. N Engl J Med 350:21, 2004

17. Cheng D, Bainbridge D, Martin J, et al: Does off-pump coronary artery bypass reduce mortality, morbidity and resource utilization when compared to conventional coronary artery bypass? A meta-analysis of randomized trials. Anesthesiology 102:188, 2005

18. Puskas JD, Williams WH, Mahoney EM, et al: Off-pump vs conventional coronary artery bypass grafting: Early and 1-year graft patency, cost, and quality-of-life outcomes: A randomized trial. JAMA 291:1841, 2004

VI

Chapter 27

Postoperative Cardiovascular Management

Jerrold H. Levy, MD • Kenichi Tanaka, MD •
James M. Bailey, MD • James G. Ramsay, MD

Biventricular dysfunction and circulatory changes occur after cardiopulmonary bypass (CPB) but can also occur in patients undergoing off-pump surgery. Pharmacologic therapy with appropriate monitoring and mechanical support may be needed for patients in the postoperative period until ventricular or circulatory dysfunction improves.

OXYGEN TRANSPORT

Maintaining oxygen transport (i.e., oxygen delivery [Do_2]) satisfactory to meet the tissue metabolic requirements is the goal of postoperative circulatory control. Oxygen transport is the product of cardiac output (CO) times arterial content of oxygen (Cao_2) (i.e., hemoglobin concentration $\times$ 1.34 mL of oxygen per 1 g of hemoglobin $\times$ oxygen saturation), and it can be affected in many ways by the cardiovascular and respiratory systems, as shown in Figure 27-1. Low CO, anemia from blood loss, and pulmonary disease can decrease Do_2. Before altering the determinants of CO, including the

643

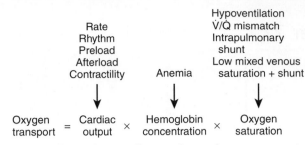

Figure 27-1   Important factors that contribute to abnormal oxygen transport.

inotropic state of the ventricles, an acceptable hemoglobin concentration (9-10 g/dL) and adequate oxygen saturation (Sa_{O_2}) should be provided, enabling increases in CO to provide the maximum available D_{O_2}.[1]

Hypoxemia from any cause reduces D_{O_2}, and acceptable arterial oxygenation (Pa_{O_2}) may be achieved with the use of an elevated inspired oxygen concentration (FI_{O_2}) or positive end-expiratory pressure (PEEP) in the ventilated patient. Use of PEEP or continuous positive airway pressure (CPAP) in the spontaneously breathing patient may improve Pa_{O_2} by reducing intrapulmonary shunt; however, venous return may be reduced, causing a decrease in CO, with D_{O_2} decreased despite an increased Pa_{O_2}.

Unexplained hypoxemia may be caused by right-to-left intracardiac shunting, most commonly by a patent foramen ovale. This is most likely to occur when right-sided pressures are abnormally elevated; an example is the use of high levels of PEEP. If suspected, echocardiography should be performed and therapy to reduce right-sided pressures should be initiated.

Patients with pulmonary disease may experience dramatic worsening of oxygenation when vasodilator therapy is started, because of release of hypoxic vasoconstriction in areas of diseased lung. Although CO may be increased, the worsening in Ca_{O_2} will result in a decrease in D_{O_2}. Reduced dosage of direct-acting vasodilators or trials of different agents may be indicated.

When D_{O_2} cannot be increased to an acceptable level as judged by decreased organ function or development of lactic acidemia, measures to decrease oxygen consumption (V_{O_2}) may be taken while awaiting improvement in cardiac or pulmonary function. For example, sedation and paralysis may buy time to allow reversible postoperative myocardial dysfunction to improve.

TEMPERATURE

Patients are often admitted to the intensive care unit (ICU) after cardiac surgery with core temperatures below 35°C (95°F), especially after off-pump cardiac surgery. The typical pattern of temperature change during and after cardiac surgery and the hemodynamic outcomes are illustrated in Figure 27-2. Decreases in temperature after CPB occur in part because of redistribution of heat within the body and because of heat loss.

The normal thermoregulatory and metabolic responses to hypothermia remain intact after cardiac surgery, resulting in peripheral vasoconstriction that contributes to the hypertension commonly seen early in the ICU. As temperature decreases, CO is decreased because of bradycardia, whereas oxygen consumed per beat is actually increased. Other adverse outcomes of postoperative hypothermia during rewarming

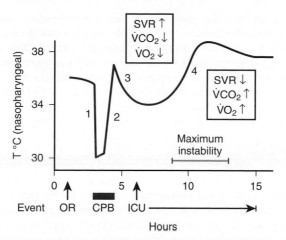

Figure 27-2 Nasopharyngeal temperature during and after cardiac surgery: (1) core (i.e., blood) cooling on cardiopulmonary bypass (CPB); (2) core warming on CPB; (3) afterdrop in temperature (T) after separation from CPB; (4) rewarming after admission to the intensive care unit (ICU). Systemic vascular resistance (SVR) is increased, and carbon dioxide production ($\dot{V}CO_2$) and oxygen consumption ($\dot{V}O_2$) are decreased on admission to the ICU because of residual hypothermia. During rapid rewarming, SVR decreases and $\dot{V}CO_2$ and $\dot{V}O_2$ increase, which can cause marked cardiac and ventilatory instability. OR = operating room. (From Sladen RN: Management of the adult cardiac patient in the intensive care unit. In Ream AK, Fogdall RP [eds]: Acute Cardiovascular Management: Anesthesia and Intensive Care. Philadelphia, JB Lippincott, 1982, p 495.)

include large increases in $\dot{V}O_2$ and CO_2 production during this process. When patients cannot increase CO (i.e., O_2 delivery), the effects of this large increase in $\dot{V}O_2$ include mixed venous desaturation and metabolic acidosis. Unless end-tidal carbon dioxide is monitored or arterial blood gases are analyzed frequently to show the increased CO_2 production and guide increases in ventilation, hypercarbia will occur, causing catecholamine release, tachycardia, and pulmonary hypertension. These effects of rewarming are most intense when patients shiver.

As the temperature rises, usually to about 36°C (96.8°F), the vasoconstriction and hypertension are replaced by vasodilation, tachycardia, and hypotension, even without hypercarbia. Often, over minutes, a patient who needs vasodilators for hypertension transforms into one requiring vasopressors or large volumes of fluid for hypotension. Volume loading during the rewarming period can help to reduce the rapid swings in blood pressure (BP) that may occur. It is important to recognize when these changes result from changes in body temperature to avoid attributing them to other processes that may call for different therapy.

ASSESSMENT OF THE CIRCULATION

Physical Examination

Surgical dressings, chest tubes attached to suction, fluid in the mediastinum and pleural spaces, peripheral edema, and temperature gradients can distort or mask information obtained by the classic techniques of inspection, palpation, and auscultation in the postoperative period. However, the physician should not be deterred from applying these basic techniques in view of the potential benefit. Physical examination may be of great value in diagnosing gross or acute pathology, such as pneumothorax,

27

hemothorax, or acute valvular insufficiency, but it is of limited value in diagnosing and managing ventricular failure. For example, in the critical care setting, experienced clinicians (e.g., internists) using only physical findings often misjudge cardiac filling pressures by a large margin. Low CO in particular is not consistently recognized by clinical signs, and systemic BP does not correlate with CO after cardiac surgery. Oliguria and metabolic acidosis, classic indicators of a low CO, are not always reliable because of the polyuria induced by hypothermia, oxygen debts induced during CPB causing acidosis, and medications or fluids given during or immediately after bypass.

Although clinicians are taught that the adequacy of CO can be assessed by the quality of the pulses, capillary refill, and peripheral temperature, there is no relationship between these indicators of peripheral perfusion and CO or calculated systemic vascular resistance (SVR) in the postoperative period. By the first postoperative day, there is a crude correlation between peripheral temperature and cardiac index (CI) ($r = -0.60$). Many patients arrive in the ICU in a hypothermic state, and residual anesthetic agents can decrease the threshold for peripheral vasoconstriction in response to this condition. A patient's extremities may therefore remain warm despite a hypothermic core or a decreasing CO. Even after temperature stabilization on the first postoperative day, the relationship between peripheral perfusion and CO is too crude to be used for hemodynamic management.

Invasive Monitoring

Despite the lack of a proven benefit with pulmonary artery (PA) catheterization, most patients in North America continue to have this monitor placed for cardiac surgery. This reflects a desire to have the information regarding myocardial performance readily at hand, and the potential difficulty in changing to PA catheterization in an emergency requiring resuscitation. Many cardiac anesthesiologists believe that the lack of evidence regarding the PA catheter may reflect the lack of a well-designed randomized trial. There can be little doubt that management of acute heart failure is facilitated by measures of filling pressures and CO. Postoperatively, many cardiac surgical centers do not have in-house physicians, and surgeons believe they can obtain more objective data over the telephone if a PA catheter is in place.

Use of the fiberoptic PA catheter to continuously monitor mixed venous oxygen saturation ($S\bar{v}o_2$) helps evaluate the adequacy of Do_2 and allows continuous assessment of the response to therapy, which may affect Do_2 or $\dot{V}o_2$ (e.g., PEEP therapy). The trend in the $S\bar{v}o_2$ may function as an early warning signal of worsening in the oxygen supply-demand relationship as Do_2 falls or $\dot{V}o_2$ increases. Catheters that continuously measure the CO are also available. A wire coil on the catheter warms the blood passing by it at time intervals determined by an algorithm, and the measured changes in temperature at the tip of the catheter are used to provide a continuous display of the CO. Although the CO displayed needs gathering of information over several minutes and is therefore not as quick as conventional thermodilution, it avoids having to give injected volumes to the patient (which can add up to a significant amount every 24 hours) and provides trends that may give earlier warning than intermittent injections.

Echocardiography

There can be little doubt that echocardiography is the technique of choice for acute assessment of cardiac function. Just as transesophageal echocardiography (TEE) has become essential for intraoperative management in a variety of

BOX 27-1   *Risk Factors for Low Cardiac Output Syndrome after Cardiopulmonary Bypass*

- Preoperative left ventricular dysfunction
- Valvular heart disease requiring repair or replacement
- Long aortic cross-clamp time and total cardiopulmonary bypass time
- Inadequate cardiac surgical repair
- Myocardial ischemia and reperfusion
- Residual effects of cardioplegia solution
- Poor myocardial preservation
- Reperfusion injury and inflammatory changes

conditions, several studies document its utility in the postoperative period in the presence and absence of the PA catheter.[2] It provides information that may lead to urgent surgery or prevent unnecessary surgery, gives important information about cardiac preload, and can detect acute structural and functional abnormalities. Although transthoracic echocardiography (TTE) can be performed more rapidly in this setting, adequate images can be obtained only in about 50% of patients in the ICU.

POSTOPERATIVE MYOCARDIAL DYSFUNCTION

Studies using hemodynamic, nuclear scanning, and metabolic techniques have documented worsening in cardiac function after coronary artery bypass grafting (CABG) surgery. All of these studies showed significant declines in left ventricular (LV) or biventricular (when measured) function in the first postoperative hours, with gradual return to preoperative values by 8 to 24 hours. Decreased ventricular performance at normal or elevated filling pressures occurs, suggesting decreased contractility. Similarly, "flattening" of the ventricular function curves is usually obvious, suggesting that preload augmentation much above 10 mmHg for central venous pressure (CVP) or 12 mmHg for pulmonary capillary wedge pressure (PCWP) is of little benefit.

Proposed factors that contribute to postoperative ventricular dysfunction include myocardial ischemia, residual hypothermia, preoperative medications such as β-adrenergic antagonists, and ischemia-reperfusion injury (Box 27-1).

POSTOPERATIVE MYOCARDIAL ISCHEMIA

Although intraoperative myocardial ischemia has often been a focus, studies have demonstrated that ischemia often occurs postoperatively and is associated with adverse cardiac outcomes. Electrocardiographic (ECG) and segmental wall motion abnormality (SWMA) evidence of ischemia occur early postoperatively in up to 40% of patients undergoing CABG surgery. Postbypass SWMAs are significantly associated with adverse outcomes (e.g., MI, death). Hemodynamic changes rarely preceded ischemia; however, postoperative heart rates (HRs) are significantly higher than intraoperative or preoperative values. Whether such changes occur because of surgery-reperfusion or events after CPB is not known. These findings do suggest that monitoring for ischemia must continue after revascularization.

27

Table 27-1 Postoperative Rate and Rhythm Disturbances

Disturbance	Usual Causes	Treatments
Sinus bradycardia	Pre/intraoperative β-blockade	Atrial pacing β-Agonist Anticholinergic
Heart block (first, second, and third degree)	Ischemia Surgical trauma	Atrioventricular sequential pacing Catecholamines
Sinus tachycardia	Agitation/pain Hypovolemia Catecholamines	Sedation/analgesia Volume administration Change or stop drug
Atrial tachyarrhythmias	Catecholamines Chamber distention Electrolyte disorder (hypokalemia, hypomagnesemia)	Change or stop drug Treat underlying cause (e.g., vasodilator, diuresis, give K^+/Mg^{2+}) May require synchronized cardio-version or pharmacotherapy
Ventricular tachycardia or fibrillation	Ischemia Catecholamines	Cardioversion Treat ischemia, may require pharmacotherapy Change or stop drug

THERAPEUTIC INTERVENTIONS

Therapeutic interventions for postoperative biventricular dysfunction include the standard concerns of managing low cardiac output states (LCOS) by controlling the HR and rhythm, providing an acceptable preload, and adjusting afterload and contractility. In most patients, pharmacologic interventions can be rapidly weaned or stopped within the first 24 hours after surgery.

Postoperative Arrhythmias

Patients with preoperative or newly acquired noncompliant ventricles need a correctly timed atrial contraction to provide satisfactory ventricular filling, especially when they are in sinus rhythm preoperatively. Although atrial contraction provides 15% to 20% of ventricular filling, this may be more important in postoperative patients, when ventricular dysfunction and reduced compliance may be present. Rate and rhythm disorders need to be corrected when possible, using epicardial pacing wires. Approaches to postoperative rate and rhythm disturbances are shown in Table 27-1.

Later in the postoperative period (days 1 through 3), supraventricular tachyarrhythmias become a major problem, with atrial fibrillation (AF) predominating. The overall incidence is between 30% and 40%, but with increasing age and valvular surgery the incidence may be in excess of 60%. There are probably many reasons for this, including genetic factors, inadequate atrial protection during surgery, electrolyte abnormalities, change in atrial size with fluid shifts, epicardial inflammation, stress, and irritation. Randomized trials of off-pump coronary artery bypass grafting (OPCAB) have found a similar incidence of postoperative AF compared with on-pump CABG.[3]

When AF or other supraventricular arrhythmias develop, treatment is often urgently required for symptomatic relief or hemodynamic benefit. The longer a patient remains in AF, the more difficult it may be to convert, and the greater is the risk for thrombus formation and embolization.[4] Treatable underlying conditions such as electrolyte disturbances or pain should be corrected while specific pharmacologic therapy is being instituted. Paroxysmal supraventricular tachycardia (uncommon in this setting) can be abolished or converted by intravenous adenosine, and atrial flutter can sometimes be converted by overdrive atrial pacing by temporary wires placed at the time of surgery. Electrical cardioversion may be required if hypotension is caused by the rapid rate; however, atrial arrhythmias tend to recur in this setting. Rate control for AF or flutter can be achieved with a variety of atrioventricular nodal blocking drugs, and conversion is facilitated by many of these drugs as well. Table 27-2 summarizes the various treatment modalities for supraventricular arrhythmias. If conversion to sinus rhythm does not occur, electrical cardioversion in the presence of antiarrhythmic drug therapy should be attempted or anticoagulation with warfarin (Coumadin) instituted.

Preload

Assessment of preload is probably the single most important clinical skill for the management of hemodynamic instability. Preload rapidly changes in the postoperative period because of bleeding, spontaneous diuresis, vasodilation during warming, the effects of positive-pressure ventilation and PEEP on venous return, capillary leak, and other causes.

Direct assessment of preload is clinically feasible using echocardiography. A fair-to-good correlation exists between echocardiographic and radionuclide measures of end-diastolic volume, and there is a good correlation between end-diastolic area by TEE and stroke volume. Although the use of echocardiography to assess preload must always be tempered by the realization that the clinician is viewing a two-dimensional image of a three-dimensional object, this is the most direct technique clinically available. Increased awareness of the value of TEE in the ICU and increased availability of echocardiography in general have made this modality a first choice in acute assessment of preload in the setting of unexplained or refractory hypotension. In the absence of echocardiography, pressure measurements are used as surrogates for volume measurements.

Afterload

Calculated SVR continues to be widely used in guiding therapy or drawing conclusions about the state of the circulation. This should only be done cautiously because SVR is not a complete indicator of afterload. Even if SVR were an accurate measure of impedance, the response to vasoactive agents depends on the coupling of ventricular-vascular function, not on impedance alone. Hemodynamic therapy should be guided based on the primary variables: BP and CO. If preload is appropriate, low BP and low CO are treated with an inotropic drug. If BP is acceptable (and preload appropriate) but CO is low, a vasodilator alone or in combination with an inotropic drug is used. If the patient is hypertensive (with low CO), vasodilators are indicated; if the patient is vasodilated (low BP and high CO), vasoconstrictors are employed (Table 27-3).

POSTOPERATIVE HYPERTENSION

Hypertension has been a common complication of cardiac surgery, reported to occur in 30% to 80% of patients.[5] The current population of older, sicker patients appears to have fewer problems with hypertension than with low-output syndromes or vasodilation. Although hypertension most commonly occurs in patients with normal preoperative ventricular function or a prior history, any patient may develop hypertension.

Table 27-2 Treatment Modalities for Supraventricular Arrhythmias

Treatment	Specifics*	Indications
Overdrive pacing by atrial wires†	Requires rapid pacer (up to 800/min); start above arrhythmia rate and slowly decrease	PAT, atrial flutter
Adenosine	Bolus dose of 6-12 mg; may cause 10 seconds of complete heart block	AV nodal tachycardia Bypass-tract arrhythmia Atrial arrhythmia diagnosis
Amiodarone	150 mg IV over 10 min, followed by infusion	Rate control/conversion to NSR in atrial fibrillation/flutter
β-Blockade	Esmolol, up to 0.5 mg/kg load over 1 min, followed by infusion if tolerated	Rate control/conversion to NSR in atrial fibrillation/flutter
	Metoprolol, 0.5-5 mg; repeat effective dose q4-6h	Rate control/conversion to NSR in atrial fibrillation/flutter
	Propranolol, 0.25-1 mg; repeat effective dose q4h‡	Rate control/conversion to NSR in atrial fibrillation/flutter
	Labetolol, 2.5-10 mg; repeat effective dose q4h‡	Conversion of atrial fibrillation/flutter to NSR
	Sotalol, 40-80 mg PO q12h	Conversion of PAT to NSR
Ibutilide	1 mg over 10 min; may repeat after 10 min	Rate control/conversion to NSR in atrial fibrillation/flutter
Verapamil	2.5-5 mg IV, repeated PRN‡	Rate control/conversion to NSR in atrial fibrillation/flutter
Diltiazem	0.2 mg/kg over 2 min, followed by 10-15 mg/hr¶	Rate control/conversion to NSR in atrial fibrillation/flutter
Procainamide	50 mg/min up to 1 g, followed by 1-4 mg/min	Rate control/conversion to NSR in atrial fibrillation/flutter Prevention of recurrence of arrhythmias Treatment of wide-complex tachycardias
**Digoxin	Load of 1 mg in divided doses over 4-24 hr§; may give additional 0.125-mg doses 2 hr apart (3-4 doses)	Rate control/conversion to NSR in atrial fibrillation/flutter
Synchronized cardioversion	50-300 J (external); most effective with anterior-posterior patches	Acute tachyarrhythmia with hemodynamic compromise (usually atrial fibrillation or flutter)

*See specific drug monographs for full description of indications, contraindications, and dosage. Doses are for intravenous administration; use lowest dose and administer slowly in patients with hemodynamic compromise.

†Verify pacer is not capturing ventricle.

‡Infusion may provide better control. This drug is less useful than diltiazem owing to myocardial depression.

§Rate of administration depending on urgency of rate control.

¶Limited experience; may cause less hypotension than verapamil.

¶When diagnosis is unclear (ventricular vs. supraventricular) and there is no acute hemodynamic compromise (i.e., cardioversion not indicated).

**Less useful than other drugs owing to slow onset and modest effect.

AV = atrioventricular; NSR = normal sinus rhythm; PAT = paroxysmal atrial tachycardia; SVT = supraventricular tachycardia.

Table 27-3 Hemodynamic Therapy Guidelines

Blood Pressure	Cardiac Output	Treatment
Low	Low	Inotrope
Normal	Low	Vasodilator ± inotrope
High	Low	Vasodilator
Low	High	Vasopressor

Table 27-4 Novel Vasodilators

Drug	Mechanism of Action	Half-Life
Nicardipine	Calcium channel blocker	Intermediate
Clevidipine	Calcium channel blocker	Ultra-short
Fenoldopam	Dopamine$_1$ agonist	Ultra-short
Nesiritide	β-Natriuretic agonist	Short
Levosimendan	K$^+$-ATP channel modulator	Intermediate

Multiple factors contribute to postoperative hypertension, including awakening from general anesthesia, increases in endogenous catecholamines, activation of the plasma renin-angiotensin system, neural reflexes (e.g., heart, coronary arteries, great vessels), and hypothermia. Arterial vasoconstriction with various degrees of intravascular hypovolemia is the hallmark.

The hazards of untreated postoperative hypertension include depressed LV performance, increased M_{VO_2}, cerebrovascular accidents, suture line disruption, MI, rhythm disturbances, and increased bleeding. Historically, pharmacologic therapy for hypertension in this setting has often been with sodium nitroprusside because of its rapid onset and short duration of action. With the introduction of alternative vasodilators, sodium nitroprusside is no longer the drug of choice.

There are many alternative drugs to sodium nitroprusside for the treatment of hypertension after cardiac surgery, including nitroglycerin, adrenergic-blocking agents such as phentolamine, β-adrenergic blockers, and the mixed α- and β-adrenergic blocker labetalol. Direct-acting vasodilators, dihydropyridine calcium channel blockers (e.g., nicardipine, clevidipine), ACE inhibitors, and fenoldopam (a dopamine-1 [D$_1$] receptor agonist) have also been used. Novel therapeutic approaches are listed in Table 27-4.

Dihydropyridine calcium channel blockers relax arterial resistance vessels without negative inotropic actions or effects on atrioventricular nodal conduction and are important therapeutic options. Dihydropyridines are artery-specific vasodilators of peripheral resistance arteries, resulting in a generalized vasodilation, including the renal, cerebral, intestinal, and coronary vascular beds. In doses that effectively reduce BP, the dihydropyridines have little or no direct negative effect on cardiac contractility or conduction. The pharmacokinetic profile of nicardipine suggests that effective administration requires variable rate infusions when trying to treat hypertension because of the half-life of 40 minutes. If even more rapid control is essential, a dosing strategy consisting of a loading bolus or rapid infusion dose with a constant-rate infusion may be more efficient. The effect of nicardipine may persist even though the infusion is stopped. Clevidipine, a new ultra-short-acting dihydropyridine, is in phase III studies, has a half-life of only minutes, and may represent a potential alternative to sodium nitroprusside in the future.[6]

POSTOPERATIVE VASODILATION

Vasodilation alone should be associated with a hyperdynamic circulatory state presenting as systemic hypotension in association with an increased CO (and a low calculated SVR). More commonly after cardiac surgery, a combination of vasodilation and myocardial dysfunction occurs, requiring vasoconstrictor and inotropic therapy. The *vasoplegic syndrome* requires very high doses of vasoconstrictors and occurs after off-pump and on-pump surgery.[7]

While underlying causes are being sought and treated, the therapeutic approach to systemic vasodilation includes intravascular volume expansion, α-adrenergic agents, and vasopressin. Administration of vasoconstrictors for more than a brief period must be guided by measures of cardiac performance, because restoration of BP may camouflage a low-output state.

CORONARY ARTERY SPASM

Coronary artery or internal mammary artery (IMA) vasospasm can occur postoperatively. Mechanical manipulation and underlying atherosclerosis of the native coronary circulation and the IMA have the potential to produce transient endothelial dysfunction. The endothelium is responsible for releasing endothelium-derived relaxing factor (EDRF), which is nitric oxide, a potent endogenous vasodilator substance that maintains normal endogenous vasodilation. Thromboxane can be liberated as a result of heparin-protamine interactions, CPB, platelet activation, or anaphylactic reactions to produce coronary vasoconstriction. Calcium administration, increased α-adrenergic tone from vasoconstrictor administration (especially in bolus doses), platelet thromboxane liberation, and calcium channel blocker withdrawal represent additional factors that may put the cardiac surgical patient at risk for spasm of native coronary vessels and arterial grafts. The therapy of choice remains empirical. Nitroglycerin is a first-line drug, but nitrate tolerance can occur. Phosphodiesterase (PDE) inhibitors represent novel approaches to this problem and have been reported to be effective. Intravenous dihydropyridine calcium channel blockers are also important therapeutic considerations.

Successful use of the radial artery as a bypass conduit have rekindled interest in this vessel. In the early days of CABG surgery, this conduit was abandoned because of its propensity to spasm. In later reports, techniques developed in the use of the IMA have been applied to the radial artery, as well as prophylactic use of diltiazem infusions.

DECREASED CONTRACTILITY

Drugs that increase contractility all result in increased calcium mobilization from intracellular sites to and from the contractile proteins or sensitize these proteins to calcium. Catecholamines, through β1-receptor stimulation in the myocardium, increase intracellular cyclic adenosine monophosphate (cAMP). This second messenger increases intracellular calcium, causing an improvement in myocardial contraction. Inhibition of the breakdown of cAMP by PDE inhibitors increases intracellular cAMP independent of the β-receptor. The "calcium sensitizers" constitute a new class of inotropic agents (Box 27-2).[8]

BOX 27-2 *Pharmacologic Approaches for Perioperative Ventricular Dysfunction*

- Inotropic agents
  - Catecholamines
  - Phosphodiesterase inhibitors
  - Levosimendan
- Vasodilator therapy
- Pulmonary vasodilators
  - Phosphodiesterase inhibitors
  - Inhaled nitric oxide
  - Prostaglandins

BOX 27-3 *Disadvantages of Catecholamines*

- Increased myocardial oxygen consumption
- Tachycardia
- Arrhythmias
- Excessive peripheral vasoconstriction
- Coronary vasoconstriction
- β-receptor downregulation and decreased drug efficacy

Table 27-5 **Catecholamines Used Postoperatively**

Drug	Infusion Dose (µg/kg/min)
Dopamine*,†	2-10
Dobutamine†	2-10
Epinephrine‡	0.03-0.20
Norepinephrine‡	0.03-0.20
Isoproterenol‡	0.02-0.10

*Less than 2 µg/kg/min predominantly "dopaminergic" (renal and mesenteric artery dilatation).
†If 10 µg/kg/min is ineffective, change to epinephrine or norepinephrine.
‡Dose to effect; may require higher dose than indicated.

27

Catecholamines

The catecholamines used postoperatively include dopamine, dobutamine, epinephrine, norepinephrine, and isoproterenol (Box 27-3). These drugs have various effects on α- and β-receptors and therefore various effects on HR, rhythm, and myocardial metabolism. Dosing recommendations for the catecholamines are provided in Table 27-5.

Epinephrine

Epinephrine is a potent adrenergic agonist with the desirable feature that, in low doses (<3 µg/min), β_1 and β_2 effects predominate. As the dose is increased, α effects (e.g., vasoconstriction) and tachycardia occur. However, in the acutely failing heart postoperatively, drugs such as epinephrine or norepinephrine provide positive inotropy and perfusion pressure. These features and its low cost make it a common first-line drug in the postoperative setting. Despite what is often stated in older literature, epinephrine causes less tachycardia than dopamine or dobutamine at equivalent inotropic doses. Because of the metabolic actions of β_2 stimulation, epinephrine infusion can cause hyperglycemia and increased serum lactate levels.

Norepinephrine

Norepinephrine, which has potent β_1- and α-receptor effects, preserves coronary perfusion pressure (CPP) while not increasing HR, actions that are favorable to the ischemic, reperfused heart. When norepinephrine is used alone without a vasodilator or PDE inhibitor, the potent β_1 effects may have variable effects on CO. Ventricular filling pressures usually increase when this drug is given, because of constriction of the capacitance vessels. Administration of a vasodilator, including the PDE inhibitors, with norepinephrine may partially oppose the vasoconstriction. End-organ ischemia would appear to be unlikely if CO can be preserved at normal levels when norepinephrine is given. PDE inhibitors in combination with norepinephrine attenuate the arterial vasoconstrictive effects.

Dopamine

A precursor of norepinephrine, dopamine probably achieves its therapeutic effects by releasing myocardial norepinephrine or preventing its reuptake, especially when administered in high doses. This indirect action may result in reduced effectiveness when given to patients with chronic congestive heart failure or shock states, because the myocardium becomes depleted of norepinephrine stores. In contrast to dobutamine, the α-agonist properties of dopamine cause increases in pulmonary artery pressure (PAP), peripheral vascular resistance (PVR), and LV filling pressure. At low doses (<2 µg/kg/min), dopamine stimulates renal dopaminergic receptors to increase renal perfusion more than can be explained by an increase in CO. Despite this action, a multicenter study in New Zealand and Australia clearly demonstrated that use of low-dose dopamine in critically ill patients confers no protection from renal dysfunction.[9] At doses higher than 10 µg/kg/min, tachycardia and vasoconstriction become the predominant actions of this drug.

Dobutamine

In contrast to dopamine, dobutamine exhibits mainly β_1-agonist properties, with decreases in diastolic BP and sometimes systemic BP being observed. Dobutamine is functionally similar to isoproterenol, with less tendency to induce tachycardia in the postoperative setting. The favorable actions of dobutamine may be limited if a tachycardia develops, and, like dopamine, its inotropic potency is modest in comparison with that of epinephrine or norepinephrine.

Phosphodiesterase Inhibitors

The PDE inhibitors are nonglycosidic, nonsympathomimetic drugs that have positive inotropic effects independent of the β_1-adrenergic receptor and unique vasodilatory actions independent of endothelial function or nitrovasodilators.[10] Patients with CHF have downregulation of the β_1-receptor, with a decrease in receptor density and altered responses to catecholamine administration. Milrinone, amrinone, and enoximone bypass the β_1-receptor, causing increases in intracellular cAMP by selective inhibition of PDE fraction III (i.e., fraction IV), a cAMP-specific PDE enzyme. In vascular smooth muscle, these agents cause vasodilation in the arterial and capacitance beds. PDE inhibitors increase CO, decrease PCWP, and decrease SVR and PVR in patients with biventricular dysfunction, and they are important therapeutic approaches in postoperative cardiac surgical patients.

BOX 27-4   *Advantages of Preemptive Phosphodiesterase Inhibitor Administration*

- Increased myocardial contractility (left and right ventricles)
- Pulmonary vasodilation
- Resolution and prevention of ischemia
- Minimal drug side effects while on cardiopulmonary bypass
- Dilation of internal mammary artery
- Avoidance of mechanical intervention
- Prevention of a "failed wean"

PDE III inhibitors have a clinical effect as inodilators; they produce dilation of arterial and venous beds, decreasing the mean arterial pressure and central filling pressures. Increases in CO are induced by multiple mechanisms, including afterload reduction and positive inotropy, but not by increasing HR. The net effect is a decrease in myocardial wall tension, representing an important contrast to most sympathomimetic agents. Catecholamine administration often needs the simultaneous administration of vasodilators to reduce ventricular wall tension. Milrinone and other PDE inhibitors also have unique mechanisms of vasodilation that may be favorable for coronary artery and IMA flow (Box 27-4).

Milrinone is a bipyridine derivative with an inotropic activity that is almost 20 times more potent than that of amrinone, and it has a shorter half-life. Milrinone is an effective inodilator for patients with decompensated CHF and low CO after cardiac surgery. Suggested dosing for milrinone is a loading dose of 50 μg/kg over 10 minutes, followed by an infusion of 0.5 μg/kg/min (0.375 to 0.75 μg/kg/min). By loading the patient with milrinone over a longer period, high peak concentrations can be prevented, and the vasodilation that is observed with rapid loading can be attenuated. A milrinone loading dose of 50 μg/kg in conjunction with an infusion of 0.5 μg/kg/min consistently maintained plasma concentrations more than 100 ng/mL. Clearance was 3.8 ± 1.7 mL/kg/min, volume of distribution was 465 ± 159 mL/kg, and terminal elimination half-time was 107 ± 77 minutes (values expressed as mean $\pm$ SD). The relationship between plasma concentration and pharmacodynamic effects produced about a 30% improvement in CI with plasma levels of 100 ng/mL, and there was a curvilinear relationship between plasma levels and improvement in CI.

Levosimendan

Levosimendan is a calcium-sensitizing drug that exerts positive inotropic effects through sensitization of myofilaments to calcium and vasodilation through opening of ATP-dependent potassium channels on vascular smooth muscle. These effects occur without increasing intracellular cAMP or calcium and without an increase in $M\dot{v}o_2$ at therapeutic doses. As would be expected with an inodilator, the hemodynamic effects include a reduction in pulmonary artery occlusion pressure (PAOP) in association with an increase in CO. β-Blockade does not block the hemodynamic effects of this drug. Levosimendan itself has a short elimination half-life, but it has active metabolites with elimination half-lives up to 80 hours. A study in patients with decompensated congestive heart failure found hemodynamic improvements at 48 hours were similar whether patients received the drug for 24 hours or 48 hours. Increasing plasma levels of the active metabolite were found for 24 hours after the drug infusion was stopped.[11] Levosimendan is in phase III clinical studies in the United States and Europe, and it has been granted fast-track status by the U.S. Food and Drug Administration (FDA).

In a study after cardiac surgery, patients were given levosimendan; of 11 patients with severely impaired CO and hemodynamic compromise, 8 patients (73%) showed evidence of hemodynamic improvement within 3 hours after the start of levosimendan infusion. Specifically, cardiac index and stroke volume were significantly increased, whereas the mean arterial pressure, indexed SVR, mean PAP, right atrial pressure, and PAOP were significantly lowered.[12] Clinical studies continue to evaluate the potential role for this new positive inotropic agent in patients with heart failure.

RIGHT-SIDED HEART FAILURE

Heart failure after cardiac surgery usually results from LV impairment. Although an isolated right-sided MI can occur perioperatively, most perioperative inferior MIs show variable involvement of the right ventricle.[13] The myocardial preservation techniques that are best for the left ventricle may not offer ideal RV protection because the right ventricle is thin walled and more exposed to body and atmospheric temperature. Cardioplegic solution given through the coronary sinus (retrograde) may not reach parts of the right ventricle because of positioning of the cardioplegia cannula in relation to the venous outflow from this chamber and because the thebesian veins do not drain into the coronary sinus. Impairment of RV function postoperatively is more severe and persistent when preoperative right coronary artery (RCA) stenosis is present. Although depression of the ejection fraction is compensated by preload augmentation, right ventricular ejection fraction (RVEF) cannot be preserved if CPP is reduced or impedance to ejection is increased.

Certain aspects of the physiology of the right ventricle make it different from the left. Normally, the RV free wall receives its blood flow during systole and diastole; however, systemic hypotension or increased RV systolic and diastolic pressures may cause supply-dependent depression of contractility when Myo_2 is increased while CPP is decreased. The normal thin-walled right ventricle is at least twice as sensitive to increases in afterload as is the left ventricle. Relatively modest increases in outflow impedance from multiple causes in the postoperative period can exhaust preload reserve, causing a decrease in RVEF with ventricular dilation. RV pressure overload may be complicated by volume overload caused by functional tricuspid regurgitation. Decreases in RV stroke volume will diminish LV filling, and dilation of the right ventricle can cause a leftward shift of the interventricular septum, interfering with diastolic filling of the left ventricle (i.e., ventricular interaction) (Fig. 27-3). A distended right ventricle limited by the pericardial cavity further decreases LV filling. RV failure has the potential to affect LV performance by decreasing pulmonary venous blood flow, decreasing diastolic distending pressure, and decreasing LV diastolic compliance. The resulting decrease in LV output will further impair RV pump function. The mechanical outcomes of RV failure in postoperative cardiac surgical patients are depicted in Figure 27-4. It can therefore be appreciated how, once established, RV failure is self-propagating; and aggressive treatment interventions may be needed to interrupt the vicious cycle.

Diagnosis

In the postoperative cardiac surgical patient, a low cardiac index with right atrial pressure increased disproportionately compared with changes in left-sided filling pressures is highly suggestive of RV failure. The PAOP may also increase because

VI

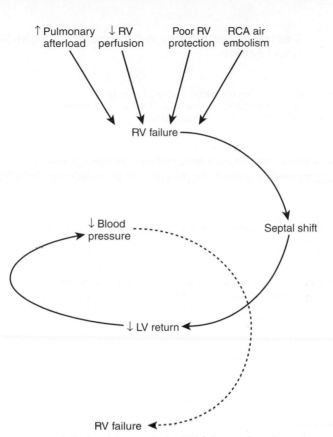

Figure 27-3 Sequence inducing right ventricular (RV) failure and causing a downward spiral of events. RCA = right coronary artery; LV = left ventricular.

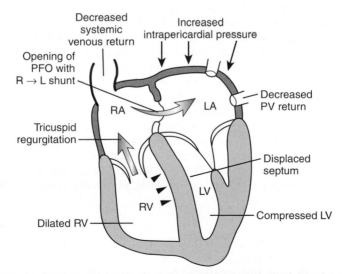

Figure 27-4 Mechanical changes produced by acute right ventricular failure. LA = left atrium; LV = left ventricle; PFO = patent foramen ovale; PV = pulmonary veins; RA = right atrium; R→L = right to left; RV = right ventricle.

Table 27-6 Treatment Approaches in Postoperative Right-Sided Heart Failure

Preload Augmentation

Volume, vasopressors, or leg elevation (CVP/PCWP < 1)
Decrease juxtacardiac pressures (pericardium and/or chest open)
Establish atrial kick (sinus rhythm, atrial pacing)

Afterload Reduction (Pulmonary Vasodilation)

Nitroglycerin, isosorbide dinitrate nesiritide
cAMP-specific phosphodiesterase inhibitors, β_2-adrenergic agonists
Inhaled nitric oxide
Nebulized PGI_2
Intravenous PGE_1 (+ left atrial norepinephrine)

Inotropic Support

cAMP-specific phosphodiesterase inhibitors, isoproterenol, dobutamine
Norepinephrine
Levosimendan

Ventilatory Management

Lower intrathoracic pressures (tidal volume < 7 mL/kg, low PEEP)
Attenuation of hypoxic vasoconstriction (high Fio_2)
Avoidance of respiratory acidosis ($Paco_2$ 30-35 mm Hg, metabolic control with meperidine or relaxants)

Mechanical Support

Intra-aortic counterpulsation
Pulmonary artery counterpulsation
Right ventricular assist devices

CVP/PCWP = central venous pressure/pulmonary capillary wedge pressure; cAMP = cyclic adenosine monophosphate; PGI_2 = prostaglandin I_2; PGE_1 = prostaglandin E_1; PEEPs = positive end-expiratory pressures.

of ventricular interaction, but the relationship of right atrial pressure to PAOP stays close to or higher than 1.0. The absence of a step-up in pressure in going from the RA to the pulmonary artery (mean), provided PVR is low, suggests that RV failure is severe and the right side of the heart is acting only as a conduit. This hemodynamic presentation is typical of cardiogenic shock associated with RV infarction. The venous waveforms are accentuated with a prominent Y descent similar to constrictive pericarditis, suggesting reduced RV compliance. Large V waves may also be discernible and may relate to tricuspid regurgitation.

Echocardiography allows a qualitative interpretation of RV size, contractility, and configuration of the interventricular septum and can provide a definitive diagnosis of RV dysfunction or failure. Because of the crescent shape of the right ventricle, volume determination is not easy but the qualitative examination and assessment for tricuspid regurgitation are very valuable. TEE is also useful to determine if the increased right atrial pressures open a patent foramen ovale, producing a right-to-left shunt.

Treatment

Treatment approaches in postoperative RV failure may differ from those used in LV failure, and they are affected by the presence of pulmonary hypertension (Table 27-6). In all cases, preload should be increased to the upper range of normal; however, the Frank-Starling relationship is flat in RV failure; and to avoid ventricular dilation, the CO response to an increasing CVP should be determined. Volume loading should be stopped when the CVP exceeds 10 mmHg and CO does not increase despite increases in this pressure. The CVP should not be permitted to exceed the PAOP, because if these pressures equalize, any increase obtained in pulmonary blood flow will be offset by decreased diastolic filling of the left ventricle by means of ventricular interdependence. The atrial contribution to RV filling is important when the ventricle is dilated and noncompliant. Maintenance of sinus rhythm and use of atrial pacing are important components of treating postoperative RV failure.

Although vasodilators may lead to cardiovascular collapse in RV infarction (as a result of decreases in RV filling and coronary perfusion), postoperative RV failure is often associated with increased PVR and pulmonary hypertension. In this context, attempts to decrease RV outflow impedance may be worthwhile. Intravenous vasodilators invariably reduce systemic BP, mandating the simultaneous administration of a vasoconstrictor. One way to reduce the pulmonary effects of the required vasoconstrictor is to administer the vasoconstrictor through a left atrial catheter. The PDE inhibitors are commonly used for their effect on the pulmonary vasculature and RV function, but this also usually requires systemic norepinephrine. In recent years, there has been an increased interest in and availability of aerosolized pulmonary vasodilators. This route of administration reduces or even abolishes the undesirable systemic vasodilation. Delivery of the drug directly to the alveoli improves pulmonary blood flow to these alveoli, potentially improving oxygenation by better matching blood flow to ventilation. Three drugs have been used: nitric oxide, prostaglandin I_2 (i.e., epoprostenol or prostacyclin), and milrinone.[14]

The intra-aortic balloon pump (IABP) may be of substantial benefit, even in patients in whom the right ventricle is mainly responsible for circulatory decompensation. This beneficial effect is mediated by increased coronary perfusion. Right-sided heart assist devices have a place as temporizing measures in severe intractable failure. Pulmonary artery counterpulsation is experimental, and its clinical role is uncertain. In cases of severe RV failure it may be necessary to leave the sternum open or to reopen the chest if it has been closed. This decreases the tamponade-like compression of the left ventricle by the distended right ventricle, right atrium, and edematous mediastinal tissues.

Effects of Mechanical Ventilation in Heart Failure

Congestive heart failure at the time of surgery is a significant predictor of postoperative respiratory complications. Maintenance of gas exchange in these situations usually mandates prolonged ventilatory support. Besides improving Pao_2, mechanical ventilation can influence Do_2 through its effects on CO. Suppression of spontaneous respiratory efforts may substantially decrease the work of breathing and improve the oxygen supply-demand relationship. Traditionally, the influence of mechanical ventilation on hemodynamics has been viewed as negative. The inevitable rise in intrathoracic pressure caused by positive-pressure ventilation or PEEP is associated with a decreased CO. However, in the presence of congestive heart failure or myocardial ischemia, raised intrathoracic pressure has the potential to favorably affect the determinants of global cardiac performance. Understanding these heart-lung interactions is essential for the integrated management of the ventilated patient with congestive heart failure after cardiac surgery. The effects of ventilation on RV and LV failure need to receive independent consideration.

Raised intrathoracic pressure may significantly improve LV performance as a result of the reduced transmural pressure required to generate an adequate systemic BP. This can be viewed as afterload reduction, a beneficial effect separate from the resistance to

27

venous return that may also help such patients. Clinically significant improvements in cardiac function have been documented in patients ventilated for cardiogenic respiratory failure produced by myocardial ischemia and after CABG surgery. High LV filling pressures may help identify a subgroup benefiting from reduced afterload with increased intrathoracic pressure.

The circulatory responses to changes in ventilation should always be assessed in patients with cardiac disease; the goal of improving or maintaining Do_2 must be kept in mind. This usually requires measurement of arterial oxygenation and CO. In right and biventricular failure the increase in the airway pressure caused by ventilatory support should be kept at a minimum compatible with adequate gas exchange. This means avoidance of high levels of PEEP and trials of decreased inspiratory times, flow rates, and tidal volumes. Breathing modes that emphasize spontaneous efforts such as intermittent mandatory ventilation, pressure support, or CPAP should be considered. Alternatively, if isolated LV failure is the reason for ventilatory therapy, improvements in cardiac performance may be achieved by the use of positive-pressure ventilation with PEEP. In particular, patients with elevated LV filling pressures, mitral regurgitation, and reversible ischemic dysfunction may improve from afterload reduction related to increased airway and intrathoracic pressures.

Effects of Ventilatory Weaning on Heart Failure

Traditional criteria for weaning of ventilatory support assess the adequacy of gas exchange and peak respiratory muscle strength. In the patient with CHF, the response of global hemodynamics to spontaneous respirations must also be considered. The changes of the loading conditions of the heart brought about by the resumption of spontaneous ventilation can induce a vicious cycle resulting in hypoxemia and pulmonary edema.

Pulmonary congestion, often present in patients with LV dysfunction, decreases pulmonary compliance. Consequently, large decreases in inspiratory intrathoracic pressure are needed to cause adequate lung inflation. These negative swings of intrathoracic pressure increase venous return. Increased diaphragmatic movements may increase intra-abdominal pressure, further increasing the pressure gradient for venous return. Decreased intrathoracic pressure also raises the ventricular transmural pressures, raising the impedance to ventricular emptying. The increased afterload causes further increases in preload, with these changes jeopardizing the myocardial oxygen balance. Accordingly, worsening of myocardial ischemia as evidenced by ST-segment deviations was demonstrated when ventilatory support was removed in patients ventilated after MI.

CARDIAC TAMPONADE

Cardiac tamponade is an important cause of the low cardiac output syndrome after cardiac surgery and occurs when the heart is compressed by an external agent, most commonly blood accumulated in the mediastinum. Hemodynamic compromise, to some degree attributable to the constraining effect of blood accumulating within the chest, is often observed in the 3% to 6% of patients needing multiple blood transfusions for hemorrhage after cardiac surgery. Postoperative cardiac tamponade usually manifests acutely during the first 24 hours after surgery, but delayed tamponade may develop 10 to 14 days after surgery and has been associated with postpericardiotomy syndrome or postoperative anticoagulation.

VI

The mechanism of hemodynamic deterioration during tamponade is primarily the result of impaired filling of one or more of the cardiac chambers. As the external pressure on the heart increases, the distending or transmural pressure (external-intracavitary pressure) is decreased. The intracavitary pressure increases in compensation lead to impaired venous return and elevation of the venous pressure. If the external pressure is high enough to exceed the ventricular pressure during diastole, diastolic ventricular collapse occurs. These changes have been documented in the right and the left sides of the heart after cardiac surgery.[15] As the end-diastolic volume and end-systolic volume decrease there is a concomitant decrease in stroke volume. In the most severe form of cardiac tamponade, ventricular filling occurs only during atrial systole. Intense sympathoadrenergic activation increases venous return by constricting venous capacitance vessels. Tachycardia helps to maintain CO in the presence of a reduced stroke volume. Adrenergic mechanisms may also explain decreased urinary output and sodium excretion, but these phenomena may also be caused by reduced CO or a reduction in atrial natriuretic factor from decreased distending pressure of the atria.

The diagnosis of cardiac tamponade depends on a high degree of suspicion. Tamponade after heart surgery is a clinical entity distinct from the tamponade typically seen in medical patients in whom the pericardium is intact and the heart is surrounded by a compressing fluid. In the setting of cardiac surgery, the pericardial space is often left open and in communication with one or both of the pleural spaces, and the compressing blood is at least in part in a clotted, nonfluid state and able to cause localized compression of the heart. Serious consideration should be given to the possibility of tamponade after cardiac surgery in any patient with inadequate or deteriorating hemodynamics, as evidenced by hypotension, tachycardia, increased filling pressures, or low CO, especially when there has been excessive chest tube drainage. A more subtle presentation of postoperative tamponade is gradually increasing requirements for inotropic and pressor support. Many of the classic signs of tamponade may not be present in these patients, partly because they are usually sedated and ventilated but also because the pericardium is usually left open, resulting in a more gradual increase in the restraining effects of blood accumulation. There may be localized accumulations that affect one chamber more than another.[16] The classic findings of elevated CVP or equalization of CVP, PAd, and PAOP may not occur.[17,18] It may therefore be difficult in the presence of a declining CO and elevated filling pressures to distinguish tamponade from biventricular failure. A useful clue may be pronounced respiratory variation in BP with mechanical ventilation in association with high filling pressures and low CO, because the additional external pressure applied to the heart by positive-pressure ventilation may further impair the already compromised ventricular filling in the presence of tamponade.

Echocardiography may provide strong evidence for the diagnosis of tamponade. Echolucent crescents between the RV wall and the pericardium or the posterior LV wall and the pericardium are discernible with transthoracic imaging or TEE. Echogenicity of grossly bloody pericardial effusions, especially when clots have been formed, may sometimes make delineation of the borders of the pericardium and the ventricular wall difficult, compromising the sensitivity of this technique. A classic echocardiographic sign of tamponade is diastolic collapse of the right atrium or right ventricle, with the duration of collapse bearing a relationship to the severity of the hemodynamic alteration, but such findings are frequently absent in the postcardiac surgery patient. In many cases, transthoracic imaging is difficult because of mechanical ventilation, and TEE is required for adequate visualization.

The definitive treatment of tamponade is surgical exploration with evacuation of hematoma. The chest may have to be opened in the ICU if tamponade proceeds to hemodynamic collapse. In the case of delayed tamponade, pericardiocentesis may be adequate. Medical palliation in anticipation of reexploration consists of reinforcing the physiologic responses that are already occurring while preparing for definitive treatment. Venous return can be increased by volume administration and leg elevation. The lowest tidal volume and PEEP compatible with adequate gas exchange should be used. Epinephrine in high doses gives the needed chronotropic and inotropic boost to the ventricle and increases systemic venous pressures. Sedatives and opioids should be given cautiously because they may interfere with adrenergic discharge and precipitate abrupt hemodynamic collapse. Occasionally, patients develop significant cardiac tamponade without accumulation of blood in the chest. Edema of the heart, lungs, and other tissues in the chest after CPB may not permit chest closure at the initial operation and necessitate staged chest closure after the edema has subsided. Similarly, it was found that some patients with inadequate hemodynamics after cardiac surgery despite maximum support in the ICU improve with opening of the chest because of relief of this tamponade effect. Reclosure of the chest in the operating room is often possible after a few days of continued cardiovascular support and diuresis.

TRANSPLANTED HEART

Postoperative circulatory control in the heart transplant recipient differs from that of the nontransplant population in three major respects. The transplanted heart is noncompliant with a relatively fixed stroke volume, acute rejection must be considered when cardiac performance is poor or suddenly deteriorates, and these patients are at risk for acute RV failure if pulmonary hypertension develops.

The fixed stroke volume combined with denervation of the donor heart means that maintenance of CO is often dependent on therapy to maintain an elevated HR (110 to 120 beats per minute). The drug most commonly used is isoproterenol, because it is a potent inotropic agent and because it causes a dose-related increase in HR. Its vasodilating β_2 effect on the pulmonary vasculature may be of benefit if PVR is above normal. Alternatively, atrial pacing may be used to maintain HR if contractility appears normal. Pacing is often used to allow the withdrawal of isoproterenol in the first postoperative days. Parasympatholytic drugs, such as atropine, do not have any effect on the transplanted heart.

Major concerns in monitoring and therapy for the transplant recipient are the potential for infection and rejection. Immunosuppressive therapy regimens include cyclosporine and usually corticosteroids or azathioprine, or both. These drugs also suppress the patient's response to infection, and corticosteroid therapy may induce elevations in the white blood cell count, further confusing the issue. Protocols for postoperative care stress strict aseptic technique and frequent careful clinical evaluations for infection.

Preoperative evaluation helps screen patients with fixed pulmonary hypertension, because the normal donor RV may acutely fail if presented with an elevated PAP in the recipient. However, patients may have progression of disease between the time of evaluation and surgery, or the right ventricle may be inadequately protected during harvest or transport. When separation from CPB is attempted, acute RV dilation and failure occur, and such patients may emerge from the operating room on multiple drug therapy, including the inhaled agents nitric oxide and prostacyclin, as described earlier. Gradual withdrawal of these drugs occurs in the first postoperative days, with close monitoring of PAPs and oxygenation.

SUMMARY

- Maintaining oxygen transport and oxygen delivery appropriately to meet the tissue metabolic requirements is the goal of postoperative circulatory control.
- Multiple parameters of cardiac function worsen after cardiac surgery.
- Myocardial ischemia often occurs postoperatively, and it is associated with adverse cardiac outcomes.
- Therapeutic interventions for postoperative biventricular dysfunction include controlling the heart rate and rhythm, providing an acceptable preload, and adjusting afterload and contractility. In most patients, pharmacologic interventions can be rapidly weaned or stopped within the first 24 hours after surgery.
- In the postoperative period, supraventricular tachyarrhythmias become a major problem, with atrial fibrillation predominating.
- Postoperative hypertension has been a common complication of cardiac surgery, and newer therapeutic interventions, including the dihydropyridine calcium channel blockers, have an expanding role in the treatment.
- Multiple drugs that increase contractility, including catecholamines, phosphodiesterase inhibitors, and levosimendan, have been studied for treating biventricular dysfunction.
- Many drugs are important for producing vasodilation in systemic, pulmonary, and other vascular beds. Phosphodiesterase inhibitors and levosimendan have clinical effects as inodilators. Vasoactive therapies often are required after cardiac surgery and are useful in understanding vasodilatory shock. Vasopressin has an expanding role.
- Right ventricular dysfunction is an important complication of cardiac surgery that warrants specific vasodilator therapy for reducing right ventricular afterload.
- Mechanical positive-pressure ventilation has multiple effects on the cardiovascular system, with complex interactions that should be considered in patients after cardiac surgery.

REFERENCES

1. Wu WC, Rathore SS, Wang Y, et al: Blood transfusions in elderly patients with acute myocardial infarction. N Engl J Med 345:1230, 2001
2. Costachescu T, Denault A, Guimond JG, et al: The hemodynamically unstable patient in the intensive care unit: Hemodynamic vs TEE monitoring. Crit Care Med 30:1214, 2002
3. Puskas JD, Williams WH, Mahoney EM, et al: Off-pump versus conventional coronary artery bypass grafting: Early and 1-year graft patency, cost, and quality of life outcomes. JAMA 291:1841, 2004
4. Hill LL, De Wet C, Hogue CW: Management of atrial fibrillation after cardiac surgery: II. Prevention and treatment. J Cardiothorac Vasc Anesth 16:626, 2002
5. Vuylsteke A, Feneck RO, Jolin-Mellgard A, et al: Perioperative blood pressure control: A prospective survey of patient management in cardiac surgery. J Cardiothorac Vasc Anesth 14:269, 2000
6. Bailey JM, Lu W, Levy JH, et al: Clevidipine in adult cardiac surgical patients: A dose-finding study. Anesthesiology 96:1086, 2002
7. Gomez WJ, Erlichman MR, Batista-Filho ML, et al: Vasoplegic syndrome after off-pump coronary artery bypass surgery. Eur J Cardiothorac Surg 23:165, 2003
8. Lehmann A, Boldt J: New pharmacologic approaches for the perioperative treatment of ischemic cardiogenic shock. J Cardiothorac Vasc Anesth 19:97, 2005
9. Bellomo R, Chapman M, Finfer S, et al: Low-dose dopamine in patients with early renal dysfunction: A placebo-controlled randomized trial: Australian and New Zealand Intensive Care Society (ANZICS) Clinical Trials Group. Lancet 356:2139, 2000
10. Levy JH, Bailey JM, Deeb M: Intravenous milrinone in cardiac surgery. Ann Thorac Surg 73: 325, 2002
11. Kivikko M, Lehtonen L, Colucci WS, et al: Sustained hemodynamic effects of intravenous levosimendan. Circulation 107:81, 2003

27

12. Labriola C, Siro-Brigiani M, Carrata F, et al: Hemodynamic effects of levosimendan in patients with low-output heart failure after cardiac surgery. Int J Clin Pharmacol Ther 42:204, 2004

13. Jacobs A, Leopold J, Bates E, et al: Cardiogenic shock caused by right ventricular infarction: A report from the SHOCK registry. J Am Coll Cardiol 41:1273, 2003

14. Meade MO, Granton JT, Matte-Martyn A et al: A randomized trial of inhaled nitric oxide to prevent ischemia-reperfusion injury after lung transplantation. Am J Respir Crit Care Med 167:1483, 2003

15. Chuttani K, Pandian NG, Mohanty PK, et al: Left ventricular diastolic collapse: An echocardiographic sign of regional cardiac tamponade. Circulation 83:1999, 1991

16. Kochar GS, Jacobs LE, Kotler MN: Right atrial compression in postoperative cardiac patients: Detection by transesophageal echocardiography. J Am Coll Cardiol 16:511, 1990

17. Bommer WJ, Follette D, Pollock M, et al: Tamponade in patients undergoing cardiac surgery: A clinical-echocardiographic diagnosis. Am Heart J 130:1216, 1995

18. Chuttani K, Tischler MD, Pandian NG, et al: Diagnosis of cardiac tamponade after cardiac surgery: Relative value of clinical, echocardiographic, and hemodynamic signs. Am Heart J 127:913, 1994

VI

Chapter 28

Postoperative Respiratory Care

Thomas L. Higgins, MD • Jean-Pierre Yared, MD

Patients undergoing cardiac surgery experience physiologic stresses from anesthesia, thoracotomy, surgical manipulation, and cardiopulmonary bypass (CPB). Each of these interventions can create transient deleterious effects on pulmonary function even with normal lungs; the effects may be exaggerated in the presence of preexisting pulmonary pathologic processes. Important pulmonary changes after cardiac surgery include diminished functional residual capacity (FRC) after general anesthesia and muscle relaxants, transient 50% to 75% reduction in vital capacity (VC) after median sternotomy and intrathoracic manipulation, atelectasis, and increased intravascular lung water. Acute FRC reduction results in arterial hypoxemia due to mismatch between ventilation and perfusion and in diminished lung compliance with increased work of breathing. This additional work of breathing, which increases oxygen consumption by up to 20% in spontaneously breathing patients, also increases myocardial work at a time when myocardial reserves may be limited. Changes in spirometric measurements and respiratory muscle strength can last up to 8 weeks postoperatively.[1]

Thus, a sizeable proportion of cardiac surgical patients can be expected to have respiratory complications. Acute lung injury, sometimes progressing to acute respiratory distress syndrome (ARDS), can occur in up to 12% of postoperative cardiac patients.

RISK FACTORS FOR RESPIRATORY INSUFFICIENCY

The lung is especially vulnerable because disturbances may affect it directly (atelectasis, effusions, pneumonia) or indirectly (via fluid overload in heart failure, as the result of mediator release during CPB, shock states, or infection, or via changes in respiratory pump function as with phrenic nerve injury). Postoperative status will be determined in part by the patient's preoperative pulmonary reserve, as well as by the level of stress imposed by the procedure. Thus, a patient with reduced VC due to restrictive lung disease, undergoing minimally invasive surgery, may have fewer postoperative pulmonary issues than a relatively healthy patient undergoing simultaneous coronary artery bypass grafting and valve replacement with its accompanying longer operative/anesthetic and CPB times. Respiratory muscle weakness contributes to postoperative pulmonary dysfunction, and prophylactic inspiratory muscle training has been shown to improve respiratory muscle function, pulmonary function tests, and gas exchange. Training reduces the percentage of patients requiring more than 24 hours of postoperative ventilation support from 26% to 5%.

Assessing Risk Based on Preoperative Status

The Society of Thoracic Surgeons (STS) National Adult Cardiac Surgery Database is widely used and offers, in addition to a mortality model, a model customized to predict prolonged ventilation.[2] Chronic obstructive pulmonary disease (COPD) might be expected to be a major risk for postoperative morbidity and mortality. However, hospital mortality with mild-to-moderate COPD is not especially high; it is the minority of patients with severe COPD, especially those older than the age of 75 years or receiving corticosteroids, who are at highest risk. Patients with preexisting COPD have higher rates of pulmonary complications (12%), atrial fibrillation (27%), and death (7%).[3] Obesity, defined by increased body mass index, does not appear to increase the risk of postoperative respiratory failure.

Studies have used multivariate regression techniques to elucidate factors specifically associated with postoperative respiratory failure (Table 28-1).[4-7] They differ in their endpoints for outcome and in their choice of preoperative versus operative versus postoperative variables. The STS model was found to be the single best predictor of mechanical ventilation support for longer than 72 hours but also identified mitral valvular disease, age, vasopressor and inotrope use, renal failure, operative urgency, type of operation, preoperative ventilation, prior cardiac surgery, female gender, myocardial infarction within 30 days, and previous stroke as contributors.[5] None of these models, general or specific for respiratory complications, is sufficiently sensitive or specific to prohibit consideration of surgery for an individual patient, but all provide the clinician with early warning for patients at high risk.

Operating Room Events

Reoperative patients are at risk, partly because of longer CPB time with reoperation, increased blood transfusion, and the additional likelihood of bleeding in this population. CPB time is repeatedly identified as a risk, and a correlation between CPB time and inflammatory cytokine release has been demonstrated. Low cardiac output (CO) states are important because prolonged periods of inadequate perfusion result in additional mediator release. Hemodynamic management when separating from CPB includes the use of vasopressors, inotropes, and potentially mechanical support (intra-aortic balloon pump [IABP], ventricular assist device [VAD]) to avoid multisystem organ failure as a consequence of persistent low CO. Patients maintained on an IABP or a VAD have borderline or insufficient CO; it makes little sense to impose the additional work of breathing until the cardiac issues have resolved. Cardiovascular collapse occasionally occurs at the time of chest closure secondary to severe distention or edema of the lungs. Physiologically, this acts much like cardiac

Table 28-1 Factors Predicting Postoperative Respiratory Outcome

Study	Endpoint	Risk Factors
Spivack et al, 1996[4]	Mechanical ventilation > 48 hr	Reduced LVEF Preexisting CHF Angina Current smoking Diabetes
Branca et al, 2001[5]	Mechanical ventilation > 72 hr	STS-predicted mortality estimate Mitral valve disease Advanced age Pressors/inotropes Renal failure Operative urgency Type of operation Preoperative ventilation Prior CABG Female gender Myocardial infarction within 30 days Previous stroke
Rady et al, 1999[6]	Extubation failure (reintubation after initial extubation)	Age ≥ 65 yr Inpatient Vascular disease COPD/asthma Pulmonary hypertension Reduced LVEF Cardiac shock Hct ≤ 34% BUN ≥ 24 mg/dL Serum albumin ≤ 4.0 mg/dL $Do_2 \le 320$ mL/mm/L^2 > 1 prior CABG Thoracic aortic surgery ≥ 10 units of blood products Total CPB time > 120 min
Canver and Chandra, 2003[7]	Mechanical Ventilation > 72 hr	CPB time Sepsis and endocarditis Gastrointestinal bleeding Renal failure Deep sternal wound infection New cerebrovascular accident Bleeding requiring reoperation

LVEF = left ventricular ejection fraction; CHF = congestive heart failure; STS = Society of Thoracic Surgeons; CABG = coronary artery bypass grafting; COPD = chronic obstructive pulmonary disease; BUN = blood urea nitrogen; Do_2 = systemic oxygen delivery; CPB = cardiopulmonary bypass; Hct = hematocrit.

tamponade, and the solution is to leave the chest open for 24 to 48 hours. An open chest delays early extubation and also has a potential to produce long-term ventilator dependency should infection or sternal osteomyelitis develop.

Postoperative Events

The expected postoperative course is a short period of ventilation support while the patient is warmed, allowed to awaken, and observed for bleeding or hemodynamic instability. Preoperative risks, issues with difficult intubation, and operating room

> **BOX 28-1** *Criteria to Be Met before Early Postoperative Extubation*
>
> - *Neurologic*: Awake, neuromuscular blockade fully dissipated; following instructions, able to cough and protect airway
> - *Cardiac*: Stable without mechanical support; cardiac index ≥ 2.2 L/min/m^2; MAP $\geq$ 70 mm Hg, no serious arrhythmias
> - *Respiratory*: Acceptable chest radiograph and ABGs (pH ≥ 7.35); MIP at least 25 cm H$_2$O; minimal secretions, comfortable on CPAP or T-piece with spontaneous respiratory rate ≤ 20 breaths per minute
> - *Renal*: Diuresing well; urine output > 0.8 mL/kg/hr; not markedly fluid overloaded from operative/CPB fluid administration or SIRS
> - *Hematologic*: Chest tube drainage minimal
> - *Temperature*: Fully rewarmed; not actively shivering
>
> ---
>
> MAP = mean arterial pressure; ABGs = arterial blood gases; MIP = maximal inspiratory pressure; CPAP = continuous positive airway pressure; CPB = cardiopulmonary bypass; SIRS = systemic immune response syndrome.

events should be communicated from the operating room team to the ICU team at the time of ICU admission. Box 28-1 outlines criteria to be met before routine extubation.

Before extubation, a quick neurologic examination should be performed to rule out new cerebrovascular events, presence of excess opioids, or residual neuromuscular blocking agents. Knowledge that the work of breathing can consume up to 20% of CO should preclude extubation in the hemodynamically unstable patient. Although patients may be successfully extubated while on IABP, the need to lie flat after balloon and sheath removal may dictate continued temporary ventilator support.

Postoperative care of low-risk cardiac surgical patients has come to resemble a recovery room model, but high-risk patients benefit from postoperative involvement of anesthesiologists, cardiologists, and critical care specialists. The presence of full-time ICU staff physicians improves outcome and is now recommended by the Leapfrog Group as a patient safety standard.[8]

Hospital-acquired infections are an important cause of postoperative morbidity, and nosocomial pneumonia is common in patients receiving continuous mechanical ventilation. The actuarial risk of ventilator-associated pneumonia appears to be around 1% per day when diagnosed using protected specimen brush and quantitative culture techniques. Strategies thought to be effective at reducing the incidence of ventilator-associated pneumonia include early removal of nasogastric or endotracheal tubes, formal infection control programs, handwashing, semirecumbent positioning of the patient, avoiding unnecessary reintubation, providing adequate nutritional support, avoiding gastric overdistention, use of the oral rather than the nasal route for intubation, scheduled drainage of condensate from ventilator circuits, and maintenance of adequate endotracheal tube cuff pressure.

DIAGNOSIS OF ACUTE LUNG INJURY AND ACUTE RESPIRATORY DISTRESS SYNDROME

ARDS may develop as a sequela of CPB, or, more commonly, in the postoperative patient with cardiogenic shock, sepsis, or multisystem organ failure. Components of ARDS include diffuse alveolar damage resulting from endothelial and type I epithelial cell necrosis, and noncardiogenic pulmonary edema due to breakdown of the endothelial barrier with subsequent vascular permeability. The exudative phase of ARDS occurs in the first 3 days after the precipitating event and is thought to be mediated by neutrophil activation and sequestration. Neutrophils release mediators, causing endothelial damage. Ultimately, the alveolar spaces fill up with fluid as a result of increased endothelial permeability.

Intravascular and intra-alveolar fibrin deposition is common. Procoagulant activity becomes enhanced in ARDS, and bronchoalveolar lavage reveals increased tissue factor levels. The clinical presentation is typically an acute onset of severe arterial hypoxemia resistant to oxygen therapy, with a Pao_2 to Fio_2 (P/F) ratio of less than 200 mmHg. ARDS is classically diagnosed only in the absence of left ventricular failure, which complicates the issue in the postoperative cardiac patient who may also be in congestive heart failure (CHF). Other findings in ARDS include decreased lung compliance (<30 mL/cm H_2O) and bilateral infiltrates on the chest radiograph.

The proliferative phase of ARDS occurs on days 3 to 7 as inflammatory cells accumulate as a result of chemoattractants released by the neutrophils. At this stage, the normal repair process would remove debris and begin repair, but a disordered repair process may result in exuberant fibrosis, stiff lungs, and inefficient gas exchange. Evidence suggests that careful medical and ventilator management may affect this process. Any precipitating factors should be addressed (e.g., draining closed-space infections). Conventional ventilator support following cardiac surgery is to maintain large tidal volumes (typically 10 to 12 mL/kg) to reopen atelectatic but potentially functional alveoli. The problem is that the compromised lung is no longer homogeneous and high pressures can further damage the remaining normal lung over time. Direct mechanical injury may occur as a result of overdistention (volutrauma), high pressures (barotrauma), or shear injury from repetitive opening and closing. "Biotrauma" may also occur as a result of inflammatory mediator release and impaired antibacterial barriers. Current clinical practice with known or suspected lung injury is to limit inflation pressures. The maximal "safe" inflation pressure is not known, but evidence favors keeping peak inspiratory pressures at less than 35 cm H_2O and restricting tidal volumes to about 6 mL/kg of ideal body weight. The landmark ARDSNet trial randomized patients to 6 mL/kg versus 12 mL/kg of ideal body weight and demonstrated a significant difference in 28-day survival with the low-tidal-volume group.[9]

Additional Therapy for Acute Lung Injury/Acute Respiratory Distress Syndrome

Maintaining a lung-protective ventilatory strategy (LPVS) can involve permissive hypercapnia if normal Pco_2 levels cannot be achieved with low tidal volumes. Prone positioning is useful in achieving oxygenation.

Cardiopulmonary Interactions

Understanding cardiopulmonary interactions associated with mechanical ventilation is essential. Hemodynamic changes may occur secondary to changes in lung volume and intrathoracic pressure even when tidal volume remains constant.[10] Pulmonary vascular resistance and mechanical heart-lung interactions play prominent roles in determining the hemodynamic response to mechanical ventilation. Because lung inflation alters pulmonary vascular resistance and right ventricular wall tension, there are limits to intrathoracic pressure that a damaged heart will tolerate. High lung volumes may

intervention in almost all patients by postoperative day 6. Alcohol or benzodiazepine withdrawal should be considered in the differential diagnosis of delirium. Initial management of agitation consists of reassurance and orientation of the patient and control of pain with opioids.

Diaphragmatic paralysis may complicate any procedure, but it is more common in patients undergoing reoperation, owing to the difficulty in identifying the phrenic nerve in fibrotic pericardial tissue. The diagnosis of diaphragmatic paralysis should be considered whenever a patient fails to wean from mechanical ventilation; it should be documented by observing paradoxical movement of the diaphragm during inspiration and by comparing vital capacity (VC) and tidal volume (V_T) in the supine and seated positions. Differences in supine and seated VC of more than 10% to 15% should prompt fluoroscopic examination of the diaphragm ("sniff" test). Bilateral paralysis may be missed by this test, because comparison of left and right diaphragmatic excursion has lower specificity when both diaphragms are involved. Transient diaphragmatic paralysis can occur secondary to cold injury to the phrenic nerve. Less often, the phrenic nerve is injured or transected during dissection of the internal mammary arteries or during mobilization of the heart in patients undergoing reoperation.

Cardiac Complications

Patients maintained on chronic amiodarone therapy are prone to postoperative respiratory failure, longer intubation times, and longer ICU stays, even with only subclinical evidence of pulmonary amiodarone toxicity.[13] Rarely, patients taking amiodarone develop life-threatening pulmonary complications, including ARDS. Histologic lung examination of these patients demonstrates marked interstitial fibrosis with enlarged air spaces ("honeycomb" appearance) and hyperplasia of type II pneumocytes.

Patients with valvular disease have significantly higher respiratory system and lung elastances and resistances than those undergoing surgery for ischemic heart disease, but these may correct with successful surgery. Thus, valve surgery patients have less work of breathing and improved respiratory function after correction of the valvular pathology, but coronary artery bypass grafting patients are less likely to show dramatic improvement postoperatively.

Infectious Complications

Mediastinitis, sternal dehiscence, or both, are complications of coronary revascularization, with an incidence of about 1% and a mortality rate of about 13% and a tendency to prolong ventilator dependency. Predisposing factors for wound complications after cardiac surgery include diabetes, low CO, use of bilateral internal mammary grafts, and reoperation for control of bleeding. Keeping blood glucose lower than 200 mg/dL in the perioperative period reduces the sternal wound infection rate from 2.4% to 1.5%. Mediastinal infection manifests as unexplained fever, an unstable sternum and, sometimes, failure to wean. In addition to selective antibiotic therapy, surgical débridement and drainage of the wound are usually necessary. Additional management of mediastinitis may include primary or delayed sternal closure using pectoralis or omental flaps.

MODES OF VENTILATOR SUPPORT

Positive-pressure ventilators employed outside the operating room have a nonrebreathing circuit, may be volume or pressure limited, and may be triggered by changes in flow or changes in pressure. All modern ventilators contain multiple modes of ventilatory support that accommodate both mandatory and patient-triggered breaths. The most common modes of positive-pressure ventilation are assist-control (A/C), synchronized intermittent mandatory ventilation (SIMV), and pressure-support ventilation (PSV). Volume-cycled support is still most common. With volume modes, the inspiratory flow rate, targeted volume, and inspiratory time are set by the clinician, and inspiratory peak pressure will vary depending on the patient's lung compliance and synchrony with the ventilator. Volume cycling ensures consistent delivery of a set tidal volume as long as the pressure limit is not exceeded. With nonhomogeneous lung pathology, however, delivered volume tends to flow to the area of low resistance, which may result in overdistention of healthy segments of lung and underinflation of atelectatic segments and consequent ventilation-perfusion mismatching.

Intermittent mandatory ventilation (IMV) and then SIMV were developed to facilitate weaning from mechanical ventilatory support. With either IMV modality, a basal respiratory rate is set by the clinician, which may be supplemented by patient-initiated breaths. In contrast to A/C ventilation, however, the tidal volume of the patient's spontaneous breaths will be determined by the patient's own respiratory strength and lung compliance rather than delivered as a preset volume. SIMV mode is appropriate for patients with normal lungs recovering from opioid anesthesia. Weaning is accomplished by reducing the mandatory IMV rate and allowing the patient to assume more and more of the respiratory effort over time.

Pressure-Support Ventilation

Pressure-support ventilation, which is primarily a weaning tool, must be distinguished from pressure-control ventilation, which is generally used during the maintenance phase of acute lung injury. PSV may be used in conjunction with continuous positive airway pressure (CPAP) or SIMV modes. Pressure support augments the patient's spontaneous inspiratory effort with a clinician-selected level of pressure. Putative advantages include improved patient comfort, reduced ventilatory work, and more rapid weaning. The volume delivered with each PSV breath depends on the pressure set for inspiratory assist as well as the patient's lung compliance. The utility of PSV in weaning from chronic ventilation support is that it allows the patient's ventilatory muscles to assume part of the workload while augmenting tidal volume, thus preventing atelectasis, sufficiently stretching lung receptors, and keeping the patient's spontaneous respiratory rate within a reasonable physiologic range.

LIBERATION FROM MECHANICAL SUPPORT (WEANING)

When terminating mechanical ventilation, two phases of decision-making are involved. First, there should be resolution of the initial process for which mechanical ventilation was begun. The patient cannot be septic, hemodynamically unstable, or burdened with excessive respiratory secretions. If these general criteria are met, then specific weaning criteria can be examined. These include oxygenation (typically a $Pao_2 > 60$ mm Hg on 35% inspired oxygen and low levels of PEEP), adequate oxygen transport (measurable by O_2 extraction ratio or assumed if the cardiac index is adequate and lactic acidosis is not present), adequate respiratory mechanics (tidal volume, maximal inspiratory pressure) and adequate respiratory reserve (minute ventilation at rest of < 10 L/min), and a low frequency/tidal volume ratio ($f/V_T < 100$) indicating adequate volume at a sustainable respiratory rate.

28

673

Weaning: The Process

The actual process of weaning from mechanical ventilatory support must be individualized. There is no "one size fits all" method. Whereas gradually lowering the rate in increments of two breaths per minute generally works for short-term ventilatory support, long-term patients often have difficulty making the transition from SIMV rates of 2 to CPAP. The time-honored method of weaning by maintaining a patient on full ventilatory support alternating with increasingly longer periods of spontaneous ventilation on a T-piece is effective but time consuming because it requires setting up additional equipment and a nurse or respiratory therapist to be immediately available at bedside during each weaning attempt. Breath-to-breath monitoring, display of tidal volumes, and ventilator alarms will not be available during a T-piece trial. More commonly, pressure support is used as an adjunct to weaning either with IMV or CPAP while still connected to the ventilator and its alarm system. The preference is to use CPAP with pressure support alone (i.e., no additional IMV rate) because mechanical ventilation introduces one more variable into the evaluation of a patient's progress. Sufficient CPAP is applied to maintain open alveoli (generally 5 to 8 cm H_2O but often higher when recovering from acute lung injury/ARDS) and then the pressure support level titrated to provide the patient with sufficient volume and a respiratory rate less than 24 breaths per minute. As the patient's exercise tolerance improves, the pressure support level can be lowered in increments of 2 to 3 cm H_2O. It is usually necessary to address fluid overload, nutritional support, and other nonpulmonary factors to achieve the pressure support reduction.

Specific Impediments to Weaning

Weaning from ventilator support affects CO due to changes in pulmonary vascular resistance (PVR). Increased PVR can lead to septal shifts and consequent changes in the efficiency of right and left ventricular function. Thus, it makes little sense to attempt weaning in the hemodynamically unstable patient. The standard approach has been to keep these patients on full ventilator support with sedation and neuromuscular blockade if necessary until the acute cardiac problem is resolved.

VI

Inability to Wean

A small percentage of patients will not be able to wean from ventilator support despite all efforts. Predictive models, however, are rarely useful for deciding which individuals with multisystem failure will not benefit from continuation of aggressive life support.

The experience has been that it is rarely a single problem, but the interaction among multiple morbidities that creates a situation in which the patient may not separate from the ventilator. At this point, a frank discussion with the patient (if he or she has decisional capacity) or the health care proxy can be helpful in defining the benefits and burdens of further therapy and the patient's desires. Consultation from the hospital's ethics team may be very helpful. Patients who remain in a low cardiac output state and who have sustained multiorgan failure rarely if ever end their dependence on high-technology support, including ventilation and hemodialysis. On the other hand, malnutrition and deconditioning in the absence of ongoing sepsis and organ system failure sometimes respond to prolonged rehabilitation, which may be better handled by a long-term ventilation facility than an acute-care hospital. Recommendations for the difficult-to-wean cardiac surgical patient are summarized in Boxes 28-3 and 28-4.

BOX 28-3 *Nonrespiratory Factors Affecting Weaning*

- Nutrition status—both malnutrition and over feeding
- Renal function
- Fluid balance, especially fluid overload
- Sepsis/infection; may be occult
- Hematologic status/anemia; optimal hemoglobin of 8–10 gm%
- Metabolic disturbance
- Cardiac function, which may deteriorate with respiratory work
- Pharmacologic therapy including long-lasting metabolites of sedatives
- Neurologic compromise including phrenic nerve injury
- Neuropsychiatric issues/delirium
- Sleep deprivation; try to have normal day-night cycle
- Endotracheal tube size
- Patients perception of breathing, may respond to opiates

BOX 28-4 *The Difficult-to-Wean Patient*

- Recognize patients at risk based on preoperative and operating room events (see Table 28-1).
- Where possible, minimize risk (see Box 28-2).
- Prioritize organ system support; without adequate perfusion, all other systems will fail.
- Maintain full ventilator support during acute phase of respiratory insufficiency or circulatory failure.
- Adopt a lung-protective ventilation strategy for patients with acute lung injury or acute respiratory distress syndrome.
- Expect and defend against common problems (see Box 28-3).
- Pay attention to general support measures and safety issues including sedation holidays and infection control.
- Prepare patient and family for involvement in rehabilitation phase.
- Have a clear weaning plan or protocol and follow it.
- Recognize when the burdens of treatment are disproportionate, and initiate appropriate discussions with the patient or health care provider.

28

SUMMARY

- Pulmonary complications after cardiopulmonary bypass are relatively common, with up to 12% of patients experiencing acute lung injury and about 1.5% requiring tracheostomy for long-term ventilation.
- Risk factors for postoperative respiratory insufficiency include advanced age, presence of diabetes or renal failure, chronic obstructive lung disease, peripheral vascular disease, prior cardiac surgery, and emergency or unstable status.
- Patients with preexisting chronic obstructive lung disease have higher rates of pulmonary complications, atrial fibrillation, and death.
- Operating room events that increase risk include reoperation, blood transfusion, prolonged cardiopulmonary bypass time, and low cardiac output states, particularly if a mechanical support device is required.
- Hospital-acquired infections are an important cause of postoperative morbidity and nosocomial pneumonia. Strategies to reduce the incidence of ventilator-associated

pneumonia include early removal of gastric and tracheal tubes, formal infection control programs, handwashing, semirecumbent positioning of the patient, and scheduled drainage of condensate from ventilated circuits.

- Patients at risk for acute lung injury and those developing acute respiratory distress syndrome should be switched to a lung-protective ventilation strategy, which involves maintaining peak inspiratory pulmonary pressure less than 35 cm H_2O and restricting tidal volumes to 6 mL/kg of ideal body weight.
- Permissive hypercapnia may be necessary to accomplish lung-protective ventilatory strategy.
- Impediments to weaning and extubation include delirium, unstable hemodynamics, respiratory muscle dysfunction, renal failure with fluid overload, and sepsis.
- Short-term weaning success can be achieved with any variety of ventilation modes. The long-term patient requires an individualized approach, which may encompass pressure-support ventilation, synchronized intermittent mandatory ventilation weaning, or T-piece trials.
- While a number of parameters exist to assess respiratory strength and endurance, the single best parameter is the frequency/tidal volume ratio.
- Long-term administration of neuromuscular blocking agents is associated with persistent muscle weakness. Possible causes include accumulation of drug metabolites, critical illness polyneuropathy, or neurogenic atrophy.
- A very small percentage of patients will not be able to be weaned from ventilation support. Characteristics of these patients include persistent low-output state with multisystem organ failure. Long-term weaning may be best accomplished in a specialized unit rather than an acute cardiovascular recovery area.

REFERENCES

1. Johnson D, Hurst T, Thompson D, et al: Respiratory function after cardiac surgery. J Cardiothorac Vasc Anesth 10:571, 1996
2. The Society of Thoracic Surgeons: 30-Day operative mortality and morbidity risk models. Ann Thorac Surg 75:1856, 2003
3. Samuels LE, Kaufman MS, Morris RJ, et al: Coronary artery bypass grafting in patients with COPD. Chest 113:878, 1998
4. Spivack SD, Shinozaki T, Albertini JJ, Deane R: Preoperative prediction of postoperative respiratory outcome. Coronary artery bypass grafting. Chest 109:1222-1230, 1996
5. Branca P, McGaw P, Light RW, et al: Factors associated with prolonged mechanical ventilation following coronary artery bypass surgery. Chest 119:537, 2001
6. Rady MY, Ryan T: Perioperative predictors of extubation failure and the effect on clinical outcome after cardiac surgery. Crit Care Med 27:340, 1996
7. Canver CC, Chandra J: Intraoperative and postoperative risk factors for respiratory failure after coronary bypass. Ann Thorac Surg 75:853, 2003
8. www.leapfroggroup.org/factsheets/ICU_factsheet.pdf accessed on April 28, 2004
9. The Acute Respiratory Distress Syndrome Network: Ventilation with lower tidal volumes as compared with traditional tidal volumes for acute lung injury and the acute respiratory distress syndrome. N Engl J Med 342:1301, 2000
10. Steingrub JS, Tidswell MA, Higgins TL: Hemodynamic consequences of heart-lung interactions. J Intens Care Med 18:92, 2003
11. http://www.AHRQ.gov/clinic/ptsafety/addend.htm. Accessed May 20, 2004
12. Milbrandt EB, Deppen S, Harrison PL, et al: Costs associated with delirium in mechanically ventilated patients. Crit Care Med 31:955, 2004
13. Nalos PC, Kass RM, Gang ES, et al: Life-threatening postoperative pulmonary complications in patients with previous amiodarone pulmonary toxicity undergoing cardiothoracic operations. J Thorac Cardiovasc Surg 93:904, 1987

VI

Chapter 29

Central Nervous System Dysfunction after Cardiopulmonary Bypass

Ivan Iglesias, MD • John M. Murkin, MD

Overt and subclinical perioperative cerebral injury remains an unresolved problem. Overall mortality for patients undergoing coronary artery bypass grafting (CABG) has decreased by 23% over the past decade despite a projected risk-adjusted mortality predicting a 33% increase in mortality, but the incidence of stroke has remained relatively unchanged.[1]

AGE-ASSOCIATED RISK OF CENTRAL NERVOUS SYSTEM INJURY

Current data show a persistent association between increased age and cerebral injury after cardiac surgery. In a review of 67,764 cardiac surgical patients, of whom there were 4743 octogenarians and who underwent cardiac surgery at 22 centers in the National Cardiovascular Network, Alexander and colleagues reported that the incidence of type I cerebral injury, defined as stroke, transient ischemic attack (TIA), or coma, was 10.2% in patients older than 80 years old versus 4.2% in patients younger than 80 years old.[2] In addition to the age-related factor, reports from Europe and North America consistently describe previous cerebrovascular disease, diabetes mellitus, hypertension, peripheral vascular disease, aortic atherosclerosis, and intraoperative and postoperative complications as all being additional factors increasing the incidence of cerebral injury in cardiac surgical patients (Box 29-1).

The impact of age-associated cerebral injury in cardiac surgery is becoming more relevant owing to the progressive increase in the average age of the general population

---

BOX 29-1   *Factors Related to Cerebral Injury in Cardiac Surgery*

- Hemodynamic instability
- Diabetes mellitus
- Age
- Combined/complex procedures
- Prolonged cardiopulmonary bypass time
- Prior stroke
- Aorta atheromatosis
- Peripheral vascular disease

---

and, in particular, of the cardiac surgical population. As overall survival and quality of life after cardiac surgery continue to improve in elderly patients, advanced age alone is no longer considered a deterrent when evaluating a patient for cardiac surgery. The presence and extent of comorbidities should be considered as being of equal or greater importance than age itself as a risk factor for cerebral injury in cardiac surgical patients.[3]

CENTRAL NERVOUS SYSTEM INJURY

Cerebral injury is classified in two broad categories: type I (focal injury, stupor, or coma at discharge) and type II (deterioration in intellectual function, memory deficit, or seizures). Cerebral injury can also be broadly classified as stroke, delirium (encephalopathy), or cognitive dysfunction.

The incidence of stroke or type I injury after closed-chamber cardiac procedures is generally considered to be 1% to 4%, increasing to 8% to 9% in open-chamber (e.g., valvular surgery) or combined/complex procedures. The incidence of cognitive dysfunction (type II) is reported as ranging in incidence from 30% to 80% in the early postoperative period.[4] To some extent there is a difference in the incidence of cerebral injury after cardiac surgery related to the type and complexity of the procedure, such as open chamber, combined valvular, and CABG.

Overall, the increased length of stay (LOS) and increased mortality rates associated with any form of cerebral complication in cardiac surgical patients are especially striking findings. Despite the relatively greater impact on mortality of stroke as opposed to cognitive dysfunction, type II injury is still associated with a fivefold increase in mortality.

Retrospective versus Prospective Neurologic Assessment

The detection of central nervous system (CNS) injury depends critically on the methodology used, and retrospective studies have been deemed insensitive by different authors. A retrospective chart review is inadequate as an assessment of the overall incidence of postoperative neurologic dysfunction. The reasons for the inability of retrospective chart audit to detect the majority of patients with neurologic dysfunction are readily apparent and include incompleteness of records, a reluctance to document apparently minor complications, and, most important, an insensitivity to subtle neurologic dysfunction. The timing, thoroughness, and reproducibility (single examiner) of the neurologic examinations, as well as the incorporation of a preoperative assessment for comparison, all determine the sensitivity and accuracy with which postoperative CNS injury can be detected.

Valvular versus Coronary Artery Bypass Graft Surgery

Increasing the complexity or undertaking open chamber-type procedures increases the risk of CNS injury. Ebert and coworkers prospectively studied 42 patients who underwent valve replacement surgery and 42 patients for CABG, with both groups matched post hoc for age, sex, and preoperative cognitive status.[5] Patients were investigated preoperatively as well as 2 and 7 days postoperatively with a comprehensive neuropsychological and neuropsychiatric assessment. Valve replacement surgery patients exhibited more severe neuropsychological deficits and showed a slower recovery than patients who underwent CABG. In a study of 64,467 patients who underwent CABG alone and 3297 patients who underwent CABG in conjunction with aortic valve replacement (CABG/AVR) or CABG in conjunction with mitral valve repair or replacement (CABG/MVR), the incidence of type I cerebral injury in patients younger than 80 years of age was 4.2% for CABG, 9.1% for CABG/AVR, and 11.2% for CABG/MVR.[2] It should be noted that the total CPB time was 96 minutes for CABG, 148 minutes for CABG/AVR, and 161 minutes for CABG/MVR.

The incidence of subtle neurologic dysfunction and cognitive abnormalities is similar in all adult patients undergoing surgical coronary artery revascularization. Increasing age has been repeatedly shown to be one of the major risk factors for stroke after CABG, likely related to the greater prevalence of severe aortic atherosclerosis in the elderly. This suggests that there may be different factors operative in the production of gross neurologic damage than in the genesis of cognitive dysfunction. Although calcific or atheromatous macroembolic debris from the ascending aorta or aortic arch appears to be a prime factor in the production of clinical stroke syndromes and it was formerly thought that microembolic elements, either gaseous or particulate, produced cognitive dysfunction, studies from beating-heart surgery in which CPB is avoided, despite a much lower incidence of embolic events, appear to have a relatively similar incidence of cognitive dysfunction to CABG using conventional CPB.[6]

Aortic Atherosclerosis

Atheroembolism from an atheromatous ascending aorta and aortic arch is recognized as a major risk factor in the patient undergoing cardiac surgery and is a widespread problem.[7]

Atheroembolism in cardiac surgery has a broad spectrum of clinical presentations, including devastating injuries and death; yet its true incidence is probably underestimated. Thoracic aorta atheromatosis is associated with coronary artery disease and stroke in the general population. Yahia and associates prospectively studied patients with diagnoses of TIA or stroke using TEE for assessment of aortic atheromatosis.[7] Thoracic aortic atheromas were present in 141 of 237 patients (59%); mild plaque (<2 mm) was present in 5%, moderate plaque (2 to 4 mm) in 21%, severe plaque (≥4 mm) in 33%, and complex plaque in 27%. Plaques were more frequently present in the descending aorta and the arch of the aorta than in the ascending aorta. Overall, atherosclerosis of the ascending aorta is present in 20% to 40% of cardiac surgical patients, with the percentage increasing with age, and it is an independent risk factor for type I cerebral injury.

Transesophageal Echocardiography versus Epiaortic Scanning

The detection of ascending aorta atheromatosis is a cornerstone of strategies to decrease cerebral injury in cardiac surgery. Despite its widespread utilization, manual palpation of the aorta has a very low sensitivity for this purpose. The association of severe thoracic

29

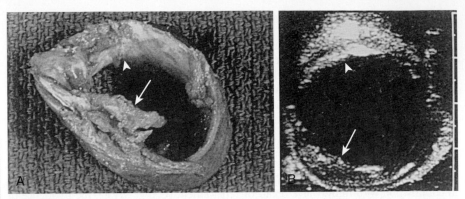

Figure 29-1 Transverse ultrasonic image of the ascending aorta and the corresponding segment of aorta in a patient with severe atherosclerosis. Note the calcification (*arrowhead*) and the projection of atheroma (*arrow*) into the lumen. (From Wareing TH, Davila-Roman VG, Barzilai B, et al: Management of the severely atherosclerotic ascending aorta during cardiac operations: A strategy for detection and treatment. J Thorac Cardiovasc Surg 103:453, 1992.)

aortic plaques (defined as 5-mm-thick focal hyperechogenic zones of the aortic intima and/or lumen irregularities with mobile structures or ulcerations) and coronary artery disease is well established. Identifying severe aortic disease has important clinical implications because surgical technique, including surgical procedure and siting of cannulation and anastomotic sites for proximal grafts, may be altered to avoid producing emboli and stroke. Intraoperative epiaortic ultrasound scanning (EAS) has emerged as a most helpful tool for the diagnosis of ascending aortic atherosclerosis and has revealed major insights into the nature and distribution of this disease.

Djaiani and colleagues performed TEE and EAS to assess the severity of aortic atherosclerosis in the ascending aorta and the aortic arch.[8] Patients were allocated to either low-risk or high-risk groups according to thickness of the intima of the aorta. Transcranial Doppler imaging was used to monitor the middle cerebral artery. Diffusion-weighted magnetic resonance imaging (MRI) was performed 3 to 7 days after surgery. The NEECHAM Confusion Scale was used for assessment and monitoring patient consciousness level. In the high-risk group (intimal thickness > 2 mm), confusion was present in six (16%) patients versus five (7%) patients in the low-risk group, and there was a threefold increase in median embolic count, 223.5 versus 70.0 ($P = .0003$). Diffusion-weighted MRI–detected brain lesions were only present in patients from the high-risk group, 61.5% versus 0% ($P < .0001$). There was significant correlation between the NEECHAM scores and embolic count in the high-risk group. Multiple studies have documented that most of the significant atherosclerotic lesions in the ascending aorta are missed by intraoperative palpation by the surgeon, and intraoperative echocardiographic studies of the aorta have been recommended (Fig. 29-1). However, the ability of TEE to reliably detect all ascending aorta and aortic arch lesions is limited.

The high acoustic reflectance attributable to the air-tissue interface resulting from overlying right main bronchus and trachea limits TEE assessment of the upper ascending aorta where cannulation is generally undertaken. Intraoperative EAS has emerged as a most helpful tool for the diagnosis of ascending aortic atherosclerosis and has revealed major insights into the nature and distribution of this disease. Konstadt and colleagues investigated 81 patients (57 male and 24 female; aged 32 to 88 years, mean age 64 years) scheduled for elective cardiac surgery.[9] A comprehensive examination of the entire thoracic aorta in both the longitudinal and transverse planes was performed by biplane TEE. After pericardiotomy, a sterile-draped 7-MHz probe was used to scan the entire ascending aorta in both long- and short-axis views. In both echocardiographic examinations, the presence and location of protruding plaques and intimal thickening greater than 3 mm were recorded. Fourteen (17%) of the 81 patients had significant atherosclerotic disease of the ascending aorta as diagnosed by EAS echocardiography. The sensitivity of TEE was 100%, the specificity was 60%, the positive predictive value was 34%, and the negative predictive value was 100%. According to the authors, if the complete biplane TEE examination is negative for plaque, it is highly unlikely that there is significant plaque in the ascending aorta. If the TEE examination is positive for plaque, there is a 34% chance that there is significant disease of the ascending aorta, and EAS should be considered. TEE is a very sensitive but only mildly specific method of determining whether ascending aortic atherosclerosis is present.

Identification of ascending aorta atheromatous disease would prompt the surgical team for strategies to either modify, decrease, or avoid aortic manipulation. Management strategies for the diseased ascending aorta range from minimally invasive aortic "no-touch" techniques to maximally invasive procedures, including ascending aorta replacement with application of deep hypothermic circulatory arrest. Operative modifications in CABG include avoidance of aortic cross-clamping, alternative methods of aortic cross-clamping, and placement of all arterial in situ bypass conduits, Y-grafts, or extra-anatomic bypass grafts.

NEUROPSYCHOLOGICAL DYSFUNCTION

Compared with stroke, cognitive dysfunction is a considerably more frequent sequela of cardiac surgery and has been demonstrated in up to 80% of patients early postoperatively.[10] The pathogenesis of cognitive dysfunction after cardiac surgery is still uncertain. Variables that have been postulated to explain the development of postoperative neurocognitive decline include advanced age, concomitant cerebrovascular disease and severity of cardiovascular disease, and intraoperative factors such as embolization, cerebral hypoperfusion or hypoxia, activation of inflammatory processes, aortic cross-clamp or CPB time, and possibly low mean arterial pressure in patients with impaired cerebrovascular autoregulation. In many instances, subtle signs of neuropsychological dysfunction are detectable only with sophisticated cognitive testing strategies. The fact that many of these abnormalities are difficult to properly assess on routine clinical work and their apparently transient nature have led to a tendency to minimize their clinical relevance. The mid- and long-term impact of cognitive dysfunction on quality of life after cardiac surgery has been addressed by different studies.

MECHANISMS OF BRAIN INJURY

Determining which factor or, more likely, which combination of factors is responsible for postoperative neurologic or behavioral dysfunction in patients undergoing cardiac surgery using CPB is problematic (Box 29-2). Based on postmortem studies, as well as correlative analysis of intraoperative events with neurologic outcomes, two primary mechanisms appear to be responsible for brain injury in otherwise uncomplicated cardiac operations: cerebral hypoperfusion and cerebral emboli.

Intraoperative cerebral embolization of particulate and microgaseous elements has been demonstrated to have a significant role in the genesis of cerebral events in postoperative cardiac surgical patients. Increasing attention is also being paid to the

29

BOX 29-2 *Risk Factors for Neurologic Complications in Cardiac Surgery*

- Hemodynamic instability
- Diabetes mellitus
- Advanced age
- Combined/complex procedures
- Prolonged CPB time
- Prior stroke
- Aortic atheromatosis
- Peripheral vascular disease

BOX 29-3 *Mechanisms and Factors for Neurologic Lesions*

- Embolization
- Hypoperfusion
- Inflammation
- Influencing factors
  - Aortic atheroma plaque
  - Cerebrovascular disease
  - Altered cerebral autoregulation
  - Hypotension
  - Intracardiac debris
  - Air
  - Venous obstruction on bypass
  - CPB circuit surface
  - Reinfusion of unprocessed shed blood
  - Cerebral hyperthermia
  - Hypoxia

role of perioperative hypoperfusion, particularly in patients with intracranial and extracranial atherosclerosis, and to the effect of inflammatory processes triggered during exposure to surgery and CPB (Box 29-3).[11]

Watershed Infarctions

Watershed, or boundary zone, infarcts are ischemic lesions that are situated along border zones between the territories of two major cerebral arteries (e.g., the middle and posterior, or the anterior and middle cerebral arteries) where terminal arteriolar anastomoses exist.

A profound reduction in systemic blood pressure is the most frequent cause of watershed infarcts. These areas are thought to be more susceptible to ischemia resulting from hypotension because of their critical dependence on a single blood supply.

These areas are also highly susceptible to ischemia due to end-artery embolization, and it is also recognized that although severe hypotension is the most common cause, showers of microemboli may lodge preferentially in these areas and cause infarcts in the underlying brain.[12] As such, although they are commonly due to profoundly hypotensive episodes, watershed lesions are not pathognomonic of a hypotensive episode and may be the result of cerebral emboli. Embolization and hypoperfusion acting together play a synergistic role and either cause or magnify the brain damage of cardiac surgical patients.

Cerebral Perfusion Pressure

Using radioisotope techniques for measurement of cerebral blood flow (CBF), and incorporating a jugular venous catheter for calculation of the cerebral metabolic rate of oxygen, it was determined that there is a profound reduction in the cerebral metabolic rate of oxygen during hypothermic CPB and that CBF is decreased proportionately and will autoregulate down to a cerebral perfusion pressure (CPP) of 20 mm Hg in the presence of α-stat pH management. Low arterial pressure during the hypothermic phase of CPB is, thus, unlikely to result in cerebral ischemia *in the absence of cerebrovascular disease.*

It should also be appreciated that during CPB cerebral venous hypertension can result from partial obstruction of the superior vena cava (SVC), particularly in the presence of a single two-stage venous cannula, and may give rise to cerebral edema, as well as producing a disproportionate lowering of CPP relative to arterial pressure. This strongly suggests that cerebral venous hypertension, as can occur during CPB with myocardial dislocation and impaired drainage of SVC, may result in cerebral ischemia and necrosis if unrecognized and untreated. It is feasible that such unrecognized cerebral venous hypertension has resulted in some of the postoperative neurologic syndromes that have been reported.

Although the association between hypotension during CPB and cerebral dysfunction remains contentious, there is some evidence that certain subsets of patients may be at particular risk. Although mean arterial pressure (MAP) and rewarming are not primary determinants of cognitive decline, hypotension and rapid rewarming contribute significantly to cognitive dysfunction in the elderly. Again, because elderly patients comprise an increasing segment of the cardiac surgical population, these aspects are becoming increasingly important clinical management issues.

The interaction of emboli, perfusion pressure, and the particular conditions of the regional cerebral circulation (e.g., preexisting cerebral intravascular lesions) will determine the final expression of brain damage in the cardiac surgical patient. Combinations of hemodynamic events from apparently normal CPB procedures are related to the development of postoperative neurologic complications and affect the impact of common clinical risk factors. A multivariate statistical procedure (cluster analysis) was applied to a dataset of automatically recorded perfusions from 1395 patients who underwent CABG.[13] The following five parameters emerged for cluster analysis: MAP, dispersion of MAP, dispersion of systemic vascular resistance, dispersion of arterial pulse pressure, and the maximum value of mixed venous saturation. Patients who underwent CPB procedures with large fluctuations in hemodynamic parameters particularly showed an increased risk for the development of postoperative neurologic complications.

Cerebral Emboli and Outcome

Two different types of cerebral emboli appear to occur during CPB and are composed of solid or gaseous matter, such as macroemboli (e.g., atherosclerotic debris) and microemboli (e.g., micro-gaseous bubbles, microparticulate matter). Overt and focal neurologic damage likely reflects the occurrence of cerebral macroemboli (e.g., calcific and atheromatous debris generated during valve tissue removal or instrumentation of an atheromatous aorta), whereas less focal neurologic dysfunction has been ascribed to cerebral microemboli. Microemboli appear to have some role in diffuse, subtle neurologic and cognitive disturbances, whereas macroemboli likely produce clinically apparent catastrophic strokes. Whatever the nature of the cerebral

> **BOX 29-4** *Clinical Strategies That May Decrease Neurologic Complications in Cardiac Surgery*
>
> - Early and aggressive control of hemodynamic instability
> - Perioperative glycemia < 200 mg/dL
> - Routine epiaortic scanning before manipulation of ascending aorta
> - Avoidance of manipulation of ascending aorta in severe atheromatosis
> - Maintenance of adequate cerebral perfusion pressure (neuromonitoring/cerebral oximetry?)
> - Full-dose aprotinin in high-risk patients (subject to regulatory agency guidelines & clinical availability)

> **BOX 29-5** *Strategies to Decrease Impact of CPB on Neurologic Complications*
>
> - Avoidance of reinfusion of unprocessed shed blood
> - Use of cell saver
> - Monitoring of cerebral venous pressure via a proximal central venous pressure catheter or the introducer port of a pulmonary artery catheter
> - Management of alpha-stat pH during moderate hypothermic CPB
> - Avoidance of arterial inflow temperature > 37°C
> - Use of CPB circuitry incorporating membrane oxygenator and 40-μm arterial line filter
> - Use of surface-modified and reduced-area CPB circuitry

insult, however, it seems that coexistent inflammatory processes can exacerbate the magnitude of injury.

Gaseous emboli are not innocuous. It has been demonstrated that the effects of air emboli on the cerebral vasculature not only are due to bubble entrapment with direct blockage of cerebral vessels but also represent the effects that such bubbles have on vascular endothelial cells.[14] Ultrastructural examinations of pial vessels exposed to cerebral air emboli demonstrated severe injury to endothelial plasmalemma, leading to loss of cellular integrity and endothelial cell swelling. Such endothelial damage produces disruptions of vasoreactivity. Air embolism also produces changes in blood elements, leading to formation of a proteinaceous capsule around the bubbles, marked dilation of pial vessels, platelet sequestration, and damage to endothelial cells. Air-induced mechanical trauma to the endothelium causes basement membrane disruption, thrombin production, release of P-selectin from intracellular vesicles, synthesis of platelet-activating factor, and a reperfusion-like injury with perturbations in inflammation and thrombotic processes. These phenomena likely impair nitric oxide production, giving rise to alterations in cerebral microvascular regulation.

CEREBROPROTECTIVE STRATEGIES

Cardiopulmonary Bypass Equipment

Early studies demonstrated increased microemboli in patients undergoing CPB using bubble oxygenators, with a reduction in cerebral embolization with the use of membrane oxygenators and arterial line filtration[15] (Boxes 29-4 and 29-5). It is apparent that emboli may be generated continuously during CPB and that equipment modification (e.g., arterial line microfiltration and preferential usage of membrane oxygenators) can decrease the generation of such emboli. Membrane oxygenators are

---

BOX 29-6 *Strategies to Improve Cardiopulmonary Bypass Influence on Outcome*

- Minimization of "blind" manipulation or clamping of the ascending aorta
- Avoidance of reinfusion of unprocessed shed blood (use of cell saver recommended)
- Monitoring of cerebral venous pressure via a proximal central venous pressure catheter or the introducer port of a pulmonary artery catheter
- Maintaining high cerebral perfusion pressure (> 60 mm Hg)
- Alpha-stat pH management
- Avoidance of arterial inflow temperature > 37°C
- Cardiopulmonary bypass circuitry incorporating membrane oxygenator and 40-μm arterial line filter
- Surface modified and reduced area cardiopulmonary bypass circuitry
- Perioperative blood glucose concentration below 200 mg/dL

---

currently recommended for CPB. It is equally evident that such equipment modifications, while decreasing the embolic load, cannot completely eliminate it.

In an attempt to decrease emboli originating from the surgical field, cell savers have been used for processing cardiotomy suction blood before returning it to the CPB circuit. Jewell and coworkers[16] reported on 20 patients prospectively randomized to either cell saver or cardiotomy suction and demonstrated that compared with cardiotomy suction, cell saver removed significantly more fat from shed blood, such that the percentage reduction in fat weight achieved by cell saver or cardiotomy suction was 87% compared with 45%.

Applied Neuromonitoring

Intraoperative neurophysiologic monitoring may be of benefit to decrease CNS injury.[17] Brain oximetry studies using noninvasive near-infrared spectrophotometry (NIRS) have shown promising results.

Intraoperative transcranial Doppler imaging has been demonstrated to detect embolic events in real time and allows modification of perfusion and surgical techniques. It has been shown that the numbers of emboli generated by perfusionist interventions (e.g., drug injection, blood return), as well as episodes of entrainment of air from the surgical field, are rapidly identified and corrected by transcranial Doppler detection of intraoperative emboli. Even during beating-heart procedures, compromised cerebral perfusion can occur relatively frequently, and, if unrecognized, may account for the relative lack of difference in CNS outcomes between CABG and off-pump CABG.[18] Combined EEG and cerebral oximetry identified episodes of cerebral ischemia in 15% of a series of 550 beating-heart patients; all were treated successfully by a combination of pharmacologically improved cardiac output, increased perfusion pressure, and cardiac repositioning.

Pharmacologic Cerebral Protection

In general, pharmacologic protection from cerebral ischemia remains an elusive goal. While results suggest that there is as yet no pharmacologic "magic bullet" that can be used to reduce neurologic injury in patients undergoing cardiac surgery, there is a combination of technical and pharmacologic measures currently available that might positively affect the outcome of these patients. In patients identified as being at risk for perioperative cerebral injury, preventive measures as outlined in Box 29-6 should

29

be instituted with organ-targeted management to guide the whole intraoperative and postoperative period. As the age and incidence of comorbid disease in the cardiac surgical population continue to rise, the importance of these issues becomes ever more acute because primary prevention continues to be the only effective measure to decrease cerebral injury in cardiac surgical patients.

SUMMARY

- Studies have shown an association between advanced age and a higher incidence of neurologic events in cardiac surgical patients.
- Neurologic events in cardiac surgical patients are associated with increased postoperative mortality, prolonged intensive care unit and hospital stay, decreased quality of life, and decreased long-term survival.
- Neurologic complications range from coma, stroke, and visual field deficits to impairments of cognitive processes (e.g., impaired memory and attention, mood alterations).
- Mechanisms for neurologic injury in cardiac surgery include some combination of cerebral embolism, hypoperfusion, and inflammation; associated vascular disease and altered cerebral autoregulation render the brain more susceptible to injury.
- Perioperative risk factors for neurologic complications include diabetes mellitus, hypertension, prior cerebrovascular disease, aortic atheromatosis, manipulation of ascending aorta, complex surgical procedures, bypass time longer than 2 hours, hemodynamic instability during and after bypass, hyperglycemia, hyperthermia, and hypoxemia.
- Routine epiaortic scanning before instrumentation of the ascending aorta is a sensitive and specific technique to detect nonpalpable aortic atheromatosis.
- In patients with significant ascending aorta atheromatosis, avoidance of aortic manipulation ("no-touch technique") can decrease perioperative stroke.
- Perioperative blood glucose concentration below 200 mg/dL may positively influence neurologic outcome.
- Strategies to decrease the impact of cardiopulmonary bypass on embolization, inflammation, and coagulation will decrease neurologic complications.

VI

REFERENCES

1. Ferguson TB Jr, Hammill BG, Peterson ED, et al: A decade of change: Risk profiles and outcomes for isolated coronary artery bypass grafting procedures, 1990-1999. A report from the STS National Database Committee and the Duke Clinical Research Institute. Society of Thoracic Surgeons. Ann Thorac Surg 73:480, 2002
2. Alexander KP, Anstrom KJ, Muhlbaier LH, et al: Outcomes of cardiac surgery in patients ≥ 80 years: Results from the National Cardiovascular Network. J Am Coll Cardiol 135:731, 2000
3. Blacker DJ, Flemming KD, Link MJ, Brown RD Jr: The preoperative cerebrovascular consultation: Common cerebrovascular questions before general or cardiac surgery. Mayo Clin Proc 79:223, 2004
4. Ahonen J, Salmenpera M: Brain injury after adult cardiac surgery. Acta Anaesthesiol Scand 48:4, 2004
5. Murkin JM, Newman SP, Stump DA, Blumenthal JA: Statement of consensus on assessment of neurobehavioral outcomes after cardiac surgery. Ann Thorac Surg 59:1289, 1995
6. Omar Y, Balacumaraswami L, Pigott DW, et al: Solid and gaseous cerebral microembolization during off-pump, on-pump, and open cardiac surgery procedures. J Thorac Cardiovasc Surg 127:1759, 2004
7. Yahia AM, Kirmani JF, Xavier AR, et al: Characteristics and predictors of aortic plaques in patients with transient ischemic attacks and strokes. J Neuroimaging 14:16, 2004
8. Djaiani G, Fedorko L, Borger M, et al: Mild to moderate atheromatous disease of the thoracic aorta and new ischemic brain lesions after conventional coronary artery bypass graft surgery. Stroke 35:e356, 2004
9. Konstadt SN, Reich DL, Kahn R, Viggiani RF: Transesophageal echocardiography can be used to screen for ascending aortic atherosclerosis. Anesth Analg 81:225, 1995

10. Knipp SC, Matatko N, Wilhelm H, et al: Evaluation of brain injury after coronary artery bypass grafting: A prospective study using neuropsychological assessment and diffusion-weighted magnetic resonance imaging. Eur J Cardiothorac Surg 25:791, 2004

11. Murkin JM: Inflammatory responses and CNS injury: Implications, prophylaxis, and treatment. Heart Surg Forum 6:193, 2003

12. Boyajian RA, Otis SM: Embolic stroke syndrome underlies encephalopathy and coma following cardiac surgery. Arch Neurol 60:291, 2003

13. Ganushchak YM, Fransen EJ, Visser C, et al: Neurological complications after coronary artery bypass grafting related to the performance of cardiopulmonary bypass. Chest 125:2196, 2004

14. Eckmann DM, Armstead SC, Mardini F: Surfactants reduce platelet-bubble and platelet-platelet binding induced by in vitro air embolism. Anesthesiology 103:1204, 2005

15. Haworth WS: The development of the modern oxygenator. Ann Thorac Surg 76:S2216, 2003

16. Jewell AE, Akowuah EF, Suvarna SK, et al: A prospective randomised comparison of cardiotomy suction and cell saver for recycling shed blood during cardiac surgery. Eur J Cardiothorac Surg 23:633, 2003

17. Murkin JM: Perioperative multimodality neuromonitoring: An overview. Semin Cardiothorac Vasc Anesth 8:167, 2004

18. van Dkijk D, Moons KG, Keizer AM, et al: Association between early and three month cognitive outcome after off-pump and on-pump coronary bypass surgery. Heart 90:431, 2004

29

Chapter 30

Long-Term Complications and Management

Dean T. Giacobbe, MD • Michael J. Murray, MD

Sedation in the Intensive Care Unit

Sedative Agents
Neuromuscular Blocking Agents

Infections in the Intensive Care Unit

Intravascular Device–Related Infections
Sternal Wound Infections
Prosthetic Valve Endocarditis
Systemic Inflammatory Response Syndrome
  and Sepsis

Hematology

Transfusion
Acute Renal Failure
Treatment and Renal Replacement Therapies

Electrolyte Abnormalities

Summary

References

In the modern era, the majority of cardiac surgical patients have brief stays in the intensive care unit (ICU) (<24 hours), and these stays follow a predictable pattern. During this time, most instability and morbidity are attributable to the cardiopulmonary organ systems, bleeding, hypothermia, and the emergence from anesthesia. A small minority of patients, however, have prolonged ICU stays characterized by multisystem complications involving both the cardiac and noncardiac systems. This group of patients consumes a disproportionate number of ICU resources, generates enormous hospital costs, and ultimately has a much worse prognosis (both in-hospital and long term).[1]

When caring for the unfortunate minority of cardiac surgical patients requiring prolonged stays in the ICU, a distinct shift in orientation of the health care providers must occur—from a "recovery room" mode, focusing primarily on the cardiovascular organ system, to a true intensive care mode, focusing on preventing and treating dysfunction in multiple organ systems. At the same time, the physician's decision to continue aggressive treatment must be tempered with a realistic view of the patient's prognosis and an assessment of the "cost" of that treatment to the patient, family, and society.

SEDATION IN THE INTENSIVE CARE UNIT

The major goals of sedation in the ICU are to provide anxiolysis and to improve the patient's perceptual experience during this physiologically and emotionally stressful period (Box 30-1). Secondarily, sedation reduces the physiologic stress response and attendant cardiovascular work, may facilitate the maintenance of circadian rhythms, and lessens delirium and agitation. These goals are distinct from those associated with analgesia, which are the alleviation of pain through nonpharmacologic and

BOX 30-1   *Sedation*

- Use specific agents targeted to therapeutic goals (e.g., sedatives for agitation; opioids for analgesia).
- Use goal-directed sedation therapy titrated to objective scoring system.
- Wean sedatives daily to assess the patient and reevaluate the need for sedation.

Table 30-1   **Range of Sedation and Agitation for 138 Patient Assessments**

Patient Category	Sedation-Agitation Scale (%)	Ramsey (%)	Harris A (%)
Agitated	62 (45)	67 (49)	74 (54)
Calm	36 (26)	30 (22)	23 (17)
Sedated	40 (29)	41 (30)	41 (30)

Reprinted with permission from Riker RR, Picard JT, Fraser GL: Prospective evaluation of the Sedation-Agitation Scale for adult critically ill patients. Crit Care Med 27:1325, 1999.

pharmacologic means and to facilitate diagnostic and therapeutic procedures. Although sedation and analgesia are separate therapeutic goals usually provided by individual drugs, there is often synergism between anxiolytic and analgesic drugs; and some newer agents provide elements of both analgesia and anxiolysis, thus blurring the distinction in clinical practice.

The Society of Critical Care Medicine (SCCM) published guidelines for sedation,[2] which emphasize the need for the goal-directed delivery of psychoactive medications. Goal-directed sedation is supported by an increasing body of literature that shows that daily interruption of sedation, intermittent sedation, and sedation protocols all reduce the duration of mechanical ventilation and in some instances decrease ICU length of stay.[3]

There are several scoring systems available to assess a patient's degree of sedation in the ICU and facilitate goal-directed therapy (Table 30-1). The Riker Sedation-Agitation Scale (SAS) was the first scale proved to be reliable and valid in critically ill adults. The SAS score is assigned by choosing a score from a seven-item scale that best matches a patient's behavior. Another scale, the Motor Activity Assessment Scale (MAAS), has seven categories to describe patients' behavior in response to stimulation. Like the SAS, it has been validated in critically ill adults. Most comparative clinical studies of sedation in critically ill patients have used the Ramsey scale. This scale is a six-point scale of motor activity that ranges from 1 ("patient anxious, agitated or restless, or both") to 6 ("no response to light glabellar tap or loud auditory stimulus") (Table 30-2). This scale was originally designed as a research tool but has been used for decades in clinical practice. Although no scientific consensus exists about which level of sedation using the Ramsey scale is optimal, recent literature frequently cites sedation goals of Ramsey 2 to 4, reflecting more realistic levels of sedation as part of goal-directed therapy. Other sedation scales that have been validated in critically ill adults include the Vancouver Interaction and Calmness Scale (VICS), the COMFORT Scale, and the Richmond Agitation-Sedation Scale (RASS). The SCCM's guidelines do not advocate one specific scoring system. Instead, they advocate defining a specific sedation goal or endpoint for each patient and then regularly assessing and documenting the patient's level of sedation in response to therapy.

30

Table 30-2   **The Ramsey Sedation Scale**

Awake levels	1 Patient anxious and agitated or restless or both
	2 Patient cooperative, oriented, and tranquil
	3 Patient responds to commands only
Asleep levels	4 Brisk response to a light glabellar tap or loud auditory stimulus
	5 Sluggish response to a light glabellar tap or loud auditory stimulus
	6 No response to a light glabellar tap or loud auditory stimulus

Reprinted with permission from Young C, Knudsen N, Hilton A, Reves JG: Sedation in the intensive care unit. Crit Care Med 28:854, 2000.

Sedative Agents

Benzodiazepines

Many drugs are available for sedating patients in the cardiothoracic ICU. The most frequently used agents for sedation include benzodiazepines (midazolam, lorazepam), propofol, and the α_2-agonist dexmedetomidine. While there are multiple medications that can be used to allay anxiety, the traditional approach has been to use benzodiazepines. These drugs act by binding to benzodiazepine receptors (subunits of the $GABA_A$ [γ-aminobutyric acid] receptors, in the limbic area of the brain). This binding enhances the effects of GABA in a dose-dependent fashion. Benzodiazepines can be titrated to effect, which can range from light sedation to coma. Side effects such as respiratory depression are also dose dependent and are more likely to appear in patients with comorbid conditions such as chronic obstructive pulmonary disease (COPD), in those at the extremes of age, and in patients receiving drugs with synergistic properties, such as opioids.

Midazolam is a short-acting benzodiazepine that can only be given parenterally. It is water soluble, its intravenous administration causes no pain or venous irritation (and therefore thrombosis), and its potency is two to four times that of diazepam. Midazolam is readily redistributed in tissues and is rapidly cleared by the liver and kidneys. It is enzymatically degraded in the liver to α-hydroxy-midazolam, which has minimal, if any, clinical sedative or hypnotic effects. The clinical effects of midazolam are short lived owing to an elimination half-life of 1.5 to 3.5 hours. These properties make midazolam ideal as an anxiolytic benzodiazepine for short-term use in the ICU. Depending on the situation, intermittent boluses of midazolam can be given or a continuous infusion of 0.5 to 5.0 mg/hr can be used. Higher doses may be required, and infusions of up to 20 mg/hr have been safely used in mechanically ventilated patients.

In patients whose condition deteriorates while in the ICU, such as the patient who develops sepsis or multiple organ dysfunction syndrome, midazolam elimination may be decreased and its clinical effect prolonged. This prolongation of effect may be due to the increased volume of distribution that occurs in patients with multiple organ dysfunction syndrome whose renal clearance is decreased.

Propofol

Propofol is an intravenous alkylphenol anesthetic agent that is chemically unrelated to other anesthetics. It has been used to provide sedation for patients in ICUs and is the preferred drug for "fast tracking" patients. Because it is so hydrophobic, it is formulated in a lipid emulsion (10% Intralipid), which must be taken into account when it is administered to patients. It is short-acting and rapidly redistributed and metabolized, making it very suitable for continuous infusion. Because of its rapid recovery and favorable side effect profile, it is an appealing drug not only to sedate patients but also for certain procedures, such as cardioversions, chest tube insertions or discontinuations, pleurodesis, and so on.

Several studies have shown that propofol, compared with midazolam, allows for more rapid weaning of patients from mechanical ventilation, and it is because of this property that it is more commonly used for "fast tracking" cardiac surgical patients.[4] When used for sedation, an initial dose of 0.5 to 1.0 mg/kg should be used, followed by an infusion of 25 to 50 μg/kg/min. Because of case reports of mortality in patients who receive excessively high doses of propofol, the maximum dose should probably be 100 μg/kg/min. This propofol infusion syndrome has been reported in patients who have received propofol for a very short period of time, indicating that this may be an idiosyncratic reaction.

Dexmedetomidine

Herr and colleagues conducted a multicenter trial comparing dexmedetomidine and propofol for sedation after coronary artery bypass grafting (CABG).[5] In their trial there was no significant difference in time to extubation between groups but the dexmedetomidine patients had significantly reduced use of supplemental analgesics, antiemetics, epinephrine, and diuretics.

Neuromuscular Blocking Agents

Occasionally, some patients are so critically ill that they cannot be adequately sedated to receive appropriate care. This most commonly happens in an agitated patient requiring mechanical ventilation in whom the level of sedation would mimic a general anesthetic and whose hemodynamic status does not tolerate this degree of deep sedation. In these circumstances, neuromuscular blocking agents (NMBAs) are used.

If these medications are used, it cannot be overemphasized that the patient must be adequately sedated before the initiation of the NMBA. Once an adequate degree of sedation (usually to include an analgesic medication such as an opioid) is achieved, the patient is administered a bolus and then a continuous infusion of an NMBA. Although there are several drugs available, the drugs most commonly used in the ICU are the aminosteroidal compounds (pancuronium, vecuronium, and rocuronium) and the benzylisoquinolinium compounds (doxacurium, atracurium, and cisatracurium). Pancuronium and doxacurium are long-acting NMBAs, whereas rocuronium and vecuronium are intermediate-duration medications and atracurium and cisatracurium are short-acting medications, at least when given by bolus. Because these drugs are infused continuously, this attribute is not as important, but it does become important when the medication is discontinued and the physician is assessing the return of the patient's neuromuscular function. When infusing these medications, a twitch monitor should be used and the physician should strive to achieve a train-of-four of one or two twitches.[6] If there are no twitches observed, then the patient may be overdosed and may be at risk for development of acute quadriplegic myopathy syndrome (AQMS), a situation that develops in patients receiving NMBAs in which, when the medication is discontinued, the patient remains flaccid for much longer than would be predicted simply based on pharmacokinetics of the medications that were infused. The etiology of this syndrome is unknown but is most likely secondary to the destruction of myosin by the NMBA or one of its metabolites. Often, it is difficult to differentiate between AQMS and critical illness polyneuropathy, but in the latter profound muscle necrosis as is seen with AQMS would not be expected to occur.

30

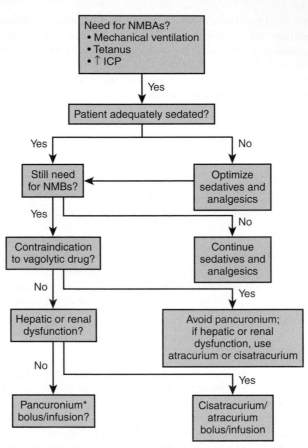

Figure 30-1   Use of neuromuscular blocking agents (NMBAs) in the intensive care unit. Monitor train-of-four ratio, protect eyes, position patient to protect pressure points, and address deep venous thrombosis prophylaxis. Reassess every 12 to 24 hours for continued NMBA indication. ICP=intracranial pressure. (Redrawn from Murray MJ, Cowen J, DeBlock H, et al: Clinical practice guidelines for sustained neuromuscular blockade in the adult critically ill patient. Crit Care Med 30:142, 2002.)

Another way to minimize the likelihood of this syndrome is to institute a daily drug holiday. Not only is this beneficial in decreasing the incidence of AQMS, but in patients receiving opioids and benzodiazepines the incidence of drug withdrawal also decreases with the discontinuation of the medication. When using NMBAs in the ICU, the algorithm as shown in Figure 30-1 is recommended.

INFECTIONS IN THE INTENSIVE CARE UNIT

Intravascular Device–Related Infections

Virtually all adult patients having cardiac surgery are monitored with invasive intravascular devices (IVDs), such as arterial, central venous, and pulmonary artery catheters. Unfortunately, these IVDs are frequently associated with bloodstream infections (BSIs). IVD-related BSIs are associated with an attributable mortality of 12% to 15%, prolonged hospitalization (mean of 7 days), and increased hospital cost of approximately $35,000.[7]

BOX 30-2 *Central Catheter Management*

- Central catheters should only be placed by practitioners with documented competency.
- Place under maximal sterile barrier precautions:
  - Chlorhexidine 2% is the skin preparation of choice.
  - Use chlorhexidine-impregnated sponge dressings.
  - Use antibiotic-impregnated catheters in high-risk patients.
- Do not "routinely" replace catheters.
- Remove as soon as clinically feasible.

Approximately 90% of all vascular catheter-related bloodstream infections (CRBSIs) occur with use of short-term central venous catheters (CVCs). CVCs that are present for a short term are most commonly colonized from the skin surrounding the insertion site. Organisms migrate along the external surface of the catheter and then the intercutaneous and subcutaneous segments, leading to colonization of the intravascular segment. Once colonized, it is difficult to eradicate organisms from the intravascular segment without catheter removal because the microbes adhere to and are covered by either a biofilm layer they produce or the thrombin layer the host forms on the device. Because the skin is the most common site of colonization, coagulase-negative staphylococci and *Staphylococcus aureus* from the host's skin and the hands of hospital personnel caring for the patient are the most common infecting pathogens. However, with long-term catheters, contamination of the catheter hub also contributes to intraluminal colonization.

Several factors have been associated with a risk of CVC-related bacteremia. These include site of insertion (femoral > internal jugular > subclavian), number of lumens (multiple > single), duration of catheter in situ, established infection elsewhere in body, bacteremia, and experience of personnel placing the catheter.

In an effort to reduce IVD-related BSIs, a Centers for Disease Control and Prevention advisory committee has formulated evidence-based guidelines pertaining to the prevention of IVD-related BSIs. These guidelines are summarized in Box 30-2.[8]

The diagnosis of central catheter infection can be challenging. The diagnosis should be suspected in patients with evidence of infection (e.g., fever, leukocytosis, positive blood cultures) when another source is not evident. Careful inspection of the catheter site is warranted, because exit site erythema or purulence strongly supports the diagnosis. If there are no visible signs of infection, then clinical suspicion and supporting data must be used to guide therapy. The most commonly used technique to culture CVCs is the semiquantitative roll-plate technique. With this technique, the most common threshold to define colonization is the growth of a colony count greater than 15.

The first clinical decision to make when managing a suspected CVC-related BSI is whether to remove the catheter. This decision is influenced by whether the risk of CVC-related BSI is low, intermediate, or high. Risk, in turn, is determined by the infecting organism and whether the CVC-related BSI is complicated or uncomplicated. Complicated infections are those associated with shock, persistence of positive blood cultures for longer than 48 hours after appropriate antibiotics, CVC-related BSIs associated with septic thrombosis, septic emboli, or deep-seated infections (e.g., endocarditis), or a tunnel or port-pocket infection (Fig. 30-2).

- A low-risk CVC-related BSI is caused by organisms of low virulence (e.g., coagulase-negative staphylococci) that are uncomplicated.
- A moderate-risk CVC-related BSI is characterized by uncomplicated infections with moderate to highly virulent organisms (*Staphylococcus aureus, Candida* species).
- A complicated CVC-related BSI is a high risk.

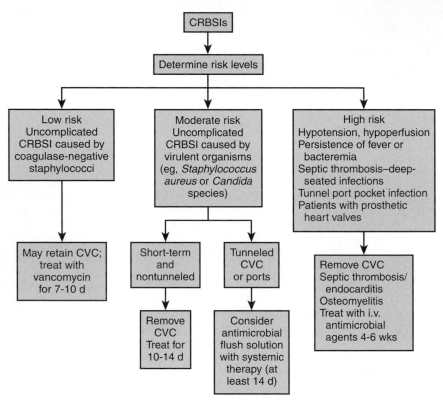

Figure 30-2 Algorithm for the management of catheter-related bloodstream infections (CRBSIs). A prelude to appropriate management involves confirming the diagnosis of a CRBSI through simultaneous blood cultures (5:1 of colony-forming units from blood cultures drawn through the catheter compared with the peripheral vein or differential time to positivity of 2 hours) or colonization of the catheter demonstrated through semiquantitative or quantitative catheter cultures with the same organism isolated from the peripheral blood culture. CVC = central venous catheter, i.v. = intravenous. (Redrawn from Raad II, Hanna HA: Intravascular catheter-related infections: New horizons and recent advances. Arch Intern Med 162:871, 2002. Copyright © 2002, American Medical Association. All rights reserved.)

Low-risk CVC-related BSIs can be treated without catheter removal. However, catheters should be removed in low-risk patients with prosthetic heart valves. In intermediate-risk patients, the catheters should be removed and the patients treated with a 10- to 14-day course of antibiotics. In high-risk patients, catheters should be removed and duration of antibiotic use based on the nature of the complication. In deep-seated infections such as septic thrombosis or endocarditis, antimicrobial agents should be administered for 4 to 6 weeks.[9]

Sternal Wound Infections

Deep and superficial surgical site infections are infrequent but morbid complications after cardiac surgery, with an incidence of 1% to 4% (Box 30-3). Deep sternal infections are defined as those infections involving muscle and fascial layers or any other organ spaces manipulated during the operation or organ involvement. They are associated with a 250% higher mortality than for matched individuals without infection, and postoperative wound infections double the length of hospitalization. A host of

BOX 30-3 *Latent Sources of Infection in the Cardiothoracic Intensive Care Unit*

- Intravascular device–related bloodstream infections
- Sternal wound infections
- Prosthetic valve endocarditis
- Sepsis
- Urinary tract infection
- *Clostridium difficile* enterocolitis
- Sinusitis

preoperative, intraoperative, and postoperative risk factors have been identified for chest wall infections[10]:

- *Host factors:* obesity, diabetes mellitus, hyperglycemia, use of internal mammary artery grafts (especially bilateral), advanced age, male gender, COPD, smoking, prolonged mechanical ventilation, corticosteroids, preoperative hospital stay longer than 5 days
- *Surgical factors:* duration of surgery and bypass, use of intra-aortic balloon pump, postoperative bleeding, reoperation, sternal rewiring, extensive electrocautery, shaving with razors, and use of bone wax
- *Postoperative factors:* postoperative bleeding, prolonged ventilation, chest reexploration, blood transfusion, and use of intra-aortic balloon pump

The diagnosis of sternal infections is based on wound tenderness, drainage, cellulitis, fever, leukocytosis, and sternal instability. *S. aureus* and coagulase-negative staphylococci account for approximately 50% of the organisms associated with post-CABG sternal wound infections. Several preventive strategies have been proposed to reduce cardiac surgical site infection rates. Martorell and colleagues reported a reduction in chest wall infections from greater than 8% to less than 2% after an intensive surveillance and intervention program that included nasal mupirocin and preoperative chlorhexidine showering. Other variables that are being investigated to reduce infection rates include perioperative antibiotics, adequacy of glycemic control, perioperative temperature control, and conservative transfusion protocols. The treatment of mediastinitis involves the prompt institution of antibiotics (empirically cover *Staphylococcus* species before culture results), débridement, open packing, and frequent dressing changes. On resolution, the chest is closed by primary closure or flap transposition in patients with large chest wall defects.

Prosthetic Valve Endocarditis

Prosthetic valve endocarditis (PVE), the infection of a prosthetic heart valve and/or the surrounding cardiac tissues, is a rare but serious source of infection in postoperative cardiac surgical patients.[11] The incidence of PVE is between 0.3% and 0.8% after valve replacement surgery. PVE cases can be clustered into two groups according to the time of infection. In early PVE (within 2 months of valve implantation), the valve and sewing ring have not yet endothelialized and hence microorganisms frequently invade the surrounding tissue planes, causing perivalvular abscess and perivalvular leak. In early PVE, the responsible microorganisms are nosocomial pathogens such as staphylococci, gram-negative bacilli, and *Candida* species that are introduced at the time of surgery or are hematogenously seeded in the immediate

30

postoperative period. The pathophysiology of late PVE probably resembles that of native valve endocarditis; that is, platelet-fibrin thrombi form on the valve leaflet and are then hematogenously seeded during episodes of transient bacteremia. In late PVE, the infecting organisms are usually streptococci, *S. aureus,* enterococci, and fastidious gram-negative organisms (the HACEK group). Infection appears to occur with equal frequency in both the mitral and aortic position and is exceedingly rare in tricuspid prosthesis (excluding intravenous drug abusers).

In the ICU, cases of early PVE present more dramatically than the often-subtle presentation of either native valve endocarditis or late PVE. The clinical signs that suggest PVE include new or changing murmurs, congestive heart failure, new ECG conduction disturbances, and systemic emboli. In fact, 40% of patients have clinically apparent central nervous system emboli. The diagnosis is confirmed by positive blood cultures and transesophageal echocardiography (TEE). If blood cultures are obtained before antibiotic therapy, more than 90% will be positive. TEE is the diagnostic imaging modality of choice because it has a sensitivity of 82% to 96% versus 17% to 36% with transthoracic echocardiography. TEE also allows the detection of abscesses, fistulas, and perivalvular leaks. The treatment of early PVE involves antibiotics directed at the cultured organism and prompt surgical intervention in cases of complicated PVE. In complicated PVE, survival is improved with both medical and surgical therapy versus with medical therapy alone.[12]

Systemic Inflammatory Response Syndrome and Sepsis

Sepsis is defined as the clinical syndrome that occurs as the result of an infection (or suspected infection) and an inflammatory response[13] (Table 30-3). Severe sepsis is sepsis that is associated with organ dysfunction, hypoperfusion, or hypotension. Septic shock is sepsis-induced hypotension and organ perfusion abnormalities that persist despite fluid resuscitation.

Sepsis is the leading cause for admission to surgical ICUs and, despite recent advances in therapy, remains the leading cause of mortality in ICUs.[14] The mortality rate increases across the inflammatory spectrum from SIRS to septic shock.

Because of the unacceptably high mortality rate associated with sepsis and the inflammatory disorders, an international group of experts in sepsis convened in 2003 and launched the "surviving sepsis campaign" with the goal of producing treatment recommendations that could be used to reduce the mortality from sepsis.[15] These recommendations were formulated from an evidence-based review of the medical literature and from expert opinion when high-level evidence was absent. They reflect the current "state of the art" in the management of critically ill, septic patients.

Initial Resuscitation (First 6 Hours)

Resuscitation should begin as soon as possible (do not delay for ICU admission). The goals of resuscitation should be the following:

- Central venous pressure 8 to 12 mm Hg (12 to 15 in mechanically ventilated patients, or if high abdominal pressure).
- Mean arterial pressure greater than 65 mm Hg.
- Urine output greater than 0.5 mL/kg/hr.
- Central venous or mixed venous oxygen saturation greater than 70%.
- If unable to increase central venous/mixed venous saturation above 70%, then transfuse to hematocrit greater than 30% and/or administer dobutamine (to maximum dose of 20 µg/kg/min) to achieve this goal.

Table 30-3   Diagnostic Criteria for Sepsis

Infection,* documented or suspected, and some of the following†:
General variables
    Fever (core temperature > 38.3°C)
    Hypothermia (core temperature < 36°C)
    Heart rate > 90 beats per minute or > 2 SDs above the normal value for age
    Tachypnea
    Altered mental status
    Significant edema or positive fluid balance (>20 mL/kg over 24 hr)
    Hyperglycemia (plasma glucose > 120 mg/dL or 7.7 mmol/L) in the absence of diabetes
Inflammatory variables
    Leukocytosis (WBC count > 12,000/μL)
    Leukopenia (WBC count < 4,000/μL)
    Normal WBC count with > 10% immature forms
    Plasma C-reactive protein > 2 SDs above the normal value
    Plasma procalcitonin > 2 SDs above the normal value
Hemodynamic variables
    Arterial hypotension† (SBP < 90 mm Hg, MAP < 70, or an SBP decrease > 40 mm Hg in
    adults or < 2 SDs below normal for age)
    $S\bar{v}o_2 > 70\%$†
    Cardiac index > 3.5 L/min/m^2
Organ dysfunction variables
    Arterial hypoxemia ($Pao_2/Fio_2 < 300$)
    Acute oliguria (urine output < 0.5 mL/kg/hr)
    Creatinine increase > 0.5 mg/dL
    Coagulation abnormalities (INR > 1.5 or aPTT > 60 sec)
    Ileus (absent bowel sounds)
    Thrombocytopenia (platelet count < 100,000/μL)
    Hyperbilirubinemia (plasma total bilirubin > 4 mg/dL or 70 mmol/L)
Tissue perfusion variables
    Hyperlactatemia (> 1 mmol/L)
    Decreased capillary refill or mottling

---

*Infection defined as a pathologic process induced by a microorganism.
† $S\bar{v}o_2 > 70\%$ is normal in children (normal, 75% to 80%), and CI 3.5 to 5.5 is normal in children.
WBC = white blood cell; SBP = systolic blood pressure; MAP = mean arterial blood pressure;
$S\bar{v}o_2$ = mixed venous oxygen saturation; INR = international normalized ratio; aPTT = activated
partial thromboplastin time.
    Reprinted with permission from Levy MM, Fink MP, Marshall JC, et al: 2001 SCCM/ESICM/ACCP/
ATS/SIS International Sepsis Definitions Conference. Crit Care Med 31:1250, 2001.

30

Diagnosis

- Appropriate cultures should always be obtained before initiating antibiotics.
- Obtain at least two blood cultures—one from the periphery and one from each vascular access device.
- Culture other sites as clinically indicated (cerebrospinal fluid, wounds, urine, respiratory secretions, other body fluids).
- Diagnostic and imaging studies should be performed promptly to identify the source of infection.

Antibiotic Therapy

- Intravenous antibiotic therapy should be started within the first hour of recognition of severe sepsis (after cultures).
- Empirical therapy with antibiotics should include one with activity against the most likely pathogen and that can penetrate the likely source.

- Empirical antibiotics should be broad spectrum until the causative organism is identified.
- The antibiotic regimen should be reassessed after 48 to 72 hours on the basis of clinical and microbiological data. The goal is to use a narrow-spectrum antibiotic to limit toxicity, cost, and development of superinfection and microbial resistance.
- Once the causative organism is identified, use monotherapy for 7 to 10 days (some experts prefer combination therapy for *Pseudomonas* infections).
- Most experts use combination therapy for neutropenic patients and treat for the duration of neutropenia.

Source Control

- Every patient should be evaluated for the presence of a focus of infection that is amenable to source control measures (e.g., drainage of abscess, removal of infected vascular access device).
- Risks versus benefits of source control procedures must be weighed. Source control with the least physiologic insult is generally best (e.g., percutaneous rather than surgical drainage of abscess).
- Source control measures should be instituted as soon as possible after initial resuscitation.

Fluid Therapy

- Use a fluid challenge with crystalloids or colloids in cases of suspected hypovolemia.
- Repeat boluses based on response (increase in blood pressure and urine output) and tolerance (evidence of intravascular volume overload).
- There is no evidence to support a preference for crystalloid or colloid.

Vasopressors

- After fluid resuscitation a vasopressor should be started to restore blood pressure.
- In life-threatening hypotension, a vasopressor and fluid resuscitation may need to be simultaneously started.
- Dopamine and norepinephrine are the vasopressors of choice.
- All patients requiring vasopressors should be monitored with an arterial catheter.
- Vasopressin may be considered in hypotension refractory to conventional vasopressors.

Inotropic Therapy

- In patients with low cardiac output despite fluid resuscitation, dobutamine is the agent of choice to increase cardiac output.
- A vasopressor can be added to raise blood pressure, once cardiac output is normalized.

Corticosteroids

- Intravenous corticosteroids (hydrocortisone, 200 to 300 mg/day for 7 days in three or four divided doses or by continuous infusion) can be used for patients with septic shock who require vasopressor therapy despite adequate fluid resuscitation.
- Some experts recommend using a 250-µg adrenocorticotropic hormone (ACTH) stimulation test to identify responders (>9 µg/dL increase in cortisol after 30 to 60 minutes) and recommend only treating nonresponders.
- Dose should not exceed 300 mg of hydrocortisone daily.
- Some experts add 50 µg of fludrocortisone orally (this is controversial because hydrocortisone has mineralocorticoid activity).

- There is no evidence to recommend fixed-duration therapy over taper or clinically guided regimen.

Recombinant Human Activated Protein C (rhAPC)

- rhAPC is recommended in patients with high risk of death (APACHE II score > 25, sepsis-induced multiple organ dysfunction syndrome, septic shock, or sepsis-induced ARDS) without any contraindications.
- Contraindications include active internal bleeding, recent (within 3 months) hemorrhagic stroke, recent (within 2 months) intracranial or intraspinal surgery or severe head trauma, trauma with increased risk of life-threatening bleeding, presence of epidural catheter, intracranial neoplasm, mass lesion, or cerebral herniation.

Blood Product Administration

- Once tissue hypoperfusion has resolved, red blood cell transfusion should only occur when hemoglobin decreases to less than 7.0 g/dL and to target a hemoglobin value of 7.0 to 9.0 g/dL.
- Erythropoietin is not recommended to treat anemia of sepsis (may use if other coexisting conditions merit treatment with erythropoietin, e.g., renal failure).
- Fresh frozen plasma should not be administered to correct laboratory abnormalities in the absence of bleeding or planned invasive procedures.
- Antithrombin administration is not recommended to treat severe sepsis or septic shock.
- Platelet transfusion: Administer if counts are less than 5000/mm^3; consider when counts are 5000 to 30,000/mm^3 and there is significant risk of bleeding; counts greater than 50,000/mm^3 are typically required for surgery or invasive procedures.

Mechanical Ventilation of Sepsis-Induced Acute Lung Injury/ARDS

- Use low tidal volumes (6 mL/kg) with goal of plateau pressure less than 30 cm H_2O.
- Permissive hypercapnia is tolerated to minimize plateau pressures and tidal volumes.
- A minimum amount of positive end-expiratory pressure (PEEP) should be set to minimize lung collapse at end-expiration.
- Prone positioning may be considered in patients requiring potentially injurious levels of plateau pressure or F_{IO_2} who are not at high risk for adverse consequences of prone positioning.
- Unless contraindicated, mechanically ventilated patients should be maintained with the head of the bed raised to 45 degrees to prevent the development of ventilator-associated pneumonia.
- A weaning protocol should be in place.
- When stable, patients should undergo daily, spontaneous-breathing trials (T-piece or 5 cm H_2O continuous positive airway pressure [CPAP]).
- If spontaneous breathing trials are successful, consideration should be given to extubation.

Sedation, Analgesia, and Neuromuscular Blockade

- Sedation protocols should be used that include the use of a sedation goal, measured by a standardized subjective sedation scale.
- Use either continuous infusion or intermittent bolus to achieve predetermined endpoints.
- Sedation should be interrupted/lightened daily to evaluate patients.
- Neuromuscular blocking agents should be avoided if possible. When used, train-of-four monitoring of depth of blockade should be used.

30

Glucose Control

- Maintain blood glucose levels less than 150 mg/dL with the use of insulin infusion.
- Blood glucose should be monitored every 30 minutes initially and then regularly (every 4 hours) once glucose concentration has stabilized.
- Glycemic control should include the use of a nutrition protocol that favors enteral feeding.

Renal Replacement

- In acute renal failure (ARF), continuous venovenous hemofiltration and intermittent hemodialysis are equivalent.
- Venovenous hemofiltration may be tolerated better in hemodynamically unstable patients.
- There is no evidence to support hemofiltration in sepsis independent of renal replacement needs.

Bicarbonate Therapy

- There is no evidence to support the use of bicarbonate therapy for treatment of hypoperfusion-induced lactic acidemia.

Deep Vein Thrombosis Prophylaxis

- Severe sepsis patients should receive deep vein thrombosis (DVT) prophylaxis with low-dose unfractionated heparin or low-molecular-weight heparin.
- Mechanical prophylaxis should be used in patients with contraindications to heparin.
- In extremely high-risk patients (history of DVT), a combination of pharmacologic and mechanical therapy is recommended.

Stress Ulcer Prophylaxis

- All septic patients should receive stress ulcer prophylaxis.
- H_2-receptor antagonists are more efficacious than sucralfate.
- No studies have directly compared the use of proton-pump inhibitors with H_2-receptor antagonists, so their efficacy is unknown.

Consideration of Limitation of Support

- Advanced care planning, including the communication of likely outcomes and realistic treatment goals, should be discussed with patients and their families.
- Less aggressive therapy and withdrawal of therapy may be in the patient's best interest.

HEMATOLOGY

Transfusion

Blood products are frequently transfused into critically ill patients. In a general ICU population, patients receive an average of 0.2 U/day, and this incidence is increased to 1.3 U/day in cardiothoracic ICUs.[16] Whereas transfusion is often necessary to either improve oxygen delivery or restore the coagulation system there is a growing body of literature that suggests that transfusion carries substantial risk for postoperative cardiac surgical patients.

Several large studies have identified transfusion as increasing the risk of infection after cardiac surgery (Box 30-4). In fact, in 17 of 19 retrospective studies that were reviewed, transfusion was found to be a significant factor and frequently the best predictor of postoperative infection. Transfusion has been cited as a risk factor for

BOX 30-4 *Transfusion Strategy in Cardiothoracic Intensive Care Unit*

- Transfusion is associated with increased morbidity and mortality.
- During first 24 to 48 hours, transfuse to target oxygen delivery and resolution of coagulopathy/bleeding.
- Long-term ICU patients have lower morbidity and mortality when a conservative transfusion strategy is used.

mediastinitis, early bacteremia, pneumonia, increased mortality rate, and length of stay after cardiac surgery. A randomized, controlled trial identified nosocomial pneumonia as the most frequent infection after cardiac surgery and that it only occurred in patients transfused more than 4 units of blood components.

In 1999, Hebert and colleagues[17] published a landmark study that has fundamentally altered the approach to transfusion in critically ill patients. Their large, multicenter, randomized, prospective trial of 838 patients admitted to Canadian ICUs found no difference in 30-day mortality between patients assigned to a liberal (hemoglobin: 10 to 12 g/dL) and conservative red blood cell transfusion protocol (hemoglobin: 7 to 9 g/dL). In fact, mortality was lower in less ill patients (APACHE II score ≤ 20) and in younger patients (≤55 years of age). Also, the restrictive strategy resulted in a 54% reduction in red blood cell transfusions. Prior to this study, red blood cell transfusion had been extensively investigated as a component of the now dated paradigm that supranormal oxygen delivery was associated with increased survival in critically ill patients. Hebert and colleagues' study showed not only that a conservative strategy was associated with no increase in mortality but also that it halved the number of transfused units with its attendant decrease in infectious risk, immunomodulation, and cost.

Acute Renal Failure

Acute renal failure (ARF), like many of the clinical syndromes frequently encountered in the ICU, has been difficult to precisely define.[18] If it is agreed that the principal functions of the kidney are to create urine and excrete water-soluble waste products of metabolism, then ARF is the sudden loss of these functions.

Renal solute excretion is a function of glomerular filtration. Glomerular filtration rate (GFR) is a convenient and time-honored way of quantifying renal function. It must be appreciated, however, that GFR varies considerably under normal circumstances as a function of protein intake. A normal GFR for men is 120 ± 25 mL/min, and it is 95 ± 20 mL/min for women. Creatinine is the most frequently used surrogate of GFR and hence solute excretion. When measured in the *steady state* and analyzed in the context of age, gender, and race, it loosely reflects renal function.

Creatinine is much less accurate in estimating renal function in non–steady-state conditions (e.g., ARF in the critically ill). Creatinine is formed from nonenzymatic dehydration of creatine (98% muscular in origin) in the liver. Because critical illness affects liver function, muscle mass, tubular excretion of creatinine, and the volume of distribution of creatinine, its limitations as a useful marker of renal function become apparent. Nonetheless, changes in serum creatinine and the rate of change in creatinine remain the most convenient and frequently used surrogates of renal dysfunction.

Urine output is the other frequently measured parameter of renal function in the ICU. Oliguria is defined by a urine output of less than 0.3 mL/kg/hr. Under a wide range of normal physiologic conditions, urine output primarily reflects changes in renal hemodynamics and volume status rather than representing renal parenchymal function and reserve. Hence, it is very nonspecific for renal dysfunction unless urine output is severely reduced or absent. And, while oliguric renal failure has a higher mortality rate than nonoliguric renal failure, no data demonstrate that the pharmacologic creation of urine in patients with renal failure reduces mortality. The pathogenesis of ARF after cardiac surgery is thought to primarily result from hypoperfusion and ischemia. Other contributing factors include nephrotoxins, nonpulsatile flow during cardiopulmonary bypass, and aortic emboli. The two most important determinants of ARF after cardiopulmonary bypass are preexisting renal insufficiency and postoperative low cardiac output states.

Several strategies for preventing perioperative renal failure have been evaluated in cardiac surgical patients. "Renal dose" dopamine has been shown to have no effect on either renal function or mortality after both cardiac and vascular surgery.[19] Similarly, the diuretics furosemide and mannitol have demonstrated no renal-protective effects.

Treatment and Renal Replacement Therapies

Just as the diagnosis and prevention of ARF remain enigmatic, so, too, does the treatment of ARF. In the critically ill patient developing ARF, the initial treatment strategy is to create an optimal "environment" for the kidney to heal, that is, to maximize oxygen delivery to the renal parenchyma via the manipulation of hemodynamics and volume status, while simultaneously avoiding nephrotoxins (e.g., contrast, aminoglycosides) and ensuring no postrenal obstruction exists. If provided this optimization and the kidney does not recover, the clinician must provide renal replacement therapy (RRT).

Many of the classic indications for RRT are noncontroversial and include the following[20]:

- Uremic symptoms (anorexia, nausea, vomiting).
- Uremic signs (uremic pericarditis, bleeding, encephalopathy)
- Hyperkalemia refractory to medical therapy
- Volume overload unresponsive to restriction and diuretics
- Metabolic acidosis
- Dialyzable intoxications (e.g., lithium, toxic alcohols, salicylate)
- Some cases of hypocalcemia/hypercalcemia, hyperphosphatemia

Once the decision to initiate RRT has been made, the mode of replacement must be chosen. In broad terms, RRT can be divided into intermittent hemodialysis or continuous RRT. The latter comes in a wide variety of forms, each associated with its own unique acronym (e.g., slow continuous ultrafiltration [SCUF], slow low-efficiency daily dialysis [SLEDD], continuous venovenous hemofiltration [CVVH], continuous venovenous hemofiltration-dialysis [CVVH-D]). The differences between these different forms of continuous RRT lie in the membrane used, the mechanism of solute transport, the presence or absence of a dialysis solution and the type of vascular access. In the United States, the majority of patients with ARF are treated with hemodialysis but the trend is toward the increased use of continuous RRT, whereas in other countries continuous RRT predominates. At present there are no studies supporting the use of one modality over another, but most intensivists prefer continuous RRT in hemodynamically unstable patients or in whom the hypotension associated with hemodialysis would be adverse. A trial of weaning of continuous RRT should be considered when the following criteria have been met:

- Criteria to initiate have resolved.
- Urine output averages 1 mL/kg/hr over 24 hours.
- Fluid balance can be maintained with present urine output.
- Complications of continuous RRT outweigh benefits.

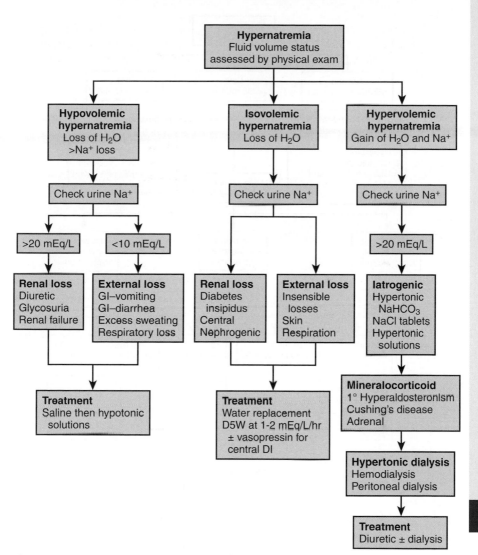

Figure 30-3 Assessment and treatment of hypernatremia. GI = gastrointestinal; D5W = 5% dextrose in water; DI = diabetes insipidus. (Modified from Torres N: Electrolyte abnormalities: Sodium. In Faust RJ [ed]: Anesthesiology Review, 2nd ed. New York, Churchill Livingstone, 1994, p 34; with permission of Mayo Foundation.)

ELECTROLYTE ABNORMALITIES

Fluid and electrolyte abnormalities are common after cardiac surgery. Diagnosis and treatment algorithms are shown in Figures 30-3 and 30-4 for hypernatremia and hyponatremia, Figure 30-5 and Table 30-4 for hyperkalemia, Figure 30-6 for hypokalemia, and Table 30-5 for hypercalcemia. Hypomagnesemia is common; and the underlying cause should be identified, if possible, and then treated with an intravenous infusion of 0.1 to 0.2 mEq/kg/day or via the oral route at 0.4 mEq/kg/day. Close monitoring is necessary with treatment of any electrolyte disorder.

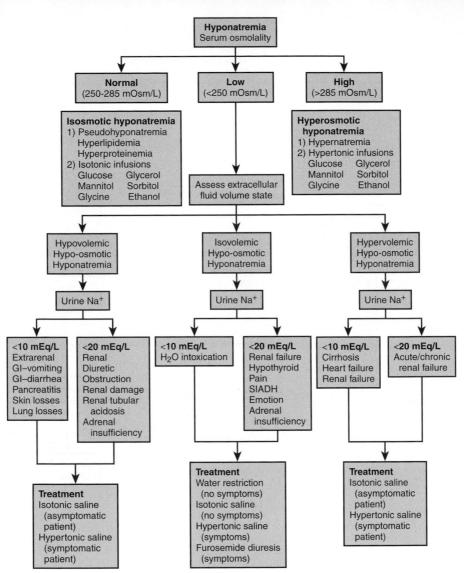

Figure 30-4 Assessment and treatment of hyponatremia. GI = gastrointestinal; SIADH = syndrome of inappropriate antidiuretic hormone. (Modified from Torres N: Electrolyte abnormalities: Sodium. In Faust RJ [ed]: Anesthesiology Review, 2nd ed. New York, Churchill Livingstone, 1994, p 35; with permission of Mayo Foundation.)

Table 30-4 Treatment of Hyperkalemia

Treatment	Dose	Mechanism	Onset	Duration
Calcium chloride	7 to 14 mg/kg	Direct antagonism	Instantly	15 to 30 min
Sodium bicarbonate	0.7 to 1.4 mEq/kg	Direct antagonism Redistribution	15 to 30 min	3 to 6 hr
Glucose + insulin	25 g + 10 to 15 units	Redistribution	15 to 30 min	3 to 6 hr
Kayexalate	30 g PO/PR	Elimination of K^+	1 to 3 hr	
Peritoneal dialysis		Elimination of K^+	1 to 3 hr	
Hemodialysis		Elimination of K^+	Rapid	

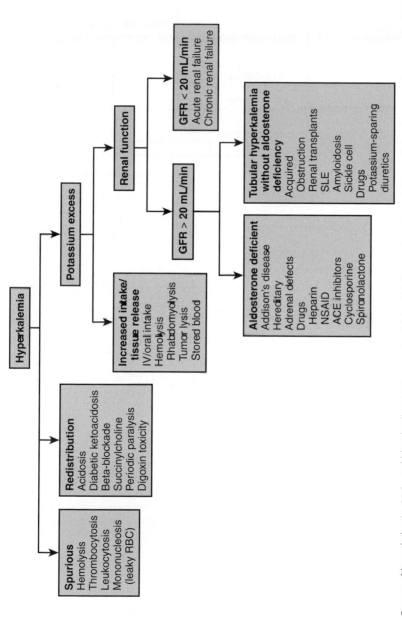

Figure 30-5   Causes of hyperkalemia. RBC = red blood cell; NSAID = nonsteroidal anti-inflammatory drug; ACE = angiotensin-converting enzyme; SLE = systemic lupus erythematosus. (Modified from Torres N: Electrolyte abnormalities: Sodium. In Faust RJ [ed]: Anesthesiology Review, 2nd ed. New York, Churchill Livingstone, 1994, p 37; with permission of Mayo Foundation.)

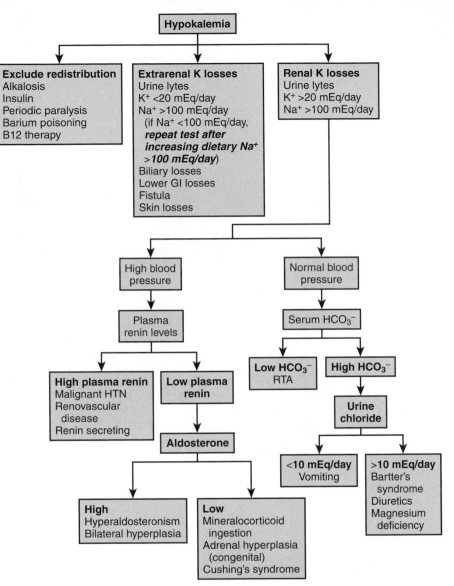

Figure 30-6 Algorithmic approach to hypokalemia. GI = gastrointestinal; HTN = hypertension; RTA = renal tubular acidosis. (Modified from Torres N: Electrolyte abnormalities: Sodium. In Faust RJ [ed]: Anesthesiology Review, 2nd ed. New York, Churchill Livingstone, 1994, p 38; with permission of Mayo Foundation.)

Table 30-5 Features of Hypercalcemia and Its Treatment

Calcium Level (mg/dL)	>13.0 <11.5	Symptoms: anorexia, nausea, vomiting, lethargy, dehydration, coma, death Asymptomatic			
Treatment	Onset of Action	Duration of Action	% Normalization	Advantages	Disadvantages
Saline (200 to 500 mL/hr) (increases urine calcium and excretion)	Hours	During infusion	0 to 10	Rehydration	Cardiac failure, electrolyte changes, hypokalemia, hypomagnesemia, intensive monitoring
Saline + loop diuretics (furosemide 40 to 80 mg every 2 hr)	Hours	During treatment (saline infusion rate = urine flow rate)	0 to 10	Enhanced calcium elimination	As above
Zoledronate (most potent bisphosphonate available, administer 4 mg IV over 15 min)	1 to 2 days	32 to 39 days	60 to 80	Potency efficacy	Increase phosphate, 3-day infusion
Calcitonin (4 units/kg SQ or IM every 12 hr) (inhibits osteoclasts and stimulates calciuresis)	Hours	2 to 3 days	10 to 20 rapid onset	Nontoxic	Only decrease calcium by 2 to 3 mg/dL, tachyphylaxis
Gallium nitrate (200 mg/m²/day in 1 L normal saline over 5 days)	2 to 3 days	10 to 14 days	70 to 80	Potent	Long infusion time, cannot use in renal failure

IM = intramuscular; IV = intravenous; SQ = subcutaneous.

30

SUMMARY

- Cardiac surgical patients usually follow a fairly predictable postoperative course that involves physiologic derangements and treatments that are routine for cardiac anesthesiologists.
- A small percentage of cardiac surgical patients have complicated postoperative courses and prolonged intensive care unit stays.
- This small subset of patients dies primarily of noncardiac organ dysfunction.
- The anesthesiologist/intensivist caring for this complex patient population must consider all organ systems when considering diagnosis and treatment.
- Meticulous attention to detail and the application of recent evidence-based treatments will result in improved survival in this complicated group of patients.

REFERENCES

1. Williams MR, Wellner RB, Hartnett EA, et al: Long-term survival and quality of life in cardiac surgical patients with prolonged intensive care unit length of stay. Ann Thorac Surg 73:1472, 2002
2. Nasraway SA, Jacobi J, Murray MJ, Lumb PD: Sedation, analgesia, and neuromuscular blockade of the critically ill adult: Revised clinical practice guidelines for 2002. Crit Care Med 30:117, 2002
3. Kress JP, Pohlman AS, O'Conner MF, Hall JB: Daily interruption of sedative infusions in critically ill patients undergoing mechanical ventilation. N Engl J Med 342:1471, 2000
4. Myles PS, Buckland MR, Weeks AM, et al: Hemodynamic effects, myocardial ischemia, and timing of tracheal extubation with propofol-based anesthesia for cardiac surgery. Anesth Analg 84:12, 1997
5. Herr DL, Sum-Ping ST, England M: ICU sedation after coronary artery bypass graft surgery: Dexmedetomidine-based versus propofol-based sedation regimens. J Cardiothorac Vasc Anesth 17:576, 2003
6. Murray MJ, Cowen J, DeBlock H, et al: Clinical practice guidelines for sustained neuromuscular blockade in the adult critically ill patient. Crit Care Med 30:142. 2002
7. Alberti C, Brun-Buisson C, Burchardi H, et al: Epidemiology of sepsis and infection in ICU patients from an international multicentre cohort study. Intensive Care Med 28:108, 2002
8. Garland JS, Henrickson K, Maki DG: The 2002 Hospital Infection Control Practices Advisory Committee Centers for Disease Control and Prevention Guideline for Prevention of Intravascular Device-Related Infection. Pediatrics 110:1009, 2002
9. Raad II, Hanna HA: Intravascular catheter-related infections. New horizons and recent advances. Arch Intern Med 162:871, 2002
10. Hollenbeak CS, Murphy DM, Koenig S, et al: The clinical and economic impact of deep chest surgical site infections following coronary artery bypass graft surgery. Chest 118:397, 2000
11. Edwards MB, Ratnatunga CP, Dore CJ, Taylor KM: Thirty-day mortality and long-term survival following surgery for prosthetic endocarditis: A study from the UK heart valve registry. Eur J Cardiothorac Surg 14:156, 1998
12. Gordon SM, Serkey JM, Longworth DL, et al: Early onset prosthetic valve endocarditis: The Cleveland Clinic experience 1992-1997. Ann Thorac Surg 69:1388, 2000
13. Levy MM, Fink MP, Marshall JC, et al: 2001 SCCM/ESICM/ACCP/ATS/SIS International Sepsis Definitions Conference. Crit Care Med 31:1250, 2003
14. Hotchkiss RS, Karl IE: The pathophysiology and treatment of sepsis. N Engl J Med 348:138, 2003
15. Dellinger RP, Carlet JM, Masur H, et al: Surviving sepsis campaign guidelines for the management of severe sepsis and septic shock. Crit Care Med 32:858, 2004
16. Leal-Noval SR, Rincón-Ferrari MD, García-Curiel A, et al: Transfusion of blood components and postoperative infection in patients undergoing cardiac surgery. Chest 119:1461, 2001
17. Hebert PC, Wells G, Blajchman MA, et al: A multicenter, randomized, controlled clinical trial of transfusion requirements in critical care. Transfusion Requirements in Critical Care Investigators: Canadian Critical Care Trials Group. N Engl J Med 340:409, 1999
18. Bellomo R, Kellum JA, Ronco C: Defining acute renal failure: Physiologic principles. Intensive Care Med 30:33, 2004
19. Lassnigg A, Donner E, Grubhofer G, et al: Lack of renoprotective effects of dopamine and furosemide during cardiac surgery. J Am Soc Nephrol 11:97, 2000
20. Bellomo R, Ronco C: Continuous renal replacement therapy in the intensive care unit. Intensive Care Med 25:781, 1999

Chapter 31

Pain Management for the Postoperative Cardiac Patient

Mark A. Chaney, MD

Adequate postoperative analgesia prevents unnecessary patient discomfort, may decrease morbidity, may decrease postoperative hospital length of stay, and thus may decrease cost. Because postoperative pain management has been deemed important, the American Society of Anesthesiologists has published practice guidelines regarding this topic.[1] Furthermore, in recognition of the need for improved pain management, the Joint Commission on Accreditation of Healthcare Organizations has developed new standards for the assessment and management of pain in accredited hospitals and other health care settings.[2] Patient satisfaction (no doubt linked to adequacy of postoperative analgesia) has become an essential element that influences clinical activity of not only anesthesiologists but also all health care professionals.

Achieving optimal pain relief after cardiac surgery is often difficult. Pain may be associated with many interventions, including sternotomy, thoracotomy, leg vein harvesting, pericardiotomy, and/or chest tube insertion, among others. Inadequate analgesia and/or an uninhibited stress response during the postoperative period may increase morbidity by causing adverse hemodynamic, metabolic, immunologic, and hemostatic alterations. Aggressive control of postoperative pain, associated with an attenuated stress response, may decrease morbidity and mortality in high-risk patients after noncardiac surgery and may also decrease morbidity and mortality in patients after cardiac surgery. Adequate postoperative analgesia may be attained via a wide variety of techniques (Table 31-1). Traditionally, analgesia after cardiac surgery has been obtained with intravenous opioids (specifically morphine). However, intravenous opioid use is associated with definite detrimental side effects (nausea/vomiting, pruritus, urinary retention, respiratory depression), and longer-acting opioids such as morphine may delay tracheal extubation during the immediate postoperative period

Table 31-1   Techniques Available for Postoperative Analgesia

Local anesthetic infiltration
Nerve blocks
Opioids
Nonsteroidal anti-inflammatory agents
α-Adrenergic agents
Intrathecal techniques
Epidural techniques
Multimodal analgesia

BOX 31-1   *Pain and Cardiac Surgery*

- Originates from many sources
- Most commonly originates from chest wall
- Preoperative expectations influence postoperative satisfaction
- Quality of postoperative analgesia may influence morbidity/mortality

---

BOX 31-2   *Potential Clinical Benefits of Adequate Postoperative Analgesia*

- Hemodynamic stability
- Metabolic stability
- Immunologic stability
- Hemostatic stability
- Stress response attenuation
- Decreased morbidity/mortality

---

via excessive sedation and/or respiratory depression. Thus, in the current era of early extubation ("fast-tracking"), cardiac anesthesiologists are exploring unique options other than traditional intravenous opioids for control of postoperative pain in patients after cardiac surgery.[3] No single technique is clearly superior; each possesses distinct advantages and disadvantages. It is becoming increasingly clear that a multimodal approach/combined analgesic regimen (utilizing a variety of techniques) is likely the best way to approach postoperative pain (in all patients after surgery) to maximize analgesia and minimize side effects. When addressing postoperative analgesia in cardiac surgical patients, choice of technique (or techniques) is made only after a thorough analysis of the risk/benefit ratio of each technique in the specific patient in whom analgesia is desired.

PAIN AND CARDIAC SURGERY

Surgical or traumatic injury initiates changes in the peripheral and central nervous systems that must be addressed therapeutically to promote postoperative analgesia and, it is hoped, positively influence clinical outcome (Boxes 31-1 and 31-2). The physical processes of incision, traction, and cutting of tissues stimulate free nerve endings and a wide variety of specific nociceptors. Receptor activation and activity are further modified by the local release of chemical mediators of inflammation and sympathetic amines released via the perioperative surgical stress response. The perioperative surgical stress response peaks during the immediate postoperative period and exerts major effects on many physiologic processes. The potential clinical benefits of attenuating the perioperative surgical stress response (above and beyond simply attaining adequate clinical analgesia) have received much attention during the past decade and remain fairly controversial. However, it is clear that inadequate postoperative analgesia and/or an uninhibited perioperative surgical stress response has the potential to initiate pathophysiologic changes in all major organ systems, including the cardiovascular, pulmonary, gastrointestinal, renal, endocrine, immunologic, and/or central nervous systems, all of which may lead to substantial postoperative morbidity.

Pain after cardiac surgery may be intense and originates from many sources, including the incision (e.g., sternotomy, thoracotomy), intraoperative tissue retraction and dissection, vascular cannulation sites, vein-harvesting sites, and chest tubes, among others. Patients in whom an internal mammary artery is surgically exposed and used as a bypass graft may have substantially more postoperative pain.

Persistent pain after cardiac surgery, although rare, can be problematic.[4] The cause of persistent pain after sternotomy is multifactorial, yet tissue destruction, intercostal nerve trauma, scar formation, rib fractures, sternal infection, stainless-steel wire sutures, and/or costochondral separation may all play roles. Such chronic pain is often localized to the arms, shoulders, or legs. Postoperative brachial plexus neuropathies may also occur and have been attributed to rib fracture fragments, internal mammary artery dissection, suboptimal positioning of patients during surgery, and/or central venous catheter placement. Postoperative neuralgia of the saphenous nerve has also been reported after harvesting of saphenous veins for coronary artery bypass grafting (CABG). Younger patients appear to be at higher risk for developing chronic, long-lasting pain. The correlation of severity of acute postoperative pain and development of chronic pain syndromes has been suggested (patients requiring more postoperative analgesics may be more likely to develop chronic pain), yet the causative relationship is still vague.

Patient satisfaction with quality of postoperative analgesia is as much related to the comparison between anticipated and experienced pain as it is to the actual level of pain experienced. Satisfaction is related to a situation that is better than predicted, dissatisfaction to one that is worse than expected. Patients undergoing cardiac surgery remain concerned regarding the adequacy of postoperative pain relief and tend to preoperatively expect a greater amount of postoperative pain than that which is actually experienced. Because of these unique preoperative expectations, patients after cardiac surgery who receive only moderate analgesia postoperatively will likely still be satisfied with their pain control. Thus, patients may experience pain of moderate intensity after cardiac surgery yet still express very high satisfaction levels.

POTENTIAL CLINICAL BENEFITS OF ADEQUATE POSTOPERATIVE ANALGESIA

Inadequate analgesia (coupled with an uninhibited stress response) during the postoperative period may lead to many adverse hemodynamic (tachycardia, hypertension, vasoconstriction), metabolic (increased catabolism), immunologic (impaired immune response), and hemostatic (platelet activation) alterations. In patients undergoing cardiac surgery, perioperative myocardial ischemia (diagnosed by electrocardiography and/or transesophageal echocardiography) is most commonly observed during the immediate postoperative period and appears to be related to outcome. Intraoperatively, initiation of CPB causes substantial increases in stress response hormones (e.g., norepinephrine, epinephrine) that persist into the immediate postoperative period and may contribute to myocardial ischemia observed during this time. Furthermore, postoperative myocardial ischemia may be aggravated by cardiac sympathetic nerve activation, which disrupts the balance between coronary blood flow and myocardial oxygen demand. Thus, during the pivotal immediate postoperative period after cardiac surgery, adequate analgesia (coupled with stress-response attenuation) may potentially decrease morbidity and enhance health-related quality of life.[5]

TECHNIQUES AVAILABLE FOR POSTOPERATIVE ANALGESIA

Local Anesthetic Infiltration

Pain after cardiac surgery is often related to median sternotomy (peaking during the first 2 postoperative days). One method that may hold promise is continuous infusion of local anesthetic (Box 31-3). In a prospective, randomized, placebo-controlled, double-blind clinical trial, White and associates[6] studied 36 patients undergoing cardiac surgery. Intraoperative management was standardized. All patients had two indwelling infusion catheters placed at the median sternotomy incision site at the end of surgery (one in the subfascial plane above the sternum, one above the fascia in the subcutaneous tissue). Patients received 0.25% bupivacaine (n = 12), 0.5% bupivacaine (n = 12), or normal saline (n = 12) via a constant rate infusion through the catheter (4 mL/hr) for 48 hours after surgery. Average times to tracheal extubation were similar in the three groups (5 to 6 hours). Compared with the control group (normal saline), there was a statistically significant reduction in verbal rating scale pain scores and patient-controlled analgesia (PCA) using intravenous morphine in the 0.5% bupivacaine group. Patient satisfaction with their pain management was also improved in the 0.5% bupivacaine group (vs. control). However, there were no significant differences in PCA morphine use between the 0.25% bupivacaine and control groups. Although tracheal extubation time and the duration of the intensive care unit (ICU) stay (30 hours vs. 34 hours, respectively) were not significantly altered, time to ambulation (1 day vs. 2 days, respectively) and duration of hospital stay (4.2 days vs. 5.7 days, respectively) were lower in the 0.5% bupivacaine group than in the control group.

The management of postoperative pain with continuous direct infusion of local anesthetic into the surgical wound has been described following a wide variety of surgeries other than cardiac (inguinal hernia repair, upper abdominal surgery, laparoscopic nephrectomy, cholecystectomy, knee arthroplasty, shoulder surgery, and gynecologic operative laparoscopy). The infusion pump systems used for anesthetic wound perfusion are regulated by the U.S. Food and Drug Administration (FDA) as medical devices. Thus, adverse events involving these infusion pump systems during direct local anesthetic infusion into surgical wounds are reported to this organization. Complications encountered with these infusion pump systems reported to the FDA include tissue necrosis, surgical wound infection, and cellulitis after orthopedic, gastrointestinal, podiatric, and other surgeries. None of these reported adverse events has involved patients undergoing cardiac surgery.

Nerve Blocks

With the increasing popularity of minimally invasive cardiac surgery, which utilizes nonsternotomy incisions (minithoracotomy), the use of nerve blocks for the management of postoperative pain has increased as well (Box 31-4).[7] Thoracotomy incisions (transverse anterolateral minithoracotomy, vertical anterolateral minithoracotomy), owing to costal cartilage trauma tissue damage to ribs, muscles, or peripheral nerves, may induce more intense postoperative pain than that resulting from median sternotomy. Adequate analgesia after thoracotomy is important because pain is a key component in alteration of lung function after thoracic surgery. Uncontrolled pain causes a reduction in respiratory mechanics, reduced mobility, and increases in hormonal and metabolic activity. Perioperative deterioration in respiratory mechanics may lead to pulmonary complications and hypoxemia, which may in turn lead to myocardial ischemia/infarction, cerebrovascular accidents, thromboembolism, and delayed wound healing, leading to increased morbidity and prolonged hospital stay. Various analgesic techniques have been developed to treat postoperative thoracotomy pain. The most commonly used techniques include intercostal nerve blocks, intrapleural administration of local anesthetics, and thoracic paravertebral blocks. Intrathecal techniques and epidural techniques are also very effective in controlling post-thoracotomy pain.

Intercostal nerve block has been used extensively for analgesia after thoracic surgery. Intercostal nerve blocks can be performed either intraoperatively or postoperatively and usually provide sufficient analgesia lasting 6 to 12 hours (depending on amount and type of local anesthetic used) and may need to be repeated if additional analgesia is required. Local anesthetics may be administered as a single treatment under direct vision, before chest closure, as a single preoperative percutaneous injection, as multiple percutaneous serial injections, or via an indwelling intercostal catheter. Blockade of intercostal nerves interrupts C-fiber afferent transmission of impulses to the spinal cord. A single intercostal injection of a long-acting local anesthetic can provide pain relief and improve pulmonary function in patients after thoracic surgery for up to 6 hours. To achieve longer duration of analgesia, a continuous extrapleural intercostal nerve block technique may be used in which a catheter is placed percutaneously into an extrapleural pocket by the surgeon. A continuous intercostal catheter allows frequent dosing or infusions of local anesthetic agents and avoids multiple needle injections. Various clinical studies have confirmed the analgesic efficacy of this technique, and the technique compares favorably with thoracic epidural analgesic techniques. A major concern associated with intercostal nerve block is the potentially high amount of local anesthetic systemic absorption, yet multiple clinical studies involving patients undergoing thoracic surgery have documented safe blood levels with standard techniques. Clinical investigations involving patients undergoing thoracic surgery indicate that intercostal nerve blockade by intermittent or continuous infusion of 0.5% bupivacaine with epinephrine is an effective method, as is continuous infusion of 0.25% bupivacaine through indwelling intercostal catheters for supplementing systemic intravenous opioid analgesia for post-thoracotomy pain.

Intrapleural administration of local anesthetics initiates analgesia via mechanisms that remain incompletely understood. However, the mechanism of action of extrapleural regional anesthesia seems to depend primarily on diffusion of the local anesthetic into the paravertebral region. Local anesthetic agents then affect not only the ventral nerve root but also afferent fibers of the posterior primary ramus. Posterior ligaments of the posterior primary ramus innervate posterior spinal muscles and skin and are traumatized during posterolateral thoracotomy. Intrapleural administration of local anesthetic agent to this region through a catheter inserted in the extrapleural space thus creates an anesthetic region in the skin. The depth and width of the anesthetic region depend on diffusion of the local anesthetic agent in the extrapleural space.

Thoracic paravertebral block involves injection of local anesthetic adjacent to the thoracic vertebrae close to where the spinal nerves emerge from the intervertebral foramina (Fig. 31-1). Thoracic paravertebral block, compared with thoracic epidural analgesic techniques, appears to provide equivalent analgesia, is technically easier, and may harbor less risk. Several different techniques exist for successful thoracic paravertebral block and have been extensively reviewed.[8] The classic technique, most commonly used, involves eliciting loss of resistance. Injection of local anesthetic results in ipsilateral somatic and sympathetic nerve blockade in multiple contiguous thoracic dermatomes above and below the site of injection (along with possible suppression of the neuroendocrine stress response to surgery). These blocks may be effective in alleviating acute and chronic pain of unilateral origin from the chest and/or abdomen. Bilateral use of thoracic paravertebral block has also been described. Continuous thoracic paravertebral infusion of local anesthetic via a catheter placed under direct vision at thoracotomy is also a safe, simple, and effective method of providing analgesia after thoracotomy. It is usually used in conjunction with adjunct intravenous medications (opioid or other analgesics) to provide optimum relief after thoracotomy.

Opioids

Beginning in the 1960s, large doses of intravenous opioids have been administered to patients undergoing cardiac surgery (Box 31-5). Because even very large amounts of intravenous opioids do not initiate "complete anesthesia" (unconsciousness, muscle relaxation, suppression of reflex responses to noxious surgical stimuli), other intravenous/inhalation agents must be administered during the intraoperative period. Analgesia is the best known and most extensively investigated opioid effect, yet opioids are also involved in a diverse array of other physiologic functions, including control of pituitary and adrenal medulla hormone release and activity, control of cardiovascular and gastrointestinal function, and the regulation of respiration, mood, appetite, thirst, cell growth, and the immune system. A number of well-known and potential side effects of opioids (nausea and vomiting, pruritus, urinary retention, respiratory depression) may limit postoperative recovery when opioids are used for postoperative analgesia.

The classic pharmacologic effect of opioids is analgesia, and these drugs have traditionally been the initial choice when a potent postoperative analgesic is required. Two anatomically distinct sites exist for opioid receptor–mediated analgesia: supraspinal and spinal. Systemically administered opioids produce analgesia at both sites.

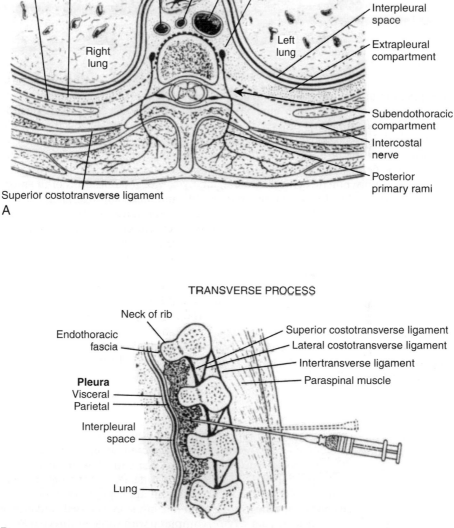

A

TRANSVERSE PROCESS

B

Figure 31-1 Anatomy of the thoracic paravertebral space (**A**) and sagittal section through the thoracic paravertebral space showing a needle that has been advanced above the transverse process (**B**). (From Karmakar MK: Thoracic paravertebral block [review article]. Anesthesiology 95:771, 2001.)

Supraspinally, the μ_1-receptor is primarily involved in analgesia whereas the μ_2-receptor is the one predominantly involved in the spinal modulation of nociceptive processing. $\varkappa$-Receptors are important in mediating spinal and supraspinal analgesia as well. δ-Ligands may have a modulatory rather than a primary analgesic role. All three types of opioid receptors (μ, $\varkappa$, and δ) have been demonstrated in peripheral

---

BOX 31-5 *Opioids*

- *Advantage:*
  - Time-tested, reliable analgesia
- *Disadvantages:*
  - Pruritus
  - Nausea and vomiting
  - Urinary retention
  - Respiratory depression

---

terminals of sensory nerves. Activation of these receptors seems to require an inflammatory reaction because locally applied opioids do not produce analgesia in healthy tissue. The inflammatory process may also activate previously inactive opioid receptors.

Morphine is the prototype opioid agonist with which all opioids are compared. Morphine is perhaps the most popular analgesic used in patients after cardiac surgery. Many semisynthetic derivatives are made by simple modifications of the morphine molecule. Morphine is poorly lipid soluble and binds approximately 35% to plasma proteins, particularly albumin. Morphine is primarily metabolized in the liver, principally by conjugation to water-soluble glucuronides. The liver is the predominant site for morphine biotransformation, although extrahepatic metabolism also occurs in the kidney, brain, and possibly gut. Extrahepatic clearance accounts for approximately 30% of the total body clearance. The terminal elimination half-life of morphine is 2 to 3 hours. In patients with liver cirrhosis, morphine pharmacokinetics are variable, probably reflecting the variability of liver disease in patients. Morphine's terminal elimination half-life in patients with renal disease is comparable to that of normal patients. While morphine is perhaps the most popular intravenous analgesic used in patients after cardiac surgery, other synthetically derived opioids have been developed and may be utilized as well. These include fentanyl, alfentanil, sufentanil, and remifentanil.

Patient-Controlled Analgesia

When intravenous opioids are used for controlling postoperative pain (most commonly morphine and fentanyl), PCA technology is generally used. Essentials in the successful use of PCA technology include "loading" the patient with intravenous opioids to the point of patient comfort before initiating PCA, ensuring that the patient wants to control analgesic treatment, using an appropriate PCA dose and lockout interval, and considering the use of a basal rate infusion. Focused guidance of PCA dosing by a dedicated acute pain service, compared with surgeon-directed PCA, may result in more effective analgesia with fewer side effects.

Nonsteroidal Anti-inflammatory Agents

The NSAIDs, in contrast to the opioids' central nervous system mechanism of action, mainly exert their analgesic, antipyretic, and anti-inflammatory effects peripherally by interfering with prostaglandin synthesis after tissue injury (Box 31-6).[9] NSAIDs inhibit cyclooxygenase (COX), the enzyme responsible for the conversion of arachidonic acid to prostaglandin. Combining NSAIDs with traditional

VI

BOX 31-6 *Nonsteroidal Anti-Inflammatory Agents*

- *Advantage:*
  - Opioid-sparing, reliable analgesia
- *Disadvantages:*
  - Gastric mucosal dysfunction?
  - Renal tubular dysfunction?
  - Inhibition of platelet aggregation?
  - Sternal wound infection?
  - Thromboembolic complications?

intravenous opioids may allow a patient to achieve an adequate level of analgesia with fewer side effects than if a similar level of analgesia was obtained with intravenous opioids alone. Numerous clinical investigations reveal the potential value (opioid-sparing effects) of NSAIDs when combined with traditional intravenous opioids during the postoperative period after noncardiac surgery. In fact, the administration of NSAIDs is one of the most common nonopioid analgesic techniques currently used for postoperative pain management. The efficacy of NSAIDs for postoperative pain has been repeatedly demonstrated in many analgesic clinical trials. Unlike opioids, which preferentially reduce spontaneous postoperative pain, NSAIDs have comparable efficacy for both spontaneous and movement-evoked pain, the latter of which may be more important in causing postoperative physiologic impairment. Certainly, NSAIDs reduce postoperative opioid consumption and accelerate postoperative recovery and represent an integral component of balanced postoperative analgesic regimens after noncardiac surgery. However, little is known regarding NSAID use in the management of pain after cardiac surgery. It is likely that concerns regarding NSAID side effects, including alterations in the gastric mucosal barrier, renal tubular function, and inhibition of platelet aggregation, have made clinicians reluctant to use NSAIDs in patients undergoing cardiac surgery. Other rare side effects of NSAIDs (from COX inhibition) include hepatocellular injury, asthma exacerbation, anaphylactoid reactions, tinnitus, and urticaria. Despite these fears, a small number of clinical investigations seem to indicate that NSAIDs may provide analgesia in patients after cardiac surgery without untoward effects (e.g., gastrointestinal ulceration, renal dysfunction, excessive bleeding).

NSAIDs are not a homogeneous group and vary considerably in analgesic efficacy as a result of differences in pharmacodynamic and pharmacokinetic parameters. NSAIDs are nonspecific inhibitors of COX, which is the rate-limiting enzyme involved in the synthesis of prostaglandins. A major scientific discovery revealed that COX exists in multiple forms. Most important, a constitutive form is present in normal conditions in healthy cells (COX-1) and an inducible form (COX-2) exists that is the major isozyme induced by and associated with inflammation. Simplistically, COX-1 is ubiquitously and constitutively expressed and has a homeostatic role in platelet aggregation, gastrointestinal mucosal integrity, and renal function, whereas COX-2 is inducible and expressed mainly at sites of injury (and kidney and brain) and mediates pain and inflammation. NSAIDs are nonspecific inhibitors of both forms of COX yet vary in their ratio of COX-1 to COX-2 inhibition. Recent molecular studies distinguishing between constitutive COX-1 and inflammation-inducible COX-2 enzymes have led to the exciting hypothesis that the therapeutic and adverse effects of NSAIDs could be uncoupled (Fig. 31-2).[10]

31

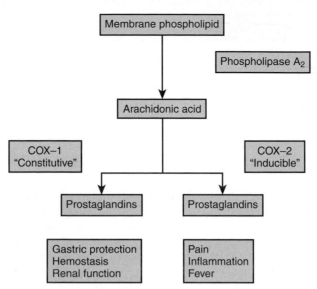

Figure 31-2 Cyclooxygenase pathways. Recent molecular studies distinguishing between COX-1 and COX-2 enzymes have led to the exciting hypothesis that the therapeutic and adverse effects of the nonspecific inhibitors (NSAIDs) could be uncoupled. (From Gajraj NM: Cyclooxygenase-2 inhibitors [review article]. Anesth Analg 96:1720, 2003.)

BOX 31-7 α_2-Adrenergic Agonists

- *Advantage:*
  - Cardiovascular stability?
- *Disadvantages:*
  - Sedation
  - Hypotension

VI

α_2-Adrenergic Agonists

The α_2-adrenergic agonists provide analgesia, sedation, and sympatholysis (Box 31-7). The potential perioperative analgesic benefits of α_2-agonists, when administered to patients undergoing cardiac surgery, were demonstrated almost 20 years ago. Most of the clinical investigations regarding perioperative use of this class of drugs remain focused on exploiting the sedative effects and beneficial cardiovascular effects (decreasing hypertension and tachycardia) associated with their use. α_2-Adrenergic agonists have been used perioperatively in patients undergoing cardiac surgery, yet the focus of such clinical investigations has been on the intraoperative period and the potential for enhanced postoperative hemodynamic stability, potentially leading to reduced postoperative myocardial ischemia (not specifically at enhanced postoperative analgesia).

Intrathecal and Epidural Techniques

It is clear from numerous clinical investigations that intrathecal and/or epidural techniques (using opioids and/or local anesthetics) initiate reliable postoperative analgesia in patients after cardiac surgery (Boxes 31-8 and 31-9). Additional potential

---

BOX 31-8 *Intrathecal Techniques*

- *Advantages:*
  - Simple, reliable analgesia
  - Stress-response attenuation
  - Less hematoma risk than epidural techniques
- *Disadvantages:*
  - No cardiac sympathectomy
  - Hematoma risk increased
  - Side effects of intrathecal opioids

BOX 31-9 *Epidural Techniques*

- *Advantages:*
  - Reliable analgesia
  - Stress-response attenuation
  - Cardiac sympathectomy
- *Disadvantages:*
  - Labor intensive
  - Hematoma risk increased
  - Side effects of epidural opioids

---

advantages of using intrathecal and/or epidural techniques in patients undergoing cardiac surgery include stress-response attenuation and thoracic cardiac sympathectomy.

Intrathecal Techniques

Most clinical investigators have used intrathecal morphine in hopes of providing prolonged postoperative analgesia. Some clinical investigators have used intrathecal fentanyl, sufentanil, and/or local anesthetics for intraoperative anesthesia and analgesia (with stress response attenuation) and/or thoracic cardiac sympathectomy. An anonymous survey of members of the Society of Cardiovascular Anesthesiologists indicates that almost 8% of practicing anesthesiologists incorporate intrathecal techniques into their anesthetic management of adults undergoing cardiac surgery.[11] Of these anesthesiologists, 75% practice in the United States, 72% perform the intrathecal injection before induction of anesthesia, 97% use morphine, 13% use fentanyl, 2% use sufentanil, 10% use lidocaine, and 3% use tetracaine.

The mid 1990s saw the emergence of fast-track cardiac surgery, with the goal being tracheal extubation in the immediate postoperative period. Chaney and associates in 1997[12] were the first to study the potential clinical benefits of intrathecal morphine when used in patients undergoing cardiac surgery and early tracheal extubation. They prospectively randomized 40 patients to receive either intrathecal morphine (10 μg/kg) or intrathecal placebo before induction of anesthesia for elective CABG. Intraoperative anesthetic management was standardized (intravenous fentanyl, 20 μg/kg, and intravenous midazolam, 10 mg) and postoperatively all patients received intravenous morphine via PCA exclusively. Of the patients who were tracheally extubated during the immediate postoperative period, the mean time from ICU arrival to tracheal extubation was significantly ($P = .02$) prolonged in patients who received intrathecal morphine (10.9 ± 4.4 hours) compared with placebo controls (7.6 ± 2.5 hours). Three patients who received intrathecal morphine had tracheal extubation substantially delayed (12 to 24 hours) because of prolonged ventilatory depression (likely secondary to intrathecal morphine). Although the mean postoperative intravenous morphine use for 48 hours was less in patients who received intrathecal morphine (42.8 mg) compared with patients who received intrathecal placebo (55.0 mg), the difference between groups was not statistically significant. No clinical differences existed between groups regarding postoperative morbidity, mortality, or duration of postoperative hospital stay (approximately 9 days in each group).

These somewhat discouraging findings (absence of enhanced analgesia, prolongation of tracheal extubation time) stimulated the same group of investigators in 1999 to try again, this time decreasing the amount of intraoperative intravenous fentanyl patients received (hoping to decrease fentanyl's effect on augmenting postoperative respiratory depression associated with intrathecal morphine).[13] Forty patients were prospectively randomized to receive either intrathecal morphine (10 μg/kg) or intrathecal placebo before induction of anesthesia for elective CABG. Intraoperative anesthetic management was standardized (intravenous fentanyl, 10 μg/kg, and intravenous midazolam, 200 μg/kg) and all patients postoperatively received intravenous morphine exclusively via PCA. Of the patients tracheally extubated during the immediate postoperative period, mean time to tracheal extubation was similar in patients who received intrathecal morphine (6.8 ± 2.8 hours) compared with intrathecal placebo patients (6.5 ± 3.2 hours). However, once again, four patients who received intrathecal morphine had tracheal extubation substantially delayed (14, 14, 18, and 19 hours) because of prolonged respiratory depression (likely secondary to intrathecal morphine). The mean postoperative intravenous morphine use during the immediate postoperative period was actually higher in patients receiving intrathecal morphine (49.8 mg) compared with patients receiving intrathecal placebo (36.2 mg), yet the difference between groups was not statistically significant. No clinical differences existed between groups regarding postoperative morbidity, mortality, or duration of postoperative hospital stay (approximately 6 days in each group). Thus, Chaney and associates, from their three prospective, randomized, double-blind, placebo-controlled clinical investigations in the late 1990s involving 140 healthy adults undergoing elective CABG, concluded that although intrathecal morphine certainly can initiate reliable postoperative analgesia, its use in the setting of fast-track cardiac surgery and early tracheal extubation may be detrimental by potentially delaying tracheal extubation in the immediate postoperative period.

Epidural Techniques

Most clinical investigators have used thoracic epidural local anesthetics in hopes of providing perioperative stress response attenuation and/or perioperative thoracic cardiac sympathectomy. Some clinical investigators have used thoracic epidural opioids to provide intraoperative and/or postoperative analgesia. An anonymous survey of members of the Society of Cardiovascular Anesthesiologists indicates that 7% of practicing anesthesiologists incorporate thoracic epidural techniques into their anesthetic management of adults undergoing cardiac surgery.[11] Of these anesthesiologists, 58% practice in the United States. Regarding the timing of epidural instrumentation, 40% perform instrumentation before induction of general anesthesia, 12% perform instrumentation after induction of general anesthesia, 33% perform instrumentation at the end of surgery, and 15% perform instrumentation on the first postoperative day.

Numerous clinical studies further attest to the ability of thoracic epidural anesthesia and analgesia with local anesthetics and/or opioids to induce substantial postoperative analgesia in patients after cardiac surgery (Table 31-2).

Many clinical investigations have proven that thoracic epidural anesthesia with local anesthetics also significantly attenuates the perioperative stress response in patients undergoing cardiac surgery. Patients randomized to receive intermittent boluses of thoracic epidural bupivacaine intraoperatively followed by continuous

Table 31-2 Reports of Epidural Anesthesia and Analgesia for Cardiac Surgery

First Author	Year	Study Design	Total No. of Patients	Drugs: Dosage Method	Intraoperative Management	Remarks
Royse	2003	Prospective, randomized	80	Ropivacaine, fentanyl infusion	Not standardized	Reliable postoperative analgesia
Pastor	2003	Prospective, observational	714	Bupivacaine or ropivacaine boluses plus infusion	Not standardized	No hematoma formation
Priestley	2002	Prospective, randomized	100	Ropivacaine, fentanyl infusion	Not standardized	Reliable postoperative analgesia
de Vries	2002	Prospective, randomized	90	Bupivacaine: bolus plus infusion Sufentanil: bolus plus infusion	Standardized	Reliable postoperative analgesia Facilitated early extubation Possible decreased hospital stay
Canto	2002	Prospective, observational	305	Ropivacaine: bolus plus infusion	Not standardized	No hematoma formation
Fillinger	2002	Prospective, randomized	60	Bupivacaine: bolus plus infusion Morphine: bolus plus infusion	Not standardized	No benefit
Jideus	2001	Prospective, randomized	41	Bupivacaine: bolus plus infusion Sufentanil: infusion	Not standardized	Stress response attenuation Thoracic cardiac sympathectomy
Scott	2001	Prospective, randomized	206	Bupivacaine: bolus plus infusion Clonidine: infusion	Standardized	Decreased postoperative arrhythmias Improved postoperative pulmonary function Decreased postoperative renal failure Decreased postoperative confusion

Table continued on following page

31

Table 31-2   Reports of Epidural Anesthesia and Analgesia for Cardiac Surgery (Continued)

First Author	Year	Study Design	Total No. of Patients	Drugs: Dosage Method	Intraoperative Management	Remarks
Dhole	2001	Prospective, randomized	41	Bupivacaine: bolus plus infusion	Not standardized	No benefit
Djaiani	2001	Retrospective	37	Bupivacaine: bolus plus infusion	Not standardized	Facilitated early extubation
Warters	2000	Retrospective	278	Not specified	Not standardized	No hematoma formation
Loick	1999	Prospective, randomized	25	Bupivacaine: bolus plus infusion Sufentanil: bolus plus infusion	Standardized	Stress response attenuation Thoracic cardiac sympathectomy Facilitated early extubation
Tenling	1999	Prospective, randomized	14	Bupivacaine: bolus plus infusion	Not standardized	Reliable postoperative analgesia Facilitated early extubation
Sanchez	1998	Prospective, observational	571	Bupivacaine: boluses	Not standardized	No hematoma formation
Fawcett	1997	Prospective, randomized	16	Bupivacaine: bolus plus infusion	Standardized	Reliable postoperative analgesia Improved pulmonary function Stress response attenuation

Table 31-2 Reports of Epidural Anesthesia and Analgesia for Cardiac Surgery (Continued)

First Author	Year	Study Design	Total No. of Patients	Drugs: Dosage Method	Intraoperative Management	Remarks
Turfrey	1997	Retrospective	218	Bupivacaine: bolus plus infusionClonidine: infusion	Not standardized	Facilitated early extubation Possible thoracic cardiac sympathectomy
Shayevitz	1996	Retrospective	54	Morphine: bolus plus infusion	Not standardized	Reliable postoperative analgesia Facilitated early extubation
Stenseth	1996	Prospective, randomized	54	Bupivacaine: bolus plus infusion	Not standardized	Facilitated early extubation Possible thoracic cardiac sympathectomy
Moore	1995	Prospective, randomized	17	Bupivacaine: bolus plus infusion	Standardized	Stress response attenuation Possible thoracic cardiac sympathectomy
Stenseth	1995	Prospective, randomized	30	Bupivacaine: bolus plus infusion	Standardized	Thoracic cardiac sympathectomy
Kirno	1994	Prospective, randomized	20	Mepivacaine: bolus	Standardized	Stress response attenuation Thoracic cardiac sympathectomy
Stenseth	1994	Prospective, randomized	30	Bupivacaine: bolus plus infusion	Standardized	Stress response attenuation Possible thoracic cardiac sympathectomy

Table continued on following page

31

Table 31-2 Reports of Epidural Anesthesia and Analgesia for Cardiac Surgery (Continued)

First Author	Year	Study Design	Total No. of Patients	Drugs: Dosage Method	Intraoperative Management	Remarks
Liem	1992	Prospective, randomized	54	Bupivacaine: bolus plus infusion Sufentanil: bolus plus infusion	Not standardized	Reliable postoperative analgesia Stress response attenuation Possible thoracic cardiac sympathectomy
Rosen	1989	Prospective, randomized	32	Morphine: bolus	Not standardized	Reliable postoperative analgesia Facilitated early extubation
Joachimsson	1989	Observational	28	Bupivacaine: boluses	Not standardized	Reliable postoperative analgesia
El-Baz	1987	Prospective, randomized	60	Morphine: infusion	Standardized	Reliable postoperative analgesia Stress response attenuation Facilitated early extubation
Robinson	1986	Prospective, observational	10	Meperidine: bolus	Standardized	Reliable postoperative analgesia
Hoar	1976	Prospective, observational	12	Lidocaine: boluses Bupivacaine: boluses	Not standardized	Reliable postoperative analgesia Possible stress response attenuation

infusion postoperatively exhibited significantly decreased blood levels of norepinephrine and epinephrine perioperatively when compared with patients managed similarly without thoracic epidural catheters.

A relatively large clinical investigation highlights the potential clinical benefits of thoracic epidural anesthesia in cardiac surgical patients. Scott and associates[14] prospectively randomized (nonblinded) 420 patients undergoing elective CABG to receive either thoracic epidural anesthesia (bupivacaine/clonidine) and general anesthesia or general anesthesia alone (control group). The two groups received similar intraoperative anesthetic techniques. In thoracic epidural anesthesia patients, the thoracic epidural infusion was continued for 96 hours after surgery (titrated according to need). In control patients, target-controlled infusion alfentanil was used for the first 24 postoperative hours, then followed by PCA morphine for the next 48 hours. Postoperatively, striking clinical differences were observed between the two groups. Postoperative incidence of supraventricular arrhythmia, lower respiratory tract infection, renal failure, and acute confusion were all significantly lower in patients receiving thoracic epidural anesthesia compared with control patients.

In contrast to the encouraging findings of the clinical investigation by Scott and associates, other prospective, randomized, nonblinded clinical investigations reveal that using thoracic epidural anesthesia techniques in patients undergoing cardiac surgery may not offer substantial clinical benefits.[15] In 2002, Priestley and associates prospectively randomized 100 patients undergoing elective CABG to receive either thoracic epidural anesthesia (ropivacaine/fentanyl) and general anesthesia or general anesthesia alone (control group). The two groups received quite different intraoperative anesthetic techniques. Postoperatively, thoracic epidural anesthesia patients received epidural ropivacaine/fentanyl for 48 hours (supplemental analgesics available if needed), whereas control patients received nurse-administered intravenous morphine, followed by PCA morphine. Patients receiving thoracic epidural anesthesia were extubated sooner than controls (3.2 vs. 6.7 hours, respectively; $P < .001$), yet this difference may have been secondary to the different amounts of intraoperative intravenous opioid administered to the two groups (intraoperative intravenous anesthetic technique not standardized). Postoperative pain scores at rest were significantly lower in patients receiving thoracic epidural anesthesia only on postoperative days 0 and 1 (equivalent on days 2 and 3). Postoperative pain scores during coughing were significantly lower in patients receiving thoracic epidural anesthesia only on postoperative day 0 (equivalent on days 1, 2, and 3). There were no significant differences between the two groups in postoperative oxygen saturation on room air, chest radiograph changes, or spirometry. Furthermore, no clinical differences were detected between the two groups regarding postoperative mobilization goals, atrial fibrillation, postoperative hospital discharge eligibility, or actual postoperative hospital discharge.

All clinical reports involving utilization of intrathecal and thoracic epidural anesthesia and analgesia techniques for cardiac surgery involve small numbers of patients and few (if any) are well designed. There are no blinded, placebo-controlled clinical studies involving thoracic epidural anesthesia and analgesia. Furthermore, none of the existing clinical studies involving intrathecal and thoracic epidural anesthesia and analgesia techniques for cardiac surgery uses clinical outcome as a primary endpoint. Thus, there are clear deficiencies in the literature that prohibit definitive analysis of the risk/benefit ratio of intrathecal and thoracic epidural anesthesia and analgesia techniques as applied to patients undergoing cardiac surgery.

A 2004 meta-analysis by Liu and associates[16] assessed effects of perioperative central neuraxial analgesia on outcome after CABG. These authors, via MEDLINE and other databases, searched for randomized controlled trials in patients undergoing

31

CABG with CPB. Fifteen trials enrolling 1178 patients were included for thoracic epidural anesthesia analysis, and 17 trials enrolling 668 patients were included for intrathecal analysis. Thoracic epidural techniques did not affect the incidences of mortality or myocardial infarction yet reduced risk of arrhythmias (atrial fibrillation and tachycardia), reduced risk of pulmonary complications (pneumonia and atelectasis), reduced time to tracheal extubation, and reduced analog pain scores. Intrathecal techniques did not affect incidences of mortality, myocardial infarction, arrhythmias, or time to tracheal extubation and only modestly decreased systemic morphine utilization and pain scores (while increasing incidence of pruritus). These authors conclude that central neuraxial analgesia does not affect rates of mortality or myocardial infarction after CABG yet is associated with improvements in faster time to tracheal extubation, decreased pulmonary complications and cardiac arrhythmias, and reduced pain scores. However, the authors also note that the majority of potential clinical benefits offered by central neuraxial analgesia (earlier extubation, decreased arrhythmias, enhanced analgesia) may be reduced and/or eliminated with changing cardiac anesthesia practice using fast-track techniques, use of β-adrenergic blockers or amiodarone, and/or use of NSAIDs or COX-2 inhibitors. These authors also note that the risk of spinal hematoma (addressed later in this chapter) due to central neuraxial analgesia in patients undergoing full anticoagulation for CPB remains uncertain.

RISK OF HEMATOMA FORMATION

Intrathecal or epidural instrumentation entails risk, the most feared complication being epidural hematoma formation. The estimated incidence of hematoma formation is approximately 1:220,000 after intrathecal instrumentation. Hematoma formation is more common (approximately 1:150,000) after epidural instrumentation because larger needles are used, catheters are inserted, and the venous plexus in the epidural space is prominent. Furthermore, hematoma formation does not occur exclusively during epidural catheter insertion; almost half of all cases develop after catheter removal.

Risk is increased when intrathecal or epidural instrumentation is performed before systemic heparinization, and hematoma formation has occurred in patients when diagnostic or therapeutic lumbar puncture has been followed by systemic heparinization. When lumbar puncture is followed by systemic heparinization, concurrent use of aspirin, difficult or traumatic instrumentation, and administration of intravenous heparin within 1 hour of instrumentation increase the risk of hematoma formation. However, by observing certain precautions, intrathecal or epidural instrumentation can be performed safely in patients who will subsequently receive intravenous heparin. By delaying surgery 24 hours in the event of a traumatic tap, by delaying heparinization 60 minutes after catheter insertion, and by maintaining tight perioperative control of anticoagulation, more than 4000 intrathecal or epidural catheterizations were performed safely in patients undergoing peripheral vascular surgery who received intravenous heparin after catheter insertion. A retrospective review involving 912 patients further indicates that epidural catheterization before systemic heparinization for peripheral vascular surgery is safe. However, the magnitude of anticoagulation in these two studies (activated partial thromboplastin time of approximately 100 seconds and activated clotting time approximately twice the baseline value) involving patients undergoing peripheral vascular surgery was substantially less than the degree of anticoagulation required in patients subjected to CPB.

Most clinical studies investigating the use of intrathecal or epidural anesthesia and analgesia techniques in patients undergoing cardiac surgery include precautions to decrease risk of hematoma formation. Some used the technique only after the demonstration of laboratory evidence of normal coagulation parameters, delayed surgery 24 hours in the event of traumatic tap, or required that the time from instrumentation to systemic heparinization exceed 60 minutes. While most clinicians investigating use of epidural anesthesia and analgesia techniques in patients undergoing cardiac surgery insert catheters the day before scheduled surgery, investigators have performed instrumentation on the same day of surgery. Institutional practice (same-day admit surgery) may eliminate the option of epidural catheter insertion on the day before scheduled surgery.

Although most investigators agree that risk of hematoma is likely increased when intrathecal or epidural instrumentation is performed in patients before systemic heparinization required for CPB, the absolute degree of increased risk is somewhat controversial; some believe the risk may be as high as 0.35%. An extensive mathematical analysis by Ho and associates[17] of the approximately 10,840 intrathecal injections in patients subjected to systemic heparinization required for CPB (without a single episode of hematoma formation) reported in the literature as of the year 2000 estimated that the minimum risk of hematoma formation was 1:220,000 and the maximum risk of hematoma formation was 1:3600 (95% confidence level); however, the maximum risk may be as high as 1:2400 (99% confidence level). Similarly, of the approximately 4583 epidural instrumentations in patients subjected to systemic heparinization required for CPB (without a single episode of hematoma formation) reported in the literature as of the year 2000, the minimum risk of hematoma formation was 1:150,000 and the maximum risk of hematoma formation was 1:1500 (95% confidence level); however, the maximum risk may be as high as 1:1000 (99% confidence level).

Certain precautions, however, may decrease the risk. The technique should not be used in a patient with known coagulopathy from any cause. Surgery should be delayed 24 hours in the event of a traumatic tap, and time from instrumentation to systemic heparinization should exceed 60 minutes. Additionally, systemic heparin effect and reversal should be tightly controlled (smallest amount of heparin used for the shortest duration compatible with therapeutic objectives) and patients should be closely monitored postoperatively for signs and symptoms of hematoma formation. An obvious economic disadvantage of intrathecal or epidural instrumentation in patients before cardiac surgery is the possible delay in surgery in the event of a traumatic tap. However, one study involving more than 4000 intrathecal or epidural catheterizations via a 17-gauge Tuohy needle indicates that the incidence of traumatic tap (blood freely aspirated) is rare (<0.10%).

Use of regional anesthetic techniques in patients undergoing cardiac surgery, while seemingly increasing in popularity, remains extremely controversial, prompting numerous editorials by recognized experts in the field of cardiac anesthesia.[18] One of the main reasons such controversy exists (and likely will continue for some time) is that the numerous clinical investigations regarding this topic are suboptimally designed and use a wide array of disparate techniques, preventing clinically useful conclusions on which all can agree.

MULTIMODAL ANALGESIA

The possibility of synergism between analgesic drugs is a concept that is nearly a century old. While subsequent research has revealed the difference between additivity and synergy, the fundamental strategy behind such combinations ("multimodal" or "balanced" analgesia) remains unchanged: enhanced analgesia with minimization of adverse physiologic effects. Use of analgesic combinations during the postoperative

31

period, specifically the combination of traditional intravenous opioids with other analgesics (e.g., NSAIDs, COX-2 inhibitors, ketamine), has been proved clinically effective in noncardiac patients for decades. Early clinical investigations simply reported analgesic efficacy, whereas more recent clinical investigations have additionally evaluated and described specific opioid-sparing effects (which should lead to a reduction in side effects). For example, in the late 1980s, initial clinical studies involving ketorolac (the first parenteral NSAID available in the United States) revealed significant opioid-sparing effects (analgesia) along with a reduction in respiratory depression. Subsequently, substantial clinical research has clearly established the perioperative analgesic efficacy and opioid-sparing effects of NSAIDs (along with reduction of side effects).

The American Society of Anesthesiologists (ASA) Task Force on Acute Pain Management in the Perioperative Setting reports that the literature supports the administration of two analgesic agents that act by different mechanisms via a single route for providing superior analgesic efficacy with equivalent or reduced adverse effects. Potential examples include (1) epidural opioids administered in combination with epidural local anesthetics or clonidine and (2) intravenous opioids in combination with ketorolac or ketamine. Dose-dependent adverse effects reported with administration of a medication occur whether it is given alone or in combination with other medications (opioids may cause nausea, vomiting, pruritus, or urinary retention, and local anesthetics may produce motor block). The literature is insufficient to evaluate the postoperative analgesic effects of oral opioids combined with NSAIDs, COX-2 inhibitors, or acetaminophen compared with oral opioids alone. The ASA Task Force believes that NSAIDs, COX-2 inhibitors, or acetaminophen administration has a dose-sparing effect for systemically administered opioids. The literature also suggests that two routes of administration, when compared with a single route, may be more effective in providing perioperative analgesia. Examples include intrathecal or epidural opioids combined with intravenous, intramuscular, oral, transdermal, or subcutaneous analgesics versus intrathecal or epidural opioids alone. Another example is intravenous opioids combined with oral NSAIDs, COX-2 inhibitors, or acetaminophen versus intravenous opioids alone. The literature is insufficient to evaluate the efficacy of pharmacologic pain management combined with non-pharmacologic, alternative, or complementary pain management compared with pharmacologic pain management alone.

CONCLUSIONS

Multiple factors are important during the perioperative period that potentially affect outcome and quality of life after cardiac surgery, including type and quality of surgical intervention, extent of postoperative neurologic dysfunction, myocardial dysfunction, pulmonary dysfunction, renal dysfunction, coagulation abnormalities, quality of postoperative analgesia, and/or extent of systemic inflammatory response, among others[19] (Table 31-3). This list of factors is presented in no particular order; obviously, depending on specific clinical situations (e.g., surgical procedure, patient comorbidity), certain factors will be more important than others. It is extremely difficult (if not impossible) to determine exactly how important attaining adequate postoperative analgesia truly is in relation to all of these clinical factors surrounding a patient undergoing cardiac surgery. A clear link between "adequate" or "high-quality" postoperative analgesia and outcome in patients after cardiac surgery has yet to be established.[20]

Table 31-3	Factors Affecting Outcome after Cardiac Surgery

Type and quality of surgical intervention
Extent of postoperative neurologic dysfunction
Extent of postoperative myocardial dysfunction
Extent of postoperative pulmonary dysfunction
Extent of postoperative renal dysfunction
Extent of postoperative coagulation abnormalities
Quality of postoperative analgesia
Extent of systemic inflammatory response

However, despite the absence of substantiating scientific evidence, most clinicians intuitively believe that attaining high-quality postoperative analgesia is important because it may prevent adverse hemodynamic, metabolic, immunologic, and hemostatic alterations, all of which may potentially increase postoperative morbidity. While many analgesic techniques are available, intravenous systemic opioids form the cornerstone of post-cardiac surgery analgesia. Opioids have been used for many years in the treatment of postoperative pain in patients after cardiac surgery with good results. NSAIDs (specifically COX-2 inhibitors) have received much recent attention, but very important clinical issues regarding their safety (gastrointestinal effects, renal effects, hemostatic effects, immunologic effects) need to be resolved. Although PCA techniques are commonly used, their clear superiority over traditional nurse-controlled analgesic techniques remains unproved. As a general rule, it is likely best to avoid intense, single-modality therapy for the treatment of acute postoperative pain. Clinicians should strive for an approach that uses a number of different therapies (multimodal therapy), each counteracting pain via different mechanisms. Preemptive analgesia, while intriguing, needs further study to determine its role in affecting postoperative analgesia and outcome.

Finally, the ASA Task Force offers sound advice. It recommends that anesthesiologists who manage perioperative pain use analgesic therapeutic options only after thoughtfully considering the risks and benefits for the individual patient. The therapy (or therapies) selected should reflect the individual anesthesiologist's expertise, as well as the capacity for safe application of the chosen modality in each practice setting. This includes the ability to recognize and treat adverse effects that emerge after initiation of therapy. Whenever possible, anesthesiologists should employ multimodal pain management therapy. Dosing regimens should be administered to optimize efficacy while minimizing the risk of adverse events. The choice of medication, dose, route, and duration of therapy should always be individualized.

SUMMARY

- Inadequate postoperative analgesia and/or an uninhibited perioperative surgical stress response has the potential to initiate pathophysiologic changes in all major organ systems, including the cardiovascular, pulmonary, gastrointestinal, renal, endocrine, immunologic, and/or central nervous systems, all of which may lead to substantial postoperative morbidity. Adequate postoperative analgesia prevents unnecessary patient discomfort, may decrease morbidity, may decrease postoperative hospital length of stay, and thus may decrease cost.
- Pain after cardiac surgery may be intense and originates from many sources, including the incision (sternotomy or thoracotomy), intraoperative tissue

31

retraction and dissection, vascular cannulation sites, vein-harvesting sites, and chest tubes, among others. Achieving optimal pain relief after cardiac surgery is often difficult, yet may be attained via a wide variety of techniques, including local anesthetic infiltration, nerve blocks, intravenous agents, intrathecal techniques, and epidural techniques.

- Traditionally, analgesia after cardiac surgery has been obtained with intravenous opioids (specifically morphine). However, intravenous opioid use is associated with definite detrimental side effects (nausea/vomiting, pruritus, urinary retention, respiratory depression) and longer-acting opioids such as morphine may delay tracheal extubation during the immediate postoperative period via excessive sedation and/or respiratory depression.

- Although patient-controlled analgesia is a well-established technique and offers potential unique benefits (e.g., reliable analgesic effect, improved patient autonomy, flexible adjustment to individual needs), whether it truly offers significant clinical advantages (compared with traditional nurse-administrated analgesic techniques) to patients immediately after cardiac surgery remains to be determined.

- Cyclooxygenase (COX)-2 inhibitors possess analgesic (opioid-sparing) effects and lack deleterious effects on coagulation (in contrast to nonselective nonsteroidal anti-inflammatory drugs [NSAIDs]). However, current evidence does not suggest that COX-2 inhibitors provide major advantages over traditional NSAIDs. Furthermore, potential links between this class of drugs and cardiovascular complications, sternal wound infections, and thromboembolic complications need to be fully evaluated.

- Administration of intrathecal morphine to patients initiates reliable postoperative analgesia after cardiac surgery. Intrathecal opioids or local anesthetics cannot reliably attenuate the perioperative stress response associated with cardiac surgery that persists during the immediate postoperative period. Although intrathecal local anesthetics (not opioids) may induce perioperative thoracic cardiac sympathectomy, the hemodynamic changes associated with a "total spinal" make the technique unpalatable in patients with cardiac disease.

- Administration of thoracic epidural opioids or local anesthetics to patients initiates reliable postoperative analgesia after cardiac surgery. The quality of analgesia obtained with thoracic epidural anesthetic techniques is sufficient to allow cardiac surgery to be performed in "awake" patients (without general endotracheal anesthesia). Administration of thoracic epidural local anesthetics (not opioids) can both reliably attenuate the perioperative stress response associated with cardiac surgery that persists during the immediate postoperative period and induce perioperative thoracic cardiac sympathectomy.

- Use of intrathecal and epidural techniques in patients undergoing cardiac surgery, while seemingly increasing in popularity, remains extremely controversial. Concerns regarding hematoma risk and the fact that the numerous clinical investigations regarding this topic are suboptimally designed and utilize a wide array of disparate techniques have prevented clinically useful conclusions.

- As a general rule, it is best to avoid intense, single-modality therapy for the treatment of acute postoperative pain. The administration of two analgesic agents that act by different mechanisms ("multimodal" or "balanced" analgesia) provides superior analgesic efficacy with equivalent or reduced adverse effects. The therapy (or therapies) selected should reflect the individual anesthesiologist's expertise, as well as the capacity for safe application of the chosen modality in each practice setting.

REFERENCES

1. American Society of Anesthesiologists Task Force on Acute Pain Management: Practice guidelines for acute pain management in the perioperative setting: An updated report by the American Society of Anesthesiologists Task Force on Acute Pain Management. Anesthesiology 100:1573, 2004
2. Joint Commission on Accreditation of Healthcare Organizations: Pain assessment and management: An organizational approach. 2000. Available at http://www.jcaho.org. Accessed October 15, 2005
3. Myles PS, Daly DJ, Djaiani G, et al: A systematic review of the safety and effectiveness of fast-track cardiac anesthesia. Anesthesiology 99:982, 2003
4. Kalso E, Mennander S, Tasmuth T, Nilsson E: Chronic post-sternotomy pain. Acta Anaesth Scand 45:935, 2001
5. Wu CL, Naqibuddin M, Rowlingson AJ, et al: The effect of pain on health-related quality of life in the immediate postoperative period. Anesth Analg 97:1078, 2003
6. White PF, Rawal S, Latham P, et al: Use of a continuous local anesthetic infusion for pain management after median sternotomy. Anesthesiology 99:918, 2003
7. Riedel BJ: Regional anesthesia for major cardiac and noncardiac surgery: More than just a strategy for effective analgesia? (editorial). J Cardiothorac Vasc Anesth 15:279, 2001
8. Myles P: Underutilization of paravertebral blocks in thoracic surgery. J Cardiothorac Vasc Anesth 20:635, 2006
9. Ralley FE, Day FJ, Cheng DCH: Pro: Nonsteroidal anti-inflammatory drugs should be routinely administered for postoperative analgesia after cardiac surgery. J Cardiothorac Vasc Anesth 14:731, 2000
10. Kharasch ED: Perioperative COX-2 inhibitors: Knowledge and challenges [editorial]. Anesth Analg 98:1, 2004
11. Goldstein S, Dean D, Kim SJ, et al: A survey of spinal and epidural techniques in adult cardiac surgery. J Cardiothorac Vasc Anesth 15:158, 2001
12. Chaney MA, Furry PA, Fluder EM, Slogoff S: Intrathecal morphine for coronary artery bypass grafting and early extubation. Anesth Analg 84:241, 1997
13. Chaney MA, Nikolov MP, Blakeman BP, Bakhos M: Intrathecal morphine for coronary artery bypass graft procedure and early extubation revisited. J Cardiothorac Vasc Anesth 13:574, 1999
14. Scott NB, Turfrey DJ, Ray DAA, et al: A prospective randomized study of the potential benefits of thoracic epidural anesthesia and analgesia in patients undergoing coronary artery bypass grafting. Anesth Analg 93:528, 2001
15. Priestley MC, Cope L, Halliwell R, et al: Thoracic epidural anesthesia for cardiac surgery: The effects on tracheal intubation time and length of hospital stay. Anesth Analg 94:275, 2002
16. Liu SS, Block BM, Wu CL: Effects of perioperative central neuraxial analgesia on outcome after coronary artery bypass surgery: A meta-analysis. Anesthesiology 101:153, 2004
17. Ho AMH, Chung DC, Joynt GM: Neuraxial blockade and hematoma in cardiac surgery: Estimating the risk of a rare adverse event that has not (yet) occurred. Chest 117:551, 2000
18. Gravlee GP: Epidural analgesia and coronary artery bypass grafting: The controversy continues [editorial]. J Cardiothorac Vasc Anesth 17:151, 2003
19. Myles PS, Hunt JO, Fletcher H, et al: Relation between quality of recovery in hospital and quality of life at 3 months after cardiac surgery. Anesthesiology 95:862, 2001
20. Wu CL, Raja SN: Optimizing postoperative analgesia: The use of global outcome measures [editorial]. Anesthesiology 97:533, 2002

31

Index

Page numbers followed by "f" refer to illustrations; page numbers followed by "t" refer to table; page numbers followed by "b" refer to boxes.

Cardiopulmonary bypass (CPB) *(Continued)*
  emergencies, 537-541, 537b, 538t
  end-organ effects of, 520-527, 520b, 521t, 525t, 526f
  equipment, 684-686, 685b
  goals/mechanics of, 513-514, 514f
  low-output syndrome and, 148-150
  management, 527-530, 528f, 529f, 530t
    fluid, 519
    temperature, 517, 518f
  organ protection during, 546
  overview of, 530-537, 531t, 532t
  perfusion
    nonpulsatile/pulsatile, 516
    pressure during, 515-516
  physiologic parameters of, 514-515, 515b
  postoperative, 665
  preparations for
    final, 607-608, 607t
    general, 603-604, 603t, 604t
  pump flow during, 516-517
  special populations associated with, 541-544, 543t
  strategies, 518-519
  summary on, 541, 544
  techniques, 96-97
  usage of, 602
  weaning from, 608-610
Cardiovascular medicine, 79
Cardiovascular testing, 6-10, 9b
CARE. *See* Cardiac Anesthesia Evaluation Score
Carvedilol, 145
CAs. *See* Cold agglutinins
CAST. *See* Cardiac Arrhythmia Suppression Trial
Catheter(s)
  -based percutaneous therapies in interventional cardiology, 46-47
  entrapment/knotting, 186
  mixed venous oxygen saturation, 188
  PA, 455-456
  pacing, 186-188, 187t, 187b
  placement/PAP, 180t, 181, 182f
  rotablator, 42
Catheterization
  complications associated with diagnostic, 21, 22t
  heart
    left-sided, 20-21, 21b
    right-sided, 21, 21b, 656-660, 657f, 658t
  reports, interpretation of, 32
Central nervous system (CNS)
  after CPB, 677
  injuries, 547, 553, 548t, 549f, 550b, 550t, 678-681, 680f
    age-associated, 677-678
  monitoring, 240, 241b
  protection of, 240
Central venous pressure (CVP), 23, 23f, 24b, 60
  monitoring, 172-173, 173f
    complications with, 177, 178b
    of external jugular vein, 176
    indications for, 177, 177b
    of internal jugular vein, 173, 174f, 176, 176f
    of subclavian vein, 176

Cerebral oximetry, 257-261, 257f, 258b, 259f,
cGMP. *See* Cyclic guanosine monophosphate
CHD. *See* Congenital heart disease
CHF. *See* Congestive heart failure
Chronic renal failure (CRF), 438-440
Ciba Corning Biotrak systems, 277
Cimetidine. *See* Histamine-2 blockers
Circumflex artery (CX), 29, 30f, 31t
Clinical Severity Score for CABG, 4
Clopidogrel (Plavix), 43b
  studies, 269
  uses for, 45
CO. *See* Cardiac output
CO_2. *See* Carbon dioxide
Coagulation. *See also* Heparin
  monitoring, 264, 289
  tests of, 276-278
Coarctation of aorta. *See* Aorta, coarctation of
Cold agglutinins (CAs), 442
Comparison of Medical Therapy, Pacing, and Defibrillation in Heart Failure. *See* CAMPANION trial
Complement system
  cardiac surgery and, 91-92, 93f, 94f
  inhibition of, 97
Congenital heart disease (CHD), in adults, 373b, 385
  cardiac issues with, 373-385, 375t, 376f, 376t, 377b, 378f, 379b, 380t, 382b
  noncardiac issues with, 373t, 374
  summary on, 385
Congenital heart surgery, 369-370
Congestive heart failure (CHF), 4, 56
Contact activation, 92, 94f
Contractility
  decreased, 652-656, 653t, 653b, 655b
  definition of, 62, 63t
  determinants of, 62-63
    ejection phase indices and, 62-63
    isovolumic contraction phase indices and, 62
    load-independent indices and, 63, 63f
Cooling, 250
Coronary anatomy, description of, 29-30
Coronary angiography, 17, 18f
Coronary arteriography, 29-31
Coronary artery, 77
  plaque rupture and, 74-75, 74b
  spasms, 652
  stenosis, 74-75, 74b
Coronary artery bypass graft (CABG), 4, 5t
  anesthesia for, 293, 299, 300b
    induction/maintenance of, 310-315, 312f, 315f
    management of, 315-319, 316b, 317b
    monitoring of, 308-310
    premedication, 299-308
    summary on, 324
  Clinical Severity Score for, 4
  PCIs v., 39-41, 40f
  surgery, 38b
Coronary artery disease (CAD), 16, 67, 294
  myocardial infarction and, 298-299, 298f
  pathophysiology of, 295, 295f, 296f, 297f
  symptoms of, 18t

Coronary collateral(s), 31, 31t
    vessels, 75
    Coronary intervention, 71
    Coronary perfusion, 191
Coronary pressure-flow relations, 71
Coronary reserve, 72
Coronary sinus, 212f, 219
Coronary steal, 76-77, 77f
Coronary vasoregulation, 101
Corticosteroid, administration of, 96
Coumadin. *See* Warfarin sodium
CPB. *See* Cardiopulmonary bypass
CRF. *See* Chronic renal failure
CVP. *See* Central venous pressure
CX. *See* Circumflex artery
Cyclic adenosine monophosphate (cAMP), 68, 84, 150
Cyclic guanosine monophosphate (cGMP), 68
Cytokines, 91

D

De-airing, 364
Deep hypothermic circulatory arrest (DHCA), 397-398
    CPB and, 402-403
    neuroprotection strategies for, 398-399
Deoxyribonucleic acid (DNA), 79
Descending thoracic aortic aneurysms
    management of, 403-404
    repair of, 399-403, 400f, 401t
        after, 404-410, 405t, 406b, 407b,
        postoperative, 410
Desflurane, 101
Dexmedetomidine, effects of, 106b
Dextran, 474
DHCA. *See* Deep hypothermic circulatory arrest
Diastolic function, 56, 57t
    determinants of, 56-58
        active/atrial filling as, 58
        myocardial relaxation as, 56-57
        passive ventricular filling as, 57
    TEE and, 58-59, 58f
    TTE and, 58-59, 58f
Diazepam, 108
Digitalis Investigators Group, 146
Digoxin, 146, 158
Dihydropyridines, 131t
Diltiazem, 127, 127t
    pharmacology of, 128, 158
Diphenhydramine, 19
Dipyridamole-thallium scintigraphy, 10
Directional coronary atherectomy (DCA), 41
Disopyramide, 81
Diuretic(s), 146
    loop, 131t
    potassium-sparing, 131t
    thiazide, 131t
DNA. *See* Deoxyribonucleic acid
Dobutamine, 150
Dobutamine stress echocardiography (DSE), 10
Dopamine, 150
Doppler techniques, 58-59, 58f

Dor procedure, 495
Drug(s)
    adjunctive, 145-146
    analgesic, 727-728
    antiarrhythmic, cardiac rhythm and, 81-82
    centrally acting, 131t
    effect of, 103
    hypertension
        combination, 131t
        oral anti-, 131t
        oral antihypertensive, 131t
    therapies
        anti-ischemic, 118-120f, 119t, 121b, 122b, 123b, 125t, 127t, 129, 160-161
        for systemic hypertension, 129-134, 130t, 131t, 161
DSE. *See* Dobutamine stress echocardiography
D-transposition. *See* Transposition of the great arteries

E

ECG. *See* Electrocardiography
EDPVR. *See* End-diastolic pressure-volume relation
EDV. *See* End-diastolic volume
EF. *See* Ejection fraction
Eisenmenger's syndrome, 380, 380t
Ejection fraction (EF)
    definition of, 65
    determination of, 27
    function of, 55-56
ELCA. *See* Excimer laser coronary angioplasty
Electrocardiography (ECG), 192-197, 192f, 193f
    postoperative, 12
    responses, 6-7, 12
Electroencephalography (EEG), 240-241
    considerations of, 241-242, 244f
    informational display of, 242-248, 244b, 245f, 246b, 247f, 247b, 248f, 248b
    for injury prevention, 248-252, 249f, 249b, 250f, 251f, 252f, 252b
    physiologic basis of, 241, 242f, 243f, 243b
Electrolyte abnormalities, 703, 704f, 704t, 705f, 706f, 708
Electromagnetic interference (EMI), 445
Embolus detection, 254
EMI. *See* Electromagnetic interference
Encainide, 81
End-diastolic pressure (EDP), 60
End-diastolic pressure-volume relation (EDPVR), 56, 65
End-diastolic volume (EDV), 27, 60
Endobronchial hemorrhage, 185-186
Endothelin, 69
Endothelium, 68-70, 77
    -derived contracting factors, 69
    -derived relaxing factors, , 68-69, 69b
    inhibition of platelets and, 69-70, 69b
Endotoxemia, 93-94
    antiendotoxin antibodies and, 95
    early tolerance, 94-95
    late tolerance, 94, 95
    normal host defenses against, 94-95

R

RAO. *See* Right anterior oblique
RAP. *See* Right atrial pressure
Rapamycin, 25
RAS. *See* Renin-angiotensin system
RAVEL trial, 44
RCA. *See* Right coronary arteries
RCP. *See* Retrograde cerebral perfusion
Receptor(s)
   α-, 85
   adrenergic, signaling pathways and, 83-85,
     83b, 84f
   angiotensin II, 83, 83b
   β
     -adrenergic, 84-85
     functioning of, 85
   cardiac functions and, 83-86, 83b, 84f
   clinical correlates of, 86
   muscarinic
     acetylcholine, 85-86
     signaling pathways and, 85-86
   protein tyrosine kinase, 85
Regional wall motion abnormalities (RWMAs),
   225b
Regurgitant stroke volume (RSV), 28
Remifentanil, 419
Renal replacement therapies, 701-702, 703f
Renin-angiotensin system (RAS), 139-145, 140f
Reoperation, 4
Reperfusion, 102, 102b, 103f, 104f
Respiratory distress syndrome, 668-670
Respiratory insufficiency, 665-668, 667t, 668b
Restenosis, 33, 48
Retrograde cerebral perfusion (RCP), 398-399
Revascularization
   of end-stage heart failure, 494
   myocardial ischemia during, 319-324, 320f,
     324f
Rewarming, 250
Right anterior oblique (RAO), 27
Right atrial pressure (RAP), 23, 60
Right atrium (RA), 56, 212f, 219
Right coronary arteries (RCA), 31t
Right ventricles, 206-211, 212f
Right ventricular function
   alterations in, 65
   /contraction, 64, 64b, 65f
Right ventricular pressure (RVP), 23-24
Risk indices, 4, 4b, 13
RSV. *See* Regurgitant stroke volume
RVP. *See* Right ventricular pressure
RWMAs. *See* Regional wall motion abnormalities

S

Sclerosis, 73
Sedation
   during cardiac catheterization procedures, 20
   effects of, 20
   in ICU, 688-692, 689t, 689b, 690t, 703f
Segmental wall motion abnormalities (SWMAs),
   27-28, 29f
Seizure detection, 252, 252b

Seldinger technique, 172
Sepsis, 696-700, 697t
Sequestration, 115
Serum biochemical markers, 12
Seventh Report of the Joint National Committee
   on Prevention, Detection, Evaluation, and
   Treatment of High Blood Pressure (JNC-7
   Report), 129
Sevoflurane, 101, 116
Shunting, 382
Shunts
   aortopulmonary, 375, 376f, 376t
   Gott, 401-402
SIRIUS trial, 44
Sirolimus, 25, 43b
   -eluting stents, 44
Society of Thoracic Surgeons, 6, 294
Sodium (Na$^+$), 82f, 87
   channel blockers, 153-155, 155t, 156t
Spinal cord
   cooling, 409
   protection of, 409-410
Splanchnic perfusion, 95-96
Stanford type A aortic dissection, 412-413
Statins, 74
Stenosis, 77
   aortic, 230b, 356
     anesthetic considerations for, 332-333, 332b
     clinical features/natural history of, 328
     low-gradient, low-output, 331, 331t
     pathophysiology of, 329, 329f
   assessment of coronary, 30
   coronary artery, 74-75, 74b
   dynamic, 76
   mitral, 347
     anesthetic considerations for, 350-352, 351b
     assessment of, 349
     clinical features/natural history of, 347-348,
      348f
     pathophysiology of, 348-349, 349f
     surgery, 350
Stenotic lesions, 27, 28f
Stent(s), 48
   Gianturco-Roubin, 43
   graft repairs, 403
   intracoronary, 43-45, 43b
   sirolimus-eluting, 44
   Taxus, 43b, 44
Stress testing, 8-10
Stroke volume (SV), 54
   definition of, 65
   systolic function and, 59-63, 61f, 61b, 63f, 63t
Sufentanil, 439
Surgery
   for atrial fibrillation, 370
   CABG, 38b
   cardiac, 89
     hematologic problems during, 440
     increased risks associated with, 4b, 13
     perioperative myocardial injury in, 10-11,
      11b
     during pregnancy, 437-438
     renal insufficiency and, 438-440